Paediatric Nephrology

T0177457

OXFORD SPECIALIST
HANDBOOKS IN PAEDIATRICS

Paediatric
Nephrology

Third Edition

Lesley Rees

Consultant Paediatric Nephrologist;
Professor of Paediatric Nephrology,
Institute of Child health,
University College London, UK;
Great Ormond Street Hospital for
Children NHS Foundation Trust, London, UK

Detlef Bockenhauer

Honorary Consultant Paediatric Nephrologist,
Great Ormond Street Hospital; and Professor of
Paediatric Nephrology, University College London, UK

Nicholas J.A. Webb

Consultant Paediatric Nephrologist,
Royal Manchester Children's Hospital, UK;
and Honorary Professor of Paediatric Nephrology,
University of Manchester, UK

Marilynn G. Punaro

Division Chief, Paediatric Rheumatology;
and Professor of Paediatrics, University of
Texas Southwestern Medical School, Texas, USA

OXFORD
UNIVERSITY PRESS

OXFORD
UNIVERSITY PRESS

Great Clarendon Street, Oxford, OX2 6DP,
United Kingdom

Oxford University Press is a department of the University of Oxford.
It furthers the University's objective of excellence in research, scholarship,
and education by publishing worldwide. Oxford is a registered trade mark of
Oxford University Press in the UK and in certain other countries

Published in the United States of America by Oxford University Press
198 Madison Avenue, New York, NY 10016, United States of America

British Library Cataloguing in Publication Data
Data available

Library of Congress Control Number: 2018963164

ISBN 978–0–19–878427–2

Printed and bound by
Ashfod Colour Press Ltd.

v

Contents

Symbols and abbreviations

➔	cross-reference
~	approximately
↓	decreased
↑	increased
↔	normal
🕸	website
±	with or without
2D	two-dimensional
3D	three-dimensional
AAV	ANCA-associated vasculitis
ABMR	acute antibody-mediated rejection
ABPM	ambulatory blood pressure monitoring
ACTH	adrenocorticotropic hormone
ACE	angiotensin-converting enzyme
AD	autosomal dominant
ADH	antidiuretic hormone
ADPKD	autosomal dominant polycystic kidney disease
AG	anion gap
aHUS	atypical haemolytic uraemic syndrome
ALP	alkaline phosphatase
ANA	antinuclear antibody
ANCA	antineutrophil cytoplasmic antibody
AP	alternative pathway or anteroposterior
APC	antigen-presenting cell
APD	automated peritoneal dialysis
APTT	activated prothrombin time
AR	autosomal recessive
ARB	angiotensin II receptor blocker
ARPKD	autosomal recessive polycystic kidney disease
ASO	antistreptolysin O
ASOT	antistreptolysin O titre
AST	aspartate aminotransferase
ATG	antithymocyte globulin
ATN	acute tubular necrosis
AV	arteriovenous
AVP	arginine vasopressin
BBS	Bardet–Biedl syndrome
BCG	bacillus Calmette–Guérin

BKV	BK virus
BP	blood pressure
BSA	body surface area
BTS	British Transplantation Society
C3	complement component 3
C3G	C3 glomerulopathy
C3NeF	C3 nephritic factor
Ca	calcium
CAA	coronary artery abnormality
CAH	congenital adrenal hyperplasia
CAKUT	congenital anomalies of the kidney and urinary tract
c-ANCA	cytoplasmic antineutrophil cytoplasmic antibody
CAPD	continuous ambulatory peritoneal dialysis
CAPS	catastrophic antiphospholipid syndrome
CaSR	calcium-sensing receptor
CF	cystic fibrosis
CFB	complement factor B
CFH	complement factor H
CFI	complement factor I
CIC	clean intermittent catheterization
CIT	cold ischaemia time
CK	creatine kinase
CKD	chronic kidney disease
CKD-MBD	chronic kidney disease–mineral and bone disorder
Cl	chloride
CLKT	combined liver–kidney transplantation
CNI	calcineurin inhibitor
CNS	congenital nephrotic syndrome or central nervous system
COX	cyclooxygenase
CRP	C-reactive protein
CRRT	continuous renal replacement therapy
CT	computed tomography
CTA	computed tomography angiography
CVD	cardiovascular disease
CVVH	continuous venovenous haemofiltration
CVVHD	continuous venovenous haemofiltration with dialysis
DBD	donation after brain death
DCD	donation after circulatory death
DCT	distal convoluted tubule
DGF	delayed graft function
DMSA	dimercaptosuccinic acid

DRI	dietary reference intake
dRTA	distal renal tubular acidosis
DSA	donor-specific antibody
DTPA	diethylenetriaminepentaacetic acid
DUI	daytime urinary incontinence
EBV	Epstein–Barr virus
ECF	extracellular fluid
ECG	electrocardiogram
ECMO	extracorporeal membrane oxygenation
eGFR	estimated glomerular filtration rate
EGPA	eosinophilic granulomatosis with polyangiitis
ELISA	enzyme-linked immunosorbent assay
EM	electron microscopy
EMG	electromyography
ENA	extractable nuclear antibody
ENaC	epithelial sodium channel
EOS	early-onset sarcoidosis
ESA	erythropoiesis-stimulating agent
ESKD	end-stage kidney disease
ESR	erythrocyte sedimentation rate
FBC	full blood count
FBG	fasting blood glucose
FeNA	fractional excretion of sodium
FFP	fresh frozen plasma
FISH	fluorescent *in situ* hybridization
FMF	familial Mediterranean fever
FSGS	focal segmental glomerulosclerosis
Gb3	globotriaosylceramide
GBM	glomerular basement membrane
GDP	glucose degradation product
GFR	glomerular filtration rate
GH	growth hormone
GI	gastrointestinal
GN	glomerulonephritis
GP	general practitioner
GPA	granulomatosis with polyangiitis
GRA	glucocorticoid-remediable aldosteronism
HBsAg	hepatitis B surface antigen
HCQ	hydroxychloroquine
HD	haemodialysis
HDF	haemodiafiltration

HDL	high-density lipoprotein
HHV	human herpesvirus
HIV	human immunodeficiency virus
HLA	human leucocyte antigen
HLH	haemophagocytic lymphohistiocytosis
HNF	hepatocyte nuclear factor
HSP	Henoch–Schönlein purpura
HSV	herpes simplex virus
Ht	height
HUS	haemolytic uraemic syndrome
ICF	intracellular fluid
ICGN	immune complex-mediated glomerulonephritis
IGAN	immunoglobulin A nephropathy
IL	interleukin
IPP	intraperitoneal pressure
ISKDC	International Study of Kidney Disease in Children
IV	intravenous
IVC	inferior vena cava
IVCYC	intravenous cyclophosphamide
IVIG	intravenous immunoglobulin
IVMP	intravenous methylprednisolone
IVU	intravenous urogram
JVP	jugular venous pressure
K	potassium
KD	Kawasaki disease
KDIGO	Kidney Disease: Improving Global Outcomes
KDOQI	Kidney Disease Outcomes Quality Initiative
LBW	low birth weight
LDH	lactate dehydrogenase
LDL	low-density lipoprotein
LFT	liver function test
LMWH	low-molecular-weight heparin
LMWP	low-molecular-weight proteinuria
LUT	lower urinary tract
MAG3	mercaptoacetyltriglycine
MAHA	microangiopathic haemolytic anaemia
MC&S	microscopy, culture, and sensitivity
MCD	minimal change disease
MCDK	multicystic dysplastic kidney
MCUG	micturating cystourethrogram
Mg	magnesium

MHC	major histocompatibility complex
MMA	methylmalonic acidaemia
MMF	mycophenolate mofetil
MN	membranous nephropathy
MODY	maturity-onset diabetes in the young
MPA	microscopic polyangiitis *or* mycophenolic acid
MPO	myeloperoxidase
MRA	magnetic resonance angiography
MRI	magnetic resonance imaging
MRV	magnetic resonance venography
mTOR	mammalian target of rapamycin
MTX	methotrexate
Na	sodium
NAPRTCS	North American Pediatric Renal Trials and Collaborative Studies
NDI	nephrogenic diabetes insipidus
NG	nasogastric
NICE	National Institute for Health and Care Excellence
NIPD	nocturnal intermittent peritoneal dialysis
NODAT	new-onset diabetes after transplantation
NPHP	nephronophthisis
NSAID	non-steroidal anti-inflammatory drug
NSIAD	nephrogenic syndrome of inappropriate antidiuresis
P	plasma
PAN	polyarteritis nodosa
p-ANCA	perinuclear antineutrophil cytoplasmic antibody
PAS	periodic acid–Schiff
PD	peritoneal dialysis
PEG	percutaneous endoscopic gastrostomy
PET	peritoneal equilibrium test *or* positron emission tomography
PH	primary hyperoxaluria
PIGN	post-infectious glomerulonephritis
PO_4	phosphate
Posm	plasma osmolarity
PPV	pneumococcal polysaccharide
pRTA	proximal renal tubular acidosis
ptc	peritubular capillaritis
PTH	parathyroid hormone
PTLD	post-transplant lymphoproliferative disease
PTT	prothrombin time

PUJ	pelviureteric junction
PUV	posterior urethral valve
RAAS	renin–angiotensin–aldosterone system
RAS	renin–angiotensin system
RCT	randomized controlled trial
rhGH	recombinant growth hormone therapy
RNI	reference nutrient intake
RPGN	rapidly progressive glomerulonephritis
RRT	renal replacement therapy
RTA	renal tubular acidosis
RVT	renal venous thrombosis
SC	subcutaneous
SCr	serum creatinine
SD	standard deviation
SDNS	steroid-dependent nephrotic syndrome
SDS	standard deviation score
SIADH	syndrome of inappropriate antidiuretic hormone secretion
SLE	systemic lupus erythematosus
SNP	single nucleotide polymorphism
SRNS	steroid-resistant nephrotic syndrome
T4	thyroxine
TA	Takayasu arteritis
TAL	thick ascending limb of Henle's loop
TB	tuberculosis
TBMN	thin basement membrane nephropathy
TCMR	acute T-cell-mediated rejection
TCO_2	total carbon dioxide
TIN	tubulointerstitial nephritis
TINU	tubulointerstitial nephritis and uveitis
TMA	thrombotic microangiopathy
TmP	tubular maximum reabsorption rate of phosphate
TMP	transmembrane pressure
TNF	tumour necrosis factor
tPA	tissue plasminogen activator
TPD	transverse pelvic diameter
TPMT	thiopurine transmethyltransfersase
TRP	tubular reabsorption of phosphate
TS	tuberous sclerosis
TSH	thyroid-stimulating hormone
TTP	thrombotic thrombocytopenic purpura
TTTS	twin-to-twin transfusion syndrome

U	urine
U&Es	urea and electrolytes
Ua:Ucr	urine albumin to creatinine ratio
Uca:Ucr	urine calcium to creatinine ratio
UF	ultrafiltration
UFH	unfractionated heparin
UK	United Kingdom
ULN	upper limit of normal
Uosm	urine osmolarity
Upr:Ucr	urine protein to creatinine ratio
Urbp:Ucr	urine retinol-binding protein to urine creatinine ratio
US	ultrasound
USA	United States of America
UTI	urinary tract infection
VUJ	vesicoureteric junction
VUR	vesicoureteral reflux
VZIG	varicella zoster immunoglobulin
VZV	varicella zoster virus
WBC	white blood cell
WHO	World Health Organization
WIT	warm ischaemia time
XD	X-linked dominant
XR	X-linked recessive

Acknowledgements

All colleagues at Gt Ormond St Hospital for Children NHS Trust, particularly:

Dr William van't Hoff
Consultant Paediatric Nephrologist

Ms Eileen Brennan
Nurse Consultant in Paediatric Nephrology

Dr Kjell Tullus
Consultant Paediatric Nephrologist

Ms Michelle Cantwell
Clinical Nurse Specialist in Peritoneal Dialysis

Dr Steven Marks
Consultant Paediatric Nephrologist

Prof Robert Kleta
Honorary Consultant Paediatric Nephrologist

Prof Neil Sebire
Consultant Paediatric Pathologist

Prof Paul Brogan
Honorary Consultant Paediatric Rheumatologist

Ms Vanessa Shaw
Paediatric Renal Dietician

Mr Chris Callaghan
Consultant Transplant Surgeon

All colleagues at Royal Manchester Children's Hospital, particularly:

Prof Bernadette Brennan
Consultant Paediatric Oncologist

Dr Nick Plant
Consultant Paediatric Nephrologist

Mr Alan Dickson
Consultant Paediatric Urologist

Dr Dean Wallace
Consultant Paediatric Nephrologist

Dr Mohan Shenoy
Consultant Paediatric Nephrologist

Dr Neville Wright
Consultant Paediatric Radiologist

Elsewhere

Dr Joanne Clothier

Consultant Paediatric Nephrologist, Evelina Children's Hospital, London

Dr Jonathan Evans

Consultant Paediatric Nephrologist, Nottingham Children's Hospital, Nottingham

Prof Bronwyn Kerr

Consultant Clinical Geneticist, St Mary's Hospital, Manchester

Dr Kay Metcalfe

Consultant Clinical Geneticist, St Mary's Hospital, Manchester

Dr Judith Worthington

Principal Clinical Scientist, Manchester Royal Infirmary, Manchester

Dr Anne Wright

Consultant Paediatrician, Evelina Children's Hospital, London

Patient assessment

History and examination in children with or with suspected renal disease

Important points in the history

Antenatal history
* *Amniotic fluid volume*: low in fetuses with low urine output due to obstruction or severe renal impairment; high in polyuric states, e.g. neonatal Bartter syndrome and congenital nephrotic syndrome (CNS).
* *Alpha-fetoprotein level*: high in CNS, but can also be high in carriers of nephrin mutations, i.e. false positive. High in spina bifida.
* *Antenatal ultrasound (US) scan*: when was an abnormality first detected? Did the abnormality worsen through pregnancy? Important anomalies may be missed without a third-trimester scan, e.g. posterior urethral valves (PUVs). Antenatal bright kidneys may be associated with hepatocyte nuclear factor-1-beta (*HNF1B*) mutations or autosomal recessive polycystic kidney disease (ARPKD) and other ciliopathies.
* *Previous pregnancies/miscarriages*: for a genetic condition.
* *Presence of fetal distress*: associated with renal venous thrombosis (RVT) and tubular and cortical necrosis.
* *Maternal drug history*.
* *Maternal diabetes*: associated with sacral agenesis and many other renal anomalies. Consider maternal *HNF1B* mutation as a potential cause.

Birth history
* *Type of delivery*: any evidence of fetal distress/hypoxia.
* *Apgar score*: evidence of fetal hypoxia.
* *Birth weight*: evidence of intrauterine problems, e.g. low birth weight (LBW) may be associated with low nephron number; high birth weight with Beckwith–Wiedemann syndrome.
* *Number of umbilical vessels*: single umbilical artery is associated with a renal abnormality in 3% of cases, e.g. aplasia, hypoplasia, and exstrophy of the bladder.
* *Gestation and birth weight*: increased incidence of intrauterine growth restriction with renal abnormalities.
* *Weight of placenta*: large placenta, >25% of birth weight, in CNS.

Neonatal history
* *Respiratory symptoms*: associated with oligohydramnios and abnormal lung development.
* *Use of umbilical catheters*: associated with renal and other vascular thromboses.
* *Timing of passage of urine after birth*.

General questions
- Consanguinity.
- Urinary stream.
- Urinary tract infections (UTIs).
- Family history, particularly of renal disease, deafness, or diabetes.
- Previous central lines.
- Polyuria and polydipsia.
- Enuresis: primary or secondary.

Examination specific to renal disease
- Number of umbilical arteries (neonate).
- Height, weight, head circumference, and pubertal stage.
- Blood pressure (BP).
- Congenital dislocation of the hips.
- Other congenital abnormalities, e.g.:
  - Eyes, e.g. aniridia, coloboma, cataract, retinitis pigmentosa, tapetoretinal degeneration, and uveitis.
  - Ear deformities.
  - Pre-auricular pits.
  - Branchial fistulas and cysts.
  - Abnormal facies.
  - Presence of abdominal muscles.
  - Cryptorchidism.
  - Spine.
  - Genital abnormalities.
- *Palpable kidneys*: enlarged with ARPKD, autosomal dominant polycystic kidney disease (ADPKD), tuberous sclerosis (TS), multicystic dysplastic kidney (MCDK), severely obstructed kidneys, RVT, and renal tumour.
- *Evidence of bone disease*: thickened wrists, rickety rosary, and lower limb deformities.
- *Oedema, jugular venous pressure (JVP), core–peripheral temperature gap, pulse, and respiratory rate*: if assessing fluid balance.
- *Pulses and evidence of collateral circulations*: if previous intravascular lines or hypertension.
- *Handedness of child*: if contemplating a fistula.
- *Markers of systemic disease*: rash and arthropathy.

Abnormalities of the urine and urinalysis

Visual inspection of urine

Red urine

* Macroscopic haematuria:
  * Causes the urine to develop a pink to red colour.
  * Only a small amount of blood may be necessary to produce discoloration.
  * Fresh heavy bleeding is more likely to be of lower urinary tract origin, particularly when haematuria is greatest at either the end or at the beginning of micturition.
  * The presence of clots makes glomerular bleeding an unlikely cause.
  * Contact with acidic urine causes haem pigment to become oxidized to a methaem derivative, giving the urine a brown (often described as cola or tea) colour. Generally, the longer the contact and the more acidic the urine, the darker the colour.
* Red urine not due to haematuria may be due to:
  * foods e.g. beetroot, fruits containing anthocyanins (e.g. blueberries, plums, cherries) and food dyes.
  * haemoglobinuria, e.g. in intravascular haemolysis.
  * myoglobinuria, e.g. in rhabdomyolysis.
  * urate crystals (a cause of pink discoloration of nappies: 'brick-red nappy').
  * drugs, e.g. rifampicin, phenothiazines, desferrioxamine, and phenindione.
  * inborn errors of metabolism, e.g. porphyria and alkaptonuria
  * in all these forms (except urate crystals), the discolouration does not settle with time or centrifugation, but stays uniform. Thus, discolouration from these pigments can be diagnosed by letting the urine stand for 30 min or by centrifugation.

Urine microscopy is therefore mandatory following the detection of red urine. This should occur promptly to avoid red blood cell (RBC) lysis.

While Munchausen syndrome by proxy is rare, deliberate contamination of the urine with blood from the offending carer can be a presentation of this disorder.

Cloudy urine

* May be secondary to the presence of pyuria (white blood cells), calcium phosphate crystals, or a combination of calcium salts, uric acid, cysteine, or struvite.
  * Precipitation of phosphates and urates is enhanced by refrigeration.

Milky white urine (chyluria)

* Due to disruption of lymph channels within the urinary tract so that lymph and fats (chyle) drain directly into the urinary tract.
* Urinary triglycerides are present and albumin may be present.
* Causes:
  * Congenital abnormalities of the lymphatics.
  * Parasitic invasion (principally filariasis) of the urinary tract lymph channels.

- Partial nephrectomy.
- Tuberculosis (TB).
- Tumours.

Dipstick examination of urine

Blood

- Haemoglobin is detected through its ability to catalyse a reaction between hydrogen peroxide and o-tolidine.
- Spotted positivity indicates intact RBCs, whereas uniform positivity may indicate free haemoglobin (e.g. in intravascular haemolysis or red cell lysis in the urinary tract).
- Causes of false-positive haematuria include:
  - myoglobinuria.
  - oxidizing agents contaminating urine specimen (e.g. hypochlorite, povidone, and bacterial peroxidases).
  - heavy bacterial contamination.
- Causes of false-negative haematuria include reducing agents in the urine (e.g. ascorbic acid).

Urine microscopy is therefore mandatory following the detection of blood on dipstick analysis. This should occur promptly to avoid RBC lysis.

Protein

- Dipsticks undergo colour change from yellow to green following binding with proteins.
- The dipsticks actually measure a change in pH, as proteins buffer hydrogen ions. False-positive results are possible with very alkaline urine that overrides the acid buffer in the chemical of the dipstick.
- Dipstick analysis is not a good quantitative test because of the effect of urinary concentration (more concentrated urine will show a higher protein concentration), and where proteinuria is detected, formal quantification with a urine protein to creatinine ratio (Upr:Ucr) or urine albumin to creatinine ratio (Ua:Ucr) is indicated.
- Approximate estimates of urine protein concentration according to the dipstick result are shown in Table 1.1.
- Albumin is better detected than other urinary proteins (globulins, tubular proteins, etc.).
- First morning samples, obtained as soon as the patient gets out of bed, should be assessed to rule out any element of orthostatic proteinuria.

Table 1.1 Approximate estimates of urine protein concentration according to the dipstick result

Dipstick result	Approximate urine protein concentration (g/L)
Trace	0.15
1+	0.3
2+	1
3+	3
4+	20

- If there is dipstick-positive but insignificant albuminuria on quantification, consider tubular proteins (e.g. retinol-binding protein or alpha-1 microglobulin; ➜ see 'Tubulointerstitial nephritis'). However, albuminuria may also be present at the same time as tubular proteins in tubular diseases, as a substantial amount of albumin is filtered and reabsorbed. Urine albumin/creatinine ratios are usually <200 mg/mmol with tubular proteinuria.
- Causes of false-positive proteinuria include:
  - concentrated urine.
  - alkaline urine.
  - gross haematuria.
  - dipstick left in urine too long or delay in reading.
  - contamination with secretions from the urinary tract (during UTI) or vagina.
  - contamination with antiseptics, chlorhexidine, or benzalkonium.
- Causes of false-negative proteinuria include:
  - dilute urine.
  - acid urine.

Glucose
- Lower limit of detection is 4–5 mmol/L.

Leucocytes
- Some sticks may detect leucocyte esterase, indicating the presence of pyuria.
- Microscopy should be used to confirm this finding.
- Pyuria is not diagnostic of UTI and may occur secondary to fever or infection of non-urinary tract origin.
- Pyuria can also occur due to flushing of the foreskin or vagina during voiding.

Nitrites
- The majority of pathogenic bacteria possess an enzyme that converts nitrates to nitrites. Nitrites can be detected on urinalysis.
- Bacteria have to be in contact with urine for a sufficient time for this process to occur. In neonates, who pass urine frequently, there may not be sufficient time between voids to allow the conversion of nitrates to nitrites to take place.
- The test has a high specificity but a low sensitivity for the diagnosis of UTI. As such, the test is of limited usefulness.
- Where UTI is suspected or needs to be excluded, a urine culture is necessary to determine the bacteriological cause and antibiotic sensitivities or to confidently rule out UTI.

Microscopy of urine

Casts
- Produced by the aggregation of Tamm–Horsfall protein with cells or cellular debris in the renal tubule, and therefore can be a normal finding.
- Best seen in unspun urine: centrifugation may damage casts. In centrifuged urine, casts are most frequently seen at the edge of the coverslip.

- Casts dissolve with time and thus can be missed, if the urine is not fresh.
- *Hyaline casts:*
  - Present in proteinuric states, though may be found in concentrated specimens of urine from normal individuals.

Cellular casts

- Red cell casts are always pathological and indicate glomerular bleeding.
- White cell casts indicate renal inflammation due to pyelonephritis or immunologically mediated disease.
- Epithelial cell casts (often present with red and white cell casts) are produced from shed tubular epithelial cells and may be seen with acute tubular necrosis (ATN).

Red blood cells

- Normal red cell excretion increases with age and after exercise.
- The persistent presence of >5 × 10⁶ RBCs/L in uncentrifuged urine is abnormal.
- Microscopy (phase contract microscopy is best, though possible with ordinary light microscopy) can distinguish anatomically normal RBCs of lower urinary tract origin from dysmorphic RBCs of glomerular origin which have been distorted during their passage through the filtration barrier.
- The presence of acanthocytes (>5% of RBC population) may indicate the presence of glomerulonephritis.
- RBCs deform and lyse in urine of high tonicity. It is therefore important that microscopy is performed on a fresh urine specimen.

White blood cells

- The presence of >10 × 10⁶ white cells/L is abnormal.
- Neutrophils are detected in UTI, but also in contamination, proliferative glomerulonephritis, and interstitial nephritis.
- Eosinophils may be detected in the urine in children with acute interstitial nephritis (➔ see 'Tubulointerstitial nephritis').

Bacteria and other organisms

- Bacteria may be clearly visible without Gram staining.
- Their detection may be enhanced by the use of phase contrast microscopy.
- Fungi (e.g. *Candida*) and *Schistosoma* species (a rare cause of haematuria) may also be detected.

Epithelial cells

- Presence may represent desquamation from urinary tract.
- Tubular cells may be seen following tubular injury (ATN, acute transplant rejection).
- Squamous cells are commonly exfoliated from the urethra and are a normal finding.

The approach to the child with haematuria

May present with

- macroscopic haematuria:
  - symptomatic with: dysuria (e.g. urethritis, UTI); renal colic (e.g. renal calculus); loin pain (e.g. pelviureteric junction (PUJ) obstruction).
  - asymptomatic.
- microscopic haematuria:
  - detected during screening (routine or because of a family history).
  - during an intercurrent infection.

Important points in the history

- Is the haematuria at the beginning or end of the stream (suggestive of a bladder or urethral cause)?
- The foreskin: ?circumcision, ?balanitis, ?urinary stream, ?vulvovaginitis.
- Is the urine red (more likely to arise from the lower urinary tract) or tea/cola coloured (more likely to be glomerular)?
- Symptoms suggestive of UTI, calculi, or acute nephritis (see relevant chapters).
- Family history of renal disease or deafness (familial haematuria) or sickle cell disease.

Causes of macroscopic and persistent microscopic haematuria

- Lower tract bleeding:
  - UTI.
  - Urethral trauma, balanitis, urethral/meatal stenosis with urethritis, polyp, vulvo vaginitis.
- Associated with pain:
  - Structural abnormalities such as PUJ obstruction.
  - Calculi.
  - Hypercalciuria (diagnosis of exclusion).
- Glomerular disorders:
  - Immunoglobulin (Ig)-A nephropathy (➔ see Chapter 9).
  - Other glomerular disorders (e.g. C3 nephropathy).
  - Familial haematuria (➔ see 'Alport syndrome and thin basement membrane nephropathy').
- Sickle cell disease (➔ see Chapter 10).
- Schistosomiasis (➔ see Chapter 12).
- Renal tumours (➔ see Chapter 15).
- Renal tract vascular malformation.
- Clotting abnormalities as a cause is very rare.

Important points on examination

- It is important to check the genitalia in all cases of macro and microscopic haematuria in order to identify local causes (e.g. trauma, meatal stenosis, vulvovaginitis).
- Abdominal examination and BP.

Investigation of macroscopic and persistent microscopic haematuria

(See Fig. 1.1.)

Asymptomatic intermittent microscopic haematuria does not need investigation.

- Urine microscopy, culture, and sensitivity (MC&S): haematuria needs to be confirmed by urine microscopy prior to any further investigation to ensure that a positive dipstick test is not false.
- Urine phase contrast microscopy for deformed red cells (glomerular bleeding).
- Ua:Ucr or Upr:Ucr and urine calcium to creatinine ratio (Uca:Ucr).
- Renal US.
- Check urine of parents and siblings for blood and protein.
- Urea and electrolytes (U&Es), creatinine, and albumin.
- Full blood count (FBC).
- Sickle cell screen (if appropriate).
- Clotting (if history of bruising).
- Antistreptolysin O (ASO) titre, C3, C4, anti-double stranded DNA binding, hepatitis B and C (if acute nephritis suspected).
- IgA levels if asymptomatic episodes.
- Urology referral if non-glomerular bleeding suspected; may need cystourethroscopy.
- Renal biopsy (or genetic analysis if available) if raised creatinine, proteinuria, a low albumin, or family history.

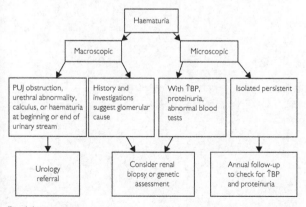

Fig. 1.1 Haematuria.

Follow-up
- Will depend on cause.
- Asymptomatic microscopic haematuria without a clear diagnosis may resolve or is likely to be benign and does not warrant biopsy. Annual follow-up is recommended to check for the development of proteinuria or hypertension.
- If proteinuria or hypertension develops, the creatinine and serum albumin should be checked.
- If there is a raised plasma creatinine, proteinuria, or a low albumin, a biopsy (or genetic analysis) may be indicated.

The approach to the child with proteinuria

Quantification of proteinuria

- 24 h urine collection remains the gold standard. This is because creatinine in the urine will be low in children with reduced muscle mass, and in young children or very dilute urines, the measurement of creatinine may be inaccurate as the machine to measure creatinine is calibrated for plasma levels.
- It is usually simpler to measure the urine protein or albumin concentration expressed as a factor of urine creatinine concentration, thus providing a correction for variation in urine concentration: Upr:Ucr or Ua:Ucr.
- A Upr:Ucr in the first urine passed after rising (to rule out any orthostatic element) should be <10 mg/mmol, which equates to <60 mg/m^2/day. However, these values may be higher in the first 2 years of life.
- 40 mg/m^2/h roughly equates to a value of 250 mg/mmol (assuming normal muscle mass), which some define as nephrotic range proteinuria.
- Microalbuminuria will not be detected by dipsticks and is defined as a Ua:Ucr >2.5mg/mmol.
- Protein/creatinine is roughly double albumin/creatinine (mg/mmol) with glomerular proteinuria, but even higher with tubular proteinuria.
- A Upr:Ucr of 100 mg/mmol, or Ua:Ucr of 70 mg/mmol, is approximately equal to 1 g of protein per 24 h.

Causes of proteinuria

It is important to decide whether proteinuria is benign, and therefore by definition isolated and not associated with abnormal BP or renal function, or pathological.

Benign proteinuria

Intermittent proteinuria is benign and does not need further investigation. Causes include the following:

- False-positive stick results (➔ see 'Abnormalities of the urine and urinalysis').
- Increased filtration of plasma proteins due to changes in renal haemodynamics:
  - Without identifiable cause or after severe exercise, cold exposure, or intercurrent febrile illnesses.
  - Orthostatic proteinuria, which occurs when the child is ambulant but not when recumbent. It can be diagnosed by giving the family Albustix® to test the very first urine passed immediately (i.e. before doing anything else) on rising. Results will be persistently negative despite positive results in the day. Alternatively, a 24 h collection can be split into a day and a night aliquot.
    - It occurs mostly in adolescents, particularly boys.
    - Proteinuria is mild.
    - It usually decreases with time and disappears.

Pathological proteinuria

Proteinuria that is persistent or associated with haematuria, hypertension, or renal dysfunction is pathological. Causes include the following:

- Glomerular disease due to:
  - glomerulosclerosis or reduced nephron mass from any cause, resulting in hyperfiltration.
  - all causes of glomerulonephritis.
  - all causes of nephrotic syndrome.
  - familial haematuria.
- Tubular disease:
  - Although there is proteinuria, quantification shows albumin excretion to be low as the majority of the urine proteins are of low molecular weight.

Investigations

- Urine microscopy and culture.
- Ua:Ucr or Upr:Ucr.
- Urine retinol-binding protein to urine creatinine ratio (Urbp:Ucr) (or another low-molecular-weight protein) if tubular disease suspected.
- Renal US.
- U&Es, creatinine, and albumin.
- FBC.
- ASO titre, C3, C4, anti-double stranded DNA binding, hepatitis B and C (if acute nephritis suspected).
- IgA levels.
- Check urine of parents and siblings for blood and protein.
- Renal biopsy or genetic assessment.

Radiological investigations

The key to obtaining successful and informative imaging of the urinary tract is close liaison between clinician and radiologist. The higher the quality of clinical information given to the radiologist, the higher the quality of the resulting report.

Ultrasound

- Radiation free, painless, easily available, and low cost.
- Can be used to measure renal lengths, for which there are normal ranges (see Fig. 1.2), though there may be considerable inter-observer error.
- Normal ranges for renal length for the solitary kidney are shown in Table 1.3 (up to 6 years of age).
- Excellent for the detection and measurement of hydroureteronephrosis, renal masses including tumours, renal cystic disease, and calculi (including non-radio-opaque calculi).
- Allows for evaluation of the bladder wall (thickness, diameter, abnormalities, e.g. trabeculation, diverticulae) and lumen including ureterocoeles and measurement of pre- and post-micturition bladder volumes (Fig. 1.3).
- May be useful in the diagnosis of acute pyelonephritis (enlarged echo-bright kidney with loss of corticomedullary differentiation).
- Its role in the detection of permanent renal parenchymal scarring is controversial (compared with the gold standard dimercaptosuccinic acid (DMSA) scan), though the large majority of series have found it to be of low sensitivity.
- May detect changes secondary to vesicoureteral reflux (VUR), ureteric or renal pelvic dilatation.
- Doppler studies allow the measurement of blood flow in the main renal artery and veins, as well as in the smaller intrarenal vessels, and are useful in the diagnosis of RVT. The resistive index measures resistance to blood flow (e.g. in renal artery stenosis). Power Doppler increases sensitivity.
- Can be used in the first 6 weeks of life to assess the position of the spinal cord to check for tethering when a neuropathic bladder is suspected.

Plain abdominal X-ray

- May detect calculi, abdominal masses, calcification (including more severe nephrocalcinosis), and sacral agenesis, though is not necessarily the modality of first choice for these.
- Will detect the presence of spina bifida occulta in ~30% of individuals: this finding is nearly always of no clinical significance.
- Should not be used for the routine diagnosis of constipation.

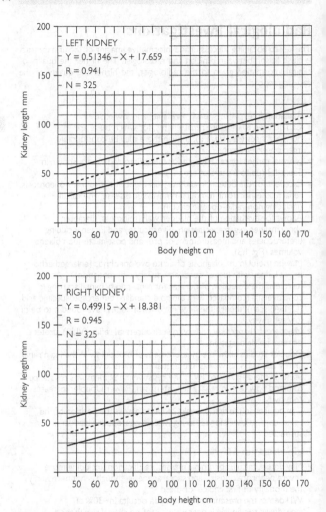

Fig. 1.2 Renal length vs height showing mean and 95th centile values. Data based on measurements performed in 325 children with no evidence of renal disease.

Reproduced with permission from Dinkel, E. et al. *Pediatric Radiology.* 15(1), 38–43. Copyright © 1985 Springer-Verlag.

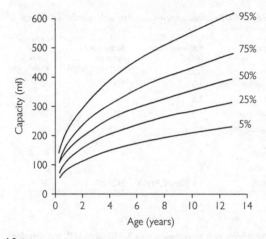

Fig. 1.3 Relationship between bladder capacity and age.

Source: data from Kaefer, M. et al. Estimating normal bladder capacity in children. *Journal of Urology*. 158(6), 2261–2264. Copyright © 1997 American Urological Association, Inc. Published by Elsevier Inc. All rights reserved.

Intravenous urogram (IVU)

- Now used very rarely, though is easy to perform and does not require specialist equipment.
- Provides information about renal anatomy including visualization of the calyces, the presence of malrotation, and may be useful in identifying the site of urinary tract obstruction e.g. congenital PUJ or VUJ obstruction and that secondary to renal calculi.
- Has been replaced by radioisotope imaging and more recently by magnetic resonance imaging (MRI).

Micturating cystourethrogram (MCUG)

- Gold standard investigation to detect and grade VUR and posterior urethral valves.
- The frequency with which this investigation is performed has fallen significantly, especially following the National Institute for Health and Care Excellence (NICE) UTI guidelines.
- Early filling films should be obtained to identify ureterocoeles, which become compressed once the bladder fills.
- Oblique or lateral films and views of the urethra without the catheter are necessary to detect a PUV.
- Requires catheterization of the bladder and can be distressing, even with experienced operators. The radiation dose is relatively high (Table 1.2).

Table 1.2 Radiation exposure associated with specific radiological investigations

Procedure	Radiation dose (mSv)	Background radiation equivalent (days)	Chest X-ray equivalents
Abdominal X-ray	1.0	161	50
IVU	2.5	403	125
DMSA scan	1.0	161	50
CT abdomen/pelvis	10	1613	500
US scan	0	0	0
MR scan	0	0	0
MCUG	1.5 (boy)/0.9 (girl)	242/145	75/45

- The procedure is associated with a 2–3% risk of UTI, and therefore should be covered with antibiotic therapy, particularly in neonates and those shown to have VUR.
  - No evidence base to guide therapy.
  - Recommendation: trimethoprim 4 mg/kg twice daily for 3 days (day before until day after procedure).

Nuclear medicine cystography

- *Direct cystography* involves the instillation of ^{99}Tc pertechnetate into the bladder.
  - The procedure is associated with a lower radiation dose than an X-ray MCUG and may have greater sensitivity. Many consider it the method of choice in girls. It does not, however, give information about posterior urethral anatomy (essential in boys to rule out a PUV) and still requires catheterization.
- *Indirect cystography* can be performed using intravenous (IV) mercaptoacetyltriglycine (MAG3; separately or as part of a dynamic investigation), thus avoiding the need for catheterization.
  - The child needs to be fully continent.
  - Scanning performed during voiding detects the presence of isotope refluxed into the ureters and renal pelvis.
  - Lower grades of VUR may be missed, and the investigation does not generate information about posterior urethral anatomy.
  - May be useful as a follow-up investigation in those with known MCUG-proven VUR.

DMSA (^{99m}Tc DMSA) scan

- DMSA is filtered by the glomeruli and reabsorbed by the proximal tubules. Therefore there is poor uptake and poor images with
  - renal tubular disease.
  - chronic kidney disease (CKD) ≥stage 3.
- The image produced is that of functioning renal cortical mass and the technique is the gold standard investigation for the detection of renal cortical defects.
- May also be helpful in identifying ectopic kidneys and confirming non-function (e.g. in the MCDK).
- Information is also generated about differential renal function (the relative contribution of each kidney to total renal function).
- Duplex kidneys (often of little clinical significance) are often detected by DMSA scans.
- Sedation is not generally necessary.
- Controversy exists over the optimum timing of DMSA scanning following UTI:
  - Early scans performed within the first few weeks post UTI will detect changes secondary to acute parenchymal inflammation in up to 50% of children with pyelonephritis which may be indistinguishable from those of cortical scarring.
  - These acute changes may persist for up to 6 months, and many advocate delaying the scan until 6 months post UTI. However, in children with recurrent UTIs, this policy may result in major delays in the investigation being performed.
- It is increasingly recognized that the congenitally dysplastic kidney (associated with intrauterine VUR and other factors) may have a DMSA scan appearance which is identical to that of acquired renal scarring:
  - Many children labelled with renal scarring may in fact have congenitally dysplastic kidneys. It is therefore preferential to use the term 'renal defects' rather than 'renal scarring'.

Dynamic renography (^{99m}Tc-diethylenetriaminepentaacetic acid (DTPA) or ^{99m}Tc-MAG3 scans)

- These scans are used to assess renal blood flow and to detect the presence and site of urinary tract obstruction.
- DTPA is excreted by glomerular filtration and therefore gives additional information about the glomerular filtration rate (GFR).
- MAG3 is excreted primarily via proximal tubular secretion; consequently, its clearance is a measurement of tubular cell function. Renal clearance of MAG3 is substantially greater than the renal clearance of DTPA so clearance curves are steeper, assisting in interpretation where obstruction is suspected.
- The child needs to be well hydrated for the scan and the isotope is injected with furosemide (there is much variation in the timing of the latter, though most give the two together to avoid multiple injections). This increases urine flow, maximally challenging the drainage system.
- Time–activity curves are generated showing uptake of the isotope by the kidneys with subsequent excretion.

- Pictures in the nephographic phase may show renal cortical scarring, though with less sensitivity than the DMSA scan.
- Renographic curves may show:
  - normal uptake and excretion.
  - reduced uptake by either or both kidneys where function is poor.
  - normal uptake but poor subsequent excretion where obstruction is present.
  - normal uptake with equivocal excretion.
  - poor clearance of isotope from very dilated pelves or ureters may give the artificial appearance of obstruction. This will be exacerbated by dehydration. The child should be sat up as a change of posture can normalize drainage.

Cross-sectional imaging

- Computed tomography (CT) scanning:
  - Excellent modality for imaging renal parenchyma.
  - Usually more readily available than MRI so often the method of choice for assessment of renal masses and renal trauma.
  - May provide additional information to US in acute pyelonephritis and pyonephrosis, particularly where drainage of the latter is being considered.
  - Renal calculi are clearly identified: these may have been missed on US examination where there is significant obesity or skeletal deformity. Conversely, dense nephrocalcinosis may have been misinterpreted as calculi on US.
  - Xanthogranulomatous pyelonephritis is one of the more significant differential diagnoses of Wilms tumour. The calculi and fatty lesions within the involved kidney are clearly identified by CT.
  - There is a significant radiation dose (Table 1.2).
  - Modern rapid image acquisition reduces motion artefact and removes the need for sedation in most cases.
- MRI:
  - Is not associated with any radiation burden.
  - Good for the evaluation of renal masses and cystic lesions.
  - Can be used for the assessment of renal parenchyma and function (magnetic resonance (MR) renography) or the drainage systems (MR urography).
  - A useful substitute for formal angiography (MRA) and venography (MRV) for the assessment of renal artery stenosis and other vascular abnormalities.
  - MR urography can produce detailed three-dimensional (3D) images of the urinary tract for the assessment of complex congenital urological anomalies.
  - The use of gadolinium-based contrast is significantly less nephrotoxic than iodine-based contrasts, though there is a risk of nephrogenic systemic fibrosis in those with CKD (➔ see 'Contrast-induced nephropathy'). This appears to occur almost exclusively in those with CKD 5 and severe CKD 4, when it should be avoided.
  - Sedation is often required for MRI.

Arteriography and venography

- Advances in MRA techniques have resulted in these investigations being performed less frequently, although MRA is still unable to reliably detect changes in medium-sized arteries (➔ see 'Investigation of primary systemic vasculitis').
- The techniques require direct arterial or venous puncture. This requires general anaesthesia in the majority of children.
- Arteriography may be used to assist in the diagnosis of the systemic vasculitides, particularly large vessel vasculitis such as Takayasu disease, but is less reliable for medium vessel vasculitis such as polyarteritis nodosa (PAN).
- Renal artery stenosis in a native or transplanted kidney may be diagnosed using formal catheter arteriography and during the same procedure it may be possible to perform angioplasty to correct the lesion.
- Interventional techniques may be used to treat arteriovenous fistulae which have occurred, e.g. after renal biopsy where these are causing bleeding or haemodynamic complications.

Table 1.3 Mean and standard deviation (SD) of renal length for age in patients with a single functioning kidney

Age range (weeks)	Mean age (weeks)	Mean length (mm)	SD	Number of patients in age group
0–4	2	51.0	5 8	13
5–15	9	56.8	6.3	40
17–34	23	62.8	5.6	25
34–52	46	69.6	6.8	18
53–94	63	71.7	7.9	33
103–153	112	78.0	8.0	32
156–207	172	79.6	8.2	17
208–258	225	86.7	9.5	14
260–312	279	91.0	7.9	12

Recommendations for ultrasound screening for renal abnormalities

Many chromosomal and genetic abnormalities and syndromes are associated with renal abnormalities of all types. Some structural abnormalities are familial. US screening is recommended when there is:

* structural renal disease, renal agenesis, or VUR with renal defects in first-degree relatives.
* single umbilical artery: this occurs in ~0.3% of births and is associated with a slightly increased risk of renal abnormalities.
* congenital external ear abnormalities with or without hearing defects.
* any of the retinal dystrophies.
* chromosomal abnormalities.
* syndromes or associations with known renal abnormalities.
* screening of children for ADPKD is discussed in → Chapter 13.
* conversely, parents (and siblings if the disease has complications that may need treatment) of children with renal cystic disease should be screened.
* screening of patients with a predisposition for Wilms tumour is described in → Chapter 15.

Percutaneous renal biopsy

Indications

Native kidney

- Nephrotic syndrome:
  - Atypical features at initial presentation (see ➔ Chapter 9).
  - Primary steroid resistance (non-response to at least 28 days of steroid therapy).
  - Secondary steroid resistance (the development of steroid resistance in a previously steroid sensitive patient).
  - To monitor calcineurin inhibitor (CNI) therapy. It is recommended that biopsy is performed after 2 years of therapy to exclude CNI nephrotoxicity: where significant interstitial damage is detected, the CNI should be discontinued.
- Acute kidney injury (AKI) of uncertain aetiology (not where diagnosis is clear cut, e.g. Shiga toxin-producing *Escherichia coli* haemolytic uraemic syndrome (STEC-HUS)) or AKI in patients in the intensive care unit with a history very suggestive of ATN).
- Rapidly progressive renal failure.
- CKD of uncertain aetiology (not if kidneys <5 cm bipolar length; increased risk of complications).
- Acute nephritic syndrome with low C3 persisting beyond 8 weeks.
- Henoch–Schönlein purpura (HSP) with heavy proteinuria, renal impairment or hypertension (➔ see Chapter 11).
- Suspected vasculitis (although beware the risk of biopsy of intrarenal artery aneurysm in polyarteritis nodosa).
- Systemic lupus erythematosus (SLE) with renal involvement.
- Macroscopic or microscopic haematuria if associated with proteinuria (urine Upr:Ucr >100 mg/mmol), hypertension, or impaired renal function. Genetic testing is replacing the renal biopsy in certain children, e.g. those with a family history of Alport syndrome.
- Sub-nephrotic proteinuria of uncertain aetiology. In general, biopsy in children with isolated proteinuria and a Upr:Ucr of <100 mg/mmol is unlikely to yield results which significantly alter clinical management.

Transplant

- Acute deterioration in graft function.
- Chronic deterioration in graft function.
- Delayed graft function.
- Stable but poor graft function.
- Proteinuria.
- Diagnosis of recurrent or *de novo* glomerular disease.
- Routine surveillance biopsies—an increasing number of centres are now performing routine protocol biopsies at, e.g. 12 months post transplantation.

Contraindications

These are all relative; assessment has to be made of the risks and benefits of the procedure. Open biopsy can be performed where the risk of complications is thought to be excessive; this is a rare occurrence. Percutaneous biopsy should not be performed in the presence of large cysts or abscesses because of the risk of spreading infection along the track of the biopsy needle.

- Abnormal clotting or low platelet count.

- Anticoagulant or antiplatelet therapy—in most centres the patient receiving aspirin post transplant will be biopsied without the aspirin being discontinued.
- Solitary native kidney.
- Horseshoe or other fused or anatomically abnormally sited native kidney.
- Severe hydronephrosis.
- Polycystic kidneys.
- Abnormal vascular supply.
- Severe CKD (need to control BP and abnormal bleeding tendency).
- Uncontrolled hypertension.
- Severe oedema.
- Obesity.

Pre-biopsy investigations

- FBC.
- Clotting studies (prothrombin time (PTT), activated prothrombin time (APTT) and fibrinogen) and history to exclude coagulopathy.
- Group and save blood.
- Renal US to confirm the presence of two kidneys, exclude hydronephrosis, etc. (may be performed at time of procedure).
- Bleeding time if urea >40 mmol/L, however this is rarely performed. In uraemic patients, desmopressin, a synthetic derivate of arginine vasopressin (AVP), has been shown to shorten the prolonged bleeding time significantly while increasing factor VIII coagulant activity. IV infusion of 0.3 g/kg diluted in 50 mL of 0.9% saline over 30 min may normalize the bleeding time for 4–8 h in most uraemic patients, so allowing renal biopsy (unlicensed indication).

Sedation/anaesthesia

- General anaesthesia may be preferable in smaller children and those in whom sedation has previously failed. Many recommend that all renal biopsies in children should be performed under general anaesthesia.
- Alternatively, sedation and analgesia may be given as per local policy. One example is an IV infusion of chlorpromazine (1 mg/kg body weight—maximum 50 mg) given over 60 min and slow IV injection of pethidine (1 mg/kg body weight, maximum 75 mg). Additional sedation, if required at the time of the biopsy with IV diazepam (0.2–0.4 mg/kg body weight) or IV midazolam (0.1 mg/kg body weight) (e.g. chlorpromazine 1 mg/kg (maximum dose 50 mg). There are NICE clinical guidelines regarding the use of sedation in children (℞ https://www.nice.org.uk/guidance/cg112).
- Older children with extraperitoneal transplants can often be biopsied with local anaesthesia ± Entonox® alone.

Procedure

- Children undergoing native renal biopsy should be placed in the prone position.
- A rolled sheet or firm sponge bolster placed under the lower ribs/upper abdomen will help to 'fix' the position of the kidneys.
- Real-time US guidance will:
  - allow pre-biopsy confirmation of the presence of two kidneys.
  - confirm the absence of severe hydronephrosis or other abnormality.

- allow the tip of the needle to be visualized, so the direction may be altered to avoid the calyceal system and major vessels.
- reduce the complication rate.
- The use of automated, spring-loaded biopsy devices (e.g. Biopty® gun) is associated with a lower incidence of complications and a smaller number of passes required to obtain an adequate tissue sample. 16–18 gauge needles are generally used in children: smaller needles are associated with a lower rate of complications, though the volume of tissue obtained is correspondingly smaller.
- Strict asepsis should be maintained.
- Local anaesthetic should be infiltrated at the biopsy site and along the proposed route of the biopsy needle to the pericapsular region.
- The biopsy needle should be passed under real-time US guidance to the site of biopsy: this should be at the lower pole of the native kidney, or the most accessible pole of a transplanted kidney, with care taken to identify and avoid the main renal vessels.
- Two adequate cores of renal tissue (➔ see following 'Tissue handling' section) should be obtained.
- More than three passes of the biopsy needle should be avoided as this increases the risk of complications.
- Fine-needle aspiration of the transplant kidney has been advocated by some for the diagnosis of acute rejection by the study of intragraft gene expression. At present, the use of this technique, which may be associated with a lower rate of complications, is generally restricted to research protocols.

Tissue handling

- The specimen should be checked under a low-power dissection microscope to ensure adequate cortical tissue has been obtained.
- The quality of a renal biopsy depends on the size, i.e. the number of glomeruli: it is generally agreed that 10–15 glomeruli are optimal; very often 6–10 glomeruli are sufficient and in some cases even 1 glomerulus is enough to make a diagnosis. However, if the percentage of glomerular involvement in a biopsy is used to determine the severity of a focal glomerular lesion, a small biopsy sample size will lead to considerable misclassification of disease severity. In addition, a small biopsy sample size will make the exclusion of focal disease difficult.
- Banff transplant biopsy criteria (1997) define adequacy as the presence in the sample of ten glomeruli and two arteries.
- The sample should be divided into three portions, for light microscopy, immunofluorescence, and electron microscopy.

Post-biopsy observations

- Bed rest for 4 h if possible.
- Encourage adequate fluid intake to ensure good diuresis (unless oliguric renal failure is present).
- Monitor pulse, BP, respiratory rate, and O_2 saturations for 6 h post procedure.
- Monitor urine for macroscopic haematuria.
- A FBC should be checked if there are abnormal observations or macroscopic haematuria.

- Activity post biopsy should be restricted as follows:
  - Stay off school for 48 h.
  - Avoiding lifting, strenuous activity, and running for 1 week after biopsy.
  - Avoid contact sports for 6 weeks.

Complications

- Pain over the biopsy site.
- Complications of analgesia/sedation.
- Macroscopic haematuria (5–7%):
  - Although transient macroscopic haematuria is seen in 0.8–12% of biopsies, massive haematuria leading to serious complications necessitating surgical intervention is not usually seen in the well-selected patient population with normal pre-biopsy screening.
  - Haematuria generally settles conservatively: bed rest and fluids are recommended to encourage a good urine output. The haemoglobin needs regular monitoring.
  - ~1–2% of cases require blood transfusion or are severe enough to cause clot colic or ureteral/bladder outlet obstruction.
- Microscopic haematuria is almost universal (and many will have had pre-biopsy microscopic haematuria).
- Asymptomatic subcapsular or perirenal haematomas can be detected in most patients if a post procedure US is performed but US is only indicated if there are clinical reasons and a routine scan is not recommended.
- Arteriovenous fistula formation:
  - Incidence depends on how hard they are looked for, but up to 15% with routine angiography.
  - Most resolve spontaneously.
  - Very rarely cause hypertension or high output cardiac failure necessitating embolization or heminephrectomy.
- Inadvertent extrarenal organ puncture.
- Mortality rate is 0.12% in adult series.
- Requirement for any surgery or interventional radiological procedure is 0.3%.
- The risk of kidney loss is <0.1%.

A recent study from the United Kingdom (UK) has proposed that a major complication rate of <5% is an acceptable standard. In this publication, major complications were defined as macroscopic haematuria requiring monitoring and/or intervention, a prolonged hospital stay due to requirement for analgesia, and hypoxia requiring intervention and/or oxygen post procedure.

Day case versus overnight stay

Most units are now performing percutaneous renal biopsy as a day-case procedure, given that most complications that develop will present within the immediate post-biopsy period. Criteria for discharge might be that:

- the observations are normal.
- the biopsy site looks satisfactory.
- the patient passes urine twice, neither sample of which is heavily blood-stained.

Renal histology: glossary of terms and examples of commonly encountered paediatric renal disease

Fig. 1.4 shows the normal human glomerulus. Figs 1.5–1.18 show examples of relatively common or classical renal pathology in children. Table 1.4 is a glossary of terms used by pathologists when describing renal biopsy material.

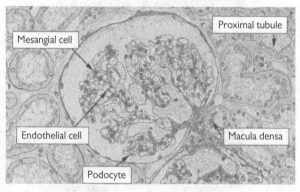

Fig. 1.4 Normal renal biopsy. See also Plate 1.

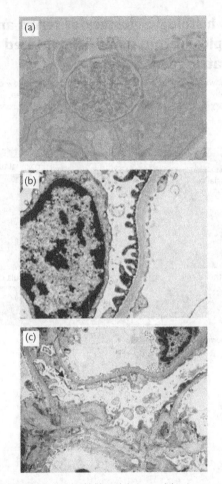

Fig. 1.5 Minimal change disease. (a) Minimal changes on light microscopy. (b) Electron microscopy (EM) of normal foot processes. (c) Minimal change disease with effacement of podocyte foot processes. See also Plate 2.

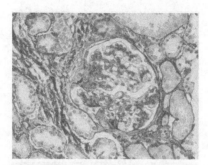

Fig. 1.6 Focal and segmental glomerulosclerosis: sclerosis of part of a glomerulus, not all glomeruli affected (silver stain). A capsular adhesion is present. There is a propensity for FSGS to affect predominantly the deep, juxta-medullary glomeruli, so cortical glomeruli may not demonstrate the lesion (false-negative renal biopsy). See also Plate 3.

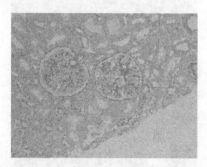

Fig. 1.7 Mesangial proliferative glomerulonephritis. Increase in mesangial cells and matrix (>4 cells/mesangial area), but without peripheral capillary loop involvement (PAS). This pattern is most characteristic of Henoch–Schönlein nephritis, IgA nephropathy, IgM nephropathy, and SLE, but may be present in many other conditions. See also Plate 4.

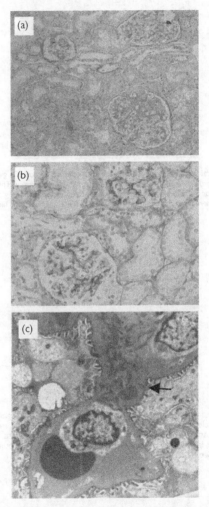

Fig. 1.8 IgA nephropathy. (a) Mesangial proliferation (PAS). (b) Granular immune complexes containing predominantly IgA in the mesangium of most or all glomeruli (immunohistochemistry). (c) EM showing electron-dense deposits in the mesangium. See also Plate 5.

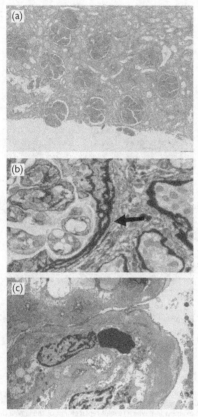

Fig. 1.9 Membranoproliferative glomerulonephritis 1. (a) Diffuse increase in glomerular cellularity with mesangial cell proliferation and lobulation of the glomerular tufts (PAS). (b) Thickening of the capillary wall caused by circumferential interposition of mesangial cells and matrix between the endothelium GBM, resulting in capillary luminal narrowing and 'double-contour' formation on silver staining (silver). (c) EM revealing separation of the endothelial cells from the GBM by interposed mesangial cell cytoplasm and subendothelial deposits, resulting in narrowing of the capillary lumen. See also Plate 6.

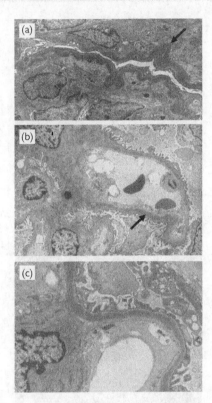

Fig. 1.10 Membranoproliferative glomerulonephritis type 2, dense deposit disease. A wide spectrum of light microscopy appearances may be seen, but the diagnosis is made on EM examination, which reveals replacement of the lamina densa of the capillary basement membrane by electron-dense material, which may also be observed in other areas.

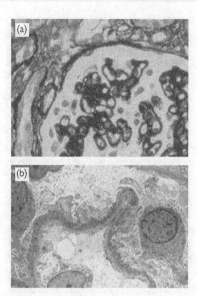

Fig. 1.11 Membranous glomerulonephritis. (a) Light microscopy demonstrating thickening of the GBMs with 'spike' formation (silver). (b) EM of membranous glomerulonephritis with thickened GBM and numerous, regular subepithelial electron-dense deposits. See also Plate 7.

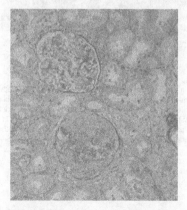

Fig. 1.12 Crescentic nephritis. Cellular crescent impinging on glomerulus (PAS). Immunohistochemistry was 'pauci-immune' compatible with antineutrophil cytoplasmic antibody (ANCA) vasculitis (in this case granulomatosis with polyangiitis). See also Plate 8.

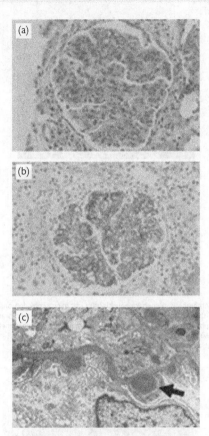

Fig. 1.13 Post-infectious glomerulonephritis (acute diffuse proliferative glomerulonephritis). (a) Glomeruli show hypercellularity. There is obliteration of the capillary lumens (endocapillary proliferation). Some polymorphonuclear leucocytes can be seen (PAS). (b) Coarse granular pattern of staining with IgG in the GBM ('lumpy bumpy' pattern), typical of post-infectious glomerulonephritis (IHC). (c) EM showing large subepithelial deposits (humps) in the GBM (arrows). See also Plate 9.

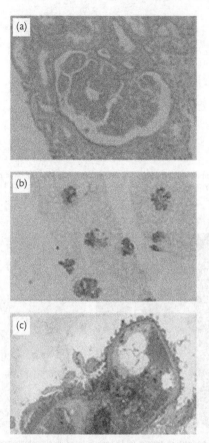

Fig. 1.14 Systemic lupus erythematosus. (a) Diffuse proliferative (World Health Organization (WHO) class 4) lupus nephritis with endocapillary cellular proliferation and massive subendothelial deposit forming 'wire-loop' and 'hyaline-drop' lesions. (b) Immunostaining in such cases often shows a 'full-house' pattern with deposition of IgG, IgM, IgA, and complement. (c) Large electron-dense deposits are seen in the subendothelial region of the GBM (arrow). See also Plate 10.

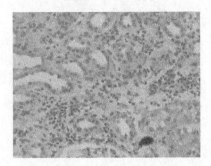

Fig. 1.15 Tubulointerstitial nephritis. Extensive interstitial infiltration of mononuclear inflammatory cells and eosinophils with tubular damage. See also Plate 11.

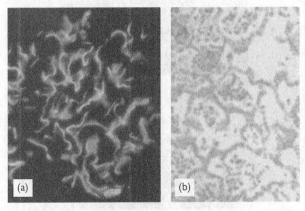

Fig. 1.16 Goodpasture disease. (a) Linear staining of immunoglobulin deposited in the glomerulus. In Goodpasture disease, the autoantibody is directed against an antigen in the GBM deposited in a linear fashion, in contrast to immune complex-mediated disease. (b) Lung of a patient with evidence of intra-alveolar haemorrhage. See also Plate 12.

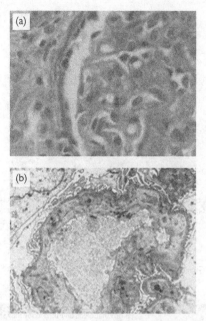

Fig. 1.17 Haemolytic uraemic syndrome. (a) A glomerulus affected by thrombotic microangiopathy with luminal reduction and double-contour formation (silver). (b) Electron micrograph demonstrating subendothelial widening containing fibrin-like material. See also Plate 13.

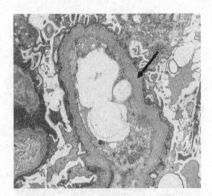

Fig. 1.18 Alport syndrome. Electron microscopy demonstrating irregularity of the basement membranes and the characteristic lamination ('basket weave') of the lamina densa.

Table 1.4 Glossary of histological terms

Term	Definition
Minimal change	Normal appearance by light microscopy. Note that electron microscopy may show fusion of podocyte foot processes, an association with glomerular proteinuria (Fig. 1.5)
Proliferation	Increase in cell numbers, may be mesangial, endocapillary, or extracapillary, (which may form crescents) E.g. mesangial proliferation = >4 cells per mesangial area (Fig. 1.7)
Exudation	Infiltrated by neutrophils, e.g. acute post-streptococcal nephritis (Fig. 1.13)
Membranous	Specific type of glomerular basement membrane thickening associated with subepithelial immune deposits, e.g. idiopathic membranous nephropathy (Fig. 1.10)
Hyalinosis	Accumulation and condensation of plasma proteins into tissues outside a blood vessel lumen, appears as homogeneous pink staining with H&E (see later in table)
Sclerosis	Scar tissue, a fibrous matrix obliterates normal structure so that capillaries collapse and normal cell nuclei are lost (Fig. 1.6)

Table 1.4 (*Contd.*)

Term	Definition
Tubular atrophy	Thickening and wrinkling of tubular basement membrane around a shrunken tubule with flattened epithelium; implies irreversible tubular damage
Crescent	Collection of cells in Bowman's space in response to glomerular damage. Initially only composed of inflammatory and epithelial cells (cellular crescent), later organizes with fibrin and collagen (fibrous crescent) (Fig. 1.12)
Diffuse	Applying to all glomeruli in a biopsy
Focal	Applying to some glomeruli, but not others
Global	Applying to the whole of a glomerulus
Segmental	Applying to part of a glomerulus, i.e. part of the glomerular capillary tuft is unaffected
'Humps'	Deposits of immunoglobulin and complement in a sub-epithelial site; typical of acute post-streptococcal nephritis (Fig. 1.13)
'Spikes'	Projections of basement membrane between regular subepithelial deposits, typical of membranous nephropathy
Foam cells	Lipid-laden cells, usually histiocytes but also mesangial or tubular cells, seen in nephrotic syndrome and Alport syndrome
Haematoxylin and eosin (H&E)	Routine histological technique which stains cytoplasm pink and nuclei blue. Allows inspection of all renal structures but is poor at distinguishing deposits or visualizing the basement membrane
Periodic acid–Schiff (PAS)	Routine histological technique which clearly delineates basement membranes and allows visualization of cellular components
Silver	Silver stains highlight connective tissue structures such as reticulin, basement membrane, and collagen, which appears black. Very useful for assessment of glomerular capillary basement membrane architecture such as 'spike formation' (see above in table)
Congo red	Stain used for the detection of amyloid, which appears red with 'apple green' birefringence using polarized light examination
Martius scarlet blue (MSB)	Stain which highlights fibrin deposits as red, collagen in blue, and erythrocytes in yellow

(*Continued*)

Table 1.4 (*Contd.*)

Term	Definition
Toluidine blue	Stain used primarily to visualize 'thin sections' prior to electron microscopic examination
Glomerulonephritis	Inflammation of the glomerulus
Tubulointerstitial nephritis	Inflammation of the tubules and interstitium
Electron dense deposits	Dark lesions identifiable on electron microscopic examination, usually corresponding to sites of immunoglobulin or complement deposition
Immunohistochemistry (IHC)	Technique for detecting and localizing specific antigens in tissue sections using a detection system visible on routine light microscopy, e.g. immunoperoxidase
Immunofluorescence (IF)	Technique for detecting and localizing specific antigens in tissue sections using a detection system visible on fluorescence microscopy. Sometimes more sensitive than IHC but requires fresh tissue and is not stable
Thin basement membrane disease	Age 3–15 years: thin glomerular basement membrane (GBM): 181–236 nm; normal: 242–333 nm. Age 9–68 years: thin GBM: 262–335 nm. Normal: 331–547 nm
'Basket weave' GBM	The disordered replication of lamina densa of the GBM in Alport syndrome Nephropathy (Fig. 1.18)

Source: data from Taylor, C.M., et al. Renal biopsy. In: Taylor, C.M. et al. (Eds) (1989) *Handbook of renal investigations in children*. London, UK: Butterworth-Heinemann Ltd. Copyright © 1989 Butterworth-Heinemann Ltd.

Reference

Taylor CM, Chapman S. Renal biopsy. In: Taylor CM, Chapman S, Eds. *Handbook of Renal Investigations in Children*. London: Wright, 1989:160–171.

Genetic testing and antenatal diagnosis

- The discovery of new disease genes has dramatically accelerated since the decoding of the human genome. Moreover, a genetic predisposition for many disorders is increasingly recognized. While the availability to test for these genes in a clinical context is lagging behind, the ongoing cost reductions through the advent of new sequencing technologies (see later in section), is improving access to testing for most genetic disorders.
- Increasingly, so-called copy number variations (CNVs) are recognized as causes of inherited diseases. In most cases it is a deletion, so that instead of the usual two copies of a gene, only one copy is present. For instance, half of all mutations identified in *HNF1B* are whole-gene deletions. But also an excess number of copies (three or more) can cause disease (e.g. trisomy 21). Bioinformatic algorithms for the interpretation of next-generation sequencing data are increasingly able to call these CNV from the 'coverage' (the number of times a stretch of DNA has been 'resequenced', see later in this section).
- Clinical genetic testing is different from research testing. Clinical genetic testing is performed in an accredited laboratory that has been demonstrated to fulfil the necessary quality criteria. In contrast, research testing is performed in a research laboratory not accredited for clinical testing. Consequently, research test results should not be used for clinical decision-making, until confirmed in an accredited laboratory.

Reasons for genetic testing

- *Precise diagnosis*: a precise diagnosis is critical to the instigation of proper treatment and counselling. While most diagnoses can be made by clinical investigations, a genetic diagnosis may obviate the need for invasive diagnostics, such as a biopsy (e.g. Alport syndrome). However, many disease genes are associated with a diverse clinical spectrum so that genetic testing may reveal a surprising diagnosis (e.g. a diagnosis of Dent disease in a patient presenting with nephrotic-range proteinuria and focal segmental glomerulosclerosis (FSGS) on biopsy). Yet most patients also report a psychological benefit of having a specific name for their disease. It also enables them to contact other patients/families affected by the same disease and find disease-specific support.
- *Supporting clinical management*: this is obviously the most important reason, although clinical examples for this are still few. The classic example is steroid-resistant nephrotic syndrome: if a patient presenting with this diagnosis is found to have underlying pathogenic mutations, then this has immediate consequences for further treatment, as it obviates the need for a kidney biopsy, influences the choice of medications (➤ see Chapter 9), and informs discussions regarding the suitability of living donor transplantation. Increased availability of genetic testing and thus more genetic diagnosis will enable correlation between genotype and phenotype, which can then inform the prognosis and management of other affected patients.
- *Precise genetic counselling*: identification of a specific mutation allows determination of carrier or affected status in other interested family members. In some conditions, early diagnosis before the development

of overt symptoms is critical for optimal outcome, e.g. cystinosis or nephrogenic diabetes insipidus. Parents can also be offered prenatal testing for selected disorders with appropriate counselling.

Concerns about genetic testing

- *Psychological burden*: presenting someone with a genetic diagnosis can be very distressing, especially if the person knows about the implications of the diagnosis from other family members. If making the diagnosis results in no therapeutic consequences, genetic testing should be very carefully considered. In children, it is advisable to wait until they are old enough to decide for themselves. A typical example is genetic testing in ADPKD (➔ see Chapter 13). Obviously, if therapeutic interventions are available, then the diagnosis should be established to allow affected patients to benefit from these interventions. As clinical diagnostic criteria based on imaging can be falsely negative in childhood, genetic testing is a more accurate way of establishing the diagnosis, if the mutation in the family is known.
- *Discrimination*: making the diagnosis of an inherited condition could stigmatize a person and affect their ability to obtain insurance, a job, or a mortgage. Some countries have legislation against this discrimination, but enforcement is difficult.

Tests used in making a genetic diagnosis

- *Karyotype*: a well-established method in which chromosomes are stained and ordered according to size from 1–23, plus the two sex chromosomes. This test can detect abnormalities in chromosome number (such as trisomy 21), as well as major structural abnormalities in a chromosome.
- *Sequencing*: this refers to the determination of the order of the nucleotide bases in a molecule of DNA. Typically, this is used to identify a mutation in a gene associated with the patient's disease. Different methods are being used:
  - *Sanger sequencing*: this is the conventional form of sequencing that can decode the nucleotide sequence for stretches of typically 500–800 base pairs. Sanger sequencing is expensive and labour intensive. To cut down on costs, sometimes only specific regions of a gene known to harbour most mutations are assessed. However, if this limited mutation screening is unsuccessful or mutations are known to be scattered throughout the whole gene, the entire gene must be sequenced. Sanger sequencing is more and more being replaced by 'next-generation' sequencing.
  - *'Next-generation' sequencing*: while various technologies for next-generation sequencing exist, they all share key features—they dramatically reduce the cost for sequencing but can only decode short stretches of DNA (20–400 base pairs, depending on the technology). To achieve sufficient accuracy these stretches need to be sequenced many times over (also called 'resequencing') and the results are then assembled by computer software. To get an idea of the cost reduction provided by these new technologies, consider these numbers: the decoding of the first human genome using Sanger sequencing was completed in 2005—it took 15 years at a cost of $2.7 billion. In 2010, a study was published in which an individual genome was sequenced in a few weeks using next-generation sequencing for less than

$50,000 and in 2017 it was available for approximately $1000 with a turnaround time of <1 week. However, these numbers apply to the bare sequencing costs, not the analysis, such as bioinformatics and, if needed, mutation confirmation by conventional methods.

- *MLPA*: this stands for multiplex ligation-dependent probe amplification and is a technique used to assess CNV (or gene dosage) of a defined stretch of DNA (e.g. an exon of a gene).
- *FISH*: this stands for fluorescent *in situ* hybridization and is another technique used to assess CNV for a defined region of DNA. It is typically used in the diagnosis of diseases caused by a defined microdeletion, such as Williams syndrome. Both MLPA and FISH are increasingly replaced by array CGH.
- *Array CGH*: this stands for comparative genomic hybridization and is a technique used to assess CNV of longer stretches of DNA (e.g. a gene or several neighbouring genes, so-called microdeletions). The advantage of this technique is that the whole genome is assessed, rather than specific stretches as in MLPA or FISH. Thus, it is in essence an extension of the karyotype with a much finer resolution. It is especially useful in patients with unclear syndromic features, but can also detect known microdeletion syndromes.
- *Linkage*: linkage analysis is a technique mostly used in research to identify new disease genes, but can also be used to assess individual patients, if other family members with the same condition are available. Rather than identifying a specific mutation, linkage analysis identifies whether an individual has inherited a given stretch of DNA that harbours the mutation. For instance, in a family with ADPKD, linkage analysis could identify whether a patient has inherited the same copy of the *PKD* gene, that all the other affected family members share. With the emergence of next-generation sequencing and thus the ability to cheaply assess even very large genes such as the *PKD* genes, linkage analysis will become less and less used for diagnostic purposes. However, it still is an important research tool in identifying disease-causing genes in single-gene disorders.
- *SNP array*: tests for single nucleotide polymorphisms, which by definition are common sequence variations (present in >1% of the population). Modern arrays can test for more than a million SNPs simultaneously. These variations have occurred over time and accumulated in the genome. It is important to understand that the vast majority of these SNPs have little or no functional effect; they are located anywhere in the genome, mostly outside of coding regions. In fact, if they had a substantial functional effect, there would have been evolutionary pressure for this variation to disappear (if it was deleterious) or to become common (if it was beneficial). Only rarely has an identified SNP actual functional significance. This is especially important in interpreting the results of the commercially offered SNP array tests, where clients can send in a buccal smear or saliva sample and then receive their 'personalized genetic information' over the Internet. Having a SNP associated with a given disease does not mean that the disease will actually develop. It only means that in previous studies, a statistically significant higher percentage of patients with the disease have this SNP compared to controls—most likely because this SNP is often inherited together (i.e. 'in linkage disequilibrium') with a functionally relevant sequence variation, which has yet to be identified. Thus, these SNPs

mainly tag a block of DNA in their immediate genomic vicinity that is commonly inherited together (a so-called haplotype), which may harbour the true disease-causing mutation. SNP arrays are used in this capacity both for linkage analysis as well as in genome-wide association studies. However, some SNPs may have a disease-modifying effect or can be causal in association with other sequence variations (often in other genes) or environmental factors. An example of this is the R229Q polymorphism in the *NPHS2* gene: patients homozygous for this variation do not develop steroid-resistant nephrotic syndrome, but in combination with certain pathogenic mutations this variation is disease causing. It is also associated with microalbuminuria in the general population.

* *GWAS*: a genome-wide association study is a research tool used to identify the genetic contribution in multifactorial diseases. Thus, in contrast to linkage analysis, which is used for single-gene disorders, a GWAS is used if a disease is thought to have a genetic contribution, but is caused by the interplay of several genes or environmental factors. Recent examples include the identification of several SNPs associated with diabetes or membranous nephropathy. Again, it is important to understand that the identified SNPs only have a statistical association with the disease, but usually are not causal themselves. Rather, they are in close vicinity to the actual underlying sequence change and thus are inherited together.

Antenatal diagnosis

A fetal abnormality may be:
* detected on US during routine screening.
* specifically looked for using US because of a family history.
* diagnosed using genetic testing.

Genetic studies are justified if early intervention or treatment improves the outcome (e.g. nephrogenic diabetes insipidus (NDI), cystinosis, X-linked hypophosphataemic rickets) or when the condition has a poor prognosis and the family would opt for termination of pregnancy.

DNA from the fetus can be obtained by:
* chorionic villus sampling:
  * is undertaken at 10–12 weeks' gestation.
  * the villi contain ample DNA for analysis.
  * there is a risk of miscarriage of 1–2%.
* amniotic fluid:
  * can be obtained from 15 weeks' gestation.
  * 3 weeks are needed for the amniotic cells to grow to obtain enough DNA.
  * there is a risk of miscarriage of 0.5%.
* maternal blood:
  * based on the fact that a small amount of free fetal DNA is found in the mother's blood.
  * obtained through a simple blood test from the mother, with no risk to the fetus.
  * testing for each individual mutation needs to be set up in advance, thus is time and labour intensive.

The neonate

The fetus and birth

Kidney development commences at 5 weeks of gestation. By week 9, the first glomeruli are formed. Over 80% of nephrons form during the third trimester. By week 34, glomerulogenesis ceases, by which time there are the definitive numbers of around 0.5–1 million glomeruli in each kidney. Thereafter, there is only tubular and vascular growth and an increase in interstitial tissue.

* The perinatal period in premature infants is crucial for the remaining nephron development.
* Therefore, the premature infant's kidneys are particularly vulnerable to insult during the period of ongoing nephrogenesis.
* Prematurity and intrauterine growth restriction is associated with reduced nephron mass and with hypertension in later life.

A bladder is detectable by week 9. By the 20th week of gestation, neonatal urine constitutes 80% of liquor volume and thereafter fetal urine contributes to >90% of liquor volume.

Important factors in the antenatal history and birth history

* ➲ See Chapter 1 for history and examination.
* 90% of infants pass urine within 24 h.
* Weight loss >10% of birth weight is significant.
* Transient proteinuria may occur in the first days of life.
* Plasma creatinine reflects maternal levels at birth.

Commonly used drugs administered during pregnancy that affect the fetal kidney

* Angiotensin-converting enzyme (ACE) inhibitors affect placental perfusion and inhibit nephrogenesis.
* Non-steroidal anti-inflammatory drugs (NSAIDs) affect fetal renal perfusion and may cause renal cysts and chronic kidney disease (CKD).

Polyhydramnios

* Polyhydramnios occurs in ~1% of pregnancies. In the majority of cases, there is no underlying fetal abnormality, but maternal problems such as diabetes may be present. If a fetal abnormality is present, the majority are in the gastrointestinal (GI) tract (decreased swallowing of liquor). Only a small proportion of polyhydramnios is caused by fetal renal disease, typically Bartter syndrome (➲ see Chapter 7).

Oligohydramnios

* Bilateral urinary tract obstruction.
* Bilateral renal agenesis.

Twin-to-twin transfusion syndrome (TTTS) can cause oligo- or polyhydramnios

- TTTS is due to imbalanced shunting of blood between monochorionic twins due to vascular anastomoses, leading to asymmetrical fetal growth, high mortality, and significant morbidity in survivors.
- Complicates 8–10% of monochorionic pregnancies.
- Polyuria and polyhydramnios are typical for the recipient and oliguria and oligohydramnios for the donor twin.
- AKI/CKD can occur in the donor twin and less commonly in the recipient twin.
- The renal histology may be renal tubular dysgenesis in the donor and haemorrhagic infarction in the recipient twin.
- There is a high incidence of neurodevelopmental abnormalities.

Raised alpha-fetoprotein

This is present in all conditions with leakage of fetal protein, such as:
- neural tube defects.
- CNS.
- epidermolysis bullosa.

Reference

Abitbol CL, DeFreitas MJ, Strauss J. Assessment of kidney function in preterm infants: lifelong implications. *Pediatr Nephrol* 2016;31:2213–2222.

'Bright' kidneys

The term 'bright' kidneys refers to kidneys whose internal structure reflects US waves more than normal renal tissue so that they appear whiter on US scans. This 'reflectivity' is compared to the liver so that if the kidneys appear 'brighter' than the liver, this represents an abnormal internal renal structure. It does not distinguish between the different potential causes. This radiological appearance is not to be confused with 'Bright disease', which refers to nephritis.

Causes of 'bright' kidneys diagnosed on antenatal US scans

* Renal dysplasia (usually small ± cysts): may be isolated, in association with VUR or obstruction, or as part of a syndrome.
* ARPKD (usually large kidneys with small cysts).
* ADPKD and TS (usually large kidneys with large cysts and may be asymmetrical).
* Glomerulocystic disease (typically *HNF1B* gene deletions/mutations; usually large).
* Beckwith–Wiedemann syndrome (visceromegaly, macroglossia, hemihypertrophy, hypoglycaemia).
* CNS.
* Congenital infection.

Causes of 'bright' kidneys diagnosed on postnatal US scans

Same causes as listed for antenatal US scans plus the following:
* Bright cortices may be normal in the neonate.
* Acute tubular necrosis.
* RVT (➔ see 'Renal venous thrombosis').
* Neonatal nephrocalcinosis:
  * Common in preterm infants, particularly if they have been on diuretics or IV feeding.
  * Distal renal tubular acidosis.
  * For other causes of nephrocalcinosis, ➔ see Chapter 8.
* Nephroblastomatosis.
* Primary hyperoxaluria.
* May be transient, due to protein precipitation in the renal tubules.
* Neonatal Bartter syndrome (➔ see Chapter 7).

The kidney in the neonate

Fluid homeostasis in the neonate is compromised because:
* at birth, the kidneys receive 2.5–4.0% of the cardiac output, increasing to 6% at 24 h of life, 10% at 1 week, and 15–18% at 6 weeks of age.
* this is in comparison to the 20–25% of cardiac output received by the adult kidney.
* the GFR is low.

There is tubular immaturity:
* Plasma creatinine may rise in the first 3 weeks of life in premature infants due to tubular reabsorption.
* Plasma bicarbonate may be lower than expected as the renal threshold for bicarbonate is 18–20 mmol/L, rising to 24–26 mmol/L by 1 year of age.
* Sodium and phosphate reabsorption is reduced.
* Maximum urine concentrating capacity is low at birth (up to 600 mOsm/kg), increasing over the first 2 months of life and then progressively over the first year of life.

A further contribution to compromised fluid balance and interpretation of it is that:
* in the first 24–48 h there may be oliguria.
* after birth, there is a contraction of extracellular water followed by natriuresis, diuresis, and weight loss of up to 10% of body weight.
* transepidermal water losses are high, between 7 and 8 mL/m²/h in the first 3 days of life, depending on maturity.

Plasma creatinine is difficult to interpret in the neonate because of:
* the presence of circulating maternal creatinine.
* varying creatinine reabsorption in the proximal tubules.
* for these reasons, some centres use cystatin C in preference to creatinine.

After birth, the GFR is dependent on gestational age, renal volume, and arterial pressure. Table 2.1 shows the mean (± SD) serum creatinine and cystatin C along with estimated GFR (eGFR mL/min/1.73m²) using both creatinine and cystatin C at different times after birth.

Table 2.1 Mean (± SD) serum creatinine and cystatin C levels at different times after birth

	Preterm	Term	3 months	6 months	12 months	24 months
Creatinine mg/dL	0.7 ± 0.3	0.5 ± 0.1	0.4 ± 0.2	0.3 ± 0.2	0.3 ± 0.1	0.3 ± 0.2
Creatinine μmol/L	62 ± 29	44 ± 9	35 ± 18	29 ± 18	29 ± 9	29 ± 18
Cystatin C mg/L	1.42 ± 0.21	1.33 ± 0.20	1.20 ± 0.26	0.98 ± 0.22	0.85 ± 0.22	0.72 ± 0.12
eGFR creatinine	24 ± 7	46 ± 10	63 ± 8	92 ± 10	105 ± 12	120 ± 17
eGFR cystatin	46 ± 10	54 ± 8	61 ± 10	78 ± 8	92 ± 12	112 ± 10

Neonatal hypernatraemic dehydration

* A complication of inadequate breast milk production which may go unrecognized, particularly in the first child who is exclusively breastfed.
* If severe, venous and/or arterial thromboses and AKI may occur.

Reference

Abitbol CL, DeFreitas MJ, Strauss J. Assessment of kidney function in preterm infants: lifelong implications. *Pediatr Nephrol* 2016;31:2213–2222.

Neonatal acute kidney injury

The diagnosis of AKI can be problematic in the neonate due to difficulty in the interpretation of creatinine levels, which can be highly variable. Novel biomarkers of renal damage that allow for the earlier identification of AKI in neonates include urine neutrophil gelatinase-associated lipocalin, cystatin C, kidney injury molecule-1, and others, but these are not of proven value or in routine clinical use.

- Incidence is up to 25% in critically ill neonates.
- Non-oliguric AKI is common (>50%).
- Is associated with increased:
  - mortality (up to 60%).
  - hypertension.
  - CKD.
  - microalbuminuria.

Predisposing factors

- Maternal exposure to NSAIDs and ACE inhibitors.
- Low birth weight (LBW)/prematurity.
- Resuscitation at birth/birth asphyxia.
- Sepsis.
- Nephrotoxic drugs (e.g. aminoglycosides, vancomycin, amphotericin, and aciclovir).
- Cardiothoracic and other surgery.
- Extracorporeal membrane oxygenation (ECMO).
- Renal diseases (usually congenital anomalies of the kidney and urinary tract (CAKUT)).

Suspect neonatal AKI if

- oliguria: newborn with no urine output noted by 48 h of age.
- urine output <1 mL/kg/h.
- increase in serum creatinine:
  - to >133 μmol/L (1.5 mg/dL).
  - by at least 17–27 mmol/L (0.2–0.3 mg/dL) per day.
  - to 150–200% from baseline.

Neonatal AKI Kidney Disease: Improving Global Outcomes (KDIGO) classification

See Table 2.2 for the neonatal AKI KDIGO classification.

Management

- The principles of management are the same as for the older child (→ see Chapter 17), except that urinary sodium <20 mmol/L, fractional excretion of sodium (FeNa) <2.5%, and urine osmolality >400 mOsm/kg suggest pre-renal AKI in neonates, compared to <10 mmol/L, <1%, and >500 mOsm/kg, respectively, in older children.
- Maintaining a normal blood sugar can be difficult in the infant who is fluid restricted.
- In neonates with perinatal asphyxia, adenosine receptor antagonists (theophylline) may prevent AKI by inhibiting the adenosine-induced vasoconstriction. The KDIGO guidelines recommend a single dose of theophylline for asphyxiated infants at risk for AKI.

Table 2.2 Neonatal acute kidney injury KDIGO classification

Stage	Serum creatinine (SCr)	Urine output
0	No change in SCr or rise <0.3 mg/dL	≥0.5 mL/kg/h
1	SCr rise ≥0.3 mg/dL within 48 h or SCr rise	
	≥1.5–1.9 × reference SCr within 7 days	<0.5 mL/kg/h for 6–12 h
2	SCr rise ≥2.0–2.9 × reference SCr	<0.5 mL/kg/h for ≥12 h
3	SCr rise >3 × reference SCr or SCr ≥2.5 mg/dL or 0.3 mL/kg/h for >24 h or receipt of dialysis	Anuria for >12 h

Reference SCr is the lowest previous SCr value.

SCr value of 2.5 mg/dL represents <10 mL/min/1.73 m^2.

* If dialysis is required, most infants are managed with peritoneal dialysis (PD) as dialysis access is easier. However, there are situation where PD is not possible and then haemodialysis (HD) can be used. The CARPEDIEM® and NIDUS® machines can be used for continuous venovenous haemofiltration (CVVH) and for 'bridging' in the very small infant until formal HD becomes possible (➔ see Chapter 20).

Outcome

* A percentage fluid overload of <20% at initiation of renal replacement therapy is associated with improved rates of survival compared with patients with a cumulative fluid balance of >20%.
* Follow-up is essential because the incidence of hypertension, microalbuminuria, and CKD is high, particularly if the renal insult is during the period of ongoing nephrogenesis (before 34 weeks of gestation).

Reference

Selewski DT, Charlton JR, Jetton JG, et al. Neonatal acute kidney injury. *Pediatrics* 2015;136:463–473.

Neonatal renal venous thrombosis

The fetus and neonate are predisposed to RVT because of their low renal blood flow. Venous thrombosis may occur wherever there is vessel wall damage, reduction in blood flow, alteration in blood composition, or an inherited procoagulant tendency. Thrombosis starts in the arcuate or interlobular veins of the kidney and then spreads to the main renal vein. This is why anticoagulation is often unsuccessful when a clot is already identified in the main renal vein, and why the term RVT rather than renal vein thrombosis should be used.

- RVT is the commonest form of venous thrombosis in neonates.
- It may develop antenatally in association with fetal stress so perinatal RVT may be a more appropriate term than neonatal RVT.
- Predisposing factors are maternal thrombotic states and diabetes, dehydration, sepsis, birth asphyxia, umbilical and femoral venous catheters, and procoagulant defects.
- RVT presents with haematuria, renal mass(es), fall in haemoglobin, and thrombocytopenia.
- AKI with a rising creatinine will occur if bilateral.
- Hypertension is common.

Investigations

- Urgent US including Doppler studies when decreased renal blood flow will be seen. It is important to look in the arcuate and interlobular veins as well as the main renal veins, inferior vena cava (IVC), and heart. Measurement of renal length at presentation is important as there is evidence that the most swollen kidneys are the ones that fare worst.
- US can be used to give ongoing information on the restoration or lack of renal blood flow and of renal length, which will show shrinkage if the kidney has died. Calcification may be seen in infarcted tissue after 6 weeks.
- Maternal blood for lupus anticoagulant and anticardiolipin antibody.
- Procoagulant screen including protein C, protein S, and antithrombin levels; lupus anticoagulant testing, dilute Russell's viper venom time (DRVVT), and anticardiolipin levels; and factor V Leiden (1691GA), methylenetetrahydrofolate reductase (*MTHFR*), and prothrombin (2021GA) mutations.
- It is important to note that clot formation, acute phase reactions, and anticoagulants may affect the protein C, protein S, and antithrombin levels. Therefore, normal levels are helpful in determining the duration of therapy but if levels are low acutely, they need to be repeated after recovery.
- Dimercaptosuccinic acid (DMSA) scan after 3–6 months for evidence of renal damage.
- CKD management is necessary in those with bilateral damage shown on DMSA scan.

Treatment

There is no evidence as to who may benefit from anticoagulation in RVT, so each case is considered on an individual basis, weighing up risks and benefits. Some suggestions are as follows:

- Before considering anticoagulation, intracranial bleeds (which may be made worse) must be excluded using intracranial US, particularly in very premature infants.

* For unilateral RVT without extension into the IVC, supportive care is with radiologic monitoring; Doppler US is used when there is extension of thrombosis.
* If extension occurs, anticoagulate with unfractionated heparin (UFH) or low-molecular-weight heparin (LMWH).
* Anticoagulate for 6 weeks to 3 months.
* For bilateral RVT, anticoagulate with UFH/LMWH or initial thrombolytic therapy with tissue plasminogen activator (tPA) (protocol below) followed by anticoagulation with UFH/LMWH (see Table 2.3).

Administration of low molecular weight heparin

This should be undertaken under the supervision of a coagulation specialist. Doses may need to be adjusted if there is AKI (see Table 2.3).

Table 2.3 Administration of subcutaneous low-molecular-weight heparin

LMWH	Age (months)	Dose/kg every 12 h
Enoxaparin	<2	1 mg
	>2	1.5 mg
Dalteparin	<3	150 units
	>3	100 units

* Monitoring is by anti-Xa levels, the first to be taken after two or three doses, 4–6 h post dose, aiming for 0.5–1 U/mL.
* The dose can be adjusted by 10–20%.
* Monitoring is daily until levels are steady in the desired range, decreasing in frequency thereafter.

Administration of recombinant tPA

* Heparin must be stopped for at least 3 h.
* Give 0.1 mg/kg over 10 min then 0.3 mg/kg/h over 3 h.
* If the treatment is not completely successful, tPA can be repeated at an increased dose of 0.4 mg/kg/h over 3 h after 12–24 h.
* All invasive procedures should be avoided.
* The fibrinogen should be maintained at ≥1.5 g/L during the infusion.
* Heparin is started at the end of the infusion at 100 U/kg/day.
* Contraindications are recent surgery, intracerebral bleeding, or other severe bleeding.
* Correct thrombocytopenia and other coagulation deficiencies.
* Normalize the BP as far as possible.

Long-term follow-up

This is required because of the risks of:
* hypertension.
* CKD (may be progressive if bilateral).
* if IVC clot, the development of collaterals may complicate the future use of the femoral veins for dialysis access and the use of the IVC for renal transplantation. Such babies will need MRI of their abdominal vessels prior to transplant.

Reference

Resontoc LP, Yap H-K. Renal vascular thrombosis in the newborn. *Pediatr Nephrol* 2016;31:907–915.

Neonatal hypertension

- BP increases rapidly during the first 5 days after birth by 2–2.5 mmHg and continues to rise over the first 4 weeks at a rate of 1–2 mmHg per week.
- BP increases with gestational and post-conceptional age, and birth weight.
- BP increases more rapidly in preterm than term infants, reaching parity with term infants by about 4 months of age.
- Hypertension occurs in ~3% of neonates admitted to intensive care units. It is less common than hypotension.

Measurement of BP

- BP should be measured in all four limbs to exclude coarctation of the aorta. Thereafter, using the right upper arm is standard procedure.
- BP may be higher by 20 mmHg if feeding and by 10 mmHg when sucking a dummy.
- BP is higher in the head-up state, during suctioning, and when restless.
- BP should therefore be measured when lying, asleep (or quiet if awake), and not feeding.

Table 2.4 provides estimated values for BPs after 2 weeks of age in infants from 26 to 44 weeks' post-conceptual age.

Presentation

- Asymptomatic.
- Non-specific symptoms: feeding difficulty, irritability, or failure to thrive.
- Congestive heart failure: tachypnoea, respiratory distress.
- Decompensated heart failure: hypotension, cardiogenic shock.
- Oliguria or polyuria: renal/renovascular causes.
- Neurological symptoms: lethargy, tremor, apnoea, seizures.

Risk factors for neonatal hypertension

- Low gestational age and LBW.
- Maternal drug ingestion and neonatal drug withdrawal.
- Bronchopulmonary dysplasia.
- Specific cardiac causes, e.g. coarctation, patent ductus arteriosus.
- Renal diseases and AKI.
- Umbilical catheter thromboembolism.
- ECMO.

Causes of severe hypertension in the newborn

- Renal:
  - CAKUT.
  - Cystic kidney disease; CNS.
  - AKI.
  - Renovascular: renal artery stenosis, mid aortic syndrome.
  - Renal arterial or venous thrombosis.
- Cardiovascular:
  - Aortic coarctation ± indometacin.
  - Umbilical catheters.

Table 2.4 Neonatal blood pressures and potential treatment parameters

Post-conceptual age	50th percentile	95th percentile	99th percentile
44 weeks			
SBP	88	105	110
DBP	50	68	73
MAP	63	80	85
42 weeks			
SBP	85	98	102
DBP	50	65	70
MAP	62	76	81
40 weeks			
SBP	80	95	100
DBP	50	65	70
MAP	60	75	80
38 weeks			
SBP	77	92	97
DBP	50	65	70
MAP	59	74	79
36 weeks			
SBP	72	87	92
DBP	50	65	70
MAP	57	72	77
34 weeks			
SBP	70	85	90
DBP	40	55	60
MAP	50	65	70
32 weeks			
SBP	68	83	88
DBP	40	55	60
MAP	49	64	69
30 weeks			
SBP	65	80	85
DBP	40	55	60

Table 2.4 (*Contd.*)

Post-conceptual age	50th percentile	95th percentile	99th percentile
MAP	48	63	68
28 weeks			
SBP	60	75	80
DBP	38	50	54
MAP	45	58	63
26 weeks			
SBP	55	72	77
DBP	30	50	56
MAP	38	57	63

DBP, diastolic blood pressure; MAP, mean arterial pressure; SBP, systolic blood pressure.

Reproduced with permission from Dionne J.M. et al. Hypertension in infancy: diagnosis, management, and outcome. *Pediatric Nephrology*. 27(1), 17–32. Copyright © 2011 Springer Science & Business Media B.V. This table includes the changes published in the Erratum, Pediatr Nephrol 2012; 27:159.

- Iatrogenic/medications:
  - Maternal steroids.
  - Inotropes.
  - Aminophylline.
  - Caffeine.
- ECMO.
- Respiratory:
  - Pneumothorax.
  - Chronic lung disease.
- Neurological:
  - Seizures.
  - Intracranial hypertension.
  - Endocrine.
  - Neonatal abstinence syndrome.
  - Neoplasms.

Investigation

Routine
- Urinalysis.
- FBC.
- U&Es, creatinine, and calcium.
- Renal US with Doppler.
- Echocardiography.

Specialized
- Renin/aldosterone.
- Head US.
- Cortisol.
- Thyroxine (T4)/thyroid-stimulating hormone (TSH).
- Angiography.

Treatment

Mild hypertension (95–99th centile)
* Asymptomatic: observe and reassess with 6-hourly BP measurements.
* Symptomatic: treat with oral medication.

Moderate to severe (>99th centile)
* Evaluate and treat with oral medications.

Hypertensive emergency
* Best managed with short-acting IV antihypertensives that can be carefully titrated with an infusion:
  * Labetalol (alpha and beta blocker) 0.2–3 mg/kg/h (use cautiously in heart failure).
  * Nitroprusside (vasodilator) 0.25–8 micrograms/kg/min.
* Avoid too rapid a reduction in BP: premature infants are at increased risk of intracranial events due to the immaturity of their periventricular circulation.
* Monitor with intra-arterial measurements or every 5–15 min manually.

Medications

Principles of treatment do not differ from those in older children but there are some differences:
* Shorter-acting drugs may be of benefit as they can be easily withdrawn if necessary.
* IV:
  * Labetalol: 0.2–1.0 mg/kg/dose IV 4–6-hourly, maximum 4 mg/kg.
  * Hydralazine: 0.2–1.0 mg/kg/dose IV 4–6-hourly.
* Oral:
  * Propranolol: 0.5–1.5 mg/kg/dose orally three times daily, but may increase bronchoconstriction in infants with lung disease.
  * Nifedipine: 0.1–0.25 mg/kg/dose orally 4–6-hourly.
  * Clonidine: 0.5–2.5 micrograms/kg/dose orally 6-hourly.
  * Captopril: 0.01–0.5 mg/kg/dose orally three times daily may be useful, but should not be used during ongoing glomerulogenesis (<34 weeks' gestation) or if renal artery stenosis is a possibility.
* Other useful oral medications:
  * Amlodipine: 0.1–0.3 mg/kg/dose orally two times daily.
  * Hydralazine: 0.25–1.0 mg/kg/dose orally two times daily.

Outcome

* May resolve spontaneously if no cause identified.
* Infants with LBW may have a low nephron number causing a high BP so they need follow-up.

Reference

Dionne JM, Flynn JT. Management of severe hypertension in the newborn. *Arch Dis Child* 2017;102:1176–1179.

Congenital abnormalities of the kidneys and urinary tract

Antenatal diagnosis of structural renal abnormalities

The majority of congenital abnormalities of the kidneys and urinary tract (CAKUT) are identified *in utero* and can be managed prospectively. They are potentially important because they may:
* be associated with abnormal renal development or function.
* predispose to postnatal infection.
* cause urinary obstruction that requires surgical treatment.
* occasionally be associated with aneuploidy or syndromes.

The antenatal detection and early treatment of urinary tract anomalies provide an opportunity to minimize or prevent progressive renal damage. A disadvantage is that minor abnormalities are also detected, most commonly mild, unilateral renal pelvic dilatation, which do not require intervention, but may lead to over-investigation, unnecessary treatment, and unwarranted parental anxiety. It must be remembered that the management of the child who presents with symptoms is not the same as that of the child who present with abnormalities on the antenatal scan.

Classification of antenatal ultrasound abnormalities

* Renal tract dilatation, which may be of the renal pelvis and/or calyces (hydronephrosis) and/or ureter (hydroureteronephrosis); see Table 3.1.
* The bladder may have diverticulae, be thick walled, and/or show poor emptying; a dilated posterior urethra may be seen.
* Absent kidney(s).
* Large, small, echogenic, or cystic kidneys.

Table 3.1 Major causes of antenatal renal tract dilatation

Transient hydronephrosis (normal postnatal scan)	50%
Hydronephrosis with no evidence of obstruction; or extrarenal pelvis	15%
PUJ obstruction	11%
VUR	9%
Megaureter (obstructed, refluxing, non-refluxing and non-obstructed or both refluxing and obstructed)	4%
Renal dysplasia	3%
MCDK	2%
Duplex kidney ± ureterocoele	2%
PUV	1%
Others	3%

Key points
- High resolution, two-dimensional (2D) US allows detailed assessment of the kidneys and urinary tract from the second trimester of pregnancy.
- The incidence of antenatal renal tract dilatation (hydronephrosis) is around 1:200 pregnancies.
- There are many causes of antenatal renal tract dilatation; detection does not necessarily indicate the presence of obstruction in the affected kidney.
- Abnormalities of other organ systems may sometimes coexist with renal anomalies.
- It is important to remember that following the detection of antenatal renal tract dilatation, ~50% of postnatal scans will subsequently be normal.
- Whenever a fetus or infant is being assessed, it is essential to take a complete antenatal history including details of all of the investigations performed to date.

Technical issues
- Antenatal US scans are usually undertaken routinely at 12–14 and 20 weeks' gestation. Many abnormalities appear early, but PUVs and others may be missed without a third-trimester scan.
- Measurement of renal length. Allow 1 mm per week of gestation, e.g. the length of the kidney in a 34-week gestation fetus is ~34 mm.
- Renal pelvic dilatation is assessed by measurement of the maximum anteroposterior (AP) pelvic diameter in the transverse plane (not including the calyces), known as the transverse pelvic diameter (TPD).
- There is much debate regarding cut-off points for isolated renal pelvic dilatation above which postnatal investigation should be initiated:
  - AP diameters of between 5 and 15 mm have been proposed as the cut-off point above which postnatal investigation should be performed;
  - There is no good evidence to support any particular measurement—this is reflected in the variation seen internationally and within countries regarding proposed cut-off points.
  - Lower cut-off points will increase the number of investigations performed postnatally (higher false-positive rate) and enhance parental anxiety. The number of abnormalities detected will increase, but these are likely to be cases of mild non-dilating VUR, which are unlikely to be of clinical significance.
- Careful assessment of the bladder and ureters should be performed:
  - Detection of calyceal and/or ureteric dilatation is of significance as their presence increases the likelihood of a significant urological abnormality being present; more intensive postnatal investigation is therefore warranted.
  - Detection of bilateral pelvic dilatation at any time must be considered significant and increases the likelihood of a significant urological abnormality being present; more intensive postnatal investigation is therefore warranted.
- Liquor volume needs careful assessment.
- It is possible to mistake the adrenal gland for the kidney in cases where the latter is absent.

Indications for antenatal referral to a fetal therapy unit

The following antenatal abnormalities need referral to a fetal therapy unit for discussion with a nephrologist/urologist (see Figs. 3.1–3.3):

- Oligohydramnios.
- Abnormal bladder: thick wall, ureterocoele, absent bladder.
- Abnormal renal parenchyma: echogenic, large or small kidneys, cystic change.
- Bilateral renal tract dilatation where the TPD is >15 mm.
- Solitary kidney where the TPD is >15 mm.
- Other major anomalies.

The management of antenatally detected renal tract dilatation is outlined in Figs. 3.1–3.3.

All infants where bilateral hydronephrosis (TPD diameter of ≥7 mm), hydronephrosis in a single kidney (TPD diameter of ≥7 mm), or hydronephrosis associated with ureteric dilatation is detected should undergo postnatal investigation (see Fig. 3.3).

Ultrasound

- The difficulty is to distinguish neonates with abnormalities who need further assessment and treatment from those who need conservative management. US is the first investigation:
  - Where unilateral hydronephrosis is present without ureteric dilatation (see Fig. 3.2), this should be performed at 1 week as the neonate is relatively oliguric for the first few days of life.
  - Where hydronephrosis is bilateral, present in a solitary kidney, or associated with ureteric dilatation or abnormal kidneys or bladder (see Fig. 3.3), this should be performed along with a MCUG within 3 days of birth if the largest TPD was >10 mm, otherwise within 7 days. This is the case in a boy even if the hydronephrosis was shown

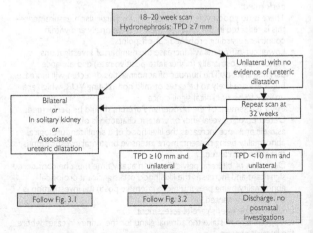

Fig. 3.1 The antenatal scan findings, indicating those that require further follow-up and investigation and those that can be discharged.

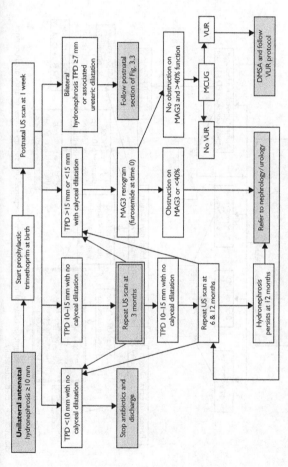

Fig. 3.2 Postnatal management for unilateral hydronephrosis diagnosed antenatally.

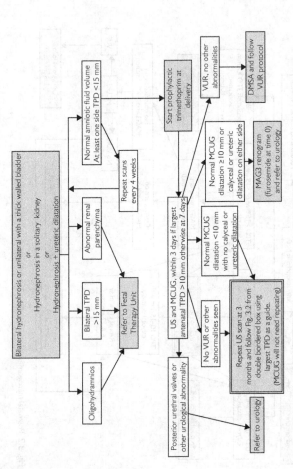

Fig. 3.3 Postnatal management for bilateral hydronephrosis, hydronephrosis in a solitary kidney, or associated ureteric dilatation detected antenatally.

to subsequently resolve during later pregnancy as the purpose is to exclude a PUV, and even if ureteric dilatation is unilateral if the bladder wall is thickened or kidneys abnormal.

- US should include:
  - measurement of renal length, and assessment of appearance and echogenicity.
  - measurement of the maximum renal pelvic diameter in the transverse plane (not including the calyces) and ureteric dilatation. A dilated renal pelvis with no dilatation of the ureter may signify a PUJ abnormality. Dilatation of the pelvis and ureter may signify a VUJ abnormality or VUR.
  - Assessment of the calyces.
  - Appearance of the bladder with measurement of wall thickness, presence of ureterocoeles, and, if the baby passes urine during the examination, post-micturition residue. Views of the posterior urethra can be obtained in boys.
  - Spinal views can be obtained if a neuropathic bladder is suspected.

MCUG

Indications for a MCUG:

- Bilateral hydronephrosis or ureteric dilatation in a solitary kidney (Fig. 3.3). This should be performed within 3 days of birth if the largest TPD was >10 mm and otherwise within 7 days.
- Distended or thick-walled bladder with or without ureteric dilatation, perform within 3 days of birth.
- Duplex kidney associated with hydronephrosis or ureterocoele.

All antenatally diagnosed scenarios whether subsequently resolved or not should have a postnatal US scan and proceed to MCUG if any of above indications present.

MAG3

The MAG3 scan can be undertaken at 1–2 months of age. It gives information on the function of each kidney relative to the total:

- Good function is >40%.
- Moderate 20–40%.
- Poor <20%.

It must be noted that the drainage curve is unreliable in the neonate and will over-diagnose obstruction because it is dependent upon:

- renal function.
- hydration and urine flow rate.
- bladder fullness.
- posture and pooling in a dilated system.

Long-term outcome studies of renal pelvic dilatation secondary to PUJ obstruction have provided the following information:

- All kidneys that showed deterioration in function had a TPD >20 mm.
- A sustained increase in dilatation may precede deterioration in function.
- There is a very high risk of deterioration in function (60%) if the TPD is >30 mm and pyeloplasty in the first 6 months of life is recommended.
- Of infants with renal pelvic measurements between 20 and 30 mm with good function, one-quarter remain stable, and some may improve by the age of 3–4 years.
- The more severe the calyceal dilatation, the greater the risk of deterioration.

Surgery is recommended:
* in infants who develop symptoms.
* when there is progressive dilatation as measured by US.
* when there is deterioration in function on MAG3 scan.
* if the renal pelvic transverse diameter is >30 mm.

Other renal anomalies

The following may also be detected and are discussed elsewhere: note that where evidence of one or more of these is detected antenatally, this should prompt referral to a fetal therapy unit:
* Cystic kidneys.
* Echo-bright kidneys.
* Multicystic dysplastic kidney (MCDK).
* Solitary kidney.
* Ectopic, horseshoe, and duplex kidneys.

Renal agenesis

Introduction

- True unilateral renal agenesis is caused by a failure of the ureteral bud to communicate with the metanephric blastema in the first few weeks of gestation.
- A number of cases of apparent renal agenesis will represent MCDKs that have undergone spontaneous regression.
- The reported incidence is 1:500 to 1:3200.
- Diagnosis is now most commonly made on antenatal renal US.
- May go undetected and be diagnosed incidentally later in life, e.g. at time of US scan for unrelated issues or urine infection, particularly if antenatal scanning was not performed.
- A 2013 systematic review of 1093 cases reported associated CAKUT of the contralateral kidney in 32% of cases:
  - VUR in 24%.
  - Megaureter in 7%.
  - PUJ obstruction in 6%.
  - Duplex kidney in 3%.
- Extrarenal anomalies were reported in 31%, including GI, cardiac, musculoskeletal, genital tract, and central nervous system.
- There is an increased incidence of asymptomatic renal malformation (9%), most frequently unilateral agenesis (4.5%), in first-degree relatives of patients with bilateral renal agenesis, bilateral severe dysplasia, or agenesis of one kidney and dysplasia of the other. US examination of first-degree relatives may therefore be warranted.

Investigation

- Ultrasound:
  - For renal size: a solitary kidney should show compensatory hypertrophy (>2 SD above the mean) (➔ see Table 1.1).
  - To search for a previously undetected ectopic kidney.
  - To detect hydronephrosis or hydroureter in the single kidney suggestive of obstruction or VUR.
  - Consider performing a DMSA scan to confirm absence of contralateral functioning renal tissue and to look for ectopically sited kidneys that have not been detected by US examination. Experienced ultrasonographers may argue that this is unnecessary and that ectopically sited kidneys can always be identified.
- If there is ureteric dilatation, this may represent VUR so the family members need to have a low threshold for seeking medical advice to exclude UTI during febrile episodes. If a UTI does occur, MCUG is needed.
- MAG3 where there is suspicion of either PUJ or VUJ obstruction because of pelvic or ureteric dilatation on US without a dilated ureter or VUR on MCUG.

* The contralateral kidney should show compensatory hypertrophy. Where compensatory hypertrophy does not occur, this suggests the presence of dysplasia, and assessment of renal function should be performed (measurement of plasma creatinine or formal measurement of GFR depending upon individual centre practice):
  * Where there is evidence of compensatory hypertrophy and no other abnormality on US examination, the outcome is likely to be very good and the child can be discharged from hospital follow-up to the care of their local doctor.
  * It is probably sensible that such children have their BP and an early morning urine dipstick for proteinuria assessed by their family doctor on an annual basis.
  * Where there is an absence of compensatory hypertrophy, with or without evidence of abnormality of renal function, the child should remain under long-term follow-up.

Outcome

Long-term outcome is dependent upon the status of the single kidney:
* Where this is entirely normal, the long-term outlook appears to be favourable; however, where dysplasia is present, it is likely that progressive deterioration in renal function will develop in the long term.
* In a 2013 systematic review of 23 studies in which data on renal injury were available, hypertension was present in 16% and microalbuminuria in 21%; 10% had an estimated or measured GFR indicating CKD stage 3 or worse.

Bilateral renal agenesis

* Rare and almost uniformly fatal. Many fetuses die *in utero*.
* Fetal anuria results in oligohydramnios from around 16 weeks' gestation, causing the Potter sequence (characteristic facial appearance with low-set malrotated ears, facial and nasal flattening, and an underdeveloped chin).
* Reduced intrauterine movement results in the development of arm and leg flexural deformities.
* Death within hours of birth usually occurs secondary to pulmonary hypoplasia.
* The small number of survivors require CKD stage 5 management from birth and have a tendency to develop recurrent pulmonary problems.
* Siblings should have a renal tract US scan.

Further reading

Westland R, Schreuder MF, Ket JC, et al. Unilateral renal agenesis: a systematic review on associated anomalies and renal injury. *Nephrol Dial Transplant* 2013;28:1844–1855.

Horseshoe kidney, renal ectopia, and duplex kidneys

These structural abnormalities may all be detected during antenatal scanning, incidentally during scanning for other reasons, or following the development of symptoms.

Horseshoe kidney

- The lower poles (95% of cases) of the kidneys are fused over the midline by an isthmus of renal parenchyma or fibrous tissue.
- The kidneys are sited more caudally than normal.
- Incidence is 1:500 live births. More common in males.
- Associated with Turner syndrome, trisomies 13, 18, 21, and 22, VATER (VACTERL) association, and oral facial digital syndrome.
- Also seen in fetal alcohol syndrome and the infant of a diabetic mother.
- The large majority are asymptomatic and are often undetected (incidental finding at postmortem).
- A small percentage may be associated with other congenital anomalies of the urinary tract and other organ systems:
  - Hypospadias or undescended testis in 4% of males and bicornuate uterus or septate vagina in 7% of females.
  - Cardiovascular, skeletal, and GI anomalies also reported.
- UTI, haematuria, and abdominal pain are the commonest presenting features.
- Complications of the horseshoe kidney can include:
  - PUJ obstruction due to the abnormal path of the ureter.
  - UTI associated with VUR (which may be present in as many as 50% of cases).
  - Renal calculi secondary to stasis and infection.
  - Trauma to the isthmus (situated anterior to the spine). The absence of protection from the ribs increases the risk of compression or fracture across the vertebral column by an abdominal blow or a car seat belt in a collision.
  - Increased risk of Wilms tumour in children and renal cell carcinoma in adults; adenocarcinoma, transitional cell carcinoma, malignant teratoma, oncocytoma, angiomyolipoma, and carcinoid have all been reported.
  - An increased incidence of hypertension is reported (this is likely to be secondary to renal cortical scarring resulting from VUR, obstruction, or dysplasia, rather than the horseshoe kidney itself).
- The identification of the isthmus and demonstration of its continuity with both lower poles may be difficult and can be missed with US.

Ectopic kidney

- Failure of ascent of the kidney during embryogenesis results in an ectopic kidney.
- Most cases are pelvic kidneys, although rare cases of thoracic kidney have been reported.
- May be unilateral or much more rarely bilateral.
- Reported incidence is 1:1000 to 1:5000.
- They are not reniform in shape and may have associated ureteric abnormalities, but are usually asymptomatic.

- The ectopic kidney may be hypoplastic and have reduced differential function.
- May be associated with VUR. Other reported genitourinary abnormalities include contralateral renal dysplasia, cryptorchidism, hypospadias, and hydronephrosis.
- Associated with extrarenal anomalies, e.g. cloacal, anorectal, cardiac, and skeletal and also as a feature in CHARGE and VACTERL syndromes.

Crossed renal ectopia

- One kidney crosses the midline and lies in an abnormally rotated position, below and medial to the normally sited one.
- There may be fusion, the upper pole being fused to the normal kidney's lower pole.
- The ureter from the ectopic kidney inserts in its normal position.
- The outcome of renal ectopia appears good. The large majority will retain normal kidney function on short- to medium-term follow-up.
- The literature contains a few reports of hydronephrosis of pregnancy developing in the maternal ectopic kidney. Pregnancy appears to be otherwise safe unless there is evidence of advanced CKD.

Duplex kidneys

- The most common congenital abnormality of the urinary tract, these occur in ~1% of the population, are familial, and usually of no significance.
- May be bilateral, although unilateral duplication is five to six times more common than bilateral.
- Duplication of the ureteric bud results in a duplex kidney and collecting system, and may be complete or partial. In both cases, the kidney is usually larger than normal.
- If duplication is complete, the kidney has two moieties, each with its own ureter: the upper pole ureter may be ectopic, draining into the vagina (causing continuous dribbling of urine) or posterior urethra, and may have a ureterocoele (which can cause obstruction); the lower pole ureter usually inserts normally into the trigone but may have VUR. Very occasionally, a PUJ obstruction may occur in the lower pole or a moiety may be dysplastic.
- Incomplete (partial) duplication results in an 'uncomplicated' duplex kidney, with either simply a divided pelvis or two ureters that join before entering the bladder.
- They may present as kidneys of different sizes during US examination. In this situation it is important to have an estimate of renal centiles in order to distinguish between a normal and a small kidney, or a large and a normal-sized kidney. If there is no dilatation of the collecting system (uncomplicated), no further imaging is necessary.

Imaging

This will depend on presentation: if asymptomatic, then US alone is usually sufficient. However, if symptoms are present, then further imaging (e.g. DMSA, CT, or MRI) is required (➔ see 'Radiological investigations').

Multicystic dysplastic kidney

Introduction

- MCDK is a developmental abnormality due to failure of union of the ureteric bud with the renal mesenchyme resulting in a non-functioning kidney that is replaced by large, non-communicating cysts of varying sizes with no renal cortex and an atretic ureter.
- Sometimes the term MCDK is used incorrectly to refer to dysplastic, yet functioning kidneys with multiple cysts. A true MCDK is always without function.
- Bilateral MCDK leads to absent fetal and neonatal renal function with associated pulmonary hypoplasia and is therefore generally considered incompatible with extrauterine life.
- Sporadic condition with an incidence of ~1:4000.
- More commonly seen in males (59%) and affecting the left kidney (53%).
- Previously presented as a unilateral abdominal mass on routine neonatal examination. Now is most frequently detected during routine antenatal US examination.

Investigation and diagnosis

- US (repeated in the early newborn period where the abnormality has been detected antenatally) shows large non-communicating cysts of varying size with no renal parenchyma.
- Further imaging (MAG3 or DMSA) may be indicated if there is concern that the diagnosis may be a severely obstructed PUJ, the apparent 'cysts' being dilated calyces or a severely dysplastic kidney with cystic change. This is not, however necessary where a confident diagnosis of MCDK is made on US.
- The contralateral kidney should show compensatory hypertrophy (defined as renal length >2 SD above the mean) (➔ see 'Radiological investigations'). Where compensatory hypertrophy does not occur, this suggests the presence of dysplasia, and assessment of renal function should be performed (measurement of plasma creatinine).
- If there is no other abnormality on US, no further imaging need be undertaken.
- Associated anomalies are seen in the contralateral kidney in 31%, most commonly VUR, which is seen in 20%. Of those with VUR, this is grade III–V in 40%. A MCUG should therefore be considered if there is UTI and/or evidence of significant calyceal or ureteric dilatation. Other reported CAKUT include PUJ obstruction (5%), ureterocoeles (1.3%), horseshoe kidney, and PUV (<1%).
- There is an increased incidence of congenital anomalies in other organ systems (15%).

Complications

- *Malignancy:*
  - While case reports of apparent malignant transformation to Wilms tumour, adenocarcinoma, and embryonic carcinoma exist, the risk of malignancy has probably previously been overstated.
  - It is not possible to calculate a precise risk of malignancy from existing data, although it has been estimated that 1600–8000 MCDKs might need to be removed to prevent one Wilms tumour.
- *Hypertension:* MCDK is associated with a slightly increased risk of hypertension which has been reported to resolve following nephrectomy.
- Infection, bleeding into, or rupture of cysts if large.

Management

Conservative

- Most authorities recommend conservative management of the MCDK. A 15-year follow-up of a large cohort of conservatively managed patients in Nottingham has shown that 62% of antenatally detected MCDKs will undergo involution by 10 years (see Fig. 3.4). Kidneys >5 cm were less likely to undergo involution (21% vs 76% in those <5 cm).
- Absence of detection on US does not necessarily equate with total disappearance of renal tissue, and the risk of hypertension and other complications may persist.
- Nephrectomy may be indicated for kidneys that have not adequately involuted by the age of 2 years if infection, hypertension, or other complications develop.
- Conservatively managed cases should be reviewed with annual BP and first morning urine stick testing for protein. US, to look for involution of the MCDK and also for growth of the contralateral kidney, which should grow above the 50th centile for height and age, should be annual until 2 years of age and then can be repeated at the age of 5 years if all is well.

Early nephrectomy

- Some have advocated elective nephrectomy for all patients at around 12 months of age.
- Advances in laparoscopic nephrectomy allow the operation to be performed as a day-case procedure.
- Surgery has a very low complication rate.
- Given what is known about the outcome of single kidneys, it is appropriate for children to remain under surveillance with annual measurement of blood pressure and monitoring for proteinuria.

(a)

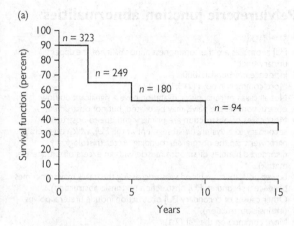

(b)

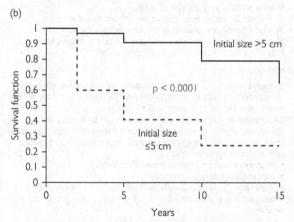

Fig. 3.4 (a) Involution of all MCDK kidneys. (b) Involution of different sized MCDK kidneys.

Reference

Schreuder MF, Westland R, Wijk JAE. Unilateral multicystic dysplastic kidney: a meta-analysis of observational studies on the incidence, associated urinary tract malformations and the contralateral kidney. *Nephrol Dial Transplant* 2009;24:1810–1818.

Pelviureteric junction abnormalities

Introduction

* PUJ anomalies are the commonest abnormality of the upper urinary tract.
* Incidence is around 1:1000.
* More common in boys (2–3:1).
* Not all cases of renal pelvic dilatation have a significant outflow obstruction; i.e. the pelvis may be dilated, but not obstructed.
* Most cases of obstruction are primary and due to obstruction secondary to a dysfunctional segment at the PUJ, which is generally narrower than the normal surrounding ureter (histologically, disordered bundles of smooth muscle with an excess of extracellular matrix).
* Lower pole aberrant blood vessels crossing the pelvis may sometimes produce a secondary PUJ obstruction (extrinsic obstruction).
* Other causes of secondary PUJ obstruction include ureteral polyps (intrinsic obstruction).
* More common on the left (2:1).
* May be bilateral in up to 40% of cases.
* The lumen is nearly always patent, albeit narrow and irregular.
* May be intermittent, depending on the rate of urine flow.
* May be associated with other renal anomalies, e.g. ectopic kidneys.
* May affect the lower pole PUJ in a duplex kidney.

Presentation

* The large majority of cases are now detected in the antenatal period during routine US assessment; significant PUJ obstruction is more likely when the antenatal hydronephrosis is >20 mm.
* Older children may present with acute loin or abdominal pain, particularly after large-volume fluid intake, haematuria, a palpable flank mass, infection (including pyonephrosis), nausea/vomiting, or pelvic rupture following minor trauma.
  * In an extreme form, this is termed Dietl's crisis.
  * Pain may subside spontaneously.
* PUJ anomalies may occasionally be detected during radiological investigation (e.g. abdominal US or CT scanning) for other clinical problems.

Investigation

The key issue is to distinguish cases of antenatally suggested PUJ obstruction, which may lead to progressive deterioration in renal function, from cases of non-obstructive hydronephrosis, which are very likely to undergo spontaneous resolution.

Ultrasound

* Older children not detected through antenatal US screening will most commonly initially undergo US assessment of the urinary tract.
* Measurements of the renal pelvis should be the AP pelvic diameter in the transverse plane (not including the calyces). A dilated renal pelvis with no dilatation of the ureter may signify a PUJ abnormality.

- The major differential diagnoses include an extra renal pelvis, a peripelvic renal cyst, non-obstructive hydronephrosis, obstructed or non-obstructed megaureter, and VUR.
- If the calyces are not dilated, obstruction is unlikely.
- US alone cannot diagnose obstruction as functional information is not provided.

MAG3 scan (dynamic renography)

- Required for confirmation of the diagnosis.
- This investigation is dependent upon a number of factors including the hydration status of the patient, the positioning of the patient, and the timing of administration of isotope and diuretic, and can be difficult to interpret.
- Produces information on differential renal function, the clearance of the isotope, and analogue pictures, which show the anatomy of the collecting system; this will allow distinction between PUJ (no isotope seen in ureters) and VUJ obstruction (isotope in ureters).
- In the presence of obstruction, isotope accumulates within the kidney and the drainage curve continues to rise even after change of posture or diuretic to encourage drainage (Fig. 3.5).

Intravenous urogram

- Traditionally has been the investigation of choice for the diagnosis of PUJ obstruction in adults and older children, but has now been replaced by radioisotope imaging.
- Provides good anatomical and some functional information (although not quantitative relative function), but the radiation dose is significantly higher than the MAG3 scan.
- Works less well in poorly functioning or immature kidneys.

Indications for surgical intervention

- The presence of clinical symptoms is always an absolute indication for surgery.
- Surgical intervention in antenatally suggested PUJ obstruction is a controversial subject:
  - Only ~25% of such cases will develop clinical problems or evidence of deteriorating renal function requiring surgical intervention.
  - There has therefore been a move away from early intervention to close monitoring with serial imaging.
  - Where the renal pelvic transverse AP diameter is <2 cm, surgery is rarely necessary.
  - Few urologists would recommend operative intervention solely on the presence of an obstructive curve on the MAG3 scan.
  - Most would operate only if (1) the differential function of the affected kidney falls to <40%, (2) there is a fall in differential function of >10% during follow-up, or (3) there is increasing dilatation of the kidney during follow-up.
- The aim of surgery is to improve the function or prevent further deterioration of the affected kidney.
- It has been suggested that the chances of improving renal function are greatest when surgery is performed in the first year of life.

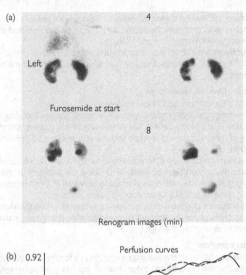

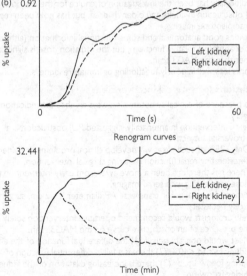

Fig. 3.5 MAG3 isotope renogram, with (a) posterior analogue images and (b) time–activity curves, showing rapid uptake of isotope in right kidney with rapid excretion, and rapid uptake but poor drainage with ongoing accumulation of isotope in the left kidney. Findings consistent with a diagnosis of a left PUJ obstruction.

- Complications associated with conservative management include:
  - potential for progressive deterioration of the function of the affected kidney.
  - haematuria.
  - loin pain.
  - urinary stasis resulting in UTI and calculus formation (the combination of obstruction and infection has the potential to rapidly destroy renal tissue).

Surgery

- In most centres laparoscopic pyeloplasty has replaced the open Anderson Hynes procedure.
- Where differential function is very poor (<10–15%), there is a case for draining the kidney via a nephrostomy to ascertain whether the kidney is viable: if function improves, a pyeloplasty is indicated; whereas if function remains poor, nephrectomy should be considered.
- Recommended follow-up: US scanning (at around 2 months) and MAG3 scanning (at around 6–12 months). These should show improvement in hydronephrosis with improved drainage with stabilization or improvement in differential renal function. It would be unusual for a US scan to return to complete normality.

Megaureter

Megaureter describes an abnormally wide ureter and is classified as obstructed, refluxing, obstructed and refluxing, or non-refluxing/non-obstructed.

Primary megaureter (PM)

- Includes cases of obstructed and non-obstructed megaureter where secondary causes (urethral obstruction, bladder outlet obstruction, etc.) have been excluded.
- More common in boys.
- More often involves the left ureter.
- 25% of cases are bilateral.
- Where unilateral, 10–15% of cases have an absent or dysplastic contralateral kidney.
- Most frequently diagnosed on routine antenatal US.
- Other cases (primarily obstructed PM) present in infancy, often with significant illness and urinary sepsis.
- Renal calculi can form within the dilated system causing pain and haematuria.

Non-obstructed primary megaureter

- The majority of PM is non-obstructed with no evidence of VUR.
- The aetiology is unclear.
- Can be managed conservatively as the risk of deterioration of renal function is very low.

Obstructed primary megaureter

- Functional obstruction occurs because of an aperistaltic section of distal ureter that cannot adequately transport urine.
- Requires surgical correction (reimplantation of distal ureter).

Investigation

- PM is most frequently detected during routine antenatal US assessment.
- Postnatal US will show and quantify the extent of hydronephrosis and hydroureter.
- A MCUG should be performed to diagnose or exclude VUR, and help eliminate secondary causes of megaureter (posterior urethral valves, bladder dysfunction). VUR may occasionally be seen in association with an obstructed PM.
- Further investigation should aim to distinguish obstructed PM from non-obstructed PM.
- MAG3 scan is the most useful investigation, although interpretation of the drainage curve may be difficult because of pooling of isotope in the dilated ureter.
- Significant obstruction is more likely where the differential function of the affected kidney is reduced to <40%.
- An obstructed PM may occasionally be associated with PUJ obstruction; an IVU may be helpful in this situation.

Treatment

The acutely sick patient presenting with pyonephrosis or pyelonephritis requires systemic antibiotic therapy and drainage of the obstructed system with the use of a percutaneous nephrostomy or a double-J stent. Following assessment of the relative function of the kidney, surgery should be performed. A nephrectomy may be necessary for a non-functioning or very poorly functioning kidney (contributing <10% of the overall GFR), although this should be assessed once the acute infection has subsided.

Non-obstructed primary megaureter

* Non-obstructed PM (➲ see 'Investigation') should be managed conservatively and the likelihood is that the dilatation will resolve with time.
* Serial US scans (6-monthly initially, then annually) should be performed to ensure there is no increase in hydronephrosis.
* Where an increase in hydronephrosis occurs, the MAG3 should be repeated to ensure that evidence of obstruction or a fall in differential function has not developed; this may occur in 1–2%.

Obstructed primary megaureter

* Severe urinary sepsis is an absolute indication for surgery.
* For other cases there is an increasing trend towards conservative management. There is widespread use of prophylactic antibiotic therapy in this clinical situation, although there is no randomized controlled trial evidence to support this.
* Regular imaging is indicated as described for the non-obstructed PM.
* During follow-up, surgery is indicated for:
  * any symptoms (infection, calculus formation, or pain).
  * worsening obstruction with increasing hydronephrosis and deteriorating relative renal function.
* Surgery involves the tapering and reimplantation of the lower ureter.
* Hydronephrosis may take several years to resolve postoperatively.

Posterior urethral valves

Introduction

- PUV is a congenital malformation of the posterior urethra occurring exclusively in male infants.
- Incidence is 1:5000 to 1:8000 pregnancies.
- Valves exhibit effects on the developing urinary tract from early in pregnancy when fetal urine production commences.
- The back-pressure produced by the valves may result in renal dysplasia, VUR, hydronephrosis, calyceal rupture (the weakest point), and urinoma.
- The bladder wall hypertrophies, becoming thickened and trabeculated in response to the obstruction. This may result in secondary VUJ obstruction.
- The effect on renal function is very variable and related to the degree of renal dysplasia, which occurs secondary to the obstruction or may be part of the abnormality itself:
  - Some infants will have normal renal function at presentation, whereas in other cases this is markedly deranged. Tubular damage predominates, leading to sodium and bicarbonate losses causing hyponatraemia, acidosis, and hyperkalaemia (sometimes leading to confusion with congenital adrenal hyperplasia).
  - The extent of improvement in renal function following relief of obstruction is also very variable: in some infants the plasma creatinine will return to normal, whereas in others, particularly where severe dysplasia is present, the plasma creatinine may remain elevated.

Presentation

- The majority of cases are diagnosed as a result of antenatal US, which may show oligohydramnios with bilateral hydronephrosis and hydroureter, bladder wall thickening, and posterior urethral dilatation. A significant proportion will be missed if there has not been a third-trimester scan.
- Not all infants have bilateral ureteric dilatation. If the bladder wall is thickened in a boy, PUV should be considered even with no ureteric dilatation.
- The oligohydramnios which may develop secondary to the urinary tract obstruction may result in pulmonary hypoplasia. This may be fatal in the newborn period.
- Oligohydramnios may also cause postural defects including dislocation of the hip, talipes, and a receding jaw (Potter-like syndrome).
- Male fetuses diagnosed with a history of bladder wall thickening ± bilateral hydronephrosis should therefore undergo urgent US assessment in the newborn period. Prophylactic trimethoprim (2 mg/kg once daily) should be commenced and an urgent MCUG organized.
- Later modes of presentation include UTI, poor urinary stream, straining to pass urine, palpable bladder, or, later in childhood, problems with daytime and night-time wetting, and CKD.

Diagnosis

- Where PUV are strongly suspected on the basis of the preliminary US findings, the infant should be catheterized (5 FG feeding tube) under broad-spectrum antibiotic cover so that any obstruction can be relieved, while radiological investigation is awaited. It should be remembered that a PUV may be destroyed by the insertion of a urethral catheter.
- The MCUG is the gold standard investigation for diagnosing PUV. Views of the urethra should be obtained without the catheter *in situ*.
  - If PUV are present: this will show posterior urethral dilatation, and the bladder is likely to be thick walled and have an abnormal trabeculated contour and diverticulae.
  - Unilateral or bilateral VUR may also be present in one-third to one-half of patients. This may resolve in around one-third following relief of obstruction.
  - It is important to consider obstruction at the VUJ if the system is dilated and there is no VUR, although this is rare.
- A DMSA scan should be arranged 3 months after relief of obstruction and resolution of infection to determine the degree of renal dysplasia, and to measure differential renal function.

Treatment

- The treatment of PUV is surgical.
- Definitive treatment is endoscopic ablation of the valve by a variety of different surgical techniques. It has been argued that ablation is the preferred initial treatment as spontaneous filling and emptying during infancy is crucial to normal bladder development.
- When primary ablation is impossible because of size or if the technique fails, urinary diversion with a vesicostomy or bilateral ureterostomies may be necessary with later elective surgical treatment of the PUV.
- Following relief of lower tract obstruction:
  - Meticulous attention should be paid to fluid balance, as there may be a marked post-obstructive diuresis. Urine output should be replaced on a millilitre-for-millilitre basis with 0.45% or 0.9% saline (depending on urinary sodium concentration) with added sodium bicarbonate as urinary sodium and bicarbonate losses will be high. Regular weighing of the child and monitoring of plasma and urine electrolytes is mandatory.
  - A secondary VUJ obstruction may develop due to the presence of the thick-walled bladder. This should be suspected where the biochemistry does not improve and a US scan shows persistent hydroureteronephrosis. It may resolve with time, but may be severe enough to necessitate nephrostomy drainage, ureterostomies, or insertion of VUJ stents; a MAG 3 scan, if renal function is adequate, may help to decide if an obstruction is present, but may be difficult to interpret when the ureters are large and tortuous.
- Early delivery of antenatally diagnosed patients has not been shown to be of benefit.

- It is technically possible to intervene *in utero* with the insertion of a vesicoamniotic shunt. However, the long-term efficacy and safety of this procedure remains uncertain. A UK randomized trial (PLUTO) comparing fetal vesicoamniotic shunt insertion with conservative management closed early because of poor recruitment and it was not possible to draw any conclusion other than the fact that survival with normal renal function was very low regardless of whether shunt insertion was performed or not. Shunt insertion should be considered an experimental procedure; the procedure may be associated with both maternal and fetal morbidity without proven benefit to renal function.

Short-term follow-up and complications

- Careful follow-up is necessary with attention to renal function and plasma biochemistry, growth (sodium deficit and acidosis will impair this and sodium bicarbonate is often routinely added to all feeds), and BP.
- Prophylactic antibiotics are given when VUR is present and UTIs should be treated promptly to prevent further renal damage. It is unclear how long antibiotics should be continued for, though some would recommend until 3–4 years of age.
- There is considerable variation in practice, though some urologists recommend a check cystourethroscopy at 3 months post ablation as further ablation of residual PUV leaflets may be necessary.

Long-term complications of posterior urethral valves

Chronic kidney disease

- The most severe long-term complication of PUV, which is the cause of ~16% of cases of CKD stage 5 in the UK.
- Around 20–30% of boys with PUV will develop CKD stage 5 during childhood.
- Clinical features predictive of a poor outcome with regards to renal function include:
  - early presentation (where antenatal diagnosis has not been made) as those with more severe urinary obstruction present earlier.
  - failure to normalize plasma creatinine following relief of urinary obstruction.
  - proteinuria.
  - daytime wetting after the age of 5 years.
- When CKD stage 5 develops, transplantation can be successfully performed; however, the bladder needs to be carefully reassessed to ensure that the success of the graft is not put at risk by abnormally high bladder pressures and poor bladder emptying.

Wetting

- Boys with PUV have bladders that may behave abnormally and there may be significant continence issues.
- Urodynamic studies may be very difficult to interpret in those who have not achieved continence: bladder dynamics will change as continence is being/is achieved.
- Urodynamic studies should be performed in all boys with daytime wetting persisting beyond 5 years of age.

- Some have argued the case for earlier routine urodynamic assessment:
  - More severe valve bladders are small, trabeculated, thick-walled, high-pressure systems with large residual volumes post micturition.
  - VUR into the upper tracts may contribute to a large proportion of the apparent bladder capacity, becoming part of the urinary storage system. This, together with the high urine output due to the decreased concentrating capacity as a result of tubular damage, may contribute to the progression of CKD, particularly when the bladder becomes very full overnight.
- Treatment options for the abnormal bladder include the use of anticholinergic agents or clean intermittent catheterization where:
  - bladder pressures are high.
  - there is concern about ongoing renal damage.
- More severe cases may require augmentation cystoplasty; a continent channel to allow catheterization of the augmented bladder can be created at the time of surgery with the use of appendix or other tissue (Mitrofanoff).

Urogenital sinus and cloacal abnormalities

Urogenital sinus abnormalities

- A disorder of females—failure of development of the urethrovaginal septum results in the urethra and vagina being a single channel and opening.
- The opening may be stenosed, causing obstruction to both uterine drainage (causing hydrocolpos) and urinary tract drainage.
- Surgical separation of the vagina and urethra is necessary. Colonic tissue may be needed to create the vagina.

Persistent cloaca

- A disorder of females—failure of development of the urorectal septum results in the urethra, vagina, and colon opening into a single channel.
- There may be obstruction of drainage of the bladder, uterus, and GI tracts.
- Relief of the obstructions is necessary (may include a colostomy), followed by reconstructive surgery.

Bladder exstrophy

- Failure of infraumbilical mesenchyme to separate the part of the cloaca that will go on to form the bladder from overlying ectoderm. This results in breakdown of the cloacal membrane causing exposure of the posterior wall of the bladder with a shortened abdominal wall, incomplete fusion of the genital tubercles, separated pubic rami, and inguinal herniae.
- The baby is born with a defective lower abdominal wall, symphysis pubis diastasis, and multiple abnormalities involving the pelvis, bladder, urethra, and external genitalia. The posterior wall of the bladder joins with the edges of the defect in the abdominal wall and has a deficient anterior wall, including the bladder neck and external urethral sphincter. There is epispadias or hemi-clitoris with a widely spaced scrotum or labia and an anterior anus.
- It is up to six times as common in males.
- Surgery is complex and in the UK is undertaken in only two hospitals: Great Ormond Street Hospital for Children and the Royal Manchester Children's Hospital. The bladder is closed in the neonatal period; this usually requires pelvic bone osteotomies. Thereafter, multiple operations are necessary to enable urinary continence and to reconstruct the genital tract.
- Early experience reported that ~10% of patients develop advanced CKD; however, with the modern surgical approach almost all patients preserve normal renal function.

Cloacal exstrophy

As well as bladder exstrophy there is omphalocoele, a rudimentary midgut with imperforate anus and lumbosacral defects.

Absent abdominal musculature syndrome

Introduction

- Previously known as Eagle–Barrett or prune belly syndrome. The latter is no longer used due to its insensitivity.
- Triad of:
  - deficiency or absence of anterior abdominal wall musculature.
  - bilateral cryptorchidism (in boys).
  - renal, ureter, bladder, and urethral abnormalities, predominantly megacystis and megaureter, secondary to dysplasia.
- Abnormalities of other organ systems occur in up to 75% of cases.
- Over 95% of cases occur in males (some consider affected females to have incomplete or pseudo-absent abdominal musculature syndrome).
- Although a genetic basis has not been established, a small number of cases have been documented in siblings and twin gestations.
- The recurrence risk is not, however, generally thought to be increased in subsequent pregnancies.
- Has been reported in association with other chromosomal abnormalities, including trisomies 13, 18, and 21.
- An abnormality of mesenchymal development has been proposed.
- Cause of 1.0% and 2.6% of cases of CKD stage 5 in the UK and USA, respectively.

Urinary tract abnormalities

Kidneys

- Varying degrees of renal dysplasia may occur and may be severe, resulting in early death from pulmonary hypoplasia.
- Severity of dysplasia is an important determinant of long-term survival.
- Acquired renal damage from UTI early in life in combination with dysplasia will accelerate progressive CKD.

Ureters

- Dilated and tortuous with associated VUR in the majority.
- Poor or ineffective peristalsis results in poor urinary drainage.
- Significant urinary stasis increases the risk of urine infection significantly.
- Kinking of ureters may result in obstruction.
- Obstruction may also occur at the PUJ and VUJ.

Bladder

- Large volume with an irregularly thick (due to fibrosis) although non-trabeculated wall.
- Multiple large diverticulae are common.
- Ureteric orifices are laterally spaced.
- Urachal cyst or patent urachus may be present.
- Has poor contractility and low voiding pressures.
- Significant post-micturition residual volume because of poor contractility and VUR into dilated upper tracts.

Urethra

- May be narrowed just below prostate gland with dilated prostatic urethra.
- Urethral atresia may occur (more common in girls).

Testes/genitals

- Cryptorchidism is universal.
- Empty, hypoplastic scrotum.
- Invariably infertile (azoospermia), although sexual function normal.
- Girls may have vaginal atresia or uterine abnormalities.

Involvement of other organ systems

Gastrointestinal tract

- Increased incidence of malrotation and malfixation.
- Constipation may be a problem.
- Increased incidence of gastroschisis.
- Imperforate anus may occur, particularly in association with urethral atresia.

Heart

- 10% incidence of congenital heart disease.
- Echocardiography screening is warranted in newborns.

Skeletal

- Increased risk of talipes equinovarus and congenital dislocation of the hip as in all infants when the pregnancy has been complicated by oligohydramnios.

Pulmonary

- Pulmonary hypoplasia may have developed in those with oligohydramnios. This is often responsible for early mortality.

Diagnosis

- Often suspected from antenatal US scans showing severely dilated urinary tract with a distended abdomen. PUV associated with urinary ascites may produce a similar appearance.
- Wrinkled and lax appearance of the neonatal abdomen wall with a palpable urinary tract and cryptorchidism (empty hypoplastic scrotum) are all clinically apparent and should lead to early diagnosis and evaluation.

Assessment

- Initial assessment should involve identifying non-renal anomalies, which may be life-threatening including significant congenital heart lesions and pulmonary hypoplasia.
- The urinary tract should initially be assessed by US.
- MAG3 scan will provide data on differential renal function and evidence of possible obstruction (although the dilated, poorly draining ureters may produce false-positive results).
- MCUG will identify VUR, although there is a significant risk of introducing infection and some have argued that this should be avoided.
- MR urography can produce further anatomical information.
- Urodynamic assessment may be helpful, particularly where there are concerns about bladder drainage.

Treatment

- There is little evidence that reconstructive surgical procedures are of benefit in this condition.
- Any instrumentation of the urinary tract may introduce infection, leading to deterioration in renal function.
- Surgery may be necessary where there is clear evidence of urinary obstruction. Ureteric and bladder drainage is the major source of problems; this may be treated with urinary diversion (cutaneous ureterostomies), clean intermittent catheterization (urethral or via a created continent channel (Mitrofanoff)), reduction cystoplasty, or tailoring followed by reimplantation of the ureters.
- There is no evidence to support the use of long-term prophylactic antibiotic therapy.
- Abdominal wall function may develop with increasing age. Reconstruction can be performed for cosmetic and psychosocial reasons
- Orchidopexy should be performed, ideally before dialysis or transplant becomes necessary.
- Renal function should be kept under review. ~50% will develop CKD stage 5 during childhood or adolescence.
- Where function deteriorates, standard CKD management should be instituted.
- Both peritoneal and haemodialysis can be successfully performed.
- Transplantation can be successfully performed, although it is essential to ensure that bladder function is satisfactory prior to transplantation.

Urinary tract infection

Background and clinical features

Background

About 3% of girls and 1% of boys have a symptomatic UTI before the age of 11 years, and 50% of them have a recurrence within a year. The highest incidence is in the first year of life. UTI may involve the kidneys (pyelonephritis), when it is associated with fever and systemic involvement, or be restricted to the bladder (cystitis), when fever is absent or low grade. Up to one-half of children with a UTI have a structural abnormality of their urinary tract. UTI is important because, if the upper tracts are involved, it may damage the growing kidney by forming a scar, predisposing to hypertension and, if bilateral, CKD.

NICE guidelines published in 2007 (℘ https://www.nice.org.uk/guidance/cg54) significantly changed clinical practice regarding the diagnosis, clinical management, and subsequent radiological investigation of the child with a UTI. The introduction to these guidelines expressed the view that 'current management—involving imaging, prophylaxis and prolonged follow up—has placed a heavy burden on NHS primary and secondary care resources, and is unpleasant for children and families, costly and not evidence-based'. As a result, investigation of UTI in children is less intensive than it was 10–20 years ago.

Important general points

The commonest error in the management of UTI in children, and especially in infants, is failure to establish the diagnosis properly in the first place. If UTI is not diagnosed, the opportunity to prevent renal damage may be missed; however, an incorrect diagnosis may lead to unnecessary invasive investigations.

NICE guidelines recommend the testing of urine in infants and children with:
* symptoms and signs of UTI
* unexplained fever of 38°C or higher (test urine within 24 h)
* an alternative site of infection but who remain unwell (consider urine test after 24 h at the latest).

Clinical features

Presentation of UTI varies with age:
* In the newborn, symptoms are non-specific and include fever, poor feeding, vomiting, failure to thrive, lethargy, and irritability; septicaemia may develop rapidly.
* The classical symptoms of dysuria, frequency, and loin pain become more common with increasing age.
* The presence of loin pain, systemic upset, and fever are suggestive of pyelonephritis.
* Dysuria without a fever is often due to vulvitis in girls or posthitis/balanitis in boys, rather than a UTI

Collection of urine samples and diagnosis

Collection of urine samples

Urine can be collected by a variety of methods in a younger child in nappies.

NICE recommended techniques

- A 'clean-catch' sample into a waiting sterile pot when the nappy is removed; this is easier in boys.
- Absorbent urine collection pads, e.g. Newcastle sterile urine collection packs, in the nappy (not cotton wool, gauze, or sanitary towels).
- Catheter sample or suprapubic aspiration (SPA), the authors' method of choice in the severely ill infant under 1 year requiring urgent diagnosis and treatment, and in cases where previous samples have suggested contamination. NICE guidelines recommend this be performed when non-invasive methods are not possible. It is recommended that US imaging should be performed to confirm the presence of urine in the bladder and to guide SPA.

Alternatives (not NICE recommended)

- An adhesive plastic bag applied to the perineum after careful washing, although there may be contamination from the skin and the false-positive rate is 85%. This method should only be used as a screening test. A negative result confidently excludes a diagnosis of UTI.

In the older child, urine can be obtained by collecting a midstream sample as in adults. Careful cleaning and collection are necessary, as contamination with both white blood cells (WBCs) and bacteria can occur from under the foreskin in boys, and from reflux of urine into the vagina during voiding in girls.

Diagnosis

- Ideally, the urine sample should undergo microscopy for organisms and WBCs, then cultured straight away.
- If not possible, refrigerate sample to prevent overgrowth of contaminating bacteria.
- Presence or absence of urinary WBCs alone is not a reliable feature of a UTI, as they are commonly present in febrile children without a UTI, and in children with balanitis or vulvovaginitis, or absent due to cell lysis during sample transport and storage.
- Positive testing of the urine with sticks for leucocyte esterase and nitrite is also suggestive of infection, but there may be both false-positive and false-negative results (sensitivity and specificity of 83% and 78% for leucocyte esterase and 53% and 98% for nitrite, respectively). This is because, as explained earlier in this section, the presence or absence of WBCs is not diagnostic of UTI and urine needs to remain in the bladder for at least an hour to allow time for the conversion of nitrate to nitrite. Sticks should therefore only be used as a screening test.
- Which urine samples should be cultured after screening is controversial. Some suggest that culture is only necessary for urine that contains organisms on microscopy. Others recommend culture if stick tests are positive and there are >5 WBCs per high power field in a spun sample, or bacteria seen in an unspun Gram-stained sample.

NICE guidelines
- Recommend urgent urine microscopy and culture, and the immediate commencement of antibiotics if:
  - age <3 months
  - specific urinary symptoms in children of 3 months to 2 years of age
  - non-specific symptoms in children of 3 months to 2 years of age at high risk of serious illness.
- If symptoms are non-specific in a child of 3 months to 2 years of age:
  - Urine should be collected and sent for urgent microscopy and culture.
  - If bacteriuria positive and pyuria positive or negative, treat as UTI with antibiotics.
  - If bacteriuria negative and pyuria positive, treat as UTI if clinically suggestive of UTI.
  - If bacteriuria and pyuria negative, do not treat as UTI.
  - If urgent microscopy is not available, treat with antibiotics if dipstick nitrites positive; urine should be sent for culture.
- In children 3 years of age and older, NICE guidelines recommend that a urine dipstick test should be used to initially diagnose UTI.
- Urine dipstick results should be interpreted as follows:
  - *If leukocyte esterase and nitrite positive:* start antibiotic treatment for UTI; send urine for culture if high or intermediate risk of serious illness or past history of UTI.
  - *If leukocyte esterase negative and nitrite positive:* start antibiotic treatment and send urine for culture.
  - *If leukocyte esterase positive and nitrite negative:* treat only if good clinical evidence of UTI; culture urine and treat depending on result.
  - *If both leukocyte esterase and nitrite negative:* do not treat as UTI or send urine for culture.
- A colony count of any Gram-negative bacilli or >10^3 colony-forming units (CFU)/mL of a Gram-positive cocci from a suprapubic aspirate of urine gives a 99% probability of infection. A colony count of >10^5 CFU of a single organism/mL in a sample obtained by catheterization gives a 95% probability of infection. A sample with ≥10^5 CFU of a single organism/mL obtained by clean catch gives an 80% probability of infection, which rises to 90% if the same result is found in a second sample. A growth of mixed organisms usually represents contamination, but if there is doubt, another sample should be collected.
- NICE guidelines recommend that acute pyelonephritis (upper UTI) is distinguished from cystitis (lower UTI) using Table 4.1. This influences which radiological investigations should subsequently be performed.

Table 4.1 Factors distinguishing between upper UTI and lower UTI

Bacteriuria and fever of 38°C or higher	Acute pyelonephritis (upper UTI)
Bacteriuria, loin pain/tenderness and fever of <38°C	Acute pyelonephritis (upper UTI)
Bacteriuria, but no systemic features	Cystitis (lower UTI)

Bacterial and host factors that predispose to infection

Infecting organism

- UTI is usually the result of bowel flora entering the urinary tract via the urethra, except in the newborn, when it is more often haematogenous.
- The commonest organism to do this is *Escherichia coli,* followed by *Proteus* and *Pseudomonas* spp.
- The virulence of *E. coli* is determined by factors including its cell wall antigens, and possession of endotoxin and cell wall appendages called P-fimbriae, which allow the organism to attach to the ureter and ascend to the kidney.
- Infecting organisms other than *E. coli* are more likely to be associated with structural abnormalities of the renal tract and one study has shown permanent damage to be more common following non-*E. coli* pyelonephritis.
- *Proteus* infection is more commonly diagnosed in boys than girls, possibly because of its presence under the foreskin, and predisposes to the formation of phosphate stones by splitting urea to ammonia and thus alkalinizing the urine.
- *Pseudomonas* infection may indicate a structural abnormality in the urinary tract affecting drainage.

Incomplete bladder emptying

Is the most important cause of UTI and may be due to:
- infrequent voiding, resulting in bladder enlargement
- vulvitis or posthitis/balanitis
- hurried micturition
- obstruction by a loaded rectum from constipation
- neuropathic bladder (➲ see Chapter 5)
- VUR.

Vesicoureteric reflux

- VUR is the retrograde passage of urine from the bladder into the upper renal tracts.
- Primary VUR is a developmental anomaly of the vesicoureteric junction (VUJ). The ureters are displaced laterally and enter directly into the bladder, rather than at an angle, with a shortened intramural course. Primary VUR is, by definition, not associated with overt bladder pathology. It occurs in ~1% of young children.
- VUR with associated ureteric dilatation is important because:
  - Refluxed urine returning to the bladder from the ureters after voiding results in incomplete bladder emptying, which encourages infection.
  - The increased work placed upon the bladder may result in bladder dysfunction and decompensation over time.
  - The kidneys may become infected (pyelonephritis), particularly if there is intrarenal reflux, resulting in renal scarring.
  - Renal scarring may lead to high BP (variously estimated at up to 10%) or to CKD if bilateral.
  - Bladder voiding pressure is transmitted directly to the renal papillae; this may contribute to renal scarring if voiding pressures are high.

- There is no evidence that primary VUR of uninfected urine at normal pressure damages the kidney.
- There may be associated renal dysplasia in severe cases; indeed, antenatal scanning has revealed that what would have been termed 'reflux nephropathy' in the past is, in fact, due to congenital renal dysplasia with or without additional acquired infection-related scar damage. The changing definition has led to a decrease in the reported incidence of 'reflux nephropathy' as a cause of CKD stage 5 and a parallel increase in the reported incidence of renal dysplasia with VUR as a cause.
- VUR is frequently familial, with a 30–50% chance of occurring in first-degree relatives.
- Secondary VUR may be due to or associated with bladder pathology, e.g. a neuropathic bladder or urethral obstruction, or occur temporarily after a UTI. High-pressure VUR associated with the neuropathic bladder or obstruction, with or without infection, may result in scar damage to the kidneys.
- The severity of VUR varies from reflux into the lower end of an undilated ureter during micturition to the severest form with reflux during bladder filling and voiding, with a distended ureter, renal pelvis, and clubbed calyces. Grading of VUR by MCUG has been popular in the past, however there are differing classifications and apparent severity can vary with the amount of contrast instilled into the bladder, and the speed and pressure applied. Also, more severe VUR occurs during filling, as well as voiding. More important is a description of the findings.
- Mild VUR is unlikely to be of significance, either in causing UTI or renal scarring, but VUR associated with a dilated ureter may be associated with intrarenal reflux, the backflow of urine from the renal pelvis into the papillary collecting ducts in compound papillae. In compound papillae, the collecting ducts fuse, making access to refluxed urine more likely than in simple, cone-shaped papillae. Compound papillae occur predominantly at the upper and lower poles of the kidney. Intrarenal reflux is associated with a particularly high risk of renal scarring if UTIs occur.
- The incidence of renal defects on scanning increases with increasing severity of VUR; however, half of children with renal defects do not have VUR.
- Overall, VUR resolves in 10% of cases each year. However, reflux into dilated ureters is less likely to resolve, particularly if associated with abnormal kidneys.
- Conversely, VUR associated with two normal kidneys is very likely to resolve.

Management

Management of the acute infection

- Prompt identification and treatment of UTI reduces the risk of renal scarring.
- Most children can be treated with oral antibiotics, but infants, children who are severely ill or vomiting, and those who are immunosuppressed require IV antibiotic therapy until their temperature has settled, when oral treatment can be substituted.
- NICE guidelines regarding antibiotic treatment are as follows:
  - *Age <3 months:* IV antibiotics—precise duration not stated, but sensible to administer for 2–3 days prior to switch to oral antibiotics if clinically improved.
  - *Age >3 months, but with upper tract UTI (pyelonephritis):* oral antibiotic with low resistance pattern (e.g. cephalosporin or co-amoxiclav) for 7–10 days; IV antibiotics (e.g. ceftriaxone or cefotaxime) for 2–4 days if vomiting, then oral antibiotics for a total duration of 10 days.
  - *Age >3 months with lower urinary tract symptoms:* oral antibiotics for 3 days (trimethoprim, nitrofurantoin, cephalosporin, or amoxicillin, depending on local guidance).
  - If aminoglycosides are chosen, they should be given using a once-daily regimen.
  - If a child on antibiotic prophylaxis develops a UTI, change the antibiotic rather than increasing the dose of the prophylactic agent.
  - Most laboratories monitor local bacterial resistance patterns and are able to advise prescribers accordingly.
  - NICE does not recommend antibiotic prophylaxis unless UTIs are recurrent.
  - Asymptomatic bacteriuria should not be treated with antibiotics, either acutely or with prophylactic therapy.

NICE guidelines (⅋ https://www.nice.org.uk/guidance/cg54) have produced a definition of atypical UTI. This is important as the presence of atypical UTI affects the subsequent radiological investigations that are recommended.

Definition of an atypical UTI

- Seriously ill child.
- Poor urine flow.
- Abdominal or bladder mass.
- Raised plasma creatinine level.
- Septicaemia.
- Failure to respond to treatment within 48 h.
- Non-*E. coli* UTI.

Investigations

The extent to which a child with a UTI should be investigated is controversial, not only because of the invasive nature and radiation burden of some of the tests (→ see 'Radiological investigations'), but also because of the lack of an evidence base to show that outcome is improved (unless urinary obstruction is demonstrated). Mild VUR usually resolves spontaneously and operative intervention to stop VUR has not been shown to decrease renal scarring. There has, therefore, been a move away from traditional protocols that use age alone to determine investigations following a UTI, to protocols that focus radiological investigations on those infants and children who are at greatest risk of developing renal scarring.

Current NICE guidelines (🖰 https://www.nice.org.uk/guidance/cg54) recommend that different investigations are performed according to whether there is a good response to antibiotic treatment within 48 h, whether there is evidence of atypical UTI (→ see 'Definition of an atypical UTI'), and whether there is evidence of recurrent UTI (two or more upper UTIs, one upper and one or more lower UTIs, or three or more lower UTIs), as well as the age of the child. Tables 4.2, 4.3 and 4.4 summarize the investigations currently recommended by NICE according to severity of UTI and age.

* The initial US will identify:
  * serious structural abnormalities and urinary obstruction
  * bladder wall thickness and emptying (note the importance of obtaining a pre- and post-micturition study as recommended by NICE)
  * renal cortical defects, although most studies that have compared US with DMSA have shown US to miss a significant proportion of renal scars. Furthermore, it has to be remembered that there is a degree of operator variability with the use of US, and experienced full-time paediatric ultrasonographers are more likely to detect more minor changes than less experienced operators.
* The DMSA scan is considered the gold standard investigation for the diagnosis of renal parenchymal damage. It should be delayed until 4–6 months after the acute UTI in order to avoid a false-positive result due to renal parenchymal inflammation that may resolve.
* The MCUG is considered the gold standard investigation for the diagnosis of urethral abnormalities and VUR.
* → See 'Radiological investigations' for further details, including recommendations for the use of prophylactic antibiotics for the MCUG.

Long-term management

Medical measures for the prevention of urinary tract infection
* High fluid intake to produce a high urine output.
* Regular voiding.
* Complete bladder emptying using double micturition to empty any residual or refluxed urine returning to the bladder.
* Prevention or treatment of constipation.
* Good perineal hygiene.
* *Lactobacillus acidophilus*, to encourage colonization of the gut by this organism.

Table 4.2 Investigations following UTI in infants under 6 months of age

	Good response within 48 h	Atypical UTI	Recurrent UTI
US at time of acute infection	No	Yes[b]	Yes
US within 6 weeks	Yes[a]	No	No
DMSA at 4–6 months	No	Yes	Yes
MCUG	No	Yes	Yes

[a] If abnormal, consider MCUG once infection adequately treated.
[b] US at 6 weeks if non-*E. coli* UTI, but responding well.

Table 4.3 Investigations following UTI in children of 6 months to 3 years of age

	Good response within 48 h	Atypical UTI	Recurrent UTI
US at time of acute infection	No	Yes[a]	No
US within 6 weeks	No	No	Yes
DMSA at 4–6 months	No	Yes	Yes
MCUG	No	No[b]	No[b]

[a] US within 6 weeks if non *E.coli* UTI, but responding well.
[b] MCUG considered if dilatation on US, poor urine flow, non *E. coli* UTI, family history of VUR.

Table 4.4 Investigations following UTI in children over 3 years of age

	Good response within 48 h	Atypical UTI	Recurrent UTI
US at time of acute infection	No	Yes[a, b]	No
US within 6 weeks	No	No	Yes[a]
DMSA at 4–6 months	No	No	Yes
MCUG	No	No	No

[a] US with full bladder (measure pre- and post-micturition volume).
[b] US at 6 weeks if non-*E. coli* UTI, but responding well.

The use of antibiotic prophylaxis is a controversial area:
* A recent Australian study (PRIVENT) was the first to show that the use of antibiotics (co-trimoxazole) reduced the incidence of UTI compared with placebo (hazard ratio 0.61) in children under 18 years with a prior history of UTI (42% had VUR). The RIVUR study (2014) from the USA similarly showed the use of prophylaxis to reduce the recurrence of UTI, however there was no reduction in the development of scarring.
* A Cochrane systematic review found evidence that long-term antibiotics did reduce the risk of more symptomatic infections but the benefit was small and must be weighed against the likelihood that future infections may be with bacteria that are resistant to the antibiotic given.
* NICE guidelines do not recommend the routine use of prophylactic antibiotics in infants and children following a first UTI, although this may be considered in those with recurrent UTI, defined as:
  * two or more upper UTIs
  * one upper UTI plus one or more lower UTIs
  * three or more lower UTIs.
* Other national guidelines (e.g. from the Canadian Pediatric Society) have stated that antibiotic prophylaxis is no longer indicated in children with UTI.
* Where prophylaxis is used, this is most often in those <2 years of age and those with ureters that are dilated up to the renal pelvis. Trimethoprim (2 mg/kg at night) is used most often, but nitrofurantoin (1 mg/kg at night) or nalidixic acid (7.5 mg/kg twice daily) may be given. Broad-spectrum, poorly absorbed antibiotics, such as amoxicillin, should be avoided.
* In children with a prior history of UTI, whether prophylactic antibiotics are used or not, there should be a high suspicion for UTI during acute illnesses. UTIs should be promptly identified and treated.

Follow-up
* NICE guidelines state that children who do not undergo radiological investigation following a UTI do not require follow-up.
* Routine urine culture in well children is not necessary.
* There is no evidence for when antibiotic prophylaxis (if used) should be stopped. This should be considered at the age of 2 years (by which time maximum renal growth has occurred) or after 1 year free of UTIs. Others will discontinue antibiotics once the child achieves daytime continence.
* Any child with a renal defect requires annual BP checks for life. Hypertension has been reported in up to 10%, but such a high incidence has been questioned.
* Regular assessment of renal function and growth using US, and early morning urine dipstick testing for proteinuria for those with bilateral renal defects, who are at risk of progressive CKD.
* No further imaging is necessary in a child with no or unilateral defects with no further infections.
* Circumcision may benefit boys with recurrent UTIs. It has been estimated that around 100 circumcisions are required to prevent one UTI.

- Antireflux surgery may be indicated if there is progression of scarring with ongoing VUR, but outcome has not been shown to be better than the use of antibiotic prophylaxis alone. More recently, open reimplantation of the ureters has been replaced by periureteric injection of bulking agents (STING procedure). However, the success rate is less for this procedure than reimplantation of the ureters, and it often needs to be repeated.
- If there are further symptomatic UTIs, investigations are required to determine whether there are new scars or continuing VUR. New scars are rare in previously unscarred kidneys after the age of 4, even in the presence of continuing VUR, and reinvestigation is rarely necessary in this group. A suggested schema for the follow-up of children with no further infections is shown in Fig. 4.1 and for those with further symptomatic UTIs in Fig. 4.2.

Asymptomatic bacteriuria

Occasionally, bacteriuria may be discovered during investigation of another problem in an asymptomatic child. Although treatment with antibiotics will eradicate the bacteriuria, recurrence is common. Asymptomatic bacteriuria should not be treated as long-term follow-up studies have shown that it does not cause renal damage in otherwise healthy children, and there is a risk of developing an infection with antibiotic resistant organisms.

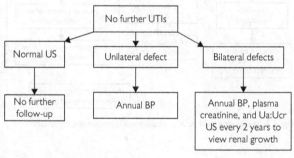

Fig. 4.1 Follow-up of children with no further UTIs.

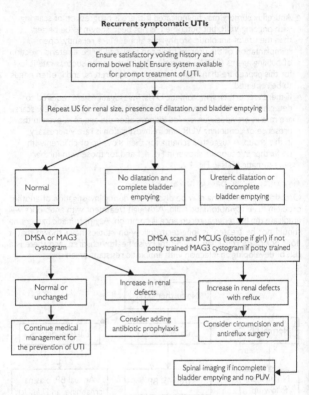

Fig. 4.2 Investigation and follow-up of children with recurrent symptomatic UTIs.

Further reading

National Institute for Health and Clinical Excellence. *Urinary Tract Infection in Children.* NICE Clinical Guideline 54. London: NICE, 2007.

The penis and foreskin

Introduction

- The foreskin is almost invariably non-retractile in the neonate. It should never be forcibly retracted for cleaning or other reasons.
- The foreskin becomes retractile with increasing age (40% at 1 year, 90% at 4 years, and 99% at 15 years). Retractility is spontaneous and does not require manipulation.

The penis should always be examined in boys with UTI because:
- infection of the foreskin (balanitis) may be misdiagnosed as UTI as there may be WBCs and bacteria in the urine
- obstruction to urine flow by the foreskin can cause UTI.

Inflammation and infection of the foreskin and glans

- Minor inflammation of the foreskin (posthitis), glans (balanitis), or foreskin and glans (balanoposthitis) is common and may be caused by soaps, bubble bath, detergents, and other factors:
  - Most cases are self-limiting.
  - Avoidance of precipitating factors, and the use of barrier or mild topical steroid ointments result in rapid resolution.
- More significant inflammation may be due to bacterial (*Streptococcus, Staphylococcus, Proteus*, and other Gram-negative organisms) or yeast infection:
  - A course of oral antibiotic therapy (amoxicillin, co-amoxiclav) will result in rapid resolution in most cases.
  - Topical antifungal therapy should be used where there is evidence of such infection (satellite lesions, etc.).
  - The inflamed foreskin will be painful and analgesia should be given.
  - Boys may find that passing urine in the bath is more comfortable.
  - Dysuria may lead to incomplete bladder emptying and the development of UTI.
- Where severe cellulitis is present, IV antibiotic therapy should be given and the patient considered for emergency circumcision.
- Elective circumcision should be considered in boys with recurrent, severe balanitis.

Phimosis (non-retractile foreskin)

- Forced retraction of the non-retractile foreskin and recurrent balanitis result in the development of scar tissue in the distal foreskin rendering it non-retractile.
- Opening of the foreskin is narrowed with visible scar tissue. Causes ballooning of the foreskin during micturition and a thin urinary stream.
- Topical corticosteroids of increasing potency may resolve matters, although circumcision should be considered when these are unsuccessful.
- Rarely this can be so severe as to cause urinary obstruction.

Paraphimosis

* Results when the tip of the foreskin is retracted behind the glans at the coronal sulcus causing oedema of the glans and foreskin and inability to manipulate the foreskin back over the glans.
* Requires reduction with or without anaesthesia.

Circumcision

* This is regularly performed in the neonate for religious reasons, most commonly by a non-medically qualified practitioner. The rate of non-religious routine circumcision varies between countries, the rate in the USA being significantly higher than in the UK.
* There is no good evidence to support an increased risk of carcinoma of the penis, HIV infection, or cervical cancer risk in partners of uncircumcised males. Circumcision to prevent UTI is essentially unproven except in boys with CAKUT.

Religious circumcision is usually performed without analgesia:
* There is significant evidence that neonates circumcised without analgesia experience pain as indicated by changes in heart rate, BP, and oxygen saturation levels.
* This can be reduced by the use of topical anaesthetic agents, such as Ametop® or EMLA®, regional anaesthesia (dorsal nerve block), or general anaesthesia.

Complications include bleeding, infection, and poor wound healing:
* Bleeding may be the first presentation of vitamin K deficiency, haemophilia, or other disorders of coagulation.
* Occasionally, severe acute problems occur including injury to the glans and urethral trauma.
* In the longer term, meatal stenosis may occur due to local trauma from rubbing on nappies and continuous exposure to urine.
* Injury can lead to incomplete bladder emptying (which can be seen on US scan) and UTIs.

Medical indications for circumcision include:
* *recurrent UTIs*: circumcision may be considered in those with CAKUT when more conventional treatment modalities have been unsuccessful
* *balanitis xerotica obliterans*: a primary non-infective aggressive inflammation of the foreskin, which results in hard fibrotic true phimosis
* severe acute or recurrent balanoposthitis
* penile malignancy
* traumatic foreskin injury where this cannot be salvaged.

Further reading

American Academy of Pediatrics. *Circumcision Policy Statement*. August 2012. Available at: ℞ http://pediatrics.aappublications.org/content/pediatrics/early/2012/08/22/peds.2012-1989.full.pdf
British Association of Paediatric Surgeons. *Consensus Statement*. 2017. Available at: ℞ http://www.baps.org.uk/content/uploads/2017/03/MANAGEMENT-OF-FORESKIN-CONDITIONS.pdf

Vulvovaginitis

Introduction

- Vulvovaginitis is a common problem in prepubertal girls.
- Clinical features include soreness, itching, discharge, and bleeding, and urinary symptoms including dysuria and frequency.
- Clinical signs include inflammation of the labia and introitus, and visible discharge.
- May cause cystitis as a result of poor bladder emptying due to pain on voiding.

Causes

- *Poor perineal hygiene:*
  - Poor wiping technique.
  - Constipation with overflow soiling.
  - Wetting.
- *Local irritation:*
  - Bubble bath/detergents.
  - Friction from wet/nylon underwear.
- *Infection (responsible for only ~20% of cases):*
  - Bacterial (group A beta-haemolytic *Streptococcus, Staphylococcus aureus, Haemophilus influenzae*).
  - Viral.
  - Fungal.
  - Sexually transmitted (rare cause though requires consideration).
  - *Enterobius vermicularis* infestation (threadworms) with associated perianal itch.
- Deficient oestrogenization of prepubertal labia.
- *Primary dermatological disease:* lichen sclerosis, eczema.
- Foreign body.
- *Sexual abuse:* rare cause though requires consideration.

Investigation

- In mild cases, no investigations are necessary
- Mid-stream urine specimen.
- *Swab from introitus:* sellotape test to collect threadworm eggs—apply sellotape to perianal region and place on glass microscopy slide to visualize eggs; test is of high specificity, but low sensitivity.

General management

- Improve perineal hygiene.
- Simple symptomatic treatment incuding:
  - front-to-back wiping
  - avoid/treat constipation
  - cotton underwear
  - salt baths
  - barrier creams e.g. Sudocrem®
  - avoid bubble bath and other chemical irritants, use mild bath soap.

- Systemic antibiotics only if swab culture results positive: sometimes one organism, e.g. group A *Streptococcus*, *Haemophilus*, *Gardnerella* has overgrown in the area and treatment with an appropriate antibiotic may help.
- Mid-stream specimen of urine may be falsely positive due to contamination.
- Consider empirical course of mebendazole (treat whole household), if *Enterobius vermicularis* is suspected.
- Some have advocated a trial of oestrogen cream (applied twice daily for 1 week) where bacterial cultures are negative.
- *Candida* infection is a relatively rare cause and empirical treatment is unlikely to be of help.
- Specific dermatological disorders require specialist advice.
- Where symptoms do not resolve or problem becomes recurrent, consider sexually transmitted infection/sexual abuse, foreign body in vagina. Suspected sexual abuse problems require consultation with appropriately trained specialists.

Enuresis

Nocturnal enuresis

Introduction

- Most children achieve night-time dryness by 5 years of age, when bladder volume exceeds nocturnal urine production.
- Nocturnal enuresis is defined as the involuntary loss of urine at night, in the absence of physical disease, at an age when the child could reasonably be expected to be dry (developmental age of 5 years by consensus):
  - Primary nocturnal enuresis is the term used when the child has never been dry.
  - Secondary or onset nocturnal enuresis is the term used where the child has previously been dry at night for 6 months or more after the age of 5 years.
  - Monosymptomatic or uncomplicated nocturnal enuresis refers to nocturnal enuresis not associated with other symptoms referable to the urinary or GI tracts;
  - Polysymptomatic or complicated nocturnal enuresis refers to bedwetting associated with symptoms suggestive of lower urinary tract (LUT) dysfunction (➋ see 'Lower urinary tract dysfunction').
- Nocturnal enuresis is common, affecting 15–20% of 5-year-olds, 5% of 10-year-olds, and 1–2% of 15-year-olds.
- The problem is socially inconvenient to the child and their family, and may result in bullying and stigmatization, with resultant low self-esteem.

Aetiology

- Remains poorly understood despite the high prevalence.
- Delay in maturation of bladder control has been proposed. Children have smaller functional bladder capacity and unstable detrusor contraction.
- There is a strong genetic component: a family history is found in most children. The gene appears to be localized on chromosome 13.
- Studies of sleep patterns have shown variable results, although it appears that children who bed wet have difficulties in waking.
- Some studies have detected loss of the normal nocturnal rise in antidiuretic hormone (ADH) production, resulting in an increase in nocturnal urine production.
- Upper airway obstruction and constipation may rarely produce wetting.

Assessment and investigation

- History of bed wetting, daytime symptoms, toileting patterns and fluid intake.
- Perform general physical examination, with particular attention to whether the bladder is palpable, and the spine and lower limb neurology.
- Routine urinalysis and culture is not necessary unless the child has started bed wetting recently, has daytime symptoms or signs of ill health, and a history suggestive of UTI or diabetes mellitus.
- Investigate the child's attitudes and motivation.
- Children with primary nocturnal enuresis should *not* be subjected to radiological or urodynamic investigation.

Management

(* Indicates evidence-based recommendation.)

General

- Primary nocturnal enuresis has a high rate of spontaneous remission: it has been estimated that 10–15% of children will see a resolution of bed wetting each year with no treatment.
- Attempts to treat children less than 7 years of age are often unsuccessful, although recent NICE guidelines recommend that younger children are not excluded from the management of enuresis on the basis of age alone.
- Specialist enuresis clinics generally provide the best service for patients. These are often run by specialist nursing staff and sited in local health centres in the community. Details of the location of such clinics are available from the charity Education and Resources for Improving Childhood Continence (ERIC: ➔ see 'Information for families').
- Management strategies are similar for both primary and monosymptomatic secondary nocturnal enuresis. In the child with secondary nocturnal enuresis, an exploration of potential psychological or social problems (marital disharmony, bullying at school, etc.) is warranted.
- In general, where daytime wetting is also occurring, this should be investigated and treated prior to addressing nocturnal enuresis.

General measures

Advise on fluid intake, diet, and toileting behaviour:

- Maintain adequate, but not excessive daytime fluid intake to develop bladder capacity and reduce evening fluid intake. NICE guidelines recommend daily fluid intakes (see Table 5.1).
- Avoid caffeine-based drinks (NB many carbonated drinks (e.g. Coca-Cola, Pepsi) contain significant amounts of caffeine).
- Healthy diet.
- Treatment and avoidance of constipation.
- Encourage regular voiding during the daytime and before sleep.
- Punitive measures should never be used.

Table 5.1 Daily recommended fluid intake

Age (years)	Total daily intake (mL)
4–8	1000–1400
9–13	1200–2100 girls
	1400–2300 boys
14–18	1400–2500 girls
	2100–3200 boys

Reward systems

This alone may be sufficient in the child who already has some dry nights:

- NICE guidelines recommend that rewards should be given for agreed behaviour (drinking recommended fluid intake, passing urine before sleep, engaging with management, etc.), rather than dry nights; however, star charts* for dry nights with or without night-time lifting or waking have been shown to reduce the number of wet nights and produce longer-term success after treatment.
- Neither lifting (carrying or walking the child to the toilet during the night without fully waking the child) nor scheduled wakings will promote long-term dryness.
- Waking should be used only as a practical measure in short-term management.
- Older children with enuresis unresponsive to treatment may find self-instigated waking (alarm clock) helpful.
- Where these measures alone are unsuccessful, there is a need to consider the use of an alarm system or drug treatment.

Alarm systems

- NICE guidelines recommend that alarm treatment be offered to children where bed wetting has not responded to advice on fluid intake, toileting, and an appropriate reward system, *and* alarm treatment is desirable and appropriate.
- A Cochrane review* has shown alarm systems to be effective, with around 50% of children achieving long-term dryness.
- Immediate alarm systems appear to be more effective than delayed alarm systems.
- Alarm systems are superior to behavioural techniques* and drug therapy.*
- There may be problems with acceptability (embarrassment with system, other family members being woken, etc.).
- Many trials involving alarm systems have had high drop-out rates.

Drug therapy

NICE guidelines recommend the use of drug treatment where rapid onset and/or short-term dryness is a priority and where alarm treatment is either undesirable or inappropriate.

Desmopressin*

200–400 micrograms orally or 120–240 micrograms sublingually at bedtime:

- NICE guidelines recommend this in the over sevens where rapid onset and/or short-term improvement in wetting is the priority of treatment and alarm is inappropriate or undesirable.
- Superior to placebo (Cochrane review), though there appears to be a high relapse rate upon stopping treatment.
- Response to therapy should be assessed at regular intervals with a dose increase where no response is seen. Where successful, treatment should be withdrawn every 3 months to assess response.
- Useful agent for short-term use to allow children to attend sleep-overs, school trips, cub or brownie camps, etc. In this situation, it is worth having a trial run at home prior to the trip to ascertain the dose required and to instil confidence in the child.

- May be used in conjunction with an alarm system.
- There are a small number of reports of hyponatraemic seizures in children; these appear to be associated with excessive water intake, which should be discouraged.
- The monitoring of weight, plasma electrolytes, BP, and urine osmolality is not necessary.

Anticholinergic agents
Oxybutynin, etc.:
- May be considered in combination with desmopressin in children with nocturnal enuresis unresponsive to desmopressin alone or in combination with an alarm system.
- May also be useful in those with both daytime symptoms and nocturnal enuresis.
- *Not* licensed for nocturnal enuresis.
- Should only be used under expert supervision.
- Should never be used in combination with a tricyclic agent.

Tricyclic agents
Imipramine, amitriptyline, viloxazine, clomipramine, and desipramine:
- NICE guidelines do not recommend the use of these agents as first-line treatment for nocturnal enuresis—use should be restricted to those who have not responded to alarm and/or desmopressin. Imipramine should be the tricyclic agent of first choice.
- Superior to placebo, with a reduction of around one wet night per week (Cochrane review).
- Similar to desmopressin, the effect is not sustained upon stopping treatment.
- These drugs have significant adverse effects. In overdose they are cardiotoxic and hepatotoxic and at therapeutic doses produce anticholinergic adverse effects (dry mouth, postural hypotension, etc.). These adverse effects and the availability of desmopressin have resulted in a very significant reduction in the use of these agents.
- If used, imipramine should be withdrawn gradually when stopping treatment.

Information for families
Education and Resources for Improving Childhood Continence (ERIC), ℘ http://www.eric.org.uk, telephone helpline (+44) (0)117 9603060, provides information and support for younger children, teenagers, parents, and professionals on nocturnal enuresis and daytime wetting.

Further reading

NICE. *Nocturnal Enuresis: The Management of Bedwetting in Children and Young People*. NICE Clinical Guidance 111. 2010. Available at: ℘ http://www.nice.org.uk/guidance/CG111
Paediatric Society of New Zealand. *Nocturnal Enuresis*. Best Practice Evidence Based Guidelines. 2005. Available at: ℘ https://www.paediatrics.org.nz/documents/guidelines/doc/File/show/nocturnal-enuresis-bedwetting-2005/

Lower urinary tract dysfunction

Daytime urinary incontinence (DUI)

Intermittent urinary incontinence (involuntary loss of urine in discrete amounts in socially inconvenient situations) when a child aged ≥5 years is awake with one or more episodes/month or three episodes in 3 months.

Enuresis

Intermittent urinary incontinence (involuntary leakage of urine in discrete amounts) that occurs in a child aged ≥5 years during sleep, with more than one episode/month or three episodes in 3 months:
- Frequent: four or more times/week.
- Infrequent: less than four times/week.

Note that the term enuresis is used in relation to nocturnal urinary incontinence rather than DUI.

Enuresis can be subclassified into:
- *monosymptomatic enuresis (MSE)*: enuresis in the absence of any LUT symptoms
- *non-monosymptomatic enuresis (NMSE)*: enuresis in the presence of LUT symptoms.

LUT symptoms may be:
- *Related to storage phase*:
  - *Frequency*: increased if eight or more times/day, decreased if three or fewer times/day.
  - *Urgency*: sudden, unexpected compulsion to void (often a sign of an overactive bladder—not applicable before achieving bladder control).
  - *Nocturia*: waking at night to void without incontinence (often young children).
  - *Holding manoeuvres/posturing*: to prevent sudden urine leak with urgency.
  - *Stress incontinence*: passage of urine with vigorous activity, coughing, or laughter, due to raising intra-abdominal pressure.
  - *Altered sensation*: strangury or absent sensation (neuropaths and Hinman bladder).
- *Related to voiding phase*:
  - *Hesitancy*: difficulty in initiating void when ready.
  - *Dysuria*: burning discomfort during micturition (source: early, urethral; terminal, bladder).
  - *Abnormal stream*: weak due to obstruction/PUV or weak detrusor, or intermittent/staccato: (weak detrusor contraction/obstruction/ dysfunctional voiding and bladder neck dysfunction).
  - *Splitting/spraying*: meatal/urethral narrowing.
  - *Straining/abdominal massage*: seen in neuropathic bladder, outlet obstruction, and dysfunctional voiders who need to increase intra-abdominal pressure to void.
- *Related to post-void phase*:
  - *Sensation of incomplete voiding*: common in dysfunctional voiding.
  - *Post-void dribbling*: common in overweight girls who have vaginal reflux of urine and syringocoele in boys.

Causes of LUT dysfunction

Commonest

- *Delayed bladder/CNS maturity*: by definition, primary in onset.
- *Overactive bladder (OAB)*: commonest clinical finding often in association with small bladder capacity.
- *Dysfunctional voiding*: associated with UTI, VUR, constipation, anxiety, and secondary overactive bladder.
- *Vaginal reflux of urine*: common cause of constant urinary dribbling in girls.
- *Constipation*: coexists with all forms of bladder dysfunction.

Less common

- Polyuria (CKD, diabetes mellitus/insipidus, tubulopathies).
- Neuropathic bladder (spina bifida, sacral agenesis, syringomyelia, cord tumours, congenital or acquired autonomic neuropathies, myelitis), primary bladder neck pathology, dyssynergia, decompensated bladder (non-neuropathic neuropathic), or 'Hinman bladder'. Ectopic ureter— causing a constant dribble of urine in girls.
- VUR (constant residual volumes of urine), PUV.

Secondary onset of LUT symptoms including DUI and enuresis

Secondary onset of DUI and enuresis is uncommon and should always be taken seriously, particularly in boys. It may be due to UTI, diabetes mellitus/insipidus, PUV, CKD, tubulopathies, and spinal cord pathology. However, discrete anatomical and medical causes are often not identified.

Assessment

1. *History and examination*: with attention to LUT symptoms as previously described including urinary stream, primary vs secondary, family history, history of obstructive sleep apnoea/sleep disordered breathing, fluid intake, UTI, and constipation.
2. *General examination*: palpate for bladder/faecal loading, examine external genitalia, urethral meatus, previous circumcision, lumbosacral spine for sacral agenesis, spina bifida, fawn's tail, haemangiomata, lower limb neurological examination, anal tone, and signs of CKD.
3. *Urinalysis*: glucose (type 1 diabetes/Fanconi proximal renal tubular acidosis (RTA)), leucocyte esterase and nitrite test (commonly positive in any condition with post-void residuals and dysfunctional voiding), MC&S if indicated/symptomatic. Proteinuria if renal impairment suspected.
4. *Renal tract US*: for all patients with NMSE and DUI symptoms (renal defects, upper tract dilatation, bladder wall, post-micturition volumes, stones, bladder capacity), assessment of rectal diameter with pelvic US if available (30 mm is upper limit of normal).
5. *Additional investigations to consider*: bloods (renal profile/FBC/glucose/gas if CKD/tubular disease is suspected), paired urine and serum osmolalities if polyuric and concentrating defect suspected, and spinal X-ray/US/MRI if lumbosacral pathology or combined bladder bowel dysfunction/neuropathic findings. DMSA/MAG3 if recurrent UTI.

Investigation of urinary tract dysfunction

* 48 h bladder and bowel diaries (mandatory assessment for clinical diagnoses).
* The following are available in specialist centres:
  * Non-invasive urodynamics: uroflowmetry ± pelvic electromyography (EMG) (time–flow pattern studies).
  * Invasive urodynamics (± video fluoroscopy): gold-standard pressure–flow studies giving information on compliance, pressure and detrusor activity in storage and voiding phases, ± video phase looking at bladder neck, outline, and upper tracts (VUR). Performed urethrally or via suprapubic route (where bladder outlet/obstruction an issue).

Management

Broadly, the issue is addressed in the following order:

1. Identification and treatment of any underlying constipation (further conservative measures unlikely to be successful if constipation remains an issue). Faecal impaction in the rectum can affect bladder filling and emptying by distortion and compression of the bladder. The bladder and bowel dysfunction cycle is established when children who hold their stool and urine by choice for long periods exhibit reduced sensation to evacuate both bladder and bowel. This is because over time there is an effect on the neural stimuli of the bladder and pelvic floor muscles, leading to a progressively decreased urge to evacuate, chronic bladder spasms, insufficient emptying, and significant post-void urine volumes.

2. Treatment of the daytime LUT symptoms with general measures such as urotherapy:
   * *Urotherapy* is a term used to describe a conservative-based management programme to improve LUT symptoms which includes:
     * education and information about the anatomy and function of the urinary tract
     * behavioural modifications such as fluid intake, voiding schedules, the use of double-voiding techniques (to empty the post void residual), toilet postures, relaxation and breathing techniques, avoidance of holding manoeuvres, diet and constipation advice, and avoidance of bladder irritants such as caffeine and blackcurrants.
   * *Specific urotherapy* is a term that now encompasses deep breathing exercises, neuromuscular re-education of the pelvic floor by biofeedback and focused pelvic floor exercises, and neuromodulation of the sacral outflow (transcutaneous electrical nerve stimulation).
   * *Drug therapy*: the mainstays of which are short- and long-acting anticholinergics such as oxybutynin, tolterodine tartrate, solifenacin, and trospium chloride. All work to relax the detrusor muscle and increase bladder compliance and capacity. The major side effects include dry mouth, blurred vision, constipation, and behavioural disturbance. The newer beta-3 agonist mirabegron is increasingly being used in paediatric settings along with the more established intravesical botulinum toxin injections for refractory LUT symptoms.

3. Treatment of the nocturnal component (enuresis) with combinations of desmopressin and anticholinergics and enuresis alarms.

Treatment of the underlying cause in the case of identified anatomical problems is also required alongside the above-mentioned measures.

Further reading

Austin PF, Bauer SB, Bower W, et al. The standardization of terminology of lower urinary tract function in children and adolescents: update report from the Standardization committee of the International Children's Continence Society. *Neurourol Urodyn* 2016;35:471–481.

Bladder function, investigation methods, and patterns of pathology

Normal bladder function

The urinary bladder is predominantly a storage organ: the detrusor muscle spends 99% of the time relaxing with a closed sphincter mechanism. During voiding, the sphincteric mechanism relaxes and the detrusor contracts to expel urine. The smooth transition between these two phases is mediated via an intact CNS. To function safely, and void when socially convenient, the bladder must have appropriate capacity, a compliant wall, maintain low pressures during storage (< 10 cmH$_2$O), and void effectively and completely.

Dysfunctional voiding occurs when there is poor coordination between detrusor contraction and sphincter relaxation in the absence of neuropathology. In the presence of neuropathology, this is termed *detrusor–sphincter dyssynergia*.

Expected bladder capacity in mL:
- <5 years = (age + 2) × 30.
- >5 years and <12 years = (age × 30) + 30.
- >12 years = 400 mL.

Bladder dysfunction (either during storage or voiding phases) can lead to

- incontinence associated with psychological morbidity
- incomplete bladder emptying with recurrent UTI, renal scarring, and hypertension
- VUR ± raised detrusor pressures with associated nephropathy and obstructive tubulopathy
- development of a decompensated state with an underactive detrusor, worsening emptying, upper tract dilatation, and UTI. This may be seen in polyuric conditions such as CKD, Bartter syndrome, diabetes insipidus, and in Hinman syndrome.

Investigation of bladder dysfunction:

Renal tract US with pre-and post-voiding volume assessment: if the bladder empties completely, primary bladder pathology is unlikely.

Non-invasive urodynamic investigations

- *48 h volume–frequency (bladder and bowel) charts*: self-completed charts, giving information on fluid intake patterns, urinary frequency, voided volumes, urgency, incontinence episodes, and bowel habit. Clinical diagnoses such as overactive bladder can be reliably made, allowing empirical therapy to be commenced.
- *Uroflowmetry with bladder scan*: usually two or three voids performed on an adapted commode onto a flow sensor (uroflowmeter): giving information on voided volume, flow curves, flow rates (volume of urine passed/unit of time), and post-void residual volumes (>20 mL or 15% of expected bladder capacity is significant). Characteristic flow curves can be seen in certain conditions (see Fig. 5.1). No information on storage or voiding pressure is given:
  - *Normal bell-shaped curve*: normal or seen in over active bladder.
  - *Tower-shaped curve*: seen in over active bladder.

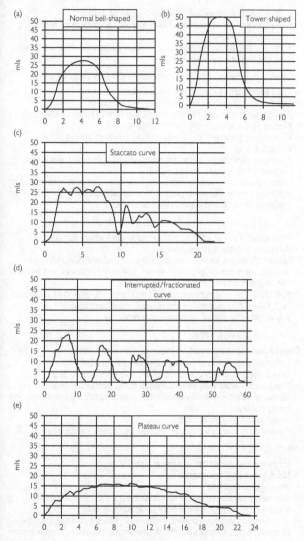

Fig. 5.1 The classical five types of uroflow curve.

Austin, P.F. et al. The Standardization of Terminology of Lower Urinary Tract Function in Children and Adolescents: Update Report from the Standardization Committee of the International Children's Continence Society. *Neurourology and Urodynamics* 2016;35(4):471–81. Copyright © 2015 Wiley Periodicals, Inc.

- *Staccato curve*: associated with dysfunctional voiding.
- *Fractionated curve*: associated with detrusor underactivity with abdominal straining.
- *Plateau long flat curve*: suggestive of fixed anatomical obstruction such as urethral/meatal stenosis/PUV.

Invasive urodynamics ± fluoroscopy (video urodynamics)

- Gold standard investigation of bladder function.
- Urethral or suprapubic catheters plus rectal catheter.
- *Artificial fill*: automated bladder-filling cycle with contrast or saline.
- *Natural fill*: i.e. ambulatory—with drinking.
- Cystometry (storage) and pressure–flow (voiding) phases occur characterizing:
  - *storage*: capacity, detrusor baseline pressures, detrusor overactivity, compliance, leakage, and sensation
  - *voiding*: detrusor voiding pressures, flow rates and post void residuals;
- *Video*: bladder and urethral outline, bladder neck position and behaviour, presence of VUR, and vaginal reflux of urine.

Additional imaging

- Plain spinal X-ray or US (up to 6 weeks of age) where spinal dysraphism/pathology is suspected.
- Spinal MRI where lumbosacral anomalies are seen/suspected/need detailed characterization, particularly if bowel disturbances also present.
- MR urogram where ectopic ureters suspected.
- MAG3/DMSA where recurrent UTI and renal scarring/VUR suspected.
- MCUG—in first year of life where anatomical obstruction/VUR suspected (also part of video urodynamics).

Patterns of pathology

Delayed onset of continence/CNS maturity—primary onset

- Common delayed potty training, aversive toileting behaviours.
- Often associated with constipation and retentive withholding.
- Can be associated with developmental delay, perinatal hypoxia, attention deficit hyperactivity disorder, autistic spectrum conditions, and family history.
- Investigations usually normal.
- *Treatment*: responds well to urotherapy and consistent routine.

Monosymptomatic enuresis

- Large volume, early/late wetting at night.
- No daytime LUT symptoms.
- Investigations normal.
- Secondary to relative nocturnal vasopressin deficit, immature CNS arousal mechanisms, ± small normal bladder capacity.
- *Treatment*: urotherapy (general measures in NICE guideline), treatment of constipation, enuresis alarms, desmopressin tablets/sublingual melts.

Non-monosymptomatic enuresis: enuresis with LUT dysfunction symptoms

- Small capacity bladder common finding (≤65% expected bladder capacity).
- Frequency, urgency, nocturia, continuous fast stream, usually normal emptying on US.
- May have features of overactive bladder on uroflow.
- *Treatment:* address constipation, urotherapy, combination of anticholinergic therapy (oxybutynin, tolterodine, solifenacin, trospium chloride) and desmopressin.

Overactive bladder (primary or secondary)

- Classical symptoms of urgency (with or without incontinence) often characterized by posturing (e.g. Vincent's curtsy), frequency, nocturia ± enuresis.
- Small bladder capacity with complete emptying.
- Constipation and UTIs common (although often over-diagnosed in primary care).
- Tower-shaped uroflows/high Q_{max} flow rate.
- *Treatment:*
  - urotherapy (including timed voiding), treat constipation, anticholinergics to improve capacity and detrusor relaxation, transcutaneous electrical nerve stimulation, parasacral neuromodulation where available as alternative/adjunct.
  - Resistant overactive bladder needs invasive urodynamics and confirmation of detrusor overactivity. This may then warrant treatment with intravesical botulinum toxin or mirabegron (beta-3 agonist).

Dysfunctional voiding (commoner in girls)

- Abnormal urinary stream including hesitancy, interrupted urine flow, sensation of incomplete voiding, bladder pain, and bladder wall thickening on US.
- High association with UTI and VUR (± constipation).
- Staccato flows with pelvic EMG activity during void.
- Significant post-void residual volume.
- Often features of frequency/urgency (overactive bladder can be secondary to dysfunctional voiding).
- *Treatment:* laxatives (if constipation present), timed, double-voiding with relaxation techniques, pelvic floor exercises, and biofeedback sessions. Clean intermittent catheterization (CIC) if no response.

Neuropathic bladder

- Bladder dysfunction secondary to an identifiable neurological cause:
  - *Congenital:* spinal dysraphism, lipomyelomeningocoele, caudal regression, and sacral agenesis.
  - *Acquired:* spinal tumours, autonomic neuropathies (e.g. Guillain–Barré syndrome), transverse myelitis/acute disseminated encephalomyelitis, and trauma. MRI spine vital in assessment.

- Clinical features vary but may be silent and must be looked for—may include symptoms of overactivity, incontinence, lack of awareness of bladder/bowel sensation, inability to achieve continence/abdominal pain, and recurrent UTI. Infancy and teenage periods are the highest risk period for presentation of tethered cords. Bladder symptoms often precede spinal signs and must be investigated with invasive urodynamics or uroflowmetry with EMG.
- Imaging features may show either a thick-walled, small-capacity bladder, or a large bladder (≥150% estimated capacity), atonic bladder, ± dilatation of the ureters and upper tracts. Invasive urodynamics may demonstrate high- or low-pressure systems. *Detrusor–sphincter dyssynergia* is a common and high-risk finding for progressive renal damage. Any pattern of bladder pathology can be found and thorough investigation to characterize and treat the appropriate pattern is required.
- *Treatment*: cord untethering, anticholinergics, and botulinum toxin for overactive, high-pressure systems, alpha blockers for sphincter relaxation with CIC, or definitive surgery for incomplete emptying (vesicostomy/ureterostomy/Mitrofanoff channel formation ± bladder augmentation). Preservation of the upper tracts and avoidance of CKD is paramount.

Non-neuropathic neuropathic bladder (Hinman bladder)

- Arises where bladder dysfunction is so severe that it appears neuropathic in the absence of any identifiable neurological cause.
- Risk factors include chronic retention, incomplete voiding, prolonged uncoordinated detrusor overactivity, polyuric conditions (CKD, diabetes insipidus, Bartter syndrome), and secondary causes of bladder outlet obstruction (dysfunctional voiding/severe constipation/tumours).
- *Treatment*: similar to neuropathic bladders in terms of establishing safe emptying first (CIC and surgical options, e.g. Mitrofanoff) then addressing overactivity and pressure with anticholinergics and botulinum toxin. Faecal retention/soiling needs parallel therapy.

True giggle incontinence (special type of urge incontinence)

- Sudden, involuntary loss of bladder control with reflex bladder neck opening and incontinence associated with deep laughter and other emotional states.
- Related to cataplexy (loss of muscle tone with strong emotions), common in young (aged 5–7 years) and pubescent females, improves with age.
- Cortical phenomenon with normal bladder investigations when not laughing.
- Treated with methylphenidate if appropriate to number of episodes and symptom severity.

Specific syndromes with bladder dysfunction

- *Ochoa syndrome*: urofacial syndrome—frown-like grimace (inverted smile) when laughing or smiling, a non-neuropathic neuropathic bladder with poor emptying, incontinence and megacystis, VUR, recurrent UTI, and constipation.
- *Absent abdominal wall musculature syndrome*: renal dysplasia, atonic megacystis, poor emptying, and VUR.
- *Megacystis–megaureter*: radiological appearance of large, thin-walled bladder with primary bilateral high-grade VUR.
- *Megacystis microcolon with intestinal hypoperistalsis*: rare congenital disease with massive abdominal distension, dilated non-obstructed urinary bladder, and microcolon with decreased or absent intestinal peristalsis (Fig. 5.2).

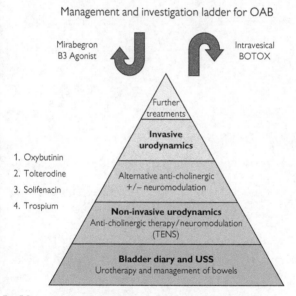

Management and investigation ladder for OAB

Mirabegron
B3 Agonist

Intravesical
BOTOX

Further
treatments

**Invasive
urodynamics**

1. Oxybutinin

2. Tolterodine

3. Solifenacin

4. Trospium

Alternative anti-cholinergic
+/− neuromodulation

Non-invasive urodynamics
Anti-cholinergic therapy/neuromodulation
(TENS)

Bladder diary and USS
Urotherapy and management of bowels

Fig. 5.2 Investigation and treatment pyramid for the overactive bladder (OAB). TENS, transcutaneous electrical nerve stimulation; USS, ultrasound scan.
Reproduced courtesy of Evelina London Children's Hospital.

Electrolyte and acid–base disorders

Disorders of sodium and water: basic principles

- Sodium (Na) and water homoeostasis are inextricably linked. Na concentration is measured in mmol/L, highlighting the fact that changes in numerator (Na) as well as denominator (water) will alter the concentration. It is impossible to assess a plasma Na measurement without considering plasma volume. Since Na constitutes the major extracellular ion, changes in plasma volume will result in the largest absolute change in Na concentration compared with the other plasma ions. For instance, when starting from a baseline of 140 mmol/L, a change in plasma water of 10% will alter the plasma Na concentration to either 154 mmol/L or 126 mmol/L.
- The kidney has no sensors for Na concentration and regulates Na reabsorption purely in response to renal perfusion.
- Changes in plasma tonicity are sensed by osmoreceptors in the brain and affect renal water handling via ADH (AVP).
- In case of conflicting signals, the most important principle is preservation or restoration of a normal plasma volume, rather than a normal Na concentration. Thus, with normal functioning kidneys, urine Na is low in hypernatraemic dehydration and elevated in syndrome of inappropriate antidiuretic hormone secretion (SIADH) or acute water intoxication. While we can easily measure Na concentration, there is no simple test for plasma water. Instead, we need to use auxiliary parameters, such as change in weight, BP, and perfusion (capillary refill) to determine whether an abnormal Na concentration is the consequence of changes in Na or water.
- In clinical practice, the vast majority of abnormal Na concentrations are due to changes in water, rather than Na. The precise aetiology can be determined by interrogating the kidneys via urine indices (Na, creatinine, osmolality). An absolute urine Na concentration is a useful first guide, but it is much better to calculate a fractional excretion of Na (FENa). FENa (%) = $100 \times (U_{Na}/U_{cr})/(P_{Na}/P_{cr})$ (where P is plasma, U is urine, and cr is creatinine; all in mmol/L).
- Normal values for FENa. With a GFR of 100 mL/min and a Na concentration of 140 mmol/L, the kidneys would filter 19,600 mmol of Na per day (filtrate is 100 mL/min, so $100 \times 60 \times 24$ mL/day = 144,000 mL or 144 L of filtrate per day. 144 L contain 140×140 mmol Na = 19600 mmol). This is equivalent to ~1.2 kg of salt (NaCl). In steady state, the kidneys need to excrete the amount of salt ingested (minus enteral and skin losses) and an average salt intake of 10 g is roughly equivalent to 1% of the filtered load. Thus, with normal GFR and normal salt intake, a normal FENa is <1% and in dehydration usually <0.3%. However, if GFR is decreased, e.g. to 50 mL/min, then the 10 g of salt is equivalent to 2% of the filtered load, so the normal range for FENa changes. In AKI, when creatinine has not reached a steady state value, normal values for FENa cannot be determined.

Disorders of sodium and water: hypernatraemia

Definition

Plasma Na >145 mmol/L.
- Caused by either a deficiency of water (common) or an excess of salt (rare).
- A diagnostic algorithm for the assessment of hypernatraemia is given in Fig. 6.1.

Clinical signs and symptoms

- *CNS dysfunction*: lethargy, irritability, nuchal rigidity, seizures, drowsiness, and coma. Intracranial haemorrhage (subdural, subarachnoid, intracerebral) may occur due to a rapid shift of water from brain cells with associated cerebral vessel distention.
- *Hypernatraemic dehydration*: signs of extracellular fluid (ECF) depletion are masked (even if very dehydrated) because water moves from cells to the extracellular compartment.
- *Salt overload*: can be associated with signs of volume overload, such as hypertension, oedema, pulmonary venous congestion, and hepatomegaly. In cases of sudden salt ingestion (e.g. deliberate salt poisoning), there is rapid progression to coma often without signs of hypervolaemia, with mortality as high as 30–60%. Note that salt is an effective emetic and the most common symptoms in patients with salt poisoning are vomiting and diarrhoea. Thus, the clinical history cannot reliably distinguish between hypernatraemic dehydration and salt poisoning. The latter should be considered if the clinical signs of dehydration and the expected weight loss (see following bullet points) are not consistent with the degree of hypernatraemia.
- The free water deficit is used to estimate the weight loss: weight (kg) × total body water ratio (0.7 in an infant; 0.65 in an older child) × (measured plasma Na − 145 [upper limit of normal])/upper limit of normal for plasma Na (145).
  - *Example*: a 6-month-old child with a previous weight of 5 kg presents with a plasma Na of 176 mmol/L. The minimal expected weight loss (loss of pure water) would be 5 × 0.7 × 31/145 = 0.748 kg. In reality, the weight loss would be even higher, as the fluids lost in diarrhoea will not be pure water, but contain some salt, as well. If no previous weight is available, the weight after rehydration should be used.
- Once considered, salt poisoning is best proved by an elevated FENa and subsequent forensic investigations.

Investigations

Plasma and urine U&Es, creatinine, glucose, and osmolality. Always consider the possibility of a urinary concentrating defect (➔ see 'Disorders of renal water handling', p. 181) as this alters management.

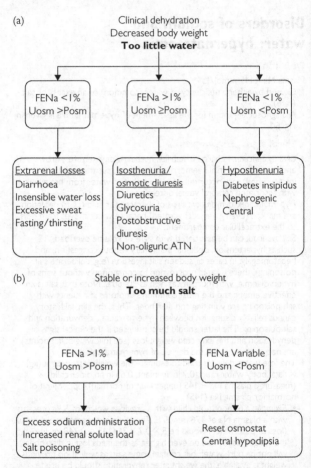

Fig. 6.1 (a) A diagnostic algorithm for hypernatraemia due to a deficiency of water. (b) A diagnostic algorithm for hypernatraemia due to an excess of salt.

Management of hypernatraemic dehydration

The general principle is that alterations that have happened acutely can be corrected relatively quickly (24–48 h), whereas chronic alterations should be treated slowly. This is because of the adaptive response of brain cells to hypernatraemia—with time, they increase intracellular osmolarity, decreasing movement of water out of cells, and preventing intracellular dehydration, by intracellular production of osmotically active low-molecular-weight organic molecules. This is important: if hypernatraemia is rapidly corrected before the brain cells have had time to adjust back to a normal intracellular osmolarity, then fluid will pass into the cells and catastrophic cerebral oedema will develop. This is the reason that the successful management of hypernatraemia depends on a gradual lowering of the Na.

- Shock should be corrected by 0.9% saline solution 20 mL/kg over 30 min and repeated if necessary.
- *Never give hypotonic fluids as a bolus!* It can lead to a rapid imbalance between extracellular and intracellular tonicity, and movement of water into cells, with the risk of fatal brain oedema and herniation. Plasma Na should decrease by <15 mmol/day.
- If IV fluids are used then 0.9% saline is usually a good initial starting point, but always consider the possibility of a renal concentrating defect. Check the urine osmolality—this should be well above plasma osmolality in hypernatraemic dehydration. The tonicity of the fluid given (not considering glucose content) should not exceed the tonicity of the urine. Thus, if the urine osmolality is 150 mOsm/kg (as in diabetes insipidus), then fluid given should be glucose with either water or 0.18% saline.
- Normal hydration should be achieved over 36–48 h and perhaps 72 h if the initial plasma Na is >170 mmol/L. Fluid volume is calculated by considering maintenance requirement, plus deficit, plus ongoing losses.
  - *Example*: a 3 kg neonate with 20% dehydration aiming for correction over 48 h: maintenance: 300 mL/day = 600 mL plus deficit of (3 [weight] × 0.2 [per cent dehydration]) = 600 mL. Thus, a total of 1200 mL should be given over 48 h = 25 mL/h. If there are ongoing losses (diarrhoea, vomiting), this needs to be added. The key is close monitoring of vital signs, weight, fluid balance, and electrolytes (6-hourly initially) to adjust treatment if needed.
- In the case of a urinary concentrating defect, administered fluids (except for boluses) should have a Na concentration equal to or lower than that of urine, otherwise hypernatraemia will worsen.
- Oral rehydration therapy in diarrhoeal-induced hypernatraemic dehydration is safe in children who are not shocked, despite a potentially faster fall in plasma Na.
- Persistent oliguria when circulatory impairment has been corrected indicates AKI, due to ATN or possible RVT.

Management of hypernatraemia due to salt excess

- Will correct spontaneously if renal function is normal (salt is excreted by kidneys).
- Avoid too rapid a correction of plasma Na (risk of cerebral oedema; ➔ see 'Management of hypernatraemic dehydration', p. 122).
- If AKI is present, dialysis may be indicated.

Disorders of sodium and water: hyponatraemia

Definition

Plasma Na <135 mmol/L. Due to:
* gain of water in excess of Na (common)
* loss of Na in excess of water (rare).

Definition of terms

* *Osmolal gap*: the difference between the calculated osmolality and the measured osmolality: $(2 \times [Na + K] + [urea] + [glucose]) - (measured osmolality)$.
* *Factitious hyponatraemia*: occurs as a result of a fluid shift between the intracellular fluid (ICF) and ECF compartments due to the presence of abnormal, relatively impermanent solutes in the ECF. Examples of such solutes are glucose in excess, mannitol, sorbitol, and maltose. In factitious hyponatraemia, the measured plasma osmolality is high despite the low plasma Na and, with the exception of hyperglycaemia, the osmolal gap will be >10 mOsm/kg.
* *Pseudohyponatraemia*: associated with a normal plasma osmolality and an increased osmolal gap may occur if there is a reduction in the fraction of plasma water (normally 93%). When indirect ion-selective electrodes are used for measurement (the most common method in paediatric hospitals due to the small plasma volume required), the sample is diluted before measurement and the measured value is corrected under the assumption of 93% plasma water (division by 0.93). In patients with marked hyperlipidaemia or hyperproteinaemia, the plasma water fraction may be substantially lower and consequently, the reported plasma Na concentration is artefactually reduced. The problem does not arise when direct ion-selective electrodes are used (e.g. bedside analysers), as the sample is not diluted.

A diagnostic algorithm for the assessment of hyponatraemia is given in Fig. 6.2.

Clinical features

* *Acute water intoxication*: low plasma osmolality will cause movement of water into cells. Most important consequences occur in the brain, as space to accommodate cell swelling is confined by the skull, causing nausea, emesis, headaches, disorientation, seizures, coma, and death.
* *Chronic hyponatraemia*: adaptive mechanisms to equilibrate intra- and extracellular osmolality (mainly excretion of osmols from cells) have had time to take place; often patients are asymptomatic or have milder, non-specific symptoms, such as malaise, anorexia, and headaches.

Investigations

* Plasma and urine U&Es, glucose, albumin, and osmolality.
* Plasma liver function tests (LFTs) and triglycerides.
* Consider adrenal and thyroid function tests.

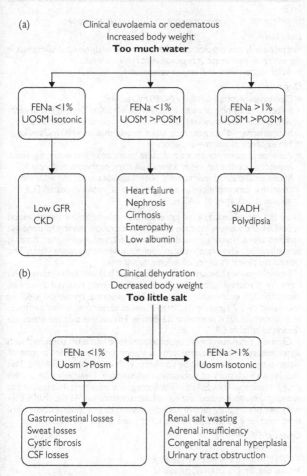

Fig. 6.2 (a) A diagnostic algorithm for hyponatraemia due to an excess of water. The limit for FENa of 1% is not absolute. Neonates have a higher FENa due to decreased GFR (➲ see 'Normal values for FENa'). In general, the lower the FENa, the better the tubular reabsorption. (b) A diagnostic algorithm for hyponatraemia due to a deficiency of salt.

Syndrome of inappropriate antidiuretic hormone

Definition
Inappropriately concentrated urine due to inappropriately elevated ADH levels in the setting of euvolaemic or hypervolaemic hyponatraemia.
* ADH is also called AVP or just vasopressin.

Diagnosis
* Decreased plasma osmolality (<280 mOsm/kg).
* Inappropriately high urine osmolality (Uosm >100 mOsm/kg). In patients with clinical water overload, urine should be maximally diluted. With normal urinary diluting capacity, Uosm should thus be <100 mOsm/kg.
* No evidence of volume depletion.
* Absence of other conditions that cause retention of free water, e.g. renal, hepatic, or cardiac failure, or adrenal, pituitary, or thyroid dysfunction.
* Stable or decreased haematocrit, plasma albumin, urea, uric acid, and creatinine concentrations as a consequence of stable/increased ECF volume is indicative of SIADH.

Note: as a consequence of the increased ECF volume from water retention in SIADH, the kidneys increase urinary Na excretion, leading to urine Na concentrations typically around 20–70 mmol/L and even higher, if salt is supplemented. This often leads to confusion with salt wasting states. The latter have clinical evidence of volume depletion.

Example: you are consulted on a 6-month-old boy with astrocytoma, who came for a routine assessment 2 weeks after having received a dose of vincristine. On examination, he is well in appearance, his weight is 4.7 kg (increased by 0.2 kg since discharge 2 weeks earlier), he is well perfused, and his systolic BP is normal at 82 mmHg. His routine biochemistries are illustrated in Table 6.1.

Clinically, this is euvolaemic hyponatraemia and thus most consistent with water excess. The urine osmolality is inappropriately high for a state of water excess, so this would be consistent with a diagnosis of SIADH. This also fits with a history of vincristine administration 2 weeks earlier, as this drug is associated with SIADH. The appropriate treatment thus is aimed at reducing the water excess and *not* salt supplementation. As the child is clinically well (the hyponatraemia has likely developed over several days), there is no need for emergency treatment. For more details see following text.

Causes of SIADH
* Pain, stress.
* *CNS disease*: meningitis, head injury.
* *Lung disease*: pneumonia, tumours.
* *Drugs*: SIADH is associated with certain drugs, sometimes with a delay of several days—exogenous vasopressin, vincristine, nicotine, chlorpropamide, carbamazepine, tricyclic antidepressants, selective

Table 6.1 Example values

	Blood	Urine
Na (mmol/L)	125	32
Osmolality (mOsm/kg)	255	625

serotonin reuptake inhibitors (SSRIs), thioridazine, cyclophosphamide, clofibrate, bromocriptine, haloperidol, tiotixene, monoamine oxidase inhibitors.
- *Inherited*: gain-of-function mutation in the vasopressin receptor type 2 gene, *AVPR2* (R137C, R137L, I130N, or F229V). Note that in this condition, ADH levels are suppressed (➔ see 'Nephrogenic syndrome of inappropriate antidiuresis', p. 185).

Emergency management

- The main concern of rapid correction of hyponatraemia is the development of pontine myelinolysis with permanent neurological sequelae. However, in an acutely symptomatic child (e.g. having seizures) with hyponatraemia, hypertonic saline is used to achieve a rapid increase in plasma Na to a level usually considered 'safe', which is 125 mmol/L.
- A bolus of 2–3 mL/kg of 3% saline over 10 min should be given. The rate of administration should be slowed as soon as symptoms improve, so that the total increase in plasma Na does not exceed 10 mmol/day. The bolus may need to be repeated once or twice if symptoms persist.

Non-emergency management

With water excess
- Restriction of water intake.
- Careful fluid balance and monitoring of weight and electrolytes are necessary, as water output must exceed water intake to achieve net water removal. This can be especially difficult in SIADH, when the urine is concentrated and thus urine volume is low.
- Especially challenging in infants where nutrition is provided in liquid form. Formulas should be maximally concentrated to allow fluid restriction without starving the baby.
- Loop diuretics can be considered, as they impair the urinary concentrating mechanism and thus enhance water excretion. They can be especially helpful in hyponatraemia associated with nephrotic syndrome, and also in SIADH.
- AVPR2 antagonists (e.g. tolvaptan) are competitive antagonists at the vasopressin receptor in the kidney and thus block the vasopressin-mediated urinary concentration. A recommended starting dose for tolvaptan is 0.1 mg/kg once daily and the dose can be up-titrated to 1.0 mg/kg daily divided in 1–2 doses, if needed. Patients should have free access to water and should be monitored closely, as pharmacologically induced nephrogenic diabetes insipidus can ensue.
- Urea increases the osmotic load and thus obligates free water excretion. Urea can be difficult to obtain as a pharmaceutical product, but may be available as a nutritional supplement. Tolerability can be difficult due to its foul taste, but is improved with formulations that mix urea with citric acid and flavourings. A reasonable starting dose is 0.25 – 0.5 g/kg/day divided into two or three doses. The dose can be increased as necessary.

With salt deficiency
Salt deficiency is usually associated with hypovolaemia. Replacement of the volume deficit and ongoing losses with normal saline is a reasonable first treatment. Again, close monitoring of the patient is necessary to avoid too rapid correction.

Disorders of potassium: basic principles

- More than 98% of body potassium (K) is intracellular, yet we measure extracellular K concentration. The plasma K level is therefore only a poor representation of total body K and levels can change because of a shift of K between compartments, as well as from changes in total K.
- In general, acute changes reflect shifts between compartments and chronic changes reflect total K. Since the ratio of extra- and intracellular K is the major determinant for the membrane potential of excitable cells, such as in heart or the neuromuscular system, acute changes in K can be life-threatening. A good indicator for the physiological relevance of a given K level is the height of the T wave in the electrocardiogram (ECG): hypokalaemia is associated with ST depression, a flat T wave, and emergence of a U wave, whereas hyperkalaemia leads to peaked T waves. If these changes are not present, the K level is unlikely to represent an emergency.
- Distribution of K between the ICF and ECF is maintained primarily by the Na^+/K^+-ATPase. Compounds that enhance the activity of this pump, such as insulin or adrenergics, can cause K alterations and be used for treatment of hyperkalaemia.
- K excretion in the kidney is determined in the collecting duct under the control of aldosterone. Excretion of K needs electrical balancing, typically by exchanging it for Na. Thus, a prerequisite for K excretion is sufficient distal delivery of Na, which is impaired in dehydration.

Disorders of potassium: hyperkalaemia

- *Pseudohyperkalaemia*: artefactually high plasma K caused by movement of K out of cells after blood taking. The commonest cause in paediatrics is a haemolysed blood sample (Fig. 6.3). Other causes include:
  - hereditary spherocytosis and familial pseudohyperkalaemia, caused by excessive tendency of K to leak from RBCs as a result of cooling of blood *ex vivo*
  - leaving the blood for a prolonged period prior to centrifugation can also cause pseudohyperkalaemia due to leakage from cells
  - improper collection or handling of blood sample (e.g. K ethylenediaminetetraacetic acid (EDTA) contamination)
  - any other cause of *in vitro* haemolysis, e.g. excessive shaking of blood bottle following collection (e.g. in pneumatic tube transport system)
  - leucocytosis or thrombocytosis.

Causes of true hyperkalaemia

Glomerular filtration rate <15 mL/min/1.73 m^2

Patients with CKD stage 5 have an intrinsic risk of hyperkalaemia, but this can be compounded by the following:

- *Decreased renal excretion*: AKI, K-sparing diuretics, ACE inhibitor, angiotensin II receptor blocker (ARB), beta blockers, non-steroidal anti-inflammatory drugs (NSAIDS), trimethoprim, heparin.
- *Increased K load*: oral/IV supplementation, blood transfusion, endogenous cell breakdown (e.g. tumour lysis syndrome, GI bleed, rhabdomyolysis, haemolysis, catabolic state).

Glomerular filtration rate >15 mL/min/1.73 m^2

The kidneys have a very high capacity to excrete K. Hyperkalaemia thus develops virtually only if other factors are present that impair distal K secretion. This can be estimated using the transtubular K gradient (TTKG):

$$TTKG = (urine\ K/urine\ osmolality)/plasma\ K/plasma\ osmolality)$$

Normal values of TTKG in children are 4.1–10.5 (median 6.0); for infants, the normal range is 4.9–15.5 (median 7.8). A decrease in TTKG suggests aldosterone deficiency or insensitivity. An increase in TTKG suggests dietary excess of K or high aldosterone activity (Table 6.2).

Table 6.2 Constituents of a 'HyperK cocktail'

Constituents	Amount
30% glucose	500 mL
Regular insulin	30 U
10% Ca gluconate	30 mL
Sodium acetate	100 mmol

Infuse at 2 mL/kg/h, preferably by central line for the first hour, then 1–2 mL/kg/h.

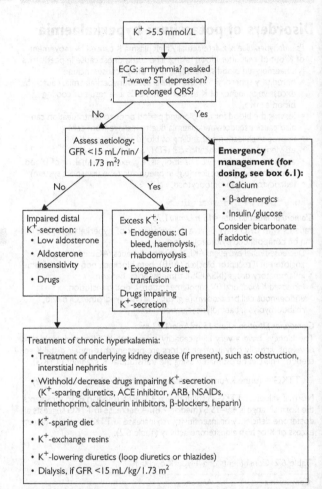

Fig. 6.3 An algorithm for hyperkalaemia.

Example: you are asked to give advice regarding a 10-day-old female neonate on the intensive care unit with the following investigation results. Na 132 mmol/L, K 8.9 mmol/L (non-haemolysed), urea 2 mmol/L, creatinine 23 μmol/L. Specifically, you have been asked whether the results may be caused by adrenocortical insufficiency (e.g. congenital adrenal hyperplasia). You request urinary electrolytes, and paired (blood and urine) osmolarity: urine K 10 mmol/L, urine osmolarity 151 mmol/L, plasma osmolarity 311 mOsm/L. This gives a TTKG of 2.3. This value would be compatible with aldosterone (mineralocorticoid) deficiency or insensitivity. The differential diagnosis would thus include congenital adrenal hyperplasia, hypoaldosteronism, pseudohypoaldosteronism, or insufficient distal Na delivery.

Causes for impaired potassium secretion

- Volume depletion/impaired distal Na delivery.
- Obstructive uropathy.
- Interstitial nephritis.
- Drugs, e.g. ciclosporin, tacrolimus, NSAIDs, ACE inhibitor, ARB, trimethoprim, K-sparing diuretics.
- Congenital adrenal hyperplasia.
- Primary hypoaldosteronism.
- Pseudohypoaldosteronism type 1 and 2.
- Sickle cell disease.
- Diabetes mellitus.

Rarely, hyperkalaemia is due to redistribution:
- Metabolic/respiratory acidosis.
- Hyperkalaemic periodic paralysis.
- Insulin deficiency (diabetic ketoacidosis: may be hyperkalaemic, but total body K depleted).
- Drugs/toxins.

Clinical features

- Muscle weakness.
- Cardiac arrhythmia.
- Hyperkalaemic RTA.

ECG changes

(See Fig. 6.4.)
- Peaked T waves ('tenting').
- Loss of P wave.
- Widened QRS.
- ST depression.
- Bradycardia, heart block, ventricular arrhythmia, cardiac arrest (K >10 mmol/L).
- See Box 6.1 for emergency treatment.

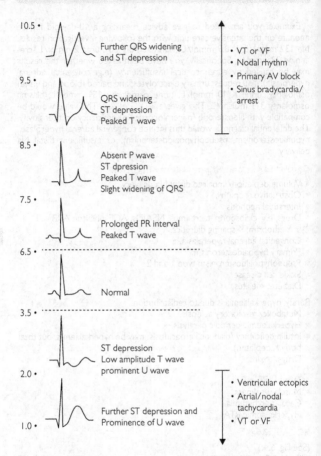

Fig. 6.4 Typical ECG patterns seen with plasma levels of K from 1.0 to 10.5 mmol/L (indicated on the left).

Box 6.1 Emergency treatment

(➔ See also Chapter 17.) Seek cause and treat appropriately. The following is a guide:

- Place on cardiac monitor.
- Salbutamol nebulizer 2.5–5 mg: repeat three times—can be given continuously, or
- Salbutamol IV 4 microgram/kg in 5 mL water given over 10–20 min.
- *Correct acidosis*: Sodium bicarbonate 1–2 mmol/kg IV over 30 min.
- *Calcium Resonium*® 1 g/kg (to a maximum 60 g), then 0.25–1 g/kg four times daily orally/rectally. If given orally, should give with lactulose 5–10 mL four times daily.
- Ca gluconate 10%: 0.5 mL/kg IV over 10 min (note: this does not lower K, but protects the myocardium against arrhythmias).
- Glucose 0.5–1 g/kg and insulin 0.1–0.2 U/kg as a bolus, or continuous infusion of 10% glucose at 5 mL/kg/h (0.5 g/kg/h) with insulin 0.1 U/kg/h. Monitor glucose at least hourly.
- Consider 'HyperK cocktail' (see Table 6.2).
- Dialysis.

Disorders of potassium: hypokalaemia

* Hypokalaemia, unless of acute onset, is rarely a clinical emergency.
* Caused by either a shift of K into the ICF or by total body K depletion.

Clinical features

* Muscle weakness, paralysis.
* *Smooth muscle involvement*: intestinal ileus, ureteric dilatation.
* *Cardiac*: myocardial cell necrosis, arrhythmia, and ECG changes (see Fig. 6.5).
* Rhabdomyolysis and myoglobinuria.
* Lethargy, confusion, tetany.
* *Autonomic insufficiency*: postural hypotension.
* Renal consequences:
  * *Decreased concentrating capacity*: polyuria, polydipsia.
  * Increased renal ammonia production.
  * Increased proton secretion in distal tubule (to allow Na reabsorption) leading to maintenance of metabolic alkalosis.

ECG changes

(See Fig. 6.4.)
* Prolonged QT and QU interval.
* Increased U-wave amplitude.
* Prolonged QRS.
* ST depression.
* Decreased T-wave amplitude.
* Increased P-wave amplitude.
* Increased PR interval.

Investigations

* Careful dietary and fluid intake history, and document extra losses, e.g. diarrhoea or vomiting.
* Careful drug history (diuretics/laxatives/chemotherapy/amphotericin).
* Measure BP (hypertension and hypokalaemia—think about Conn, Liddle, and Cushing syndromes).

Laboratory and radiological investigations guided by clinical suspicion

* *Plasma chemistry*: look for evidence of tubulopathy (acidosis or alkalosis, dehydration, hypophosphataemia, hypocalcaemia, hypomagnesaemia).
* Blood gas.
* *Urine chemistry*: consider Na, K, Ca, magnesium (Mg), creatinine, osmolality, pH, and excessive urinary losses of K.
* Plasma glucose and urine glucose/ketones.
* Plasma renin activity, aldosterone.
* Plasma cortisol; (24 h) urine corticosteroid profile.
* Renal US (nephrocalcinosis).
* Consider X-ray knee or wrist for associated rickets.

Assessment

(See Fig. 6.5.)

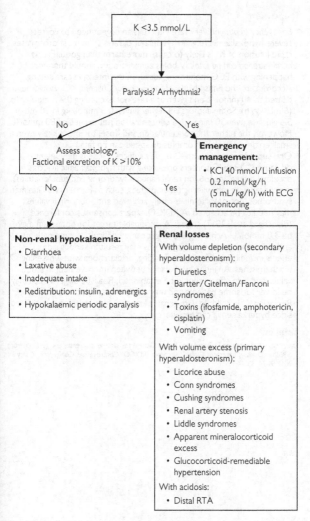

Fig. 6.5 An algorithm for the assessment of hypokalaemia.

Treatment

- *Emergency treatment*: very rarely there is an urgent need to correct severe hypokalaemia (e.g. arrhythmia or paralysis). In most other cases, rapid infusion of K^+ is likely to cause more harm than good. *Excess administration can be fatal!* IV bolus administration should therefore be happening with ECG monitoring, ideally in the intensive care setting. According to the *British National Formulary for Children*, KCl should be diluted to 40 mmol/L and given at a rate not exceeding 0.2 mmol/kg/h (5 mL/kg/h). Some authors set higher limits: 0.5 mmol/kg in 20 mL of 5% glucose over 30 min with a concentration not exceeding 80 mmol/L. However, the higher the concentration and dose, the more likely even a small error in calculation or infusion speed can be fatal!
- Oral supplementation with K^+ usually suffices. Dose is dependent on cause (➲ see 'Disorders presenting with hypokalaemic acidosis: proximal tubule', p. 166, on renal Fanconi syndrome and tubulopathies).
- In children with salt-wasting tubulopathies, such as Bartter and Gitelman syndromes, normokalaemia is rarely achieved and subnormal values may need to be accepted. A KDIGO expert consensus conference (Blanchard et al. 2017) stated: 'A reasonable target for potassium may be 3.0 mmol/L. Achieving this target can be difficult in some patients and supplementation with large doses may result in serious side effects including gastric ulcers, vomiting, or diarrhoea with worsening biochemistries. An individual balance between improvement in blood values and side effects should be established. Realistic target values may be lower for some patients and may also change with time'.
- Replacing K^+ in children with renal failure should be carefully considered since hyperkalaemia can easily occur.

Reference

Blanchard A, Bockenhauer D, Bolignano D, et al. Gitelman syndrome: consensus and guidance from a Kidney Disease: Improving Global Outcomes (KDIGO) Controversies Conference. *Kidney Int* 2017;91:24–33.

Disorders of calcium: basic principles

- Calcium (Ca) is the most abundant mineral in the body with >98% stored in bone.
- Plasma Ca is tightly regulated with a normal range of 2.1–2.6 mmol/L. However, normal ranges vary with age and infants typically have higher Ca levels than older children (→ see Chapter 18).
- ~40% of plasma Ca is protein bound (mainly albumin) and 10% complexed to anions, such as bicarbonate and phosphate. The remaining 50% represents the biologically active ionized or free Ca. Thus, total Ca levels vary with those of the binding partners and the following formula is commonly used to 'correct' total Ca levels for albumin levels:

$$\text{Corrected Ca (mmol/L)} = \text{measured total Ca (mmol/L)} + 0.02 (40 - \text{albumin (g/L)})$$

- Each mmol/L Ca is equivalent to 2.5 mg/dL.
- Measurement of ionized Ca is a better indicator of physiologically active Ca, but can be acutely altered by technique, such as the use of a tourniquet, which may cause intracellular Ca release and acidosis. The proportion of free Ca varies with pH, as protons compete with Ca for albumin binding sites: thus, alkalosis decreases and acidosis increases free Ca.
- Functions of Ca include:
  - stabilization of cell membranes
  - intra- and intercellular signalling, e.g. muscle contraction
  - neurotransmitter release, hormone secretion (PTH)
  - co-factor in enzymatic processes, especially clotting
  - stabilization of skeletal and dental structure.
- Key organs involved in Ca homoeostasis are:
  - *gut (absorption)*: active (transcellular) and passive (paracellular) transport. Active transport is regulated by vitamin D
  - *bone (storage)*: Ca can be stored in (stimulated by vitamin D) or released from (stimulated by PTH) bone
  - *kidney (excretion)*: ~65% of filtered Ca is passively reabsorbed in the proximal tubule and another 25% in the thick ascending limb of Henle's loop (→ see 'Tubulopathies: basic principles', p. 162). The remaining 10% is actively (transcellularly) reabsorbed in the distal convoluted tubule under control of PTH
  - filtered vitamin D (bound to vitamin D-binding protein) is reabsorbed and 1-alpha hydroxylated in the proximal tubule
  - *parathyroid glands (regulation)*: the parathyroid glands produce the key regulatory hormone PTH, secretion of which is controlled by direct feedback from Ca levels (via the Ca-sensing receptor), phosphate, and vitamin D (via vitamin D receptor) (→ see Chapter 18).

Disorders of calcium: hypercalcaemia

Definition

Total Ca (corrected) >2.6 mmol/L, ionized Ca >1.3 mmol/L. Severe, if total Ca (corrected) >3.0 mmol/L, ionized Ca >1.5 mmol/L.

Causes

- Hyperparathyroidism (primary, tertiary, not secondary).
- Familial hypocalciuric hypercalcaemia (FHH) is an autosomal dominant disorder of Ca regulation. Based on the underlying genetics three subforms can be distinguished: (1) FHH1—caused by loss of function mutations in the Ca-sensing receptor (CaSR). Hypercalcaemia in this disorder is usually asymptomatic and thus requires no treatment. In contrast, loss of function in both alleles (recessive inheritance) causes neonatal severe hyperparathyroidism, which results in rickets, extraosseous calcifications, and neurodevelopmental delay. Treatment is early parathyroidectomy; (2) FHH2—caused by mutations in the G-protein Gα_{11} (encoded by *GNA11*), which associates with CaSR. Like FHH1, the hypercalcaemia is usually asymptomatic; and (3) FHH3—due to mutations in *AP2S1*, which is involved in endocytosis of G-protein coupled receptors such as CaSR. Plasma Ca values tend to be highest in this subtype and associated symptoms (➔ see 'Clinical features') are more common. Syndromic features, such as cognitive impairment and atrial septal defects have been observed.
- Idiopathic infantile hypercalcaemia (IIH). IIH is characterized by infantile onset of hypercalcaemia, which can be asymptomatic and just noted incidentally, but can also be severe with total plasma Ca levels >3.0 mmol and associated symptoms. Two genetic causes have been identified in a substantial subset of patients with IIH, both with autosomal recessive inheritance: (1) mutations in *CYP24A1*. This enzyme is involved in the metabolism of vitamin D and is thus typically associated with high-dose vitamin D treatment; and (2) mutations in *SCL34A1*, encoding the phosphate transporter NaPiIIa.
- CKD (➔ see Chapter 18)—hypercalcaemia can be a complication of CKD. Risk factors include:
  - hyperparathyroidism
  - Ca-containing phosphate binders
  - activated vitamin D supplementation
  - adynamic bone disease
  - after transplantation when tertiary hyperparathyroidism is present.
- Malignancy-associated hypercalcaemia:
  - Synthesis of PTH-related peptides by the tumour.
  - Calcitriol-producing lymphoma.
- Vitamin D intoxication.
- *Extrarenal 1-alpha-hydroxylase activity*: TB, sarcoidosis, lymphoma, cat-scratch fever, and other granulomatous diseases (phosphate usually normal).
- Leprosy.
- Milk-alkali syndrome.
- Vitamin A toxicity.

- *Immobilization*: particularly after fracture.
- After BMT for osteopetrosis (transplanted osteoclasts remove excess bone).
- Subcutaneous fat necrosis.
- *Other endocrine causes*: hyperthyroidism and hypothyroidism, phaeochromocytoma, adrenal insufficiency, islet cell pancreas tumour, VIPoma.
- *Drugs*: aminophylline, oestrogen, thiazide diuretics, prostaglandin E infusion.
- *Syndromic*:
  - Williams syndrome (→ see 'Williams syndrome', p. 379).
  - Jansen syndrome (autosomal dominant—neonates with hypercalcaemia, rickets, metaphyseal dysplasia, low PTH).
  - *hypophosphatasia*: alkaline phosphatase (ALP) low or absent, hypercalcaemia, hypercalciuria, rickets.

Clinical features

Often asymptomatic, depending on severity and rapidity of onset.
- 'Stones', renal calculi; 'Bones', bone pain; 'Moans', depression; and 'Groans', (abdominal) due to constipation.
- Failure to thrive.
- Nephrocalcinosis/lithiasis.
- Decreased GFR.
- Short corrected QT-interval (QTc), arrhythmias.
- Hyporeflexia.
- Polyuria (nephrogenic diabetes insipidus).
- Venous thromboses.
- Metastatic calcification.

Investigation

Investigations to be considered in all cases
- U&Es, creatinine, Ca (total) and phosphate, and venous bicarbonate.
- LFTs including albumin and ALP.
- Ionized Ca.
- PTH.
- Daytime spot Uca:Ucr.
- US kidneys for nephrocalcinosis.

Investigations to be considered in select cases
- *Vitamin D levels*: 25-OH cholecalciferol levels are usually more informative than 1,25-OH cholecalciferol levels, due to the very short half-life of the latter.
- *Blood gas*: pH, pCO_2, pO_2, bicarbonate, base excess.
- Thyroid function tests.
- US of parathyroid glands.
- FBC and blood film/bone marrow aspirate and trephine/lymph node biopsy if suspected malignancy.
- CT or MRI of abdomen and chest.
- Mantoux test and/or QuantiFERON®-TB Gold test (or similar gamma interferon release assay for *Mycobacterium* tuberculosis).
- Serum ACE.

- C7q FISH for Williams syndrome.
- X-ray knee and wrist for rickets.
- X-ray skeletal survey (occult fracture or syndromic skeletal dysplasia, e.g. Jansen syndrome).
- ECG.
- Serology for cat scratch fever.
- *Endocrine tests*: urine vanillylmandelic acid (VMA)/homovanillic acid (HVA); plasma and urine adrenaline and noradrenaline; other (e.g. VIPOMA- seek expert advice).
- Genetic tests for FHH and IIH.

Assessment

(See Fig. 6.6.)

Treatment

In asymptomatic cases, identification and removal of the underlying cause is usually sufficient, e.g. stopping vitamin D supplementation. In acute symptomatic cases, the following can be used:

- Hyperhydration (e.g. 3 L/m^2/24 h IV 0.9% saline): Ca reabsorption in the proximal tubule passively follows Na reabsorption. As volume expansion diminishes proximal Na reabsorption, urinary Ca excretion will be increased.

In severe hypercalcaemia that does not respond, there is the occasional need for the following:

- *Loop diuretic* (furosemide 1 mg/kg/IV): 6–8-hourly (may need to replace K and Mg) to minimize Ca reabsorption in Henle's loop.
- *Corticosteroid*: occasionally for chronic hypercalcaemia (e.g. in sarcoid).
- *Calcitonin infusion* (salcatonin, derived from salmon): 5–10 U/kg IV followed by 4 U/kg IV or subcutaneously (SC) 12–24-hourly.
- *Dialysis*: if concomitant oliguric renal failure.

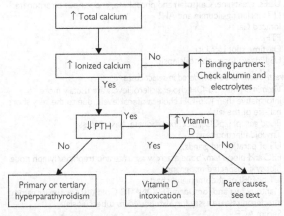

Fig. 6.6 An algorithm for the assessment of hypercalcaemia.

- *Bisphosphonate* (e.g. pamidronate infusion)—usually for hypercalcaemia of malignancy (especially if bone pain) or immobilization:
  - The dose of pamidronate is 1 mg/kg/day to a maximum of 60 mg, usually on three successive days.
  - Dilute pamidronate initially in water, but infuse in saline or 5% glucose.
  - Final concentration should not exceed 12 mg/100 mL of diluent.
  - Give infusion over 4 h on first occasion; thereafter, pamidronate can be given over 2–4 h.
  - calcimimetics in cases with hyperparathyroidism
    (➜ see 'Management: mineral and bone disorder').

Disorders of calcium: hypocalcaemia

Definition

Total Ca (corrected) <2.1 mmol/L, ionized Ca <1.2 mmol/L. Severe hypocalcaemia, if total Ca (corrected) <1.75 mmol/L, ionized Ca <0.8 mmol/L.

Causes

Neonatal

* Birth trauma, perinatal asphyxia.
* Prematurity.
* Respiratory distress syndrome.
* Infants of diabetic mothers.
* Iatrogenic: Sodium bicarbonate therapy; exchange transfusion; increased free fatty acids (intralipid).
* Congenital hypomagnesaemia with secondary hypocalcaemia.
* Transient neonatal hypoparathyroidism:
  * After operation or in severe infection.
  * Maternal hyperparathyroidism.
  * Maternal osteomalacia.
  * High phosphate intake (cow's milk formula).
  * Persistent idiopathic hypoparathyroidism.
  * Di George syndrome.
  * Intestinal malabsorption.

Older children

* Lack of PTH effect (hypoparathyroidism, pseudohypoparathyroidism).
* Vitamin D deficiency:
  * Nutritional rickets, malabsorption syndrome, chronic liver disease, anticonvulsants.
  * Renal rickets; AKI.
  * Vitamin D-dependent rickets/resistant rickets.
  * Nephrotic syndrome (increased loss of vitamin D with binding protein).
* Osteoblastic metastases.
* Hypomagnesaemia: Mg is required co-factor for PTH release from parathyroid gland.
* Hypercalciuria: usually compensated by increased Ca absorption in the gut, but will compound nutritional Ca/vitamin D deficiency.
* Hyperphosphataemia.
* Tumour lysis syndrome.
* Rhabdomyolysis.
* Acute pancreatitis.
* Hungry bones syndrome: healing of bones when there is an increased requirement for Ca, e.g. after initiation of vitamin D treatment in rickets.
* Activating mutations of the CaSR (autosomal dominant hypoparathyroidism).
* Drug induced: phosphate enemas/infusion, laxatives, calcitonin, colchicine, citrate, Ca-free albumin, furosemide, aminoglycosides.
* Alkalosis (leads to a decrease in ionized Ca).
* Massive blood transfusion (containing citrate).
* Acute leukaemia.

Clinical features

- *Neuromuscular*:
  - Paraesthesia and tetany.
  - Seizures.
  - Myopathy.
  - Psychosis.
  - Dementia.
  - Depression.
  - Laryngospasm (hypocalcaemic stridor).
  - Extrapyramidal disorders.
  - Chvostek sign (twitching of the facial muscles in response to gentle tapping over the facial nerve anterior to the earlobe).
  - Trousseau sign: carpal spasm following inflation of sphygmomanometer over upper arm above systolic BP.
- Skin and ectoderm:
  - Dry skin and eczema.
  - Hair loss, brittle nails, candidiasis.
  - Lenticular cataracts.
  - Tooth enamel hypoplasia.
- Hypotension, prolonged QT, heart block, ventricular arrhythmias, congestive cardiac failure (chronic hypocalcaemia).

Assessment

(See Fig. 6.7.)

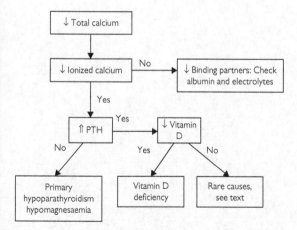

Fig. 6.7 An algorithm for the assessment of hypocalcaemia.

Treatment

Acute symptomatic hypocalcaemia

- 0.3 mL/kg 10% Ca gluconate IV over 10–30 min (monitor heart rate for bradycardia); can repeat until normal. Ensure good vascular access as extravasation causes severe skin injury.
- Correct hypomagnesaemia if present. 0.2 mL/kg of 50% magnesium sulfate IV over 30 min; repeat as necessary.
- Consider ongoing replacement therapy after the acute episode, e.g. maintenance infusion of 10% Ca gluconate (0.2–1 mmol/kg/day) or oral Ca supplements (50–75 mg/kg/day of elemental Ca in four doses).

Chronic hypocalcaemia

- In patients with CKD (➲ see Chapter 18).
- 1,25-dihydroxycholecalciferol (calcitriol) and l-α-hydroxycholecalciferol (alfacalcidol) are used to treat chronic hypocalcaemia resulting from hypoparathyroidism and pseudohypoparathyroidism. Aim to maintain the plasma Ca concentration in the low normal range and monitor Uca:Ucr (risk of hypercalciuria and nephrocalcinosis; ➲ see 'Renal calculi', p. 204 stones for normal ranges).
- *Calcitriol*: started at the initial oral dose of 15 ng/kg (maximum dose 1.5 microgram/day) usually in a split twice daily dose.
- *Alfacalcidol*: initial starting dose of 10–25 ng/kg/once daily (maximum dose usually 2 microgram/day). Alfacalcidol is usually administered as a single daily dose.

Disorders of magnesium: basic principles

* Mg is the second most abundant cation in the body, localized mainly in bone and intracellular compartments. Less than 1% is present in the ECF, of which ~30% is protein bound (mainly albumin) and 10% is complexed to other anions (e.g. bicarbonate, phosphate). The rest is in the biologically active, ionized form. Total Mg levels can be corrected for hypoalbuminaemia with the following formula:

$$\text{Corrected Mg(mmol/L)} = \text{total Mg (mmol/L)}$$
$$+ 0.005 \times (40 - \text{albumin(g/L)})$$

* 1 mmol/L of Mg is equivalent to 2.43 mg/dL.
* Functions of Mg include:
  * co-factor in many biological processes, including DNA synthesis and translation, provision of cellular fuel in the form of nucleotide triphosphates and metabolism of glucose, fatty acids, and protein
  * stabilization of cell membrane
  * intra- and intercellular signalling.
* Necessary co-factor for stimulation of CaSR.
* Magnesium is transported in gut and kidney using both passive (paracellular) and active (transcellular) pathways. A common component of the transcellular pathway in both gut and kidney is TRPM6 (➔ see also 'Disorders of renal magnesium handling', p. 187).

Disorders of magnesium: hypermagnesaemia

The kidneys can increase fractional Mg excretion to almost 100%, thus hypermagnesaemia is exceedingly rare without concomitant renal failure.

Definition

Plasma Mg >1.0 mmol/L.

Causes

- *Impaired renal excretion*: CKD; lithium.
- *Increased Mg uptake*: Mg infusions, use of Mg-containing antacids or laxatives.
- *Intracellular release*: cell necrosis.
- *Impaired regulation*: the CaSR is also important in the regulation of Mg and loss of function as in familial hypocalciuric hypercalcaemia (➜ see 'Disorders of calcium: hypercalcaemia', p. 138) is also associated with hypermagnesaemia.
- *Other*: hypothyroidism, Addison's disease.

Clinical features

Clinical symptoms are usually only seen if the plasma Mg exceeds 2.0 mmol/L. These can include:
- lethargy, drowsiness, nausea, flushing, loss of deep tendon reflexes
- ileus, urinary retention
- ECG changes (prolongation of PR and QT, widening of QRS) and arrhythmia
- coma, paralysis, apnoea if levels >5.0 mmol/L.

Investigations

- *History*: use of Mg-containing medications.
- U&Es and creatinine to assess kidney function.
- Urine Mg and creatinine to assess fractional excretion of Mg (expect >5% as appropriate renal response).

Disorders of magnesium: hypomagnesaemia

Definition

Plasma Mg <0.7 mmol/L.

Causes

Increased renal excretion

- *Inherited disorders*: ➔ see 'Disorders of renal magnesium handling', p. 192.
- *Acquired*:
  - *Tubular damage*: ATN, tubulointerstitial nephritis (TIN), postobstuctive.
  - *Drugs*: thiazides, tacrolimus, ciclosporin, loop diuretics, aminoglycosides, amphotericin, cisplatin, foscarnet, pentamidine.

Decreased intestinal absorption

- *Inherited disorders*: familial hypomagnesaemia with secondary hypocalcaemia (➔ see 'Disorders of renal magnesium handling', p. 192); primary intestinal hypomagnesaemia (Paunier disease).
- Malabsorption syndrome.
- Short bowel syndrome.
- Ileostomy.
- Coeliac disease.
- Inflammatory bowel disease.
- Prolonged diarrhoea and laxative use.

Decreased intake

- Prolonged vomiting or nasogastric suction.
- Malnutrition.
- Parenteral nutrition.

Endocrine causes

- Hypoparathyroidism.
- Hyperthyroidism.
- Infant of diabetic mother.
- Hyperaldosteronism.

Miscellaneous

- Hungry bone syndrome. Hypomagnesaemia can occur as a part of the 'hungry bone' syndrome in which there is increased uptake of Mg (and Ca) into bones as a result of bone healing, e.g. following parathyroidectomy or treatment of rickets with vitamin D.
- Hypercalcaemia.
- Phosphate depletion.
- Volume expansion (mild hypomagnesaemia).
- Intrauterine growth retardation (first 3–5 days of life).

Clinical features

Hypomagnesaemia is usually asymptomatic, unless plasma levels are severely depressed (<0.5 mmol/L):
- Weakness, tremor, tetany, and seizures.
- Positive Chvostek and Trousseau signs.
- ECG changes, ventricular arrhythmias (torsade de pointes).
- Hypokalaemia. This can be due to the same underlying aetiology, e.g. Gitelman syndrome, ➔ see Chapter 7). However, Mg is an intracellular blocker of ROMK and thus can exacerbate hypokalaemia.
- *Hypocalcaemia*: Mg is a required co-factor for PTH release.

Investigations

- History (drugs, kidney disease, family history).
- U&Es with urine Mg, Ca, creatinine. In the presence of hypomagnesaemia, a fractional excretion of Mg (FEMg) >4% is consistent with renal Mg wasting. However, with severely decreased plasma levels and thus decreased filtered load of Mg, the FEMg may well be <4% in renal Mg wasting disorders. In those cases, normalization of plasma levels with IV infusion of Mg may be necessary to establish aetiology.

Treatment

- *Acute symptomatic hypomagnesaemia*: 0.1–0.2 mmol/kg of 10% magnesium sulfate (i.e. 0.25–0.5 mL/kg) IV over 30 min; repeat as necessary. Consider ongoing replacement.
- *Chronic asymptomatic hypomagnesaemia*: oral Mg (e.g. Mg glycerophosphate) 0.2 mmol/kg/day three times daily. In renal Mg wasting, it is usually impossible to achieve normal plasma levels and excessive oral supplementation may cause diarrhoea, and thus worsen hypomagnesaemia. Levels >0.5 mmol/kg are usually acceptable. In patients with impaired intestinal absorption, intermittent IV supplementation may need to be considered.

Disorders of phosphate: basic principles

- Each mmol/L of phosphate is equivalent to 3.097 mg/dL.
- Phosphate is the most abundant anion in the body, mostly stored in bones and teeth.
- Less than 0.1% of total body phosphate is in plasma, where we measure it.
- Phosphate levels vary with age and are highest in the neonate (➔ see Chapter 18).
- Functions of phosphate include:
  - energy storage (ATP)
  - component of lipids (phospholipids) and nucleic acids
  - signalling (protein phosphorylation)
  - acid–base buffering.
- Key organs involved in phosphate homoeostasis are:
  - *gut (absorption), mostly duodenum and jejunum*: active (transcellular) and passive (paracellular) transport. Active transport is regulated by vitamin D, similar to Ca
  - *bone (storage)*: phosphate can be stored in (stimulated by vitamin D) or released from bone (stimulated by PTH), similar to Ca
  - *kidney (excretion)*: under normal circumstances, >80% of filtered phosphate is actively reabsorbed in the proximal tubule by Na/phosphate co-transporters (NaPi) under control of PTH
  - *parathyroid glands (regulation)*: the parathyroid glands produce the key regulatory hormone PTH, which mobilizes Ca phosphate from bone and enhances renal phosphate excretion.
- A key regulatory factor for phosphate excretion is fibroblast growth factor (FGF23). Other important factors, such as PHEX and Klotho, likely work through FGF23 (➔ see Chapter 18).

Disorders of phosphate: hyperphosphataemia

Definition

Plasma phosphate level above the age-appropriate upper limit of normal (2.1 mmol/L in infants, decreasing to 1.4 mmol/L in adults (➔ see Chapter 18).

Causes

Decreased renal excretion

* Renal impairment: hyperphosphataemia most commonly occurs with decreased GFR.
* Hypoparathyroidism.
* Pseudohypoparathyroidism.
* Nephrotic syndrome.

Intracellular release

* Tumour lysis, rhabdomyolysis.
* Acidosis.

Increased absorption

* Phosphate enemas.

Endocrine causes

* Thyrotoxicosis.
* Acromegaly.
* Glucocorticoid deficiency.
* Artefactual in vitro haemolysis.

Clinical features

* No specific symptoms, unless accompanying hypocalcaemia.
* Chronic hyperphosphataemia may induce ectopic calcifications, including in blood vessels.

Investigations

* Plasma: U&Es and creatinine, including Ca, albumin, ALP, PTH.
* Lactate dehydrogenase (LDH), uric acid, creatine kinase (CK) in suspected rhabdomyolysis or tumour lysis.
* Urine: phosphate and creatinine to calculate tubular reabsorption of phosphate (TRP) = (1 − (urine phosphate/urine creatinine) × (plasma creatinine/plasma phosphate)) × 100. TRP is expected to be <70% as evidence for appropriately increased renal excretion.

Management

* In CKD: ➔ see Chapter 18.
* In acute tumour/rhabdomyolysis: saline infusion can enhance renal phosphate excretion with an intact GFR. With a decreased GFR, consider haemodialysis.

Disorders of phosphate: hypophosphataemia

Definition

Plasma phosphate level below the age-appropriate lower limit of normal (1.2 mmol/L in infants, decreasing to 0.8 mmol/L in adults).

Causes

Increased renal excretion
- Hyperparathyroidism.
- Vitamin D deficiency.
- *Renal tubular dysfunction*: renal Fanconi syndrome, TIN.
- *Increased phosphaturic factors*: hypophosphataemic rickets, post-renal transplantation, tumour related.

Increased intracellular uptake
- Refeeding syndrome (insulin release with feeding of malnourished patients results in intracellular uptake of glucose and phosphate).
- Treatment of diabetic ketoacidosis.
- Alkalosis.

Decreased absorption
- Vitamin D deficiency.
- Malabsorption.
- Phosphate-binding antacids.

Endocrine causes
Glucocorticoid excess.

Clinical features

- No specific symptoms acutely, although severe hypophosphataemia (<0.5 mmol/L) may be associated with signs of decreased energy (ATP) availability, including weakness, lethargy, and paraesthesia.
- Long-standing hypophosphataemia will result in rickets.

Investigations

- *Plasma*: U&Es and creatinine, including Ca, albumin, ALP, and PTH.
- *Urine*:
  - *Phosphate and creatinine to calculate TRP*: 1 − (urine phosphate/urine creatinine)/(plasma phosphate/plasma creatinine). TRP is expected to be >80% as evidence for appropriately increased renal excretion.
  - *Note*: with severely decreased plasma phosphate and/or GFR, the filtered load may be so low that TRP is within the reference range. A better way is to calculate the threshold for tubular maximum reabsorption of phosphate (TmP) per GFR: plasma phosphate − ((urine phosphate/urine creatinine) × plasma creatinine).
- Skeletal X-ray in case of suspected rickets.

Management

Depends on the underlying cause:
* Ensure sufficient phosphate supplementation in cases of increased intracellular uptake.
* Normalize PTH by vitamin D supplementation in cases of rickets.
* With a fixed renal leak (e.g. hypophosphataemic rickets), persistent normalization of plasma phosphate is virtually impossible and phosphate supplementation is limited by side effects such as diarrhoea. Treatment should aim to minimize the associated rickets by vitamin D supplementation.

Disorders of acid–base balance: basic principles

The pH of plasma is tightly calibrated around 7.4 to enable optimal function of most enzymes in our body. This occurs mainly through regulation of bicarbonate (HCO_3^-) and CO_2 concentrations, which are related via the following equations:

Equation 1: $H_2O + CO_2 \leftrightarrow H_2CO_3 \leftrightarrow HCO_3^- + H^+$

Equation 2 (Henderson – Hasselbalch):
$pH = pKa + \log \left(HCO_3^- / CO_2 \right)$

CO_2 is regulated by the lungs and bicarbonate by the kidneys (directly via reabsorption and indirectly via excretion of H^+). Therefore, we separate respiratory (ventilation of CO_2) from metabolic disorders (excretion of bicarbonate or H^+), but the two processes can occur simultaneously (mixed acid–base disorders). The individual contributions can be assessed by plotting pH, CO_2, and bicarbonate on a nomogram (see Fig. 6.8).

- Bicarbonate concentration on a blood gas analysis is calculated, not measured. For most accurate assessment, bicarbonate concentration is best measured in plasma.
- Steady-state pH homeostasis is maintained in the kidney by excreting acid in the urine equivalent to the acid load.
- Acid load consists mainly of sulphur-containing amino acids in the diet (methionine, cystine), which are metabolized to sulphuric acid. Animal proteins contain a higher amount of sulphur amino acids compared with plant proteins. Conversely, plant protein contains a higher amount of basic amino acids (lysine, arginine), thus vegetarians have a lower acid load than the average Western diet which is high in animal protein.

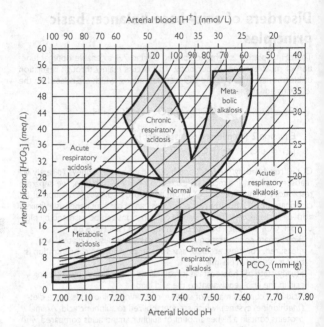

Fig. 6.8 A nomogram for the assessment of mixed acid–base disorders.
Source: data from Cogan, MG (ed.) (1992). *Fluid and Electrolytes: Physiology and Pathophysiology*. Stamford, UK: Appleton & Lange. Copyright © 1992 Appleton & Lange.

Disorders of acid–base balance: acidosis

Definition

A disorder leading to increased acidity. Because of buffering ability, plasma pH can remain normal and the acidosis manifests only in a decreased plasma bicarbonate concentration. A fall of plasma pH to <7.35 is referred to as acidaemia.

- The anion gap (AG) is a useful tool to assess whether a metabolic acidosis is due to loss of bicarbonate (most common) or accumulation of acid. It is calculated by subtracting the two main plasma anions from the main cation:

$$\text{Equation 3}: \text{AG} = \left[Na^+\right] - \left\{\left[Cl^-\right] + \left[HCO_3^-\right]\right\}$$

- A normal value for the AG is between 8 and 12. This represents the unmeasured anions, which consist mostly of proteins, such as albumin, which have an excess of negative charges. Thus, in hypoproteinaemic states, such as nephrotic syndrome, the usual normal values for AG are decreased (AG decreases roughly by 2.5 for each 10 g/L of serum albumin below 40 g/L).
- *Normal AG acidosis (bicarbonate loss)*: bicarbonate is lost in either the GI tract (e.g. diarrhoea) or the urine together with a cation, mostly Na, to maintain electroneutrality. Because of this concurrent loss of Na and bicarbonate, the AG is unchanged.
- *Increased AG acidosis*: excess accumulation of acid (e.g. lactic acid or ketones) leads to a decrease in bicarbonate (to buffer the acid) without changing Na^+ or CL^- concentration, therefore increasing the AG.
- Causes of AG acidosis are often memorized with the mnemonic MUDPILES:
  - M = metabolic disease, metformin
  - U = uraemia
  - D = diabetic ketoacidosis
  - P = paraldehyde, propylene glycol, phenformin
  - I = isoniazid, iron
  - L = lactic acidosis
  - E = ethanol, ethylene glycol
  - S = starvation, salicylates.
- A common and misleading cause of low plasma bicarbonate is exposure of blood sample to air, for instance, when it is obtained by fingerprick.
  - Example: CO_2 diffuses immediately into the air, shifting the equilibrium described in equation 1 to the left, leading to a decrease in both bicarbonate and H^+ concentration. Thus, if both a blood gas and bicarbonate are determined, this falsely low bicarbonate concentration is recognized by the simultaneous presence of elevated pH (low H^+ concentration). However, if only bicarbonate was determined in the context of an electrolyte panel, a low bicarbonate concentration with increased AG (Na and Cl^- concentrations are unaffected by CO_2 diffusion) in the absence of an obvious cause (MUDPILES), should raise suspicion of this artefact.

- It is important, that blood samples for pH and bicarbonate are analysed promptly, as they otherwise decrease due to ongoing metabolic activity of the blood cells.
- Similar problems occur in the assessment of urine pH, as exposure of the sample to air can artificially increase urine pH, so a pragmatic solution is to determine pH by urine dipstick analysis immediately after obtaining the sample. Ideally, urine is collected under oil for subsequent proper lab analysis. In clinical practice, this is difficult, especially with non-toilet-trained children. Samples obtained by urine bag or cotton balls in the nappy are unreliable for pH determination.

Diagnosis

A diagnostic algorithm for the assessment of a metabolic acidosis is shown in Fig. 6.9, based on the key diagnostic information provided by history, and plasma and urine biochemistry

Treatment

- Diagnose and treat underlying cause (e.g. give oxygen, correct shock with volume replacement, treat sepsis) and avoid lactate-containing replacement fluids.
- Role of acute alkali replacement is controversial—potential harmful effects include:
  - worsening of intracellular acidosis despite improvement of extracellular acidosis due to diffusion of CO_2 into cells (bicarbonate administration shifts the equilibrium in equation 1 to the left with increased formation of CO_2, which is membrane permeable)
  - volume overload
  - hypernatraemia
  - hypercapnia (especially in patients with respiratory insufficiency).
- In acidosis, due to chronic bicarbonate loss (e.g. CKD, renal Fanconi syndrome, chronic diarrhoea, GI stoma), bicarbonate obviously needs to be replaced (➲ see also 'Distal renal tubular acidosis', p. 158).

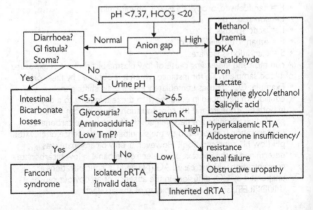

Fig. 6.9 A diagnostic algorithm for the diagnosis of renal tubular acidosis.

- In cases of severe intractable acidosis, dialysis or haemofiltration may be indicated.

Clinical features

- Failure to thrive, vomiting, anorexia, and variable degrees of muscle weakness are common to all subtypes of RTA.
- Since bone is a major buffer of acid, chronic metabolic acidosis (from any cause) can have a major impact on the developing skeleton, and poor growth is an important consequence of acidosis. Correction of the acidosis is thus important to restore growth.
- Buffering of acid by the bone leaches Ca from the bone, which needs to be excreted by the kidney with consequent nephrocalcinosis and possibly stones.
- Signs of renal Fanconi syndrome (polyuria, polydipsia, dehydration, rickets, glycosuria, hypophosphataemia, aminoaciduria) in proximal RTA.
- Some forms of distal RTA are associated with sensorineural deafness.

Renal tubular acidosis

Historically, RTA has been classified into four subtypes, numbered according to the chronological sequence of the descriptions:

- Classical (hypokalaemic) distal RTA.
- Proximal RTA (pRTA).
- Mixed proximal distal RTA.
- Hyperkalaemic RTA.

For practical purposes, we will only separate proximal from distal RTA, as the mixed form is extremely rare and easily recognizable due to its association with osteopetrosis (see Table 6.3); hyperkalaemic RTA is primarily a disorder of distal salt reabsorption with secondary acidosis.

Table 6.3 Recognized genetic causes of primary renal tubular acidosis

Gene	Function	Inheritance	Type	Extrarenal manifestation
SLC4A4 (NBC1)	Basolateral Na⁻ bicarbonate cotransporter	AR	Proximal	Eye and teeth abnormalities, short stature, developmental delay
CA2	Carbonic anhydrase	AR	Mixed	Osteopetrosis
SLC4A1 (AE1)	Basolateral Cl⁻ bicarbonate exchanger	AD or AR	Distal	Ovalocytosis (in some)
ATP6V1B1	Apical proton pump subunit	AR	Distal	Sensorineural deafness (infantile onset)
ATP6V0A4	Apical proton pump subunit	AR	Distal	Sensorineural deafness (in some)
FOXI1	transcription factor	AR	Distal	Sensorineural deafness

AD, autosomal dominant; AR, autosomal recessive.

Proximal renal tubular acidosis

pRTA is caused by an impaired ability to reabsorb bicarbonate in the proximal tubule, resulting in urinary bicarbonate wasting. Isolated proximal bicarbonate wasting is extremely rare (see Table 6.3). Instead, pRTA occurs in the context of generalized proximal tubular dysfunction, also called renal Fanconi syndrome, characterized by glycosuria, phosphaturia, amino aciduria, organic aciduria, and low-molecular-weight proteinuria. The consequent biochemical abnormalities (see also Table 6.3 and Fig. 6.9) establish the diagnosis of pRTA. Because distal urinary acidification is intact, urinary pH can be <5.5.

Distal renal tubular acidosis

This form of RTA is caused by an impaired ability to secrete protons in the collecting duct. As can be seen in Fig. 6.10, Na (and thus volume), K, and acid–base homoeostasis are linked together: Na is reabsorbed in the collecting duct in exchange for either protons or K to maintain electroneutrality. Thus, with proton secretion impaired in distal RTA (dRTA), more K needs to be secreted to allow a similar amount of Na reabsorption, resulting in hypokalaemia. In dRTA, urine pH is always >5.5, because of the impaired distal acidification.

dRTA may develop as a secondary complication of other diseases:

* Disorders affecting salt reabsorption in the collecting duct (➔ see Chapter 7). Because salt reabsorption through the epithelial Na channel ENaC (see Fig. 6.10) provides the favourable electrical gradient for proton and K secretion, impairment of this pathway results in hyperkalaemic acidosis (type 4 RTA).
* CKD (➔ see Chapter 18).
* Autoimmune diseases.
* Toxins/drugs involving the distal tubule and collecting duct.

Genetics of renal tubular acidosis

For pRTA, ➔ see also 'Disorders presenting with hypokalaemic acidosis: proximal tubule', p. 166.

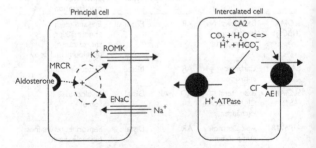

Fig. 6.10 The molecular basis of dRTA showing a principal cell and an intercalated cell. Salt reabsorption via the epithelial Na channel ENaC in the principal cell creates a favourable electrical gradient for proton secretion from the intercalated cell via the H-ATPase. Protons are generated by the action of the carbonic anhydrase 2 (CA2) and the remaining bicarbonate re-enters the bloodstream via the basolateral anion exchanger AE1.

Treatment of dRTA

Despite the often severe symptoms at presentation, the acidosis of dRTA is easily treatable:

- Correction of the acidosis allows normal growth and development and prevents worsening of the nephrocalcinosis, but does not correct extrarenal manifestations, such as deafness.
- Treatment consists of administration of alkali, equal in amount to the acid load (usually 1–3 mmol/kg/day), such as bicarbonate or citrate, ideally as K salt or mixed K/Na salt (e.g. Polycitra® or tricitrate). This allows supplementation of both alkali and K.
- Citrate may also alleviate the nephrocalcinosis.
- 1 mmol of citrate is converted in the liver to 2 mmol of bicarbonate, thus half the amount of citrate is necessary for correction of alkalosis compared with bicarbonate.
- Patients with dRTA need to have regular clinical and biochemical monitoring for adjustment of their supplementation. In the beginning, more frequent visits are necessary; once established, longer intervals (every 6 months) are usually sufficient.
- Plasma pH and bicarbonate can vary quickly, e.g. depending on the time of the last dosage.
- Urinary Ca, as a reflection of acid-buffering by the bone, may be a good long-term indicator of acidosis control.

Disorders of acid–base balance: alkalosis

Definition

* A primary elevation of plasma bicarbonate (>28 mmol/L) with a rise in arterial pH (>7.40).
* Note: normal range for bicarbonate is lower in infants.

Causes

As seen in Fig. 6.10, Na reabsorption in the collecting duct (under the control of aldosterone) is molecularly linked with K and acid–base homoeostasis. To maintain electroneutrality, Na is reabsorbed in exchange for K or protons. Thus, with enhanced distal Na reabsorption there will be increased K and proton secretion, resulting in a hypokalaemic metabolic alkalosis, the classical electrolyte pattern seen with aldosterone activation.

There are many potential causes for enhanced distal Na reabsorption:

* With volume contraction:
  * GI losses, including laxative use and congenital Cl⁻-losing diarrhoea.
  * Loop diuretics and thiazides.
  * Bartter and Gitelman syndromes.
  * Cystic fibrosis due to excess of chloride loss in the sweat.
* With excess volume:
  * Renal artery stenosis.
  * Mineralocorticoid excess (e.g. Conn syndrome).
  * Pseudo-mineralocorticoid excess (liquorice, Liddle syndrome, 11-beta-hydroxysteroid dehydrogenase deficiency; high dose glucocorticoids).
* Acid loss (usually from the stomach—if losses of fluid are not replaced, alkalosis will be further compounded by aldosterone activation):
  * Vomiting, e.g. pyloric stenosis.
  * Gastric suction.
  * Excess alkali administration.

Tubular disorders

Tubulopathies: basic principles

* A key task of the tubules is to reabsorb filtered sodium (Na). The adult kidneys filter on average ~150 L of plasma per day containing 22.5 mol of Na, the equivalent of roughly 1.25 kg of salt (NaCl). Since Na constitutes the major ion in ECF, Na homoeostasis determines volume homoeostasis and all recognized inherited causes of long-term BP dysregulation affect renal Na handling.
* Disorders in Na handling affect BP: Na-losing disorders lead to lowered BP and, conversely, disorders of increased Na reabsorption lead to increased BP.
* The kidneys have no sensor for Na concentration. This is regulated by osmoreceptors in the brain via ADH and renal water handling. Thus, disorders of renal salt handling typically have normal plasma Na concentrations.
* Usually, >99% of filtered Na is reabsorbed, so that the final excretion is <1% and equivalent to salt intake (1–10 g, depending on diet). ~80% of salt reabsorption occurs in the proximal tubule (PT), 10–15% in the thick ascending limb of Henle's loop (TAL), 5–10% in the distal convoluted tubule (DCT), and the remaining 1–5% in the collecting duct (CD) (see Fig. 7.1). The driving force is created by the basolateral Na^+/K^+-ATPase, present in all cells, which generates a favourable electrochemical gradient for Na entry into the cell. This gradient also enables co-transport of other substances (such as glucose, amino acids, and phosphate (PO_4)) into the cell or counter-transport (such as Na–hydrogen (H) exchange).
* Since Na is the main determinant of intravascular volume, fractional excretion of Na is normal in almost all renal salt-wasting disorders (<1%). This is due to activation of compensatory mechanisms, such as up-regulation of the renin–angiotensin axis (hyperaldosteronism), which enhances distal Na reabsorption in exchange for K and protons. However, if this compensatory mechanism is impaired, as in pseudohypoaldosteronism (PHA) type 1, fractional excretion of Na is elevated and the disorder is life-threatening because of progressive volume depletion.
* An overview of clinical and molecular features of inherited disorders of renal salt handling is given in Table 7.1.
* Most disorders affecting the PT cause global PT dysfunction with wasting of all substances usually reabsorbed in the PT, i.e. a renal Fanconi syndrome. Some disorders affect predominantly isolated PT reabsorption pathways, such as Lowe syndrome and Dent disease, which present mainly with low-molecular-weight proteinuria (LMWP) and hypercalciuria.
* Many of the renal salt-wasting disorders also affect renal handling of water, Ca, and Mg.
* There are also isolated disorders of renal water handling which typically present with either hyper- or hyponatraemia.
* Isolated disorders of renal Mg handling (Mg wasting) typically present with hypomagnesaemia.

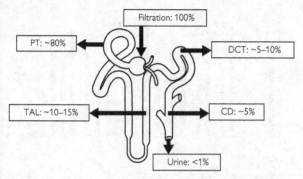

Fig. 7.1 Na reabsorption along the nephron. CD, collecting duct; DCT, distal convoluted tubule; PT, proximal tubule; TAL, thick ascending limb of Henle's loop.

Table 7.1 Clinical and molecular characteristics of renal salt-handling disorders*

Disorder	OMIM	Gene	Mode	Protein	Renin	Aldo	K+	Cl-	HCO3-	Other features/comments
Renal Fanconi	*	*	*	*			↓	↑	↓	*
Type I Bartter	601678	SLC12A1	AR	NKCC2 co-transporter (furosemide-sensitive)	↑	↑	↓	↓	↑	Nephrocalcinosis, often pre- or neonatal onset
Type II Bartter	241200	KCNJ1	AR	K channel ROMK	↑	↑	↓	↓	↑	Nephrocalcinosis, often pre- or neonatal onset
Type III Bartter	607364	CLCNKB	AR	Cl channel CLCKNB	↑	↑	↓	↓	↑	Often hypomagnesaemia Mostly childhood onset
Type IV Bartter	602522	BSND	AR	Bartin	↑	↑	↓	↓	↑	Often hypomagnesaemia deafness. Usually neonatal onset
Type V Bartter	300971	MAGED2	XR	MAGED2	↑	↓				
Gitelman syndrome	263800	SLC12A3	AR	NCC (thiazide-sensitive)	↑	↑	↓	↓	↑	Hypomagnesaemia, hypocalciuria Mostly childhood onset
EAST / SeSAME syndrome	612782	KCNJ10	AR	KCNJ10/Kir4.1	↑	↑	↓	↓	↑	Epilepsy, ataxia, sensorineural deafness, tubulopathy with hypomagnesaemia, hypocalciuria
CAH type I	201910	CYP21A2	AR	21-hydroxylase	↑	↓			↓	Virilization

Disorder	OMIM	Gene	Inheritance	Protein				Notes
CAH type II	201810	HSD3B2	AR	3-B-hydroxysteroid dehydrogenase	↑	↑	↑	Hypospadias, male pseudohermaphroditism
PHA1	264350	SCNN1A, SCNN1B, SCNN1G	AR, AR, AR	EnaC sodium channel subunits A,B,G	↑	↑	↑	Symptoms are severe in recessive form, milder in dominant form
	177735	NR3C2	AD	Mineralocorticoid receptor		↑	↑	
PHA2	614492, 614491, 614496, 614495	WNK1, WNK4, CUL3, KLHL3	AD, AD, AD, AD, AR	WNK-kinases, Ubiquitin E3 ligase components	→	↑	↑	
Liddle syndrome	177200	SCNN1B, SCNN1G	AD, AD	EnaC sodium channel subunits B,G	→	↓	↓	
AME	218030	HSD11B2	AR	11-B-hydroxysteroid dehydrogenase	→	↓	↑	Intrauterine growth retardation
GRA	103900	CYP11B1	AD	11-B-hydroxylase	↓	↓	↑	
CAH type IV	202010	CYP11B1	AR	11-B-hydroxylase	↓	↑	↑	Virilization
CAH type V	202110	CYP17A1	AR	17-alpha-hydroxylase	→	↑	↑	Ambiguous genitalia

Listed are disorders of tubular salt handling. The upper 11 rows list disorders of salt wasting (hypovolaemia/low BP), whereas the lower 6 rows list disorders of salt retention (hypervolaemia/hypertension). Aldo, aldosterone. AME, apparent mineralocorticoid excess; AR, autosomal recessive, AD, autosomal dominant, XR, X-linked recessive.

* For details of disorders in the PT, ⊙ see "Disorders presenting with hypokalaemic acidosis: proximal tubule p. 166".

Disorders presenting with hypokalaemic acidosis: proximal tubule

- Hypokalaemic acidosis as a presenting feature of disorders affecting salt reabsorption in the PT (proximal renal tubular acidosis (RTA)) are usually associated with other abnormalities, such as hypophosphataemia, reflecting a more generalized dysfunction of the PT.
- Isolated proximal RTA is only seen in the very rare AR disorder 'proximal RTA with ocular abnormalities' due to mutations in *SLC4A4*, encoding a basolateral sodiumbicarbonate transporter in the PT. Associated eye abnormalities provide the clue to this diagnosis and include band keratopathy, cataract, and glaucoma. Mental impairment and tooth enamel defects are also common features of this disorder.
  - There is also a mixed proximal/distal form due to mutations in *CA2*, encoding the carbonic anhydrase expressed in proximal and distal tubule (➔ see table 6.3, p. 157). This disorder is associated with osteopetrosis.
- Hypokalaemia is due to impaired K reabsorption in the PT and the secondary hyperaldosteronism from salt losses.
- Acidosis is due to the molecular coupling of Na and bicarbonate reabsorption in the PT.
- Renal Fanconi syndrome is a collective term used for dysfunction of the PT, of which there are many causes, both congenital and acquired.
- Substances reabsorbed by the PT include water, Na, K, Ca, PO_4, bicarbonate (proximal RTA in children is almost always associated with a renal Fanconi syndrome), urate, glucose, amino acids, and low-molecular-weight proteins.
- In classical renal Fanconi syndrome, all of these substances are wasted, while in some disorders, such as Lowe syndrome (➔ see 'Lowe syndrome') and Dent disease ((➔ see 'Dent disease') only selective proximal reabsorption pathways are affected. Causes of renal Fanconi syndrome are listed in Table 7.2.

Presentation

- Presentation in the first year of life is usually with non-specific symptoms, such as irritability, poor feeding, vomiting, and failure to thrive, as the classical symptoms of polydipsia and polyuria can be difficult to detect at this age.
- Polydipsia and polyuria are the classical symptoms. However, most children with histories of 'always being thirsty' do not have a tubular disorder—on the whole, this is a behavioural phenotype of young children. It is useful to ask whether the child would still drink excessively if only water is offered, and in the older child, whether they wake at night for a drink.
- The selective proximal tubular dysfunction seen in Dent disease usually does not result in failure to thrive and polyuria. Therefore, presentation is typically in later child- or adulthood with rickets and/or stones.
- Clinical signs of rickets.
- Poor growth.

- Constipation due to dehydration.
- Nephrocalcinosis/stones (especially Dent disease).
- Extrarenal manifestations, such as cataracts, cryptorchidism, and developmental delay (Lowe syndrome), or photophobia (from corneal crystals (cystinosis).

Investigations

- *Plasma*: Na, K, bicarbonate, chloride (Cl), Ca, PO_4, urate, pH, creatinine, urea, ALP, and PTH. The typical constellation of results is listed in Table 7.3. PTH and ALP may be elevated secondary to urinary Ca/vitamin D loss or CKD.
- *Urine*: Na, K, Cl, Ca, PO_4, urate, pH, glucose, amino acids, low-molecular-weight proteins (e.g. retinol-binding protein (RBP), beta-2-microglobulin).
- *Fractional excretion of Na*: usually normal (<1%), because of the importance for volume homoeostasis and compensation from more distal Na transporters. Fractional excretion of K is usually elevated (>15%), as is that of Ca (>1%) and PO_4 (>20%). In cases of very low plasma PO_4 and thus low amounts of filtered PO_4, the tubular reabsorption of PO_4 may be falsely normal. Calculation of the transport maximum for PO_4 (TmP/GFR) is more accurate to determine renal PO_4 wasting (see 'Disorders of phosphate: hypophosphataemia', p. 151).
- The most sensitive indicator for proximal tubular dysfunction is LMWP, such as RBP or beta-2-microglobulin.
- US for renal size and echogenicity, and to look for the presence of nephrocalcinosis, which may be present due to hypercalciuria.
- Bone X-rays for changes of rickets.
- White cell cystine and formal ophthalmology review (for corneal cystine crystals) for all cases of suspected renal Fanconi syndrome as cystinosis is the commonest cause (see 'Cystinosis', p. 302).

Treatment

- Treatment should target the underlying problem, if possible (see Table 7.2 for differential diagnosis).
- Replacement of electrolyte losses orally. It can be very difficult to replace these adequately, and very large doses of Na, Cl, K, PO_4, and bicarbonate may be required. IV rehydration with normal saline and added electrolytes (e.g. K, PO_4, etc.) is often needed, both at diagnosis and during intercurrent illness to correct biochemical disturbance. Normalization of plasma bicarbonate is usually not achievable in proximal RTA with ocular abnormalities sue to the enormous renal bicarbonate losses.
- Activated vitamin D (alfacalcidol, or calcitriol if liver dysfunction).
- Free access to water.

Acquired causes of renal Fanconi syndrome

Drugs/toxins

- Aminoglycosides.
- Ifosfamide.
- Outdated tetracyclines.
- Sodium valproate.

Table 7.2 Genetic causes of renal Fanconi syndrome

Onset	Disorder	Gene	Features	Diagnostic test
Neonatal	Galactosaemia	GALT	Liver dysfunction, encephalopathy, sepsis	Red cell galactose-1-phophate uridyl transferase
	Mitochondrial cytopathy	Various mitochondrial and nuclear genes	Multisystemic: 'illegitimate associations'	Mitochondrial DNA (blood); muscle enzymology
	Tyrosinaemia	FAH	Poor growth, hepatomegaly, and hepatic dysfunction	Plasma amino acids, urine organic acids (succinyl acetone)
Infancy	Fructosaemia	ALDOB	Rapid onset after fructose given—vomiting, hypoglycaemia, hepatomegaly	Hepatic fructose-1-phosphate aldolase B
	Cystinosis	CTNS	Poor growth, rickets, corneal cystine crystals	White cell cystine; mutational analysis
	Fanconi–Bickel syndrome	GLUT2	Failure to thrive, hepatomegaly, hypoglycaemia, rickets, severe glycosuria, galactosuria	Mutational analysis
	Lowe syndrome	OCRL	Males (X-linked), cataracts, hypotonia, developmental delay	Mutational analysis
Childhood	Cystinosis	CTNS	As cystinosis in infancy	As cystinosis in infancy
	Dent disease	CLCN5	Males (X-linked), nephrocalcinosis, hypercalciuria	Molecular diagnosis
	Wilson disease	ATP7B	Hepatic and neurological disease, Kayser–Fleischer rings	Plasma copper, caeruloplasmin

Source: data from Webb, N.J.A. and Postlethwaite, R.J. (Eds). (1994) *Clinical Paediatric Nephrology*, 2nd Ed. Oxford, UK: OUP. Copyright © 1994 OUP.

Table 7.3 Typical constellation of biochemistries in proximal tubular dysfunction

Parameter	Renal Fanconi syndrome	Lowe syndrome	Dent disease
Plasma			
Na	↔	↔	↔
K	↓	↓↔	↔
Cl	↑	↑↔	↔
HCO₃	↓	↓↔	↔↓
PO₄	↓	↓↔	↔↓
Urine			
TmP/GFR	↓	↓↔	↔↓
Ca/Cr	↑	↑	↑
FEK	↑	↑↔	↔
LMWP	↑↑↑	↑↑↑	↑↑↑
Glucose	↑	↑↔	↔

FEK, fractional excretion of potassium; LMWP, Low-molecular-weight proteinuria.

- 6-mercaptopurine.
- Heavy metal poisoning.
- Toluene.
- Paraquat.

Renal causes
- Post renal transplant (ischaemic damage).
- Recovery phase of acute tubular necrosis.
- Tubulointerstitial nephritis.
- Nephrotic syndrome (FSGS).

Fig. 7.2 represents an epithelial cell in the PT. Na is reabsorbed either in exchange with substances that need to be secreted (such as protons via the Na–H exchanger (NHE3)) or in co-transport with substances that need to be reabsorbed (such as PO₄ or glucose). The epithelial cells in the PT all express the water channel AQP1, so that solutes are reabsorbed isotonically with water.

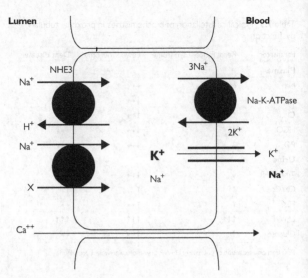

Fig. 7.2 Diagram of a PT cell.

Further reading

Klootwijk E, Dufek S, Issler N, et al. Pathophysiology, current treatments and future targets in heredi-tary forms of renal Fanconi syndrome. *Expert Opin Orphan Drugs* 2017;5:45–54.

Lowe syndrome and Dent disease

Lowe syndrome and Dent disease are X-linked disorders with a proximal tubulopathy.

Lowe syndrome

- *Clinical features*: the oculocerebrorenal syndrome of Lowe is defined by the triad of congenital cataracts and/or glaucoma, mental impairment, and a proximal tubulopathy.
- *Eyes*: patients are typically recognized in the neonatal period due to congenital cataracts. Glaucoma is another common feature. Severity can vary widely and patients without apparent eye abnormalities have been described.
- *Brain*: muscular hypotonia and hyporeflexia are typically the first recognized neurological symptoms. If measured, IQ is typically ~50, although 25% of patients have an IQ >70, indicating again a spectrum of severity. Seizures occur in about a third of patients. Most challenging for the families are typically the behavioural abnormalities, including repetitive and obsessive behaviour with temper tantrums, as well as auto-aggression.
- *Kidney*: a proximal tubulopathy predominated by LMWP and hypercalciuria is the key kidney manifestation. PO_4 and bicarbonate wasting is commonly seen. Urolithiasis is a less common complication. Untreated, rickets can develop. Patients typically have a slow progression of CKD with ESKD towards the fourth decade of life.
- *Other*: elevated muscle enzymes (CK, LDH) are typically seen. A debilitating arthropathy can develop in older patients.
- *Genetics*: virtually all patients have mutations in the underlying gene, *OCRL*.
- *Treatment*: treatment of the renal manifestations is supportive, typically involving supplementation with alfacalcidol or calcitriol, citrate and/or bicarbonate, and PO_4 if needed.

Dent disease

- *Clinical features*: Dent disease is a proximal tubulopathy, predominated by LMWP and hypercalciuria with nephrocalcinosis and stones. In addition, most patients have progressive CKD with ESKD in the fourth to fifth decades of life.
- *Genetics*: ~60% of patients have mutations in *CLCN5*, and ~15% in *OCRL*, the gene underlying Lowe syndrome. In the remaining patients, no causative mutations have so far been identified, suggesting further genetic causes. Why mutations in *OCRL* cause a kidney-specific disorder (Dent disease) in some patients and a multiorgan disorder in others is unclear, but observations suggest that mutations in *OCRL* are associated with a spectrum of clinical manifestations that always include a proximal tubulopathy plus other organ involvement in variable severity.
- *Treatment*: supportive. Citrate may reduce the risk of stone formation and thiazides can reduce calcium excretion at least in the short term. Whether this is associated with reduced stone formation is unclear.

Further reading

Bökenkamp A, Ludwig M. The oculocerebrorenal syndrome of Lowe: an update. *Pediatr Nephrol* 2016;31:2201–2212.

Disorders presenting with hypokalaemic acidosis: collecting duct

- Hypokalaemic acidosis is the typical presentation of distal RTA, i.e. of impaired acid secretion in the CD (➔ see Fig. 6.10, p. 158).
- Currently, four genes are recognized to cause inherited distal RTA (➔ see Table 6.3, p. 157).
- As untreated acidosis is buffered by the bones with consequent release of Ca, patients typically have hypercalciuria and nephrocalcinosis at presentation. In the AD form, patients may present later in life and often with urolithiasis.
- The most common presenting feature is faltering growth.
- The acidosis is treated with alkali, typically K citrate or bicarbonate (➔ see Chapter 6).
- Correction of the acidosis allows normal growth and development and normalizes urinary calcium excretion. It does not affect the potentially associated sensorineural deafness.

Disorders presenting with hypokalaemic alkalosis

- Hypokalaemic alkalosis is the biochemical fingerprint of enhanced Na reabsorption in the CD, as it is linked with K and proton secretion.
- Enhanced Na reabsorption in the CD is typically due to hyperaldosteronism. This can be primary (Conn syndrome or salt-retaining forms of congenital adrenal hyperplasia, CAH), in which case there is clinical hypervolaemia. Conversely, if hyperaldosteronism is secondary, due to salt losses elsewhere, then there is evidence of hypovolaemia.

Hypokalaemic alkalosis with hypovolaemia

- Due to the different molecular links between Na and Ca reabsorption in the TAL and DCT, urinary Ca assessment can help distinguish between salt-wasting disorders of TAL (e.g. Bartter syndrome) and DCT (e.g. Gitelman syndrome).
- Salt reabsorption in the TAL is mediated by the furosemide-sensitive Na co-transporter NKCC2 (Fig. 7.3). In Bartter syndrome, the function of this transporter is either directly or indirectly compromised, and thus its symptoms are best compared with the effects of loop diuretics, such as furosemide.
- Salt reabsorption in the DCT is mediated by the thiazide-sensitive NaCl co-transporter NCC (➔ see Fig. 7.4, p. 174). Gitelman syndrome is thus best compared with the effects of thiazides.
- Four genes underlying Bartter syndrome have been identified so far and more are expected (Table 7.1). In addition, isolated patients with AD hypocalcaemia can also have Bartter-like symptoms.
  - A transient form of Bartter syndrome, presenting with severe polyhydramnios and neonatal Bartter syndrome, is associated with recessive mutations in the gene *MAGED2*. As this gene is located on the X-chromosome, this form has so far been described only in boys. This disorder spontaneously resolves in the first few months of life.

Clinical features: Bartter syndrome
Key symptoms
- Hypokalaemic, hypochloraemic metabolic alkalosis with elevated renin and aldosterone levels, and normal to low BP.
- Polyuria, polydipsia, and salt craving to replace renal losses.

Additional symptoms
- Salt reabsorption in the TAL is a critical step in the renal concentration/ dilution system. Therefore, patients with Bartter syndrome have impaired urinary concentration (hypo- to isosthenuria). Because of this, patients with Bartter syndrome have high renal water losses and are prone to hypernatraemic dehydration.
- The combined actions of the NKCC2 co-transporter and subsequent 'recycling' of K back into the tubular lumen through the K channel ROMK provide the driving force for reabsorption of Ca and Mg in the TAL (Fig. 7.3). Therefore, patients with mutations in the genes encoding

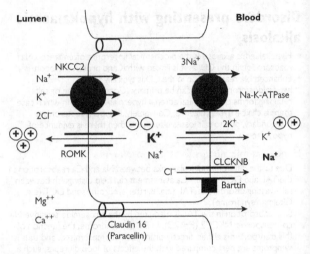

Fig. 7.3 Diagram of a TAL cell.

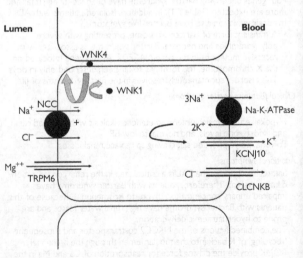

Fig. 7.4 Diagram of a DCT cell.

NKCC2 or ROMK typically have hypercalciuria, hypermagnesuria, and nephrocalcinosis. Conversely, patients with mutations affecting the Cl channel CLCKNB or its subunit Barttin typically have normocalciuria and no nephrocalcinosis.

- The Barttin subunit is also expressed in the inner ear and patients with Barttin mutations have Bartter syndrome associated with sensorineural deafness (very rare).
- The Cl channel CLCKNB is also expressed in the DCT and patients with mutations in the encoding gene may have an overlap of Bartter and Gitelman syndromes (➔ see 'Clinical features: Gitelman syndrome') features.
- The spectrum of severity can vary widely in Bartter syndrome with the most severe cases showing an antenatal presentation with polyhydramnios, premature delivery, severe and life-threatening dehydration, and failure to thrive (neonatal Bartter syndrome). These patients also have highly elevated levels of urinary prostaglandins, especially prostaglandin E2 (PGE2). Many of these patients also experience progression to CKD over time, which may be at least partially related to prematurity. Other patients with Bartter syndrome are asymptomatic and incidentally identified in adulthood during a routine blood test and have no other apparent symptoms.

Clinical features: Gitelman syndrome

- Gitelman syndrome is usually diagnosed during adolescence or later.
- Hypomagnesaemia is due to an increased urinary Mg excretion and can be associated with tetany, muscle weakness, or cramps.
- Other symptoms include hypotension and dizziness, joint pains, and nocturnal enuresis.
- Systemic calcifications, such as chondrocalcinosis, are unusual in childhood.
- Prolongation of the QT interval on ECG occurs in 10% of patients and severe arrhythmias have been described.
- The prognosis is generally excellent.

Clinical features: EAST/SeSAME syndrome

- Characterized by seizures, sensorineural deafness, ataxia, intellectual deficit, and electrolyte imbalance.
- Patients typically present in infancy because of the neurological manifestations (seizures, ataxia, developmental delay).
- The tubulopathy is identical to Gitelman syndrome, i.e. a salt-losing disorder of the DCT.
- Patients also have sensorineural deafness.

Hypokalaemic alkalosis with hypervolaemia

- Patients have hypertension, often marked.
- Hypercalciuria with/without nephrocalcinosis is typically present, presumably due to suppressed reabsorption in the PT.
- Polyuria due to impaired urinary concentrating ability (presumably related to hypercalciuria) can be present and sometimes severe.
- Mineralocorticoid excess in babies is typically due to salt-retaining forms of CAH.

- Conn syndrome is rare in childhood, but an early-onset form with underlying mutations in *KCNJ5* has been identified. Aldosterone is elevated, but renin is suppressed.
- Pseudohyperaldosteronism (apparent mineralocorticoid excess and liquorice intoxication) is due to activation of the mineralocorticoid receptor (MCR) by hormones other than mineralocorticoids. The MCR is not specific for mineralocorticoids, but can also be activated by cortisol, which is usually present in blood in a 1000-fold higher concentration than aldosterone. The enzyme HSD11B2 converts cortisol to cortisone in the principal cells of the CD and thus protects activation of MCR by cortisol. If the enzyme is dysfunctional, either due to a genetic defect (apparent mineralocorticoid excess) or blockade (liquorice), there is inappropriate activation of the MCR. Both aldosterone and renin are suppressed.
- A rare form of a gain-of-function mutation in the MCR has also been described with activation by gestagens and thus worsening hypertension during menses and pregnancy. Both aldosterone and renin are suppressed.
- Liddle syndrome is due to dominant gain-of-function mutations in the epithelial sodium channel ENaC (➔ see Fig. 7.5). Both aldosterone and renin are suppressed
- In glucocorticoid-remediable aldosteronism (GRA), an unequal crossover in meiosis creates a fusion gene from the highly homologous genes *CYP11B1* and *CYP11B2*, which are adjacent on chromosome 8 and encode key enzymes in glucocorticoid (CYP11B1) and aldosterone (CYP11B2) synthesis. In the fusion gene, the *CYP11B1* promoter is fused to the coding sequence of *CYP11B2*, so that adrenocorticotropic hormone (ACTH) now drives aldosterone, rather than glucocorticoid synthesis.

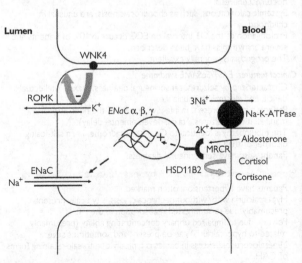

Fig. 7.5 Diagram of a principal cell.

Investigation

- Clinical examination and BP: to distinguish between salt-wasting (hypovolaemia) and salt-retaining disorders (hypervolaemia)
- *Urine*: Na, K (fractional excretion >15%), Cl (fractional excretion >0.5%), Ca (variable: high in TAL and hypervolaemic disorders, low in DCT disorders), Mg (high, fractional excretion >4% in some forms), creatinine (to calculate fractional excretions), and osmolality.
- *Plasma*: Na (variable), K, Cl (both low), Mg (normal or low in Gitelman/ EAST/SeSAME syndromes), Ca (usually normal), bicarbonate (high), urea, creatinine, albumin (as indicators of renal function and hydration), renin (suppressed in hypervolaemic disorders), and aldosterone (suppressed in hypervolaemic disorders, except Conn syndrome).
- Renal US for nephrocalcinosis.
- ECG: some patients with marked hypokalaemia and/or hypomagnesaemia may benefit from cardiological assessment of the risk of long QT syndrome.
- Genetic analysis.

Differential diagnosis

- *Extrarenal salt and water losses ('pseudo-Bartter')*: distinguished by low urinary Cl concentration (fractional excretion <0.5%). This can be difficult in Cl-losing diarrhoea as the stool may be so watery it is indistinguishable from urine. Catheterization may be necessary.
- *Hypomagnesaemia–hypercalciuria–nephrocalcinosis syndrome*: in this condition there is marked hypercalciuria, nephrocalcinosis, calculi, and progression to CKD stage 5 (➔ see 'Disorders of renal magnesium handling', p. 187).
- Surreptitious diuretic use (history and toxicology).
- Some patients with hypokalaemia and hypercalciuria have marked hyposthenuria and have been misdiagnosed as having primary nephrogenic diabetes insipidus (NDI).

Treatment: salt-wasting disorders

- First-line treatment of salt-wasting disorders involves replacement of fluid and electrolyte losses.
- Severely affected children may initially require IV saline rehydration, milder cases can simply be started on K and/or NaCl, ideally divided into three or four doses per day.
- It is usually very difficult to achieve adequate K supplementation to restore the K level to the normal range, and most patients tolerate hypokalaemia of 2.5 mmol/L with no obvious ill effects.
- There may be a role for amiloride or spironolactone in some cases with severe hypokalaemia and/or acidosis. Beware that this inhibits the physiological compensatory mechanisms and may lead to severe hypotension and even hypovolaemic shock and it must be accompanied by adequate salt supplementation (aim for 10 mmol/kg/day).
- Inhibitors of prostaglandin synthesis, the cyclooxygenase (COX) inhibitors (e.g. indometacin, ibuprofen, celecoxib), are typically of major benefit in Bartter syndrome, but of questionable benefit in Gitelman and EAST/SeSAME syndromes.

- indometacin is usually given at a dose of 0.5–1 mg/kg/day, divided into four doses, with stepwise increases to a maximum of 2–4 mg/kg/day.
  - indometacin should be given with food (or milk) and parents counselled regarding GI side effects including ulceration, and benign intracranial hypertension; concurrent use of a gastric acid inhibitor, such as ranitidine, or a proton pump inhibitor is recommended.
  - Use of indometacin in the neonatal period may increase the risk of necrotizing enterocolitis.
- Chronic use of inhibitors of prostaglandin synthesis is associated with progressive CKD. It is unclear whether this concern is relevant in patients with Bartter syndrome, as unlike other patients, who take these drugs for indications such as chronic pain and thus suppress prostaglandin levels below the normal range, in Bartter syndrome they are taken to bring prostaglandin levels closer to the normal range.
- Ibuprofen is usually given in doses of 5–10 mg/kg three times daily with similar concerns of GI side effects as with indometacin. Consider concurrent use of a gastric acid inhibitor.
- Selective COX-2 inhibitors (e.g. celecoxib) have a lower risk of GI side effects, but have been associated with long-term cardiovascular side effects in adults. Whether these risks are relevant for children with Bartter syndrome remains to be determined.
- Celecoxib is typically given in doses of 1–2 mg/kg twice daily, but can be increased up to 5 mg/kg twice daily with a maximum dose of 200 mg daily.

Treatment: salt-retaining (hypervolaemic) disorders

- These disorders are treated with blockers of the ENaC (e.g. amiloride) and/or blockers of the MCR (e.g. spironolactone).
- With adequate treatment, the electrolyte abnormalities and associated complications (such as hypertension and polyuria) completely resolve.
- Conn syndrome may need additional treatment by surgery and/or oncology.
- GRA may benefit from cortisol replacement to reduce ACTH levels which in this disorder drive the aldosterone production.

Fig. 7.3 represents an epithelial cell in the TAL. Font size represents relative concentrations for K and Na (not to scale) and (+) and (−) signs represent electric charges (not to scale).

Na is reabsorbed via NKCC2 (defective in Bartter type 1), together with one K and two Cl ions. The transporter can only function with all four ions bound and K binding is the rate-limiting step. Therefore, K is recycled through the K channel ROMK (defective in Bartter type 2) to ensure an adequate supply of K. This also leads to a relative excess of positive charges in the tubular lumen, providing the driving force for paracellular absorption of Ca and Mg.

Na can exit the cell on the basolateral (blood side) via the Na/K-ATPase, while Cl exits through the Cl channel CLCKNB (defective in Bartter type 3). CLCKNB requires Barttin (defect in Bartter type 4) for proper membrane localization.

Further reading

Seyberth HW. Pathophysiology and clinical presentations of salt-losing tubulopathies. Pediatr Nephrol 2016;31:407–418.

Disorders presenting with hyperkalaemic acidosis

Hyperkalaemic acidosis is the biochemical fingerprint of impaired Na re-absorption in the CD, which is coupled to K and proton secretion (see Fig. 7.5). As with the mirror image of hypokalaemic alkalosis, it can occur both with salt-wasting (hypovolaemic) and salt-retaining (hypervolaemic) disorders.

Clinical features

Pseudohypoaldosteronism

- A salt-wasting form (PHA1) must be distinguished from the salt-retaining form (PHA2)
- PHA1 can be further divided into a severe recessive form (PHA1A) and a milder dominant form (PHA1B).
- The recessive form is due to mutations in one of the three subunits constituting the ENaC in the CD (see Fig. 7.5).
- PHA1A typically presents in the first few days with severe, often life-threatening hypovolaemia, hyperkalaemia, and acidosis.
- Since ENaC is also expressed in the lungs and sweat glands, patients with PHA1A can also experience cystic fibrosis-like respiratory complications and a rash from obstructed sweat glands.
- PHA1B also presents with hypovolaemia and hyperkalaemic acidosis, but signs and symptoms are typically milder and often resolve spontaneously during the first months to years of life.
- An acquired form of PHA1 can be seen with urinary obstruction and in young children with pyelonephritis.
- PHA2 is a rare, AD inherited disorder. Not to be confused with PHA1, which is a salt-wasting disorder, PHA2 is a disorder of Na retention, due to mutations in the genes WNK1 or WNK4, CUL3, or KLHL3. Inheritance is AD, except for mutations in KLHL3, which can also be recessively inherited. WNK1 and WNK4 encode kinases, which regulate salt reabsorption in the distal tubule, and CUL3 and KLHL3 are involved in degradation of WNK1 and WNK4. The common downstream consequence is an overactivity of the thiazide-sensitive Na transporter in the DCT. Consequently, the signs and symptoms are the mirror image of Gitelman syndrome: patients have hypertension, hyperkalaemic, hyperchloraemic metabolic acidosis, and hypercalciuria. The hypertension often develops during adolescence and thus may not be apparent in younger children.
- An acquired form of PHA2 can be seen as a complication of tacrolimus treatment.

Fig. 7.4 represents an epithelial cell in the DCT. Na is reabsorbed via NCC and can exit towards the blood side via the Na-K-ATPase, while Cl can pass through the Cl channel CLCKNB. NCC is regulated by the WNK-kinases WNK1 and WNK4. KCNJ10 is necessary to supply sufficient K to the Na-K-ATPase and build up a voltage gradient over the basolateral membrane that promotes Cl reabsorption.

Investigations

* Clinical examination and BP: to distinguish between the salt-wasting (PHA1) and salt-retaining forms (PHA2).
* *Urine*: Na, K (fractional excretion <15%), Cl, Ca (high in PHA2), creatinine (to calculate fractional excretions), and osmolality (to calculate transtubular K gradient). Urine culture to exclude acquired form of PHA1.
* *Blood*: Na, K, Cl, bicarbonate (low), urea, creatinine, albumin (as indicators of renal function and hydration), osmolality, renin (elevated in PHA1, usually suppressed in PHA2), and aldosterone (elevated in PHA1, variable in PHA2).
* Renal US to assess for obstruction.

Treatment: PHA1

* Salt! Patients with severe PHA1 need to be resuscitated with IV 0.9% saline and sodiumbicarbonate until they are stable enough to be converted to oral forms. These patients often require a central line for reliable emergency access. Na-exchange resins (such as sodium polystyrene sulfonate) provide a good form for sustained Na administration and K removal.
* Na-exchange resins can provide a steady source of Na, while ameliorating the hyperkalaemia ('using the gut as CD') in severe forms of PHA1.
* Patients with PHA1B can often be weaned off the salt supplements over time (Fig. 7.5).

Treatment: PHA2

* Thiazides! Adequate treatment with thiazides completely reverses the hypertension and electrolyte abnormalities.

Further reading

O'Shaughnessy KM. Gordon syndrome: a continuing story. *Pediatr Nephrol* 2015;30:1903–1908.
Zennaro MC, Hubert EL, Fernandes-Rosa FL. Aldosterone resistance: structural and functional considerations and new perspectives. *Mol Cell Endocrinol* 2012;350:206–215.

Disorders of renal water handling

Basic principles

- The kidneys in an adult filter about 150 L of plasma per day. ~80% of this is passively reabsorbed in the PT, which is water permeable due to the presence of water channels (AQP1) in both apical and basolateral membranes. Thus, as solutes such as Na, bicarbonate, and PO_4 are reabsorbed in the PT, water follows passively.
- Final urine osmolality and thus water excretion is determined by the water permeability of the CD:
  - Urine is diluted in the preceding water-impermeable nephron segments, the TAL and the early DCT.
  - Salt reabsorption in THE TAL (by the furosemide-sensitive NKCC2) not only dilutes the urine, but also generates the medullary interstitial concentration gradient.
  - When the dilute urine enters the medullary CD, a concentration gradient between urine (osmolality as low as 50 mOsm/kg) and interstitium (up to 1200 mOsm/kg) exists.
  - The osmotic force is enormous (19.2 mmHg/mOsm/L) and water will move out of the tubule, if water channels are provided.
- The availability of water channels is regulated by AVP, which binds to its receptor (AVPR2), located in the principal cells of the CD. When activated by binding of vasopressin, AVPR2 causes an increase in cAMP, which in turn causes movement of intracellular vesicles containing water channels (AQP2) to the apical membrane, thereby increasing water permeability.

Disorders of renal water handling presenting
with hypernatraemia: nephrogenic diabetes insipidus

- NDI is a renal disorder characterized by tubular unresponsiveness to ADH (AVP) resulting in the excretion of an increased volume of dilute urine. Congenital (usually severe) and acquired (usually milder) forms are recognized.
- In complete and untreated NDI, the urine osmolality is typically <100 mOsm/kg. The total volume excreted depends on the osmotic load (osmotically active substances in the diet) that needs to be excreted by the kidney. A typical Western diet presents about 500 mOsm/day to the kidney. With a urine osmolality of 50 mOsm/kg, this will require 10 L water to be excreted. An extra gram of salt (~18 mmol of Na and Cl, each ~36 mOsm) in the diet thus would increase urine output by ~700 mL.
- A simple, but often confused point is the difference between osmolarity and osmolality: these are numerically similar, although osmolarity is expressed as number of osmotically active substances per volume of analysed fluid (mOsm/L), while osmolality is per weight (mOsm/kg).

Genetics of nephrogenic diabetes insipidus

- The *AVPR2* gene is located on the X-chromosome and accounts for ~90% of inherited cases of NDI, while *AQP2* is located on chromosome 12. Mutations in *AQP2* cause AR NDI. Some very rare mutations in *AQP2* can also cause AD NDI.

- Some gene mutations in *AVPR2* disrupt protein function completely, while others only decrease affinity of the receptor to AVP, resulting in a milder phenotype (partial NDI).
- Female carriers of an *AVPR2* mutation are generally asymptomatic, but skewed X-inactivation may cause various degrees of symptoms.
- In addition to genetic forms of NDI, there are many causes of secondary NDI (➔ see 'Acquired (secondary) nephrogenic diabetes insipidus', p. 184).

Clinical features (primary nephrogenic diabetes insipidus)
- Present in infancy (no prenatal symptoms, no polyhydramnios).
- Polyuria and polydipsia with episodes of hypernatraemic dehydration.
- Episodes of pyrexia, irritability, and vomiting.
- Failure to thrive (patients are only interested in drinking, but not eating).
- Females carrying an *AVPR2* mutation may be asymptomatic or present at a later age with milder symptoms. Rarely, more prominent symptoms are encountered (depending on X-inactivation).

Complications of NDI include:
- developmental delay/learning problems (due to repeated episodes of hypertonic dehydration)
- renal cortical necrosis during episodes of severe dehydration
- hydronephrosis and dilatation of the lower urinary tract (due to high urine volume, especially with urinary withholding).

Investigations
- Basic biochemistry and haematological screen: U&Es, creatinine, Ca, PO₄, LFTs, FBC (increased haematocrit as a sign of intravascular water depletion).
- *Paired urine (Uosm)/plasma osmolarity (Posm)*: inappropriately dilute urine (Uosm <Posm) in the presence of elevated plasma osmolarity establishes a diagnosis of diabetes insipidus. To differentiate central diabetes insipidus from NDI, a DDAVP® test is performed (➔ see 'DDAVP® test', p. 683).
- US kidneys and bladder (the high urine flow in NDI can cause hydronephrosis, but gross dilatation of the urinary tract and/or altered echogenicity or nephrocalcinosis should prompt investigations into secondary NDI due to underlying nephropathy (➔ see 'Acquired (secondary) nephrogenic diabetes insipidus', p. 184).

Water deprivation test and DDAVP® test
- Never undertake a water deprivation test in the presence of hypernatraemia and/or increased plasma osmolarity. In this situation, paired plasma and urine osmolarities are sufficient. Thus, children presenting with hypernatraemia do not need another water deprivation test, if Uosm had been measured at presentation.
- In normonatraemic children suspected of having diabetes insipidus, a first morning Uosm is often sufficient as an informal water deprivation test, unless the child gets up at night to drink. A Uosm >Posm rules out a severe form of diabetes insipidus.
- A formal water deprivation test, if needed, should be carried out in the early morning. The patient is weighed, and plasma and urine osmolarities measured. The test is stopped if >3% of body weight is lost

or if Posm is >300mOsm/kg. If the plasma osmolality is 300 mOsm/kg or higher, and the urine is dilute (<Posm), then the diagnosis of diabetes insipidus is confirmed. If the urine concentration is >800 mOsm/kg (or >600 mOsm/kg in infants), a normal urinary concentrating ability is established and diabetes insipidus has been ruled out. If the Uosm is <800 mOsm/kg (<600 mOsm/kg in infants), DDAVP® (desmopressin) should be given to further assess renal concentrating ability.

- *DDAVP® test*: various protocols, using oral, nasal, intramuscular, or IV administration of DDAVP® exist. The main risk of a DDAVP® test is hyponatraemia. This can only occur in patients who respond to desmopressin, but continue drinking water or who ingested a large bolus of water immediately prior to the test. In patients with an intact thirst mechanism, the risk of dysnatraemias is very low (as they will stop drinking), but patients with suspected psychogenic habitual polydipsia (or Munchhausen by proxy) are at risk. It is paramount that patients do not drink for an hour before desmopressin and are closely observed so that fluid intake during the test does not exceed urine output. The half-life of desmopressin depends on the mode of administration. The shortest is after IV administration, where only a 2 h observation period is required. This mode also eliminates questions about incomplete absorption, which is possible with oral or nasal doses.
- A well-established protocol (➔ see 'DDAVP® test', p. 683) uses 0.3 micrograms/kg desmopressin (maximum 15 micrograms) dissolved in 1 mL/kg (maximum 50 mL) of 0.9% saline as an IV bolus (this is the same dose given to patients with von Willebrand disease to promote platelet aggregation). The bladder should be emptied before the administration of desmopressin to avoid admixture of urine. As many aliquots of urine as possible should be obtained during the 2 h test and individually sent for urine osmolality. Paired plasma and urine samples are obtained at the beginning and the end of the test.
- In central diabetes insipidus, the urine will concentrate to >800 mOsm/ kg (>600 mOsm/kg in infants) following desmopressin; in complete NDI the urinary concentration will be unchanged (<Posm) or mildly increased (300–600 mOsm/kg) in partial NDI.

Management of primary nephrogenic diabetes insipidus
Diet
The mainstay of treatment is to reduce the osmotic load, which mainly con-sists of salts and protein (as it is metabolized to urea):

- Salt is restricted as much as possible, but enough protein must be given to allow proper growth. This is most challenging during infancy, when caloric and fluid intake is coupled and the input of an experienced dietician is very important.
- The general aim is to provide adequate nutrition to meet recommended intakes, but this limits the osmotic load to 15 mOsm/kg/day.
- As a general rule, each 1 g of protein provides 4 mOsm and each 1 mmol of Na or K provide 2 mOsm (because of the accompanying anion).
- Fat and carbohydrates provide calories, but no osmotic load.
  - *Example*: the importance of osmotic load reduction becomes apparent when you consider an adolescent NDI patient, who enjoys a

large steak containing 200 g of protein seasoned with 2 g of salt: the total osmotic load from the steak is 800 mOsm (200 × 4) and from the salt 34 mOsm (1 g of salt contains ~17 mmol of Na and Cl each). With an average urine osmolality of 100 mOsm/kg, the patient will need to drink almost 9 L of water in order to be able to excrete the osmotic load provided by this meal.
- The child needs free access to water and infants should be offered fluid frequently (every 1–2 h).

Drug therapy
- *Thiazides (e.g. chlorothiazide 10–20 mg/kg/day, or bendroflumethiazide 0.1 mg/kg/day):*
  - The administration of a diuretic in a polyuric disorder is counterintuitive but effective. Thiazides impair the urinary diluting mechanism in the distal tubule. Moreover, they increase urinary Na excretion, which leads to intravascular volume depletion. This enhances Na (and thus water) reabsorption in the PT. Less water is then presented to the defective portion of the tubule.
  - Watch for hypokalaemia and use K supplements if needed (however, these will present an additional osmotic load). Amiloride can sometimes be used in combination with chlorothiazide to achieve K sparing.
- *Inhibitors of prostaglandin synthesis, e.g. indometacin 0.75–2 mg/kg/day* (divided into two or three doses). Helpful in the management of infants, but often not necessary in older children. Counsel patients regarding GI bleeding. Concomitant use of an acid blocker is recommended. Alternatively, a COX-2 inhibitor, e.g. celecoxib (1–2 mg/kg twice daily) can be used. The mechanisms of action are unclear, but probably include reduction of GFR and stimulation of proximal Na (and thus water) reabsorption. Plasma creatinine usually remains stable or even decreases (reflecting improved hydration) after indometacin, arguing against GFR reduction as a mode of action

Management of NDI during intercurrent illness, and perioperatively
- During intercurrent infection, when patients are unable to drink or before elective surgery, children with NDI require IV fluids, as they have ongoing water losses in the urine.
- Unlike the usual paediatric situation, IV fluids should be given as 5% glucose without saline. The inclusion of saline will increase the solute load and thus promote hypernatraemia. The 5% dextrose in water should not be given as a bolus, however, as this can lead to rapid lowering of plasma Na, but at a rate that compensates for the urinary losses.
- Patients should be closely monitored with a strict input/output balance, daily weights, and for the development of dysnatraemias with adjustment of the rate of IV fluids accordingly. As soon as the patient is able to drink, IV fluids should be discontinued so that the thirst mechanism of the patient can regulate his/her intake.

Acquired (secondary) nephrogenic diabetes insipidus
Inherited primary NDI is a rare disease, and secondary forms occur more commonly (and often have only moderately impaired urinary concentrating ability—isosthenuria):

- Amyloidosis.
- Analgesic nephropathy.
- CKD (particularly renal dysplasia and nephronophthisis).
- Drug induced:
  - Lithium.
  - Tetracycline.
- Hypercalcaemia/hypercalciuria.
- Chronic hypokalaemia.
- Post-obstructive uropathy.
- Bartter syndrome.
- Apparent mineralocorticoid excess.
- Sarcoidosis.
- Sickle cell anaemia.

Further reading

Bockenhauer D, Bichet DG. Pathophysiology, diagnosis and management of nephrogenic diabetes insipidus. *Nat Rev Nephrol* 2015;11:576–588.

Disorders of renal water handling presenting
with hyponatraemia: SIADH and nephrogenic syndrome
of inappropriate antidiuresis

- SIADH is due to inappropriately high levels of ADH (◯ see Chapter 6).
- SIADH is traditionally treated by fluid restriction (adjusting the fluid load to the low urine output) or increasing the osmotic load (urea or protein). Na supplementation also increases the osmotic load, but is typically complicated by hypertension. Patients with SIADH have increased thirst and thus in patients with free access to water, fluid restriction is often unsuccessful.
- Specific treatment is available in the form of so-called aquaretics. These are blockers of AVPR2 and thus prevent activation by ADH. Tolvaptan is an oral aquaretic (starting dose 0.1 mg/kg once daily, can be titrated up to 0.6 mg/kg (maximum 60 mg) once daily). Patients should have free access to fluids to prevent sudden increases in plasma Na concentration.
- Nephrogenic syndrome of inappropriate antidiuresis (NSIAD) is the mirror image of NDI: in NDI water is lost, whereas in NSIAD water is inappropriately retained. Thus, NSIAD is a genetic form of SIADH.
- NSIAD is caused by gain-of-function mutations in *AVPR2* (loss of function of which cause NDI, ◯ see 'Nephrogenic diabetes insipidus', p. 181). Accordingly, NSIAD is an X-linked dominant disorder, with men typically more severely affected than women.
- Initially two mutations in the AVPR2 protein were identified in NSIAD, both affecting the same amino acid, arginine 137: R137C and R137L. Interestingly, mutation of this residue to histidine (R137H) results in NDI. Two further mutations have since been described: I130N and F229V
- Affected patients present with hyponatraemia, with no evidence of hypovolaemia and inappropriately high urine osmolality (Uosm >100 mOsm/kg).
- NSIAD can be differentiated from SIADH by the presence of a family history (usually), and very low or absent levels of ADH.

- Treatment is similar to that in SIADH, and consists of water restriction and/or increasing the osmotic load. Importantly, aquaretics are not effective (as NSIAD is not ADH mediated):
  - Older patients will typically refrain from drinking automatically, as the resulting decrease in plasma osmolality suppresses thirst, but in infants this is more difficult, as fluid and calorie intake are coupled.
  - Feeds should be concentrated as much as possible and solids introduced early to minimize fluid intake.
  - Protein and/or urea supplementation (to increase osmotic load) can be helpful.

Disorders of renal magnesium handling

Basic principles

While most other ions are predominantly reabsorbed in the PT, the key sites for Mg reabsorption are the TAL and DCT (Fig. 7.6). Consequently, all disorders associated with abnormal renal Mg handling affect transport in these two segments (Table 7.4). Clinically, they can be roughly separated into three groups, based on urinary Ca excretion (Table 7.4). In addition, hypomagnesaemia can occur in mitochondrial cytopathies.

Hypomagnesaemia associated with hypercalciuria

The molecular pathway for Mg reabsorption in TAL is paracellular, includes claudin-16 and -19, and is shared with Ca. The voltage gradient driving absorption is generated by the combined actions of NKCC2 and ROMK (mutations in which cause Bartter syndrome). Therefore, loss of function in any of these four proteins leads to wasting of both Mg and Ca.

- Inherited causes:
  - Familial hypomagnesaemia with hypercalciuria and nephrocalcinosis (AR mutations in CLDN16 or CLDN19).
  - Bartter syndrome type 1 or 2 (AR mutations in SLC12A1 (encoding NKCC2) or KCNJ1 (encoding ROMK)).
- Acquired causes:
  - Loop diuretics.
  - Amphotericin, cisplatin, foscarnet, and pentamidine (usually associated with more generalized tubular dysfunction).

Hypomagnesaemia associated with hypocalciuria

Impaired Na reabsorption in the DCT indirectly affects Mg reabsorption. Thus, disorders of Na reabsorption (e.g. Gitelman and EAST/SeSAME syndromes) are associated with renal Mg wasting. The resulting volume loss from impaired Na reabsorption leads to up-regulation of proximal Na transport, which is paralleled by Ca reabsorption. Thus, these disorders are associated with hypocalciuria.

- Inherited causes:
  - Gitelman syndrome (AR mutations in SLC12A3 (encoding NCC)).
  - Bartter syndrome type 3 and 4 (AR mutations in CLCKNB or BSND (encoding Barttin)).
  - EAST/SeSAME syndrome (AR mutations in KCNJ10).
  - HOMG2 (AD mutations in FXYD2).
  - HNF1B nephropathy (AD).
  - Transient neonatal hyperphenylalaninaemia (AR mutations in PCBD1). Aside from being involved in phenylamine transport, PCBD1 serves as a dimerization factor for HNF1B and patients thus can have hypomagnesaemia and diabetes (MODY).
- Acquired causes: thiazides.

Hypomagnesaemia associated with normocalciuria

Magnesium reabsorption in the DCT is transcellular and the key entry step for Mg into the epithelial cell is through the ion channel TRPM6. Disorders that directly or indirectly impair this entry step affect renal Mg excretion only. The excretion of other salts, such as Ca, Na, Cl, and K, is unaffected. The basolateral exit pathway for Mg remains still to be identified.

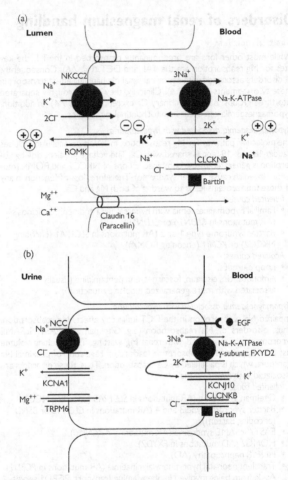

Fig. 7.6 (a) Schematic of salt transport in the TAL. (b) Schematic of salt transport in the DCT.

Table 7.4 Inherited disorders and genes associated with renal Mg wasting

Gene	Protein	Phenotype							Extrarenal	Disease
		Plasma					Urine			
		Mg	Ca	K	Cl	HCO₃	Ca	K		
Hypercalciuric hypomagnesaemias										
SLC12A1	NKCC2	↔↓	↕	↓	↓	↑	↑	↑		Bartter 1
KCNJ1	ROMK	↔↓	↕	↓	↓	↑	↑	↑		Bartter 2
CLDN16	Claudin-16	↓	↕	↕	↕	↕	↑	↕		FHHNC, HOMG3
CLDN19	Claudin-19	↓	↕	↕	↕	↕	↑	↕	Eye problems	FHHNC, HOMG5
CaSR	Calcium-sensing receptor	↓	↓	↕↑	↕↓	↔↑	↑	↔↑	Hypocalcaemia	Familial hypocalcaemia
Hypocalciuric hypomagnesaemias										
CLCKNB	CLCKNB	↓↔	↕	↓	↓	↑	↓↓	↑		Bartter 3
BSND	Barttin	↓↔	↕	↓	↓	↑	↓↓	↑	Deafness	Bartter 4
FXYD2	Na⁺/K⁺-ATPase, G-subunit	↓	↕	↕	↕	↕	↓	↕		HOMG2
PCBD1	Pterin-4-alpha-carbinolamine dehydratase 1	↓	↕	↕	↕	↕	↓	↕	Hyperphenylalaninaemia, MODY	Transient neonatal hyperphenylalaninaemia and primapterinuria

(Continued)

Table 7.4 (Contd.)

Gene	Protein	Phenotype							Extrarenal	Disease
		Plasma					Urine			
		Mg	Ca	K	Cl	HCO₃	Ca	K		
HNF1B	HNF1B	↓↓	↔	↔↑	↔↓	↔↑	↔	↔↑		RCD
SLC12A3	NCC	↓	↔	↓	↓	↑	↓	↑		Gitelman syndrome
KCNJ10	Kir4.1	↓	↔	↓	↓	↑	↓	↑	Epilepsy, ataxia, deafness, DD	EAST/SeSAME syndrome
Hypomagnesaemias with normocalciuria										
TRPM6	TRPM6	↓	↔	↔	↔	↔	↔	↔	Epilepsy, DD	HSH, HOMG1
EGF	EGF	↓	↔	↔	↔	↔	↔	↔	DD	HOMG4
EGFR	EGFR	↓	↔	↔	↔	↔	↔	↔	Skin and bowel inflammation	Neonatal skin and bowel disease type 2
KCNA1	KV1.1	↓	↔	↔	↔	↔	↔	↔	Episodic ataxia, myokymia	HOMG
CNNM2	Cyclin M	↓	↔	↔	↔	↔	↔	↔	Seizures, mental impairment	HOMG6
FAM111A	FAM111A	↓	↔↑	↔	↔	↔	↔	↔	Short stature, bone and eye anomalies, hypocalcaemia	Kenny-Caffey syndrome type 2

Hypomagnesaemias with mitochondrial cytopathies							
MT-TI	tRNA	↓	↔	↔↓	↑↔↑	↓↔↑	↔↑	Mitochondrial cytopathy
SARS2	Seryl-tRNA synthetase	↓	↔	↔↓	↑↔↑	↓↔↑	↔↑	Hyperuricaemia, CKD, pulmonary hypertension	Mitochondrial cytopathy
POLG1	Polymerase, DNA, gamma	↓	↔	↔↓	↑↔↑	↓↔↑	↔↑	Ataxia, ophthalmoplegia	Mitochondrial cytopathy

Listed are known inherited disorders of renal Mg handling. The hypercalciuric disorders concern Na and Mg handling. The hypocalciuric disorders concern Na and Mg handling in the TAL, the hypocalciuric disorders affect Mg handling in the DCT only (i.e. not salt handling). The normocalciuric hypomagnesaemias typically affect Mg handling in the DCT. Hypomagnesaemia can also occur with mitochondrial cytopathies.

DD, developmental delay; FHHNC, familial hypomagnesaemia with hypercalciuria and nephrocalcinosis; HSH, hypomagnesaemia with secondary hypocalcaemia; HOMG, hypomagnesaemia, renal; RCD, renal cysts and diabetes syndrome; MODY, maturity-onset diabetes in the young.

- *Inherited causes*:
  - Familial hypomagnesaemia with secondary hypocalcaemia (AR mutations in *TRPM6*); this disorder typically has marked hypomagnesaemia, as TRPM6 is not only important for renal Mg transport, but also for absorption of Mg from the gut. Hypocalcaemia is a common complication of hypomagnesaemia, as Mg is an important co-factor at the CaSR in the parathyroid, necessary for PTH release. Due to the severity of the hypomagnesaemia in this disorder, hypocalcaemia is commonly seen.
  - Hypomagnesaemia HOMG (AD mutations in *KCNA1*).
  - Hypomagnesaemia HOMG4 (AD mutations in *EGF*).
  - HOMG6 (AD or AR mutations in *CNNM2*). This disorder is associated with seizures and mental impairment. The pathophysiological role of CNNM2 itself is poorly understood, but it may serve as an intracellular Mg sensor.
  - Kenny–Caffey syndrome type 2 (AD mutations in *FAM111A*). Kenny–Caffey syndrome is defined by short stature, hypoparathyroidism, and skeletal and eye abnormalities. Affected patients were found to be hypomagnesaemic, but the role of FAM111A in renal Mg handling remains to be elucidated.
- *Acquired causes*: tacrolimus, ciclosporin, and proton pump inhibitors.

Hypomagnesaemia associated with mitochondrial cytopathies

Since the active, transcellular transport of Mg in the kidney requires energy, renal Mg wasting can also be seen in mitochondrial cytopathies. Since these disorders can affect any other transport pathway, the associated abnormalities can be highly variable. Hypomagnesaemia has been described in a variety of inherited mitochondrial cytopathies (see Table 7.4). Drugs affecting mitochondrial function, such as aminoglycosides, can also cause hypomagnesaemia.

Investigations and treatment

→ See 'Disorders of magnesium: basic principles'.

Further reading

Viering DH, de Baaij JH, Walsh SB, et al. Genetic causes of hypomagnesemia, a clinical overview. *Pediatr Nephrol* 2017;32:1123–1135.

Rickets

General principles

- Rickets refers to impaired mineralization at the epiphyseal growth plate, with deformity and impaired linear growth.
- Rickets occurs due to a deficiency in one of the two key components of bone: Ca and/or PO_4. This deficiency can be primary or secondary.
- Broadly speaking, the rickets syndromes can be classified by:
  - deficiency of vitamin D (with secondary deficiency of Ca and P)
  - nutritional deficiency of Ca
  - primary renal PO_4 wasting (hypophosphataemic rickets)
  - CKD (➔ see Chapter 18).
- Occasionally, more generalized proximal tubular dysfunction (e.g. glycosuria, aminoaciduria, acidosis, and LMWP) can be seen in vitamin D deficiency or Ca deficiency rickets. These findings thus do not always indicate a primary renal tubular problem such as renal Fanconi syndrome and should be reassessed when rickets is controlled.
- Glycosuria can also be seen with hypophosphataemic rickets.
- Table 7.5 summarizes the major clinical and biochemical features of the rickets syndromes, including therapy.
- PTH and ALP are elevated in all forms of rickets, reflecting the body's attempts to normalize plasma Ca and PO_4 levels by mobilization from the bone. These two parameters can thus be used as markers of rickets activity and treatment should aim at normalization of their levels.
- FGF23 has been identified as a major phosphaturic factor and is elevated in hypophosphataemic rickets.
- At presentation, it may be difficult to distinguish between vitamin D-deficient and hypophosphataemic rickets (unless plasma levels of vitamin D are available), as the elevated PTH induces renal PO_4 wasting. The initial treatment goal is thus to normalize PTH by vitamin D supplementation. Persistent renal PO_4 wasting with normal PTH argues for a primary renal defect in PO_4 transport.
- Attempts at normalization of plasma PO_4 levels in states of primary renal PO_4 wasting are usually futile: the more PO_4 is supplemented, the more is lost in the urine. Occasionally, plasma levels may return to normal, if obtained shortly after intake of PO_4 supplement.
- To avoid large swings in plasma PO_4 levels, supplementation should be spread throughout the day in four or more doses. It may be helpful to dissolve the daily dose of PO_4 supplement in a bottle of water and advise the patient to drink from this throughout the day.
- Table 7.6 lists PO_4 preparations available in the UK. At high doses, all PO_4 supplements can cause diarrhoea.
- Vitamin D supplementation with the goal of normalizing PTH and ALP in hypophosphataemic rickets is, in the authors' experience, key to optimizing growth and minimize skeletal deformities. However, ~50% of patients develop nephrocalcinosis. A good fluid intake should be encouraged to minimize urine Ca concentration.
- New treatments suppressing FGF23 levels (FGF23 antibodies) are currently being trialled in hypophosphataemic rickets.

Table 7.5 Rickets: causes and biochemical findings

Type	Cause	Biochemistry						Treatment
		Ca	PO$_4$	PTH	ALP	25 (OH) vit D	1,25 (OH) vit D	
Vitamin D related								
Nutritional/ deprivational	Lack of dietary vitamin D and/or lack of sunlight	↓↔	↓↔	↑	↑	↓	↓	Vitamin D2 or D3 at 1500–3000 IU/day (RDA in health is 7–10 micrograms/day or 280–400 IU/day) for 6–8 weeks, followed by prophylactic doses of 300–400 IU/day
Malabsorption	Malabsorption of vitamin and/or calcium	↓↔	↓↔	↑	↑	↓	↓	Treat underlying cause. Vitamin D supplements may be required
Pseudovitamin D deficiency (PDDR, VDDR type 1)	Mutations in 25-hydroxyvitamin D-1-alpha-hydroxylase genes	↓↔	↓↔	↑	↑	↔	↓	alfacalcidiol or calcitriol
Hypocalcaemic vitamin D resistant (HDRR, VDDR type II)	Mutations in the vitamin D receptor (VDR) gene. Inability of cells to respond to 1,25(OH)$_2$D	↓↔	↓↔	↑	↑	↔	↑	No satisfactory treatment. Nocturnal IV calcium infusions?

Calcium deficiency							
Calcium deficiency	Lack of calcium in diet	↓	↓↔	↑	↔	↔	Calcium supplement.
Hypophosphataemia							
Renal Fanconi syndrome	Loss of PO_4 in urine	↔	↓	↑	↔	↓↔	As per X-linked (see 'X-linked dominant', in this table)
Oncogenic	Tumour production of FGF23	↔	↓	↑	↔	↓↔	Treat tumour
Inherited hypophosphataemia							
X-linked dominant	Mutations in the *PHEX* gene causing phosphaturia plus inadequate synthesis of $1,25(OH)_2D$	↔	↓	↑	↔	↔	alfacalcidol at 25–50 ng/kg/day (maximum 2 micrograms/day) once daily. Oral PO_4 supplements: neutral PO_4 at 1–4 g/day (30–120 mmol/day) divided into 4–6 doses
Autosomal dominant	Mutation of the *FGF23* gene	↔	↓	↑	↔	↓↔	PO_4 supplementation
Autosomal hypercalciuric hypophosphataemic rickets	Recessive mutations in *SLC34A3* (NaPi-IIc). Also reported with dominant mutations in *SLC34A1* (NaPi-IIa).	↔	↓↔	↑	↔	↑↔	PO_4 supplementation

Table 7.6 Phosphate supplements

Preparation	P	K	Na
Phosphate-Sandoz® (also contains 800 mg per tablet of citrate), UK licensed	16.1 mmol	3.1 mmol	20.4 mmol
Na acid (di-hydrogen) phosphate, unlicensed special (special products)	1 mmol/mL	None	1 mmol/mL
K acid (di-hydrogen) phosphate, unlicensed special (special products)	1 mmol/mL	1 mmol/mL	None
K-Phos® neutral, film-coated tablet, 250 mg (Beach, US) import	8 mmol	1.1 mmol	13 mmol
Neutra-Phos® powder sachets (makes solution), Baker Norton, US	7.125 mmol	7.125 mmol	7.125 mmol
Neutra-Phos® K, powder sachets (makes solution), Baker Norton, US	7.125 mmol	14.25 mmol	None
K-Phos® original (Na free) tabs, Beach, US	4 mmol	3.7 mmol	None
K-Phos® MF tablet, Beach, US	4 mmol	1.1 mmol	2.9 mmol
K-Phos® No. 2, tablet, Beach, US	8 mmol	2.3 mmol	5.8 mmol

Further reading

Allgrove J, Shaw NJ. A practical approach to vitamin D deficiency and rickets. *Endocr Dev* 2015;28:119–133.

Tubulointerstitial nephritis

Basic principles

- In contrast to glomerular disorders, which typically present with oliguria, fluid retention, and hypertension, tubulointerstitial disorders usually maintain good, even increased urine output with low–normal BP and thus the possibility of kidney disease may not be considered initially.
- Presenting symptoms are often non-specific, such as malaise, fatigue, and polyuria.
- Clinical features are very similar to nephronophthisis (➔ see 'Nephronophthisis', p. 363), which is an important differential diagnosis.
- Renal dysfunction is revealed by severe uraemia. The reasons for the secondary decrease in glomerular filtration are complex and probably include tubuloglomerular feedback to limit fluid and electrolyte losses.
- TIN in children is usually acute (history of weeks to months), but chronic TIN (history of months to years) can be seen typically in the context of systemic diseases (➔ see 'Causes of chronic tubulointerstitial nephritis', p. 198).
- Acute TIN accounts for ~7% of AKI in children.
- In adults, ~70% of all cases of TIN are due to drug reactions and another 15% are infection associated. No good epidemiological data exist for children. In the authors' experience, idiopathic (presumed autoimmune) TIN, often associated with uveitis (TINU) is the most common aetiology of biopsy-proven TIN. Thus, the clinical experience from adult cases has limited relevance for paediatric patients.
- TIN can be a cause of renal transplant dysfunction, particularly with polyoma virus and *Cytomegalovirus* (CMV) infection.

Clinical features of acute tubulointerstitial nephritis

- Non-oliguric or polyuric.
- Oliguria may develop in more severe forms with advanced kidney impairment.
- Acute and progressive rise in plasma urea and creatinine.
- Laboratory parameters can reflect the whole spectrum of tubular dysfunction, including glycosuria, tubular proteinuria, acidosis, and isosthenuria.
- Normochromic normocytic anaemia may be observed in long-standing TIN, affecting the erythropoietin-producing peritubular cells.
- Haemolytic anaemia can accompany acute TIN caused by drugs.
- Uveitis is a common associated problem (TINU), which may be asymptomatic or show only minor symptoms, such as light sensitivity. In some children, uveitis precedes the TIN, in others, uveitis may develop later.
- Rarely, sensorineural deafness is observed as part of the TINU spectrum, which may respond to corticosteroid/immunosuppressant therapy.

Causes of acute tubulointerstitial nephritis

* *Idiopathic*: typically associated with uveitis and thought to be due to an autoimmune reaction against a common antigen in eye and kidney.
* *Drugs*—usually develops 1–3 weeks after exposure:
  * NSAIDs.
  * Rifampicin (TIN may occur much faster).
  * Meticillin.
  * Phenytoin.
  * Ciclosporin.
  * IV immunoglobulin.
  * Omeprazole.
  * Herbal medicines.
  * *Toxins*: heavy metals.
  * *NB*: anti-tubular basement membrane antibodies can occur in drug-induced TIN (➔ see 'Causes of chronic tubulointerstitial nephritis').
* *Infection*:
  * Viral (including HIV), bacterial (including TB), protozoal (including malaria), and fungal (including histoplasmosis).
  * Acute pyelonephritis.
* *Autoimmune disease*:
  * Complicating glomerulonephritides, e.g. SLE, IgA nephropathy.
  * *Vasculitis*: including Kawasaki disease (feature of the disease or complication of IV immunoglobulin therapy).
  * Henoch–Schönlein purpura (HSP).
  * Juvenile idiopathic arthritis.
  * Sarcoidosis.
  * Inflammatory bowel disease.
* In association with immunodeficiency or post bone marrow transplant.
* *Malignancy*: lymphoma.

Causes of chronic tubulointerstitial nephritis

This is uncommon as usually acute TIN resolves.
* Idiopathic.
* Autoimmune: ➔ see 'Autoimmune disease' bullet in 'Causes of acute tubulointerstitial nephritis'; may also be associated with anti-tubular basement membrane antibodies, sometimes in association with autoimmune enteropathy.
* Urate nephropathy: must examine renal biopsy under polarized light to detect urate crystals.
* Associated with cholestatic liver disease.
* Obstructive uropathy.
* Balkan nephropathy (non-inflammatory, chronic, slowly progressive interstitial kidney disease, frequently associated with urinary tract tumours in endemic areas).

Laboratory features

Blood
* Elevated urea and creatinine.
* Hyperchloraemic metabolic acidosis (normal anion gap) disproportionate to glomerular dysfunction.

- Hyperkalaemia (with severe uraemia); but hypokalaemia (due to renal wasting) is more commonly observed.
- Hypernatraemia with insufficient water intake.
- Hyperphosphataemia (with severe uraemia) or more typically hypophosphataemia.
- Hyperuricaemia.
- Elevated IgE.
- Eosinophilia.
- Anaemia.
- Leucocytosis, high erythrocyte sedimentation rate (ESR), and high C-reactive protein (CRP).

Urine
- Proteinuria (tubular): e.g. RBP:creatinine ratio.
- Microscopic haematuria.
- Elevated white cells in urine (eosinophiluria = >1% of all white cells in urine). Request Wright stain of urine to assess eosinophiluria.
- Isosthenuria.
- Glycosuria.
- Phosphaturia and decreased TRP: measure plasma and urine PO_4 simultaneously for this test.
- Bicarbonaturia.
- Aminoaciduria.

Renal ultrasound
- Increased renal size with loss of corticomedullary differentiation (acute TIN).
- Small kidneys in chronic TIN.

Ophthalmology review
- In view of the recognized association of TIN with uveitis (TINU), screening for uveitis is recommended for all children with biopsy-proven TIN, since uveitis may be asymptomatic until blindness occurs.
- If symptoms do occur, they include photophobia, eye pain, redness, eyelid oedema, and progressive loss of vision. Pupillary reaction may be sluggish. Changes are unilateral in 20%.
- Recurrence occurs in 40% and may progress in severity.
- This assessment is also important to screen for tapetoretinal degeneration, which can be observed as part of nephronophthisis.
- Since uveitis can develop after TIN, patients should be told to watch out for symptoms of light sensitivity or visual problems and ophthalmological follow-up for at least a year after presentation with TIN is recommended, even if no uveitis was present.

Renal biopsy
- Light microscopy in both acute and chronic TIN shows the presence of diffuse or patchy interstitial deposits consisting of activated lymphocytes, macrophages, plasma cells, polymorphonuclear leucocytes, and eosinophils in acute TIN and mainly lymphocytes in chronic TIN. Inflammatory cells can cause granulomas.
- Cortical tubules separated by expanded interstitium (oedema) in acute TIN.
- Interstitial fibrosis in chronic TIN.

- Tubular epithelial injury varying from degeneration to necrosis and focal loss of tubular basement membrane may be present in acute TIN. Tubular lumen may contain casts made of desquamated cells or blood.
- In chronic TIN, tubular atrophy and thickening of the tubular basement membrane are prominent.
- If high intratubular pressure is present (as in obstruction), renal tubules may be dilated.
- Generally kidneys are enlarged in acute TIN, and contracted and scarred in chronic TIN.
- Blood vessels and glomeruli are normal in acute TIN and in the early stages of chronic TIN, but periglomerular fibrosis and sclerosis develop during the course of chronic TIN.
- Inflammatory cells infiltrating the interstitium can cause granulomas, which ultimately become fibrotic.
- Immunofluorescence studies are generally negative for immune deposits.
- These biopsy findings can be confused with those of nephronophthisis.

Treatment of tubulointerstitial nephritis

- Supportive.
- Remove offending agent if possible (stop all drugs, ask about herbal medicines).
- Treatment for uveitis is with topical steroids and cycloplegics, and oral immunosuppression if this fails.
- There are no randomized controlled trials (RCTs) showing that corticosteroids are of benefit in TIN, and recovery may occur spontaneously or with removal of an identified cause. However, idiopathic TIN(U) typically responds well to treatment with corticosteroids. Typical dose—2 mg/kg prednisolone (maximum 60 mg) daily for 4–8 weeks, tapering over subsequent months once symptoms have improved.
  • If there is no clinical improvement with corticosteroids over 1–2 months, these should be discontinued and the differential diagnosis (especially nephronophthisis) revisited.
  • Immunosuppressants such as azathioprine and mycophenolate mofetil (MMF) have been used for TINU in combination with corticosteroids. MMF has been used more recently for steroid-resistant patients and where disease relapses occur with steroid withdrawal

Prognosis of tubulointerstitial nephritis

- The degree of interstitial fibrosis has been correlated with outcome in some studies, but in other studies there is no such relationship. These conflicting observations may be due to the patchy nature of the disease and the random sampling on renal biopsy.
- Prognosis is usually excellent for acute TIN.
- The prognosis for chronic TIN is guarded, with risk of progression to CKD stage 5.

Further reading

Joyce E, Glasner P, Ranganathan S, et al. Tubulointerstitial nephritis: diagnosis, treatment, and monitoring. *Pediatr Nephrol* 2017;32:577–587.

Renal calculi and nephrocalcinosis

Renal calculi

Types of calculi

- *Metabolic (~50%)*: supersaturation of stone-forming ions (Ca, phosphate, urate, oxalate, cystine) due to increased excretion, increased urinary concentration, alteration of ion solubility due to urine pH, or lack of normally produced inhibitors of crystal formation.
- *Infective (~25%)*: may occur in association with structural abnormalities of the urinary tract that cause stasis of urine; or with urease-producing organisms (particularly *Proteus* spp.) that break down urea to ammonia, resulting in an alkaline urine, and the precipitation of Ca phosphate and Mg ammonium phosphate (struvite) (Table 8.1).
- Idiopathic (~25%): no predisposition identified.

Presentation

- UTI.
- Pain: diffuse abdominal and/or ureteric colic (pain often absent/not perceived in children <5 years of age).
- Macroscopic or microscopic haematuria.
- AKI.
- Chronic ill health and anaemia.
- Dysuria or strangury (slow and painful micturition) due to bladder/ureteric calculi. Risk factors for bladder stones include cystinuria and augmented bladders.
- Incidental finding causing no symptoms.

Metabolic disorders that cause calculi

- *Hypercalciuria*: the commonest cause.
  - Idiopathic (majority).
  - Hypercalcaemic (rare as a cause of stones in children).
  - Can be associated with renal tubular dysfunction (e.g. RTA, Dent disease, Bartter syndrome, familial hypomagnesaemia with hypercalciuria).
- *Hyperoxaluria*: ➔ see 'Specific causes of calculi: investigation and management', p. 206.
  - Primary types 1, 2, and 3 (the association of nephrocalcinosis and renal/ureteric calculi is highly suggestive of primary hyperoxaluria (PH) type 1).
  - Enteric (associated with short-gut and malabsorption syndromes).
  - Idiopathic.
- Cystinuria.
- *Disorders of purine metabolism*:
  - Uric acid overproduction, e.g. following chemotherapy.
  - Renal hypouricaemia.
  - Xanthinuria.
  - 2,8-dihydroxyadenine calculi.
  - Lesch–Nyhan syndrome.

Table 8.1 Drugs/intoxications associated with stones

Drugs/intoxications associated with stones	Mechanism
Ampicillin	Precipitation of drug/metabolite in the urine
Triamterene	
sulfonamides	
Aciclovir	
Indinavir, lopinavir	
Ceftriaxone	
Furosemide	Increase in urinary Ca
Calcium	
Vitamin D	
Glucocorticoids	
Ethylene glycol	Metabolization to oxalate
Vitamin C	
Probenecid	Increasing urinary uric acid
Acetazolamide and other carbonic anhydrase inhibitors	Altering urinary pH

Environmental factors facilitating stone formation

- Low fluid intake due to urinary concentration and supersaturation. Stones can form after a single episode of severe dehydration.
- Diet: high salt, high protein.
- Immobilization: reduction of bone mass leads to increased Ca excretion.
- Augmented bladders: risk factor for bladder stones, presumably due to retention of mucus and bacterial colonization.

Investigations for all causes of calculi

- *An obstructive stone is an emergency.* Persistent obstruction and the potentially associated infection can cause permanent kidney damage.
- If an obstructive stone is suspected, perform immediate imaging and liaise with a urologist.
- Aetiological investigations (→ see 'Specific causes of calculi: investigation and management', p. 206) can be delayed until after the obstruction has been dealt with.

Radiological

- *US*: usually the first imaging modality. Acoustic shadowing and 'twinkle artefact' (on Doppler) are consistent with the presence of a stone. US will also help assess for obstruction. However, if obstruction has been present for longer and AKI has developed, hydronephrosis may not be obvious in the absence of urine production.
- *CT (helical, non-contrast)*: use for complex cases and where a ureteric stone is suspected.

- *Abdominal X-ray* (*beware:* purine stones are radiolucent).
- *DMSA:* in order to determine the extent of renal involvement.
  - DMSA can be combined with CT (single-photon emission computed tomography (SPECT)-CT) to combine functional and anatomical data.

Stone/gravel analysis

This is the most important tool to discover the underlying cause—the composition of the stone will give strong clues towards the aetiology (e.g. oxalate vs struvite). Any fragment excreted should be sent for analysis and patients may need to sieve their urine for a while to enhance the chances of stone recovery.

Urine

If no underlying disorder is known and if no stone analysis was done, a full metabolic screen should be performed; otherwise, only selected tests will be necessary. The metabolic screen can be started with random urine tests (in small children) but abnormalities should best be confirmed via a 24 h urine collection, if possible. A concurrent urine creatinine should always be performed to assess completeness of collection (expected creatinine excretion 0.1–0.2 mmol/kg/day, depending on muscle mass).

- Microscopy and culture (spot sample) to assess for infective aetiology.
- Ca (normal <0.1 mmol/kg/day): for incomplete collections, the Ca/creatinine ratio can be used, which varies with age (Table 8.2).
- Oxalate (normal <460 µmol/day/1.73m²). Alternatively, the oxalate/creatinine ratio can be used for a spot urine (Table 8.3).
- Urate (normal <0.1 mmol/kg/day)/creatinine ratio (Table 8.4).
- Urine amino acids (assess for cystinuria—increased excretion of dibasic amino acids).
- Citrate normal range for all ages: female—0.11–0.55 mmol/mmol creatinine; male—0.04–0.33 mmol/mmol creatinine (Tables 8.2–8.4).

Blood

- U&Es, creatinine.
- Ca, Mg, phosphate, albumin.
- Total carbon dioxide (TCO_2) (or bicarbonate).
- Urate and specific purine metabolic investigations if necessary.
- PTH.
- Genetics: to be considered in patients with features suggestive of an inherited predisposition to stones (→ see 'Specific causes of calculi: investigation and management', p. 206).

Table 8.2 Age-dependent normal values for urine Ca to creatinine ratios

Age (years)	Ca:Cr (mmol/mmol)	Ca:Cr (mg/mg)
<1	0.09–2.2	0.03–0.78
1–2	0.07–1.5	0.02–0.53
2–3	0.06–1.4	0.02–0.50
3–5	0.05–1.1	0.02–0.39
5–7	0.04–0.8	0.01–0.28
7–17	0.04–0.7	0.01–0.25

Table 8.3 Age-dependent normal values for urine oxalate to creatinine ratios

Age (years)	Oxalate:Cr (μmol/mmol)
<1 year	4–98
1–4 years	4–72
5–12 years	3–71
>12 years	1–38

Table 8.4 Age-dependent normal values for urine urate to creatinine ratios

Age	Urate:Cr (mmol/mmol)
0–7 days	0.12–1.96
7 days–2 years	0.42–1.53
2–6 years	0.57–1.35
6–10 years	0.39–0.85
10–18 years	0.15–0.67

Treatment of calculi

- *Medical*:
  - High fluid intake. This is obviously the most important and effective measure, as it dilutes the urine and thus the substances at risk of precipitation; aim for >1.5 L/m²/day. Advise to minimize or prevent/take action during episodes of dehydration.
  - Treatment of specific underlying metabolic disorder, if present (➲ see 'Specific causes of calculi: investigation and management', p. 206).
- *Surgical*: small stones (<5 mm) that are not causing any symptoms and are in peripheral areas of the kidney may not require intervention.
- *Extracorporeal shock wave lithotripsy*: often first-line therapy but not good for multiple stones. Rarely, fragments may cause obstruction.
- Percutaneous nephrostomy may be needed as a temporary measure if there is obstruction to urine flow.
- *Percutaneous nephrolithotomy*: particularly for complex stones.
- *Ureteroscopy*: for ureteric stones.
- *Open surgery*: very rarely needed, e.g. associated with PUJ obstruction.

Further reading

Hernandez JD, Ellison JS, Lendvay TS. Current trends, evaluation, and management of pediatric nephrolithiasis. *JAMA Pediatr* 2015;169:964–970.

Specific causes of calculi: investigation and management

Hyperoxaluria

Primary hyperoxalurias are inherited metabolic disorders with increased production of oxalate (➜ see 'Primary hyperoxaluria').

Secondary hyperoxaluria is due to increased enteric oxalate absorption. Oxalate absorption is increased if there is not enough Ca to bind oxalate in the gut. It occurs in:

- malabsorption syndromes (e.g. inflammatory bowel disease, cystic fibrosis, short-gut syndrome)
- low-Ca diets.

Specific treatment
A low-oxalate diet, oral citrate, or bicarbonate.

Primary hyperoxaluria

- AR disorders of increased oxalate production.
- Based on the underlying genetics, three types are recognized (see Fig. 8.1): (1) PH type 1: loss of function of the peroxisomal enzyme alanine-glyoxylate transferase (AGXT); (2) PH type 2: loss of function of the cytoplasmic enzyme glyoxylate reductase/hydroxypyruvate reductase (GR/HPR); and (3) PH type 3: loss of function of the mitochondrial enzyme 4-hydroxy-2-oxoglutarate aldolase 1 (HOGA1).
- Epidemiology: PH1 has an estimated incidence of 1:100,000 live births, PH2 is exceedingly rare, and PH3 somewhere in between.

Clinical features
Age at presentation and severity of symptoms is highly variable even within families with an identical genotype.

PH type 1
- Most commonly presents in childhood with recurrent nephrolithiasis or nephrocalcinosis.
- Associated symptoms include polyuria, dysuria, and haematuria.
- Rarely, diagnosed in late adulthood based on occasional stone passage.
- In the most severe form, PH1 presents in infancy with rapidly progressive kidney failure, strikingly echo-bright kidneys, and extrarenal oxalosis, especially in bones, leading to pain and erythropoietin-resistant anaemia. Other organs may be affected including:
  - heart: arrhythmias, heart block
  - nerves: neuropathy
  - retina: flecked retinopathy.

PH type 2
Typically presents during adolescence with recurrent oxalate stones. Progressive CKD occurs in ~10% of patients.

PH type 3
Appears to have the mildest phenotype, presenting with oxalate stones. Progressive CKD is uncommon.

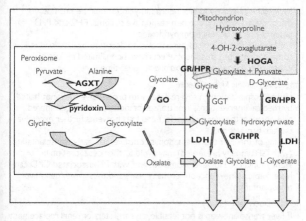

Fig. 8.1 Simplified diagram of a hepatic cell with metabolic pathways pertinent for the different types of primary hyperoxaluria. Decreased metabolism of glyoxylate by either AGXT or GR/HPR leads to increased conversion to oxalate. AGXT, alanine-glyoxylate aminotransferase (PH1); GGT: gamma-glutamyl transpeptidase; GR/HPR, glyoxylate/hydroxypyruvate reductase (PH2); HOGA: 4-hydroxy-2-oxoglutarate aldolase 1 (PH3); LDH, lactate dehydrogenase.

Diagnosis

- Elevated urinary oxalate levels without apparent cause
  (➔ see 'Hyperoxaluria') suggest PH1.
- Plasma oxalate levels typically remain normal (<10 μmol/L), unless there is impaired GFR (<30 mL/min/1.73 m²).
- In all patients with ESKD, plasma oxalate levels are elevated, but usually <50 μmol/L. Thus, a plasma oxalate level >50 μmol/L is highly suggestive of PH in a patient with unexplained ESKD and compatible clinical features
- A definitive diagnosis requires genetic testing.

Treatment

Nephrolithiasis and normal GFR

- High fluid intake (>1.5 L/m²/day) is recommended.
- Citrate can be used to inhibit crystal formation (0.5–1 mmol ~0.1–0.2 g/kg/day).
- Dietary modification is less helpful, as the oxalate is derived from internal metabolism.
- Pyridoxine, the cofactor of AGXT, in supraphysiological doses (2–5 mg/kg starting dose, can be increased up to 20 mg/kg) should be tried early in patients with PH1. Approximately one-third of patients experience reduction of oxalate levels with pyridoxine, sometimes back to the normal range. Typically, these are patients with a particular mutation, G170R, but there is no complete genotype–phenotype concordance.

Pyridoxine can rarely induce neuropathy and should be promptly discontinued in pyridoxine non-responsive patients. PH2 and PH3 patients do not benefit from pyridoxine.

* *Oxalobacter formigenes* has been shown to decrease oxalate load in some patients, but treatment effects have been limited by loss of intestinal colonization with *Oxalobacter* over time.

Progressive chronic kidney disease

* Liver transplantation: in severe cases with progressive CKD not halted by medical interventions, liver transplantation should be considered, as it corrects the metabolic defect and thus prevents further excessive oxalate production.
* Timing of the liver transplantation is controversial: early transplantation (with GFR mostly preserved) may avoid further deterioration in kidney function. However, some patients with PH-associated CKD can have stable kidney function for many years and thus avoid/delay liver transplantation.

Renal replacement therapy

* If liver transplantation is not feasible, an early start of renal replacement therapy (GFR 30–40 mL/min/1.73 m²), may ameliorate systemic oxalosis.
* Plasma oxalate levels need to be monitored and should be kept below the saturation level of ~40 μmol/L.
* Unfortunately, oxalate is cleared poorly by dialysis. Haemodialysis with high-flux membranes has the highest oxalate clearance, but even with daily sessions is typically not sufficient to maintain plasma oxalate levels in the desired range. Occasionally, a combination of haemo- and peritoneal dialysis has been used.
* Isolated renal transplantation improves oxalate clearance, but carries the high risk of graft failure due to recurrent oxalosis. Thus, combined (or sequential) liver and kidney transplantation is the preferred option in patients with advanced renal failure.

Future outlook

An approach of 'substrate reduction' by knocking down glyoxylate oxidase (using 'RNA interference'), the enzyme upstream of AGXT, appears a promising novel treatment for PH1 based on early-phase trials.

Further reading

Cochat P, Rumsby G. Primary hyperoxaluria. *N Engl J Med* 2013;369:649–658.

Cystinuria

* AR or AD disorder causing ~10% of childhood stones.
* Epidemiology: incidence estimated at 1:10,000 live births.
* Typical hexagonal crystals are present in the urine sediment.
* Often presents with bladder stones. In fact, cystine was first isolated from a bladder stone (hence the name 'cystine').
* Diagnosis is by measurement of urinary cystine >100 μmol/mmol creatinine (normal <30 μmol/mmol). Some mutation carriers may have an elevated urinary cystine concentration, but be asymptomatic.

- Can be caused by mutations in two genes, *SLC3A1* (encoding rBAT, a necessary transporter subunit) and *SCL7A9* (encoding the actual transporter).
  - SLC7A9 transports dibasic amino acids: cystine, ornithine, lysine, and arginine. Thus, the excretion of all these amino acids is increased in cystinuria, but only cystine is clinically relevant.
  - Cystine is poorly soluble at a pH between 5 and 7 and stone formation is higher with concentrations >1 mmol/L.
- Can be categorized according to genetics into three types:
  - *A*: recessive mutations in *SLC3A1* (45% of patients, heterozygotes unaffected).
  - *B*: recessive mutations in *SLC7A9* (>50%: heterozygotes have moderately increased cystine excretion).
  - *AB*: heterozygote mutations in both *SLC3A1* and *SLC7A9* (2%).

Specific treatment
- At pH >8, solubility increases threefold so treatment is by alkalinization of the urine (potassium citrate start at 0.5 mmol/kg/day in three divided doses).
- Some complex patients require chelating agents such as penicillamine and tiopronin, which cleave the disulphide bond of cystine to form complexes with cysteine, which are better soluble. Dose of penicillamine is 20–30 mg/kg given in two doses/day. Potential side effects include proteinuria, rash, hair loss, arthralgia, anaemia, and pyridoxine deficiency. Patients need to be monitored regularly. Side effects may be minimized by starting at lower doses with gradual increase. Pyridoxine supplementation may be required with long-term treatment.

Purine stones

- High urate levels may occur due to rapid cell turnover in leukaemia or lymphoma, particularly after commencement of chemotherapy (➔ see 'Tumour lysis syndrome', p. 446).
- Lesch–Nyhan syndrome is an AR disorder due to deficiency of hypoxanthine-guanine phosphoribosyltransferase. Presentation may be with choreoathetosis, self-mutilation, urate calculi, and CKD.
- Glycogen storage disease type 1 may increase urate excretion.
- Xanthinuria is an AR disorder due to deficiency of xanthine oxidase, which converts xanthine to uric acid. There is, therefore, hypouricaemia and xanthine stones.
- Adenine phosphoribosyltransferase deficiency (AR disorder) results in 2,8-dihydroxyadenine rather than adenine. 2,8-dihydroxyadenine is relatively insoluble, resulting in calculi formation.
- Renal hypouricaemia can be caused by mutations in the renal urate transporter genes *SLC2A9* or *SLC22A12*; the consequent high urine urate levels predispose to stones.

Specific treatment
Allopurinol is used, monitor with urine and blood purine metabolite analyses.

Hypercalciuria

* The commonest metabolic abnormality found in paediatric stone formers.
* Ca excretion is affected by Na intake: Ca reabsorption in the proximal tubule (PT) parallels Na reabsorption. Consequently, changes that lead to an expansion of the extracellular volume, such as a high Na intake, will decrease Na and thus Ca reabsorption in PT, and vice versa. This is used for therapeutic purpose, when thiazide diuretics are prescribed (see following section on specific treatment): the resulting volume depletion enhances Na, and thus Ca reabsorption in the PT.

For causes, see 'Nephrocalcinosis', p. 211.

Specific treatment
* Low salt intake (to reduce urinary Ca):
  * Thiazide diuretics (in combination with a low salt diet) reduce urinary Ca excretion and can be helpful in persistent hypercalciuric stone formers.
* Potassium supplements also inhibit distal sodium reabsorption and thus reduce urinary Ca excretion.
* Citrate forms soluble complexes with Ca. A typical treatment dose is 0.5 mmol/kg/day of potassium citrate. Care needs to be taken, as excess alkalinization of urine enhances phosphate precipitation. Consider dose reduction if urine pH >7.5.
* Bicarbonate supplementation increases urinary citrate and can thus be substituted. The same concern about urinary alkalization applies.

Further reading

Oliveira B, Kleta R, Bockenhauer D, et al. Genetic, pathophysiological, and clinical aspects of nephrocalcinosis. *Am J Physiol Renal Physiol* 2016;311:F1243–F1252.

Nephrocalcinosis

An increase in the Ca content of the cortex or medulla. Typically associated with (previous) hypercalciuria. US shows a typical pattern of hyperechoic medullae, which can be graded according to severity. If there is doubt, a single-slice CT scan can confirm that this is due to Ca.

Causes of medullary nephrocalcinosis

- Prematurity (presumed to prolonged furosemide use).
- Inherited disorders with increased Ca excretion (➔ see also 'Tubular disorders'), e.g. Bartter syndrome, Dent disease, Lowe syndrome, dRTA, familial hypomagnesaemia–hypercalciuria–nephrocalcinosis.
- Hyperparathyroidism.
- Hyper- and hypothyroidism.
- Idiopathic hypercalciuria.
- Immobilization.
- Lesch–Nyhan syndrome.
- Malignancy with paraneoplastic calciotropic hormone production.
- *Medications*: furosemide, dexamethasone, thus very commonly seen in premature babies.
- *Nutrition*: parenteral vitamins A, C, or D intoxication.
- Enamel–renal syndrome (amelogenesis imperfecta and nephrocalcinosis; inherited dental disorder associated with hypocalciuria, yet patients develop nephrocalcinosis).

Cause of cortical nephrocalcinosis

Cortical necrosis.

Causes of both cortical and medullary nephrocalcinosis

- Hyperoxaluria:
  - Primary types 1, 2, or 3 (the association of nephrocalcinosis and calculi is highly suggestive of primary hyperoxaluria).
  - Enteric.
  - Idiopathic.
- Hypercalcaemia.
- Lipoid (fat) necrosis.
- Sickle cell disease.

Glomerular disease

Overview of inherited glomerular diseases

Basic principles

The glomerular barrier consists of three layers:
* *Endothelium*: formed by vascular endothelial cells. No inherited kidney disease has yet been localized to this layer.
* *Basement membrane*: defects in this layer are typically associated with haematuria (e.g. Alport syndrome (AS)), except Pierson syndrome, a form of congenital nephrotic syndrome due to mutations in the basement membrane protein laminin-B2.
* *Epithelium*: formed by podocytes. Inherited diseases affecting podocyte function result in proteinuria/nephrotic syndrome (→ see 'Nephrotic syndromes: definitions').

Nephrotic syndrome

* In up to 30% of patients with steroid-resistant nephrotic syndrome (SRNS) an underlying genetic basis can be identified.
  * >30 disease genes have been described (see Table 9.1) and the list is constantly expanding.
* Nephrotic syndrome can occur in the context of mitochondrial cytopathies and these should always be considered as they are potentially treatable, e.g. in cases of coenzyme Q10 (ubiquinone) deficiencies.
* Recessive mutations in *EMP2* have been identified in 3 families with steroid-sensitive nephrotic syndrome (SSNS) in one study, but further patients have not yet been reported, nor has this gene been identified in GWAS of SSNS, making it unlikely that it is a common cause of SSNS.
* Recessive mutations in *MAGI2, TNS2, DLC1, CDK20, ITSN1, ITSN2* have been associated with partially treatment sensitive nephrotic syndrome.

The identification of a genetic cause should prompt careful consideration of further management:
* A biopsy is unlikely to provide important information.
* There are no data to support the use of aggressive immunosuppression such as high-dose methylprednisolone or cyclophosphamide in most Mendelian forms of SRNS.
* There are reports of patients with SRNS due to mutations in the *WT1* gene, who experienced partial or even complete remission with ciclosporin, which may be due to effects beyond immunosuppression, as calcineurin inhibitors have been shown to stabilize the podocyte actin skeleton. Use of an immunosuppressive drug in patients with *WT1* mutations must be carefully considered, however, as it would likely increase the already high cancer risk.
* There is also anecdotal evidence of patients with mutations in other Mendelian forms of SRNS, who have improved with immunosuppression (see Table 9.1).
* Mutations in *NPHS1* are the most common cause of congenital nephrotic syndrome and the clinical course is usually severe. However, there appears to be some genotype–phenotype correlation: a few patients homozygous for the R1160X mutation have an initial severe presentation, but then spontaneous improvement and even resolution

Table 9.1 Known disease genes in steroid-resistant nephrotic syndrome

Gene	OMIM	Inheritance	Onset	Disease
NPHS1	602716	AR	Infant/child	SRNS only
NPHS2	604766	AR	Infant to adult	SRNS only[a]
PLCE1	608414	AR	Infant	SRNS only[a]
CD2AP	604241	AD (AR)	Adult/(infant)	SRNS only
TRPC6	603652	AD	Adult/child	SRNS only
ACTN4	604638	AD	Adult	SRNS only
INF2	610982	AD	Adult/child	SRNS only
CRB2	616220	AR	Infant/child	SRNS only or ventriculomegaly with cystic kidneys
PTPRO	614196	AR	Child	SRNS only
ARHGDIA	615244	AR	Infant	SRNS ± neurological problems
ANLN	616032	AD	Adult/child	SRNS only
NUP85, 107, 133, 160	616730	AR	Child	SRNS
NUP93	616892	AR	Child	SRNS
NUP205	616893	AR	Child	SRNS
MYO1E	614131	AR	Child	SRNS only
FAT1		AR	Child	Glomerulotubular nephropathy ± neurological problems
SYNPO	616032	AD	Adult/child	SRNS only
ITGA3	614748	AR	Infant	Pulmonary fibrosis, epidermolysis bullosa and congenital NS
DGKE	615008	AR	Child	SRNS[a] or atypical HUS
Syndromes				
WT1	607102	AD	Infant	Denys–Drash syndrome, Frasier syndrome[a]
Lamb2	150325	AR	Infant	Pierson syndrome
ITGB4	147557	AR	Infant	Epidermolysis bullosa
LMX1B	602575	AD	Adult/child	Nail-patella syndrome
SCARB2	602257	AR	Child	Action-myoclonus renal failure syndrome
SMARCAL1	606622	AR	Child	Schimke immuno-osseous dysplasia

(Continued)

Table 9.1 (Contd.)

Gene	OMIM	Inheritance	Onset	Disease
WDR73	251300	AR	infant	Galloway–Mowat syndrome
COL4A3, -4, -5	301050	AR, AD, XR, XD	Child/adult	Alport syndrome
Mitochondrial cytopathies				
ADCK4	615573	AR	Child	COQ10 deficiency[b]
COQ2,9	609825	AR	Infant	COQ10 deficiency[b]
PDSS2	610564	AR	Infant	COQ10 deficiency[b]
MTTL1	590050	Mitochondrial	Infant	MELAS

NS, nephrotic syndrome; MELAS, myopathy, encephalopathy, lactic acidosis, and stroke-like episodes.

[a] Anecdotal evidence of response to immunosuppression; [b] may improve with ubiquinone supplementation.

of the nephrotic syndrome later in childhood. This needs to be considered before embarking on aggressive therapy in infancy, such as nephrectomies. Moreover, some cases of childhood-onset SRNS are due to NPHS1 mutations and these patients have at least one 'milder' mutation with presumed residual nephrin function.

• Mutations in COL4A3, -4, or -5, the genes underlying AS, can sometimes present with nephrotic syndrome and FSGS on light microscopy (➔ see 'Alport syndrome and thin basement membrane nephropathy').

• Mutations in genes involved in tubular protein reabsorption, such as CUBN (Immerslund–Grasbeck syndrome) and CLC5 (Dent disease), are sometimes identified in patients with nephrotic-range proteinuria. These patients typically do not have oedema and analysis of urine protein excretion will show predominantly LMWP.

Further reading

Lovric S, Ashraf S, Tan W, et al. Genetic testing in steroid-resistant nephrotic syndrome: when and how? Nephrol Dial Transplant 2016;31:1802–1813.

Alport syndrome and thin basement membrane nephropathy

Definitions

- *Alport syndrome (AS)*: this is a multisystem disorder including nephritis, sensorineural deafness, and often eye abnormalities. The severity of the individual symptoms is variable. Classical AS is due to mutations in type IV collagen (see Table 9.2).
- *Thin basement membrane nephropathy (TBMN)*: this is a histological diagnosis, defined by attenuation of the basement membrane. It is often equated with benign familial haematuria, but this has been shown to be incorrect. Patients with AS can initially have a picture of TBMN and a substantial portion of patients with TBMN experience progressive CKD. Thus, the finding of TBMN on biopsy in a child does not allow an accurate prediction of prognosis.

Genetics

- AS is due to structural abnormalities of the basement membrane:
  - A key component of the basement membrane is type IV collagen, which in itself is a composite of so-called alpha chains.
  - There are six genes encoding these alpha chains, COL4A1–COL4A6, and chains come together to form a trimer, which then assembles with another trimer to form type IV collagen.
  - These chains have specific assembly partners, as well as tissue and developmental expression.
  - Collagen 4 formed by the alpha-3, -4, and -5 chains is the major collagenous constituent of mature basement membranes in the glomerulus, cochlea, cornea, lens, and retina. Mutations in the genes encoding these three chains cause AS (Table 9.2).
- The most common underlying gene (80%) is COL4A5, which is located on the X-chromosome and thus affected patients are almost exclusively males.
- Heterozygous mutations in the COL4A genes are often associated with TBMN. However, in >5% of patients with AS, only heterozygous mutations in COL4A3 or COL4A4 are found (AD AS). Females, carrying COL4A5 mutations can have a broad spectrum of severity, presumably due to random X-inactivation (➤ see 'Female carriers of X-linked Alport syndrome').

Table 9.2 Genes underlying Alport-like syndromes

Gene	OMIM	Inheritance	Extrarenal symptoms
COL4A5	301050	X-linked	Eye, ear
COL4A3	120070	AR (AD)	Eye, ear
COL4A4	120131	AR (AD)	Eye, ear
MYH9	160775	AD	Ear, platelets, leucocytes

Heterozygous mutations in COL4A3, 4, and 5 can be associated with both AS and TBMN.

* A substantial portion of cases with TBMN have no identifiable mutation in the *COL4A* genes.
* A different form of hereditary nephritis and deafness is due to mutations in *MYH9*, a gene encoding a myosin heavy chain, and is further associated with macrothrombocytes (Epstein syndrome) and leucocyte inclusions (Fechtner syndrome).

Histology

* Light microscopic changes are only seen in advanced stages of AS. The characteristic changes are seen on electron microscopy—thickening of the capillary wall and lamellation of the basement membrane ('basket weave pattern') in AS and only thinning of the basement membrane in TBMN. However, there is no clear distinction between these two entities.
* The diagnostic role of the biopsy is increasingly being replaced by genetic testing.

Clinical features

* A child presenting with haematuria, particularly if intermittent macroscopic and persistent microscopic, should be assessed for symptoms associated with AS, particular if there is a family history of:
  * sensorineural deafness (with *COL4A* mutations)
  * eye abnormalities (with *COL4A* mutations): anterior lenticonus, dot-fleck retinopathy, recurrent corneal erosions
  * leiomyomatosis (appears to be restricted to individuals carrying an X-chromosomal deletion involving *COL4A5* and *COL4A6*)
  * giant platelets and leucocyte inclusions (with *MYH9* mutations).
* 100% of males and ~95% of female carriers of *COL4A5* mutations have microscopic haematuria, often with intermittent gross haematuria.
* Proteinuria in AS is usually a later feature, typically occurring in late childhood. However, some patients initially present with nephrotic syndrome and FSGS on biopsy.
* CKD stage 5 occurs in virtually all males with X-linked AS, typically between 20 and 60 years of age.

Treatment

* Angiotensin blockade is considered the standard of care in AS with overt proteinuria.
* There is an increasing amount of clinical data suggesting that blockade of the renin–angiotensin–aldosterone system (RAAS) with an ACE inhibitor or ARBs delays the progression of CKD in AS, even before the onset of pathological proteinuria, and should thus be strongly considered in patients with genetically confirmed AS, even before there is overt proteinuria.
* Transplantation in AS can be complicated by anti-GBM disease, caused by antibodies against type 4 collagen, typically the alpha-3 chain. This causes a crescentic nephritis, which is associated with a very high incidence of graft loss. Prognosis is very poor for recurrence after a second transplant.
* Live donors from the family must have AS excluded.

Further reading

Kashtan C. Alport syndrome: facts and opinions. F1000Res 2017;6:50.

Female carriers of X-linked Alport syndrome

- Female carriers of X-linked AS have a widely variable disease outcome with some having normal urinalysis and kidney function while others develop progressive CKD and deafness.
- There is also inconsistency in the disease in females within the same family so looking in detail at the genetic mutation is not always helpful. This may be due to differences in inactivation in the X-chromosome: early in development either the maternal or paternal X-chromosome is randomly switched off so that a girl has a mixture of cells with either the maternal or paternal X-chromosome. Usually, therefore, 50% of the active X-chromosomes would be of maternal origin while the remaining 50% would be of paternal origin. However, this can be skewed and it is likely that severe skewing of X-inactivation in favour of a genetic defect may be responsible for the different phenotypes in females.
- Up to 12% of females require renal replacement therapy by the age of 40 compared to 90% of males. By the age of 60, 15–30% of women need renal replacement therapy.
- For this reason, female relatives of a boy with X-linked AS who are assessed for kidney donation should have genetic testing performed. Mutation carriers should be discouraged from donation.
- The risk of hearing loss increases with age and is ~10% by the age of 40.
- Hearing loss and CKD progression are linked.
- RAAS blockade can slow progression of CKD and has been recommended in those with microalbuminuria, hypertension, or biopsy evidence of AS (lamellated basement membrane).

Further reading

Rheault MN. Women and Alport syndrome. *Pediatr Nephrol* 2012;27:41–46.

Acute nephritis (acute nephritic syndrome)

Definition

Acute glomerular injury with:
* AKI (oliguria, uraemia, elevated creatinine)
* hypertension (salt and water retention)
* haematuria (microscopic or macroscopic) with red cell casts on microscopy
* peripheral and/or pulmonary oedema
* proteinuria, which can reach nephrotic range (>200 mg/mmol) ('nephritic/nephrotic syndrome').

Differential diagnosis of acute nephritis in children

* Post infectious: usually post streptococcal, accounting for ~80% of cases.
* Other post-infectious causes:
  * Bacteria: *Staphylococcus aureus; Streptococcus pneumoniae; Mycoplasma pneumoniae, Escherichia coli, Yersinia, Campylobacter, Salmonella, Syphilis*, TB.
  * Viruses: Epstein–Barr virus (EBV), CMV, herpes simplex virus (HSV), varicella zoster virus (VZV), parvovirus B19, hepatitis B and C.
  * Rickettsiae: Rocky Mountain spotted fever, Q fever (*Coxiella burnetii*), *Legionella pneumophila*.
  * Fungi: *Candida; Aspergillus*; histoplasmosis, *Cryptococcus, Pneumocystis jirovecii, Nocardia*.
  * Parasites: malaria, schistosomiasis, leishmaniasis, trypanosomiasis, filariasis, trichinosis, *Echinococcus*, toxoplasmosis.
* Henoch–Schönlein purpura.
* IgA nephropathy.
* SLE.
* C3 glomerulopathy (C3G), ANCA-associated vasculitides (granulomatosis with polyangiitis (GPA) formerly known as Wegener's granulomatosis; microscopic polyangiitis; eosinophilic granulomatosis with polyangiitis (EGPA) formerly known as Churg–Strauss syndrome; renal limited vasculitis).
* Ventriculoatrial shunt nephritis.
* HUS.
* Goodpasture syndrome (idiopathic and after transplantation in AS).
* Thrombotic thrombocytopenic purpura.

Post-streptococcal glomerulonephritis

This is the commonest cause of acute glomerulonephritis (GN):
* May follow 1–2 weeks after infection of the throat or up to 6 weeks after infection of the skin (typically in the child with eczema) with group A beta-haemolytic *Streptococcus*.
* Presentation is with haematuria (urine tea or coca-cola coloured), proteinuria, oliguria, hypertension, and oedema.
* Antistreptolysin O (ASO) titre is raised in the majority of pharyngeal infections but may not be after a skin infection. It may be positive in up to 20% of healthy children.

- The streptozyme assay detects antibodies to other streptococcal antigens (e.g. DNAse B), therefore improving the chance of detection of infection.
- C3 is low and deposits can be seen in the glomeruli as 'humps' in the subepithelium (➔ see 'C3 glomerulopathy'). This leads to an inflammatory infiltrate ('exudative' GN).
- C4 is usually normal (unlike SLE, endocarditis, and shunt nephritis).
- C3 returns to normal by 6–8 weeks so if a low level persists, consider C3G or SLE.
- Treatment with penicillin is necessary to prevent spread to contacts, but will not help the nephritis.
- Hypertension may respond to furosemide as it is principally due to fluid overload.
- Severity and duration of nephritis is variable, but mostly resolves within 2–3 weeks.
- Renal biopsy is indicated:
  - in the acute phase if there is nephrotic syndrome and a rapidly rising creatinine, which is suggestive of a rapidly progressive (crescentic) glomerulonephritis (RPGN; ➔ see Chapter 11)
  - for prognosis and to ensure that the diagnosis is correct, where there is:
    - abnormal creatinine at 6 weeks
    - low C3 >3 months
    - proteinuria >100 mg/mmol for 6 months. Use the first urine of the morning whenever possible to exclude any orthostatic element.
- Microscopic haematuria alone may persist for 1–2 years and is of no long-term relevance.
- Immunosuppression is only to be considered if there is crescentic nephritis on biopsy. However, even then its use is controversial. There are well-documented descriptions of patients with very significant crescentic changes who have been treated conservatively (without corticosteroids) with good renal outcome, whereas there are also many reports of patients who have been given pulsed IV methylprednisolone in this situation.
- Based on the overall excellent prognosis of children with post-infectious glomerulonephritis (PIGN; <1% will develop CKD) the vast majority will be treated with supportive care, and antibiotics to eradicate the offending organism to prevent further spread. For the rare case where there is RPGN and severe crescentic change, steroids may have a role but such cases should be considered individually.

Causes of hypocomplementaemic nephritis

- PIGN.
- C3G and immune complex-mediated glomerulonephritis (ICGN).
- SLE.
- Shunt nephritis:
  - Nephritis due to infection of vascular access and ventriculoatrial shunts and infective endocarditis.
  - Commonest bacterium is *Staphylococcus*.

- May all present with fever, arthralgia, hepatosplenomegaly, AND lethargy
- Treatment is with antibiotics and removal of the infected shunt or line.
- C3 and C4 levels:
  - C3 alone is often decreased in infectious causes and C3G.
  - C3 and C4 are often both decreased in SLE.
  - C4 alone is characteristically decreased in immune complex diseases particularly vasculitis and hepatitis B and C.

Investigation of acute nephritis: generic investigations for all patients

- FBC, blood film, and ESR.
- CRP.
- Blood culture.
- U&Es, creatinine, albumin, bicarbonate, LFTs, Ca, PO_4, glucose.
- ASO titre, anti-DNaseB.
- Urine culture, microscopy for casts, and Ua:Ucr.
- Throat swab.
- C3/C4, ANA, ds-DNA, and ANCA.
- Renal US.

Specific tests for certain patients

- Blood film and LDH if HUS is suspected.
- Direct Coombs test and T-antigen (if available) if pneumococcal HUS is suspected.
- Stool culture and *Escherichia coli* 0157:H7 serology if STEC-HUS is suspected.
- Blood cultures if sepsis is suspected.
- Chest X-ray if pulmonary oedema or sepsis is suspected.
- C3 nephritic factor (C3NeF) if C3 low and C3G is suspected.
- Immunoglobulins (particularly IgA), if post-infectious causes excluded and IgA nephropathy could be a cause (➔ see 'IgA nephropathy').
- Anti-GBM antibodies if haemoptysis and Goodpasture syndrome are suspected:
  - Goodpasture syndrome is one of the 'pulmonary-renal syndromes' characterized by pulmonary haemorrhage (usually alveolar haemorrhage) and crescentic nephritis. Other causes of pulmonary-renal syndromes include SLE, GPA, microscopic polyangiitis, and HSP.
  - Goodpasture syndrome typically occurs at adolescence but can occur in younger children in whom haemoptysis may not be a feature.
  - Goodpasture syndrome is an autoimmune immune complex-mediated disease. GN and pulmonary haemorrhage occur with little or no involvement of other systems.
  - The presence of anti-GBM antibodies in peripheral blood confirms the diagnosis.
  - Treatment comprises early corticosteroids, cyclophosphamide, and plasmapheresis.

- The prognosis appears to be good if treatment is started early, although published data relating to long-term outcomes in children are lacking.
- Anti-GBM antibodies can also form following renal transplantation for AS, and are a cause of graft loss in this context (➔ see 'Alport syndrome and thin basement membrane nephropathy').

Indications/considerations for renal biopsy

- RPGN: defined as glomerular disease (proteinuria, haematuria, and red cell casts) accompanied by rapid loss of renal function with rising creatinine over days to weeks.
- C3 depressed for >3 months since in post-infectious stage the C3 will have returned to normal by then.
- Nephrotic-range proteinuria (spot Ua:Ucr of >200 mg/mmol).
- Immunology suggestive of cause other than post-infectious, e.g. C3G, SLE, ANCA-associated vasculitis.
- Family history of glomerular disease.
- Atypical age for PIGN <4 years or >15 years.
- Recurrent nephritis.
- Moderate proteinuria (>100 mg/mmol persisting > 6 months).
- Microscopic haematuria persisting >12 months (optional).
- Extra-renal symptoms: ?suggestive of vasculitis/SLE.

Management of acute nephritis

(➔ See also Chapter 17.)
- The following management section concentrates on the emergency renal management of the child with acute nephritic syndrome but does not describe the detailed management of the individual and varied causes of nephritis. The reader is referred to the individual chapters for these entities.
- As discussed previously, the indication for immunosuppression in the management of PIGN is controversial, and usually not warranted.

General management of acute nephritis

- Assess fluid balance/volume status: is the patient oliguric because of pre-renal failure, or established renal failure?
- Fluid restriction: insensible fluid losses (200–400 mL/m^2/24 h; or 20–40 mL/kg/24 h) plus previous hour's urine output, plus any additional losses (vomitus, diarrhoea). Usually given as 0.45% saline/2.5% dextrose; 0.45% saline/5–10% dextrose in infants.
- Consider diuretic challenge if severe fluid overload (cardiac failure): furosemide 2–5 mg/kg IV by slow (10 min for bigger doses) infusion/injection, usually give 2 mg/kg first then if no response after 1–2 h give 4 mg/kg. Provide calories (which reduces catabolism and improves acidosis and hyperkalaemia): this can be achieved in acutely unwell children by giving enteral Maxijul® (10–20%) via a nasogastric tube.
- For management of AKI, ➔ see Chapter 17.
- For management of RPGN, ➔ see Chapter 11.

Immunoglobulin A nephropathy

Background

- Male preponderance, mainly presenting in second and third decades.
- Adult studies show differing geographical incidences. Immunoglobulin A nephropathy (IgAN) accounts for 18–40% of all GN in Japan, France, Italy, and Australia, but only 2–10% of GN in the UK and USA. This is likely due to a combination of environmental and genetic factors, and to differing rates of pickup related to screening for haematuria in different countries.
- Familial in ~10% of cases.
- Defined by the deposition of IgA-containing immune complexes in the kidney.

Aetiology

- Current 'multi-hit' hypothesis proposes the following sequence of events:
1. IgA is produced in two forms, IgA1 and IgA2, and is secreted from mucosal surfaces. Only IgA1 is present in immune complexes involved in IgAN.
2. There is a hinge region between the alpha heavy chains of the IgA molecule, where glycosylation can occur with so-called O-glycans. The IgA1 in immune deposits is poorly glycosylated. There are associated genetic causes for this decreased glycosylation, e.g. variations in the gene *C1GALT1*, which encodes an involved galactosyltransferase.
3. Poorly glycosylated IgA1 appears in the circulation, which usually is only on the mucosal surfaces. This may be due to an aberrant immune response with mistrafficking of mucosal-type B cells to the bone marrow, rather than the mucosal surface, with resultant release of mucosal type poorly glycosylated IgA1 into the circulation.
4. IgG (and IgM) autoantibodies bind to poorly glycosylated IgA1. Somatic mutations, potentially triggered by exposure to environmental antigens in genes encoding immunoglobulins, have been demonstrated in patients with IgAN. These mutations lead to increased affinity of the antibody to poorly glycosylated IgA1.
5. Circulating immune complexes of IgA1–IgG/IgM deposit in the mesangium in susceptible individuals, triggering glomerular inflammation and injury. Inflammation involves the complement system.
- Thus, key events in the development of IgAN is the presence of poorly glycosylated IgA1 and its complex formation with O-glycan-specific antibodies.

Clinical and laboratory findings

Five main presentations:
- Macroscopic haematuria.
- Asymptomatic microscopic haematuria with or without proteinuria.
- Acute nephritis (haematuria, proteinuria, renal insufficiency, hypertension).
- Nephrotic syndrome (<10%).
- Mixed nephritic/nephrotic state.

The commonest mode of presentation is macroscopic haematuria following an upper respiratory tract infection. The time interval between infection and haematuria is 1–2 days, in contrast to PIGN where the time interval is typically 10–14 days post pharyngitis or 3–6 weeks following skin infection.

Diagnosis

- Only by renal biopsy—deposits of IgA are found in the glomerular mesangium. C3 is also usually present and IgG and IgM are seen in ~50% of biopsies. The Oxford classification of IgAN has been used and validated in adults to identify risk factors for progression based on histology. The presence of mesangial hypercellularity (M), endocapillary proliferation (E), segmental glomerulosclerosis (S), and tubular atrophy/interstitial fibrosis (T) are independent predictors of outcome.
- 30–50% of children will have elevated serum IgA, but this has poor specificity. Measurement of poorly glycosylated IgA1, if available, is more specific and elevated in ~75% of patients.
- Serum complement levels are normal.
- The course in the majority of patients is benign, including spontaneous resolution. Yet, up to 20% of paediatric patients progress eventually to CKD stage 5, although the rate of progression is usually very slow. Features associated with CKD progression are:
  - nephrotic-range proteinuria
  - hypertension
  - decreased GFR at biopsy
  - biopsy findings of glomerulosclerosis, fibrous crescents, tubular atrophy, and interstitial fibrosis.

Treatment

A RCT of first-line treatment in children with IgAN with either prednisolone or fish oil vs no treatment did not show any benefit of treatment. Empiric treatment is usually guided by the severity of the disease and its likelihood of progression.

- *Isolated microscopic haematuria and/or recurrent macroscopic haematuria*: are not of clinical significance. Tonsillectomy has been recommended by some investigators. Some reports suggest that vitamin E may be effective.
- *Proteinuria*: patients may benefit from renin–angiotensin system (RAS) blockade (ACE inhibitors or ARBs). In adults with persistent proteinuria >1 g/day despite 3–6 months of RAS blockade, a 6-month course of corticosteroid has been suggested by a KDIGO expert consensus statement. However, a subsequent trial in adults (STOP-IgAN) showed no evidence of benefit from added immunosuppression.
- *Children with adverse risk factors*: first line of treatment is for hypertension (to maintain below the 50th percentile) and proteinuria. Immunosuppressive regimens have been used, including steroids, azathioprine, cyclophosphamide, MMF, and mizoribine. Although some studies suggest a benefit, there is no conclusive evidence, so most

would recommend starting with antihypertensives and antiproteinurics, with consideration for immunosuppression if there is further progression.

- The involvement of the complement system in the inflammation of IgAN has suggested a potential benefit of complement-directed therapy, such as eculizumab in IgAN.
- *Crescentic nephritis*: ➔ see 'The standard treatment of childhood vasculitis'.

Omega-3 fatty acids may be of benefit, based on a RCT in adults. Available preparations are:

- Omacor®, one capsule (1 g) contains 460 mg eicosapentaenoic acid (EPA) and 380 mg docosahexaenoic acid (DHA).
- Maxepa® one capsule (1 g) and liquid (1.1 mL) contains 170 mg EPA and 115 mg DHA.
- Children unable to swallow the capsules can be given the liquid preparation of Maxepa®.

Doses

- 920 mg EPA and 760 mg DHA twice daily for children >50 kg.
- 460 mg EPA and 380 mg DHA twice daily for children <50 kg.

In practice, children may not adhere to therapy with fish oil as it has a large capsule burden and side effects include halitosis.

Further reading

Coppo R. Biomarkers and targeted new therapies for IgA nephropathy. *Pediatr Nephrol* 2017;32:725–731.

Nephrotic syndromes: definitions

- *Nephrotic syndrome*: triad of heavy proteinuria (protein/creatinine ratio >200 mg/mmol), hypoalbuminaemia (<25 g/L), and generalized oedema.
- *Congenital nephrotic syndrome (CNS)*: presentation of nephrotic syndrome during the first 3 months of life (often present before or at birth).
- *Infantile nephrotic syndrome*: presentation of nephrotic syndrome between 3 and 12 months of age.
- *Idiopathic nephrotic syndrome*: nephrotic syndrome in the absence of other glomerular pathology mediated by systemic disease (e.g. SLE), structural glomerular changes (e.g. AS), vasculitis, and immune complex deposition (e.g. PIGN).
- *Urinary remission*: urine Albustix® negative or trace for three consecutive days.
- *Relapse*: urine Albustix® ++ or more for three consecutive days is the International Study of Kidney Disease in Children (ISKDC) definition. However, most will use +++ or more for three consecutive days.
- *Frequently relapsing nephrotic syndrome*: children who relapse two or more times in the first 6 months after presentation or four or more times within any 12-month period.
- *Steroid-dependent nephrotic syndrome (SDNS)*: children who relapse while on steroid therapy or within 14 days of discontinuation of steroid therapy. These children will almost invariably also have frequently relapsing nephrotic syndrome, though the additional presence of steroid dependency indicates the presence of a more significant tendency to relapse.
- *Steroid-resistant nephrotic syndrome (SRNS)*: failure of proteinuria to resolve following at least 28 days of prednisone at a dose of 60 mg/m^2/day. There is some variability in this definition:
  - The ISKDC defined non-responders as those children who failed to achieve remission following 8 weeks of the standard ISKDC oral prednisone regimen (60 mg/m^2 daily for 4 weeks followed by 40 mg/m^2 on alternate days for 4 weeks).
  - Other reported definitions include failure to achieve remission following 4 weeks of daily oral prednisone at a dose of 60 mg/m^2 and 4 weeks of daily oral prednisone at a dose of 60 mg/m^2 followed by three doses of IV methylprednisolone. The latter is widely accepted in Western Europe.
- The terms *minimal change disease (MCD)/nephrotic syndrome* and *steroid sensitive/responsive nephrotic syndrome* are often used interchangeably. This is not strictly correct, as a small proportion of cases of MCD will not exhibit steroid sensitivity and ~20% of cases of FSGS will respond to steroids. In general, response to steroids is of greater prognostic significance than histology.

Congenital and infantile nephrotic syndromes

Definitions

Congenital nephrotic syndrome (CNS): children presenting with nephrotic syndrome during the first 3 months of life (often present before or at birth).

Infantile nephrotic syndrome refers to those presenting between 3 and 12 months of age.

In contrast to idiopathic nephrotic syndrome presenting in children >12 months of age, the renal outcome of CNS and infantile nephrotic syndrome is generally poor with the majority developing CKD stage 5, although the age at which this develops can be variable. An exception is with secondary CNS, e.g. due to placental transfer of anti-PLAR2 antibodies or infectious aetiology; here proteinuria generally resolves spontaneously or with treatment of the causative infection.

Congenital nephrotic syndrome

Many of the non-infection-related causes of CNS and infantile nephrotic syndrome have a genetic origin with mutations in genes affecting the integrity of the glomerular filtration barrier.

NPHS1 (Finnish type) CNS

Mutations in *NPHS1* (nephrin) result in the so-called Finnish type CNS because of its relatively high incidence in Finland (1:8200 live births). Inherited in an AR manner. Almost invariably results in the development of CKD stage 5. In Finland, it is due to two severe truncating nonsense mutations in >90% of the patients. Worldwide, >200 mutations have been identified in the *NPHS1* gene (℘ http://www.ncbi.nlm.nih.gov/gene/4868) and most patients have individual mutations. This is the commonest form of CNS.

Alpha-fetoprotein is raised in pregnancy in blood and amniotic fluid (secondary to proteinuria), but caution—raised alpha-fetoprotein levels may also be present in heterozygotes, so an elevated plasma level does not necessarily equate with an affected fetus.

In Finland, the phenotype includes:
* prematurity
* placental weight > 25% of the weight of the newborn
* severe proteinuria commencing in utero with oliguria and oedema soon after birth
* widely spaced fontanelles and cranial sutures
* postural elbow and knee deformities.

Most other non-Finnish mutations also have a severe phenotype with an early onset of nephrotic syndrome, but a milder course of disease and/or later onset of nephrotic syndrome have also been described.

Spontaneous improvement in some females with the R1160X mutation has been reported.

Other primary causes of CNS

* Diffuse mesangial sclerosis secondary to mutations in *WT1*, *PLCE1*, and *LAMB2*.
* FSGS secondary to mutations in *NPHS2*, *PLCE1*, *WT1*, and others.
* MCD.

Diffuse mesangial sclerosis

- Characteristic histological changes on light microscopy include thickened GBM and increased mesangial matrix without hypercellularity. Capillary loops are usually collapsed and dilated Bowman's spaces are seen.
- Early-onset hypertension and CKD develop.
- May be isolated renal disease or as part of Denys–Drash syndrome:
  - Denys–Drash syndrome describes the association of male pseudohermaphroditism (females have normal genitalia), early-onset nephrotic syndrome secondary to diffuse mesangial sclerosis, and mutations in the *WT1* gene which predispose the child to an increased risk of Wilms tumour. Because of this risk and the fact that CKD is almost inevitable, it is important to consider early bilateral nephrectomies. This should certainly be performed prior to transplantation as immunosuppression will further increase the risk of malignancy.
  - All apparently phenotypic females presenting with diffuse mesangial sclerosis should therefore undergo chromosomal analysis to ensure that they are not in fact male with severe pseudohermaphroditism.
  - Diffuse mesangial sclerosis does not appear to recur post transplantation.
  - Diffuse mesangial sclerosis has also been associated with mutations in *PLCE1* and *LAMB2*.

Minimal change disease and focal segmental glomerulosclerosis

- MCD rarely presents in infancy and may be steroid responsive as in cases presenting during later childhood life.
- Both familial and sporadic forms of idiopathic FSGS may present during infancy. A number of these cases will be associated with *NPHS2* and other podocyte gene mutations.

Secondary causes of CNS

- *Infectious*:
  - Congenital CMV.
  - Hepatitis B and C.
  - HIV.
  - Congenital syphilis.
  - Congenital toxoplasmosis.
  - Congenital Rubella.
  - Malaria.
- *Syndrome associated*:
  - Denys–Drash syndrome.
  - Nail–patella syndrome.
  - Lowe syndrome.
  - Galloway–Mowatt syndrome.
  - Frasier syndrome.
  - Pierson syndrome (microtia and CNS).
- *Other*:
  - Membranous nephropathy (MN; transplacental antibody transmission).
  - SLE.
  - HUS.
  - Nephroblastoma.
  - Drug reaction.
  - Mercury toxicity.

The role of renal biopsy in CNS and infantile nephrotic syndrome

* Biopsy is relatively infrequently performed in typical CNS because of the risk of the procedure in small infants and the fact that light microscopy findings are frequently normal in the first few months of life. The constellation of clinical features accompanied by genetic testing is generally sufficient to make the diagnosis.
* The cardinal histological feature after the first few months of life is tubular dilatation resulting in diffuse microcystic change (cysts of 0.1–0.5 mm).
* Progressive glomerular sclerosis and interstitial fibrosis develop by 6–12 months of age; this is associated with deterioration in renal function.
* There may be a role for biopsy in the child with infantile nephrotic syndrome, where the differential diagnosis is wider and includes, e.g. diffuse mesangial sclerosis and MCD. This and appropriate genetic tests will help to establish the diagnosis.

Management of NPHS1 (Finnish type) CNS

The advice provided here applies to children with a clinical diagnosis of Finnish type CNS as well as those with proven mutations in the NPHS1 gene. The aim of treatment is to enable growth and development to allow the child to reach a size where transplantation is possible. Various approaches are possible:

Reduction of urinary protein losses

* Nephrectomy:
  * The Helsinki group advocate insertion of a PD catheter at around 4 months of age, with bilateral nephrectomies at around 5 months of age following confirmation of catheter function. The ultimate goal is transplantation once the child has reached ~9–10 kg.
  * An alternative approach, used in some centres, is to perform early unilateral nephrectomy at around 3 months of age in conjunction with medical therapy (see below), with the second nephrectomy and subsequent transplantation being performed at 3–4 years of age when the child is significantly larger and the risk of early graft loss is lower.
* Another approach is to manage with medical therapy alone. ACE inhibitors (e.g. captopril up to 5 mg/kg divided into three doses and prostaglandin inhibitors e.g. indometacin up to 4 mg/kg divided into three doses) will reduce GFR and thus protein loss.
* This may not be effective in those children with very heavy proteinuria.

Replacement of albumin

* Children with symptomatic oedema, particularly if signs of intravascular fluid depletion or difficulty in feeding and/or growth, need IV albumin.
* 20% albumin infusions can be built up to 4 g/kg daily, usually as a single daily infusion.
* This dose (or frequency of administration) may be reduced as the GFR falls.
* A central venous catheter is usually required to provide long-term vascular access to deliver this.
* Albumin may be given less frequently in children who are receiving medical therapy or who have undergone unilateral nephrectomy.

Symptom treatment

- Intensive treatment as proposed by the Helsinki group involves a strong commitment from families and carers: patients are typically hospitalized for most of their first year of life, have multiple interventions (central venous line placements, dialysis access, nephrectomies), and a high risk of infectious complications.
- Despite the intensive treatment, mortality is high (10–20%).
- If the child does not receive a transplant early on, dialysis access can become a serious problem due to infectious complications and thrombosis of central veins.
- Some families feel that such intensive treatment is too great a burden for the child and the family, especially, if there are siblings needing care and attention.
- An alternative for these families is medical treatment. Parents can be taught to administer the IV albumin at home if needed. Admission to hospital is often needed during acute illnesses.
- Recent retrospective reviews suggest that mortality is comparable between the Helsinki and the symptomatic approach. Yet, there may be a selection bias with the symptomatic approach used in clinically less severely affected infants.

Transplantation

- The child needs to be of adequate size to undergo transplantation (9–10 kg).
- The high risk of thrombosis in this condition, especially if central lines have been used for albumin infusions, mandates that the major abdominal vessels are assessed prior to transplant (US or MRA) to ensure patency.
- Following transplantation, recurrent nephrotic syndrome may occur in up to 25% of children with Finnish type CNS:
  - Related to the production of anti-nephrin antibodies following exposure to normal nephrin in transplanted kidney.
  - May respond to treatment with cyclophosphamide ± plasma exchange.
  - Up to 50% graft loss may occur due to recurrence.

Other important factors

- Diuretics, e.g. furosemide and/or amiloride to reduce oedema (alone and/or in conjunction with albumin infusions).
- If there is neonatal hyperbilirubinaemia, the risk of kernicterus is increased due to the low plasma albumin. More aggressive phototherapy starting at a lower serum bilirubin level is therefore warranted.
- Close attention to nutrition and growth—high-calorie and high-protein diet (4 mg/kg/day).
- Children with heavy proteinuria are hypercoagulable and at a significantly increased risk of arterial and venous thrombosis:
  - May be decreased by anticoagulation with warfarin.
  - Warfarin must be stopped 4 days before surgery and antithrombin given.
  - Aspirin may have a role.

- Infection is a significant problem in the nephrotic child:
  - Low threshold for the empiric aggressive treatment of suspected infection.
  - The Helsinki group have found that the use of prophylactic antibiotics and IV immunoglobulin do not reduce the infection risk and have abandoned this practice.
- Thyroid function should be checked. Thyroxine is usually necessary from birth.
- Administration of childhood vaccines:
  - Should be completed prior to transplantation.
  - Efficacy is increased if performed after nephrectomy when the child is no longer heavily proteinuric, but it is preferable to progress normally through immunizations (checking for an antibody response) so that transplantation is not delayed.

Management of other forms of CNS

- Where nephrotic syndrome has occurred secondary to congenital infection, then treatment of the specific infection, where possible, leads to resolution of proteinuria.
- Children presenting with MCD in infancy should be treated with corticosteroids in an identical manner to older children (➔ see 'Steroid-sensitive nephrotic syndrome: presenting episode')
- Those with FSGS should be treated in line with protocols for children with SRNS. Genetic testing is mandatory and may guide therapy (➔ see 'Steroid-resistant nephrotic syndrome')
- There are no specific therapies for diffuse mesangial sclerosis or the FSGS associated with Frasier syndrome.

Transient neonatal nephrosis (congenital membranous nephropathy)
- Induced by circulating maternal antibodies which cross placenta.
- Caused by maternal deficiency of a podocyte antigen (neutral endopeptidase), which is present in the podocytes of the developing fetus.
- A history of transient neonatal nephrosis in successive pregnancies is suggestive.

Steroid-sensitive nephrotic syndrome: presenting episode

Introduction

Nephrotic syndrome describes the clinical triad of:
- heavy proteinuria (protein/creatinine ratio >200 mg/mmol, albumin/creatinine >200 mg/mmol)
- hypoalbuminaemia (<25 g/L)
- generalized oedema.

~80% of cases have MCD on histological examination (no abnormality seen on light microscopy).

Foot process fusion is seen on electron microscopy, as in all conditions with heavy proteinuria.

Key points about minimal change disease
- Commonest glomerular disorder of childhood.
- Median age of presentation 2–3 years.
- More common in boys (2:1).
- Incidence 2–4/100,000 child population in the UK.
- Six times more common in the UK South Asian population.
- >90% will respond to corticosteroid therapy.
- >80% of those who respond to corticosteroids will subsequently develop a relapsing course.
- 80% will enter long-term remission during childhood; the remainder will continue to have relapses into adulthood, although the frequency of these tends to decrease and a substantial proportion will enter long-term remission in early adult life.
- Steroid responsiveness is the most important factor in determining prognosis: where the presenting episode of nephrotic syndrome responds to steroids and the disease remains steroid sensitive, there is an extremely low risk of developing CKD. This very rare outcome is linked to the development of late (secondary) steroid resistance.
- Published series report mortality rates of 1–7% (sepsis and vascular thrombosis), though the current rate is thought to be much lower.
- A small number (<1–2%) of cases are familial.

The remaining 20% of cases, who do not respond to initial corticosteroid therapy, have a variety of histological diagnoses, including FSGS and C3 glomerulopathy and immune complex-mediated glomerulonephritis. These histological findings and the clinical presentation may inform ongoing further treatment. These pathologies tend to present in older children and the majority of cases do not respond to oral steroid therapy alone. Their prognosis is correspondingly poorer. The likelihood of an alternative histological diagnosis increases with increasing age of the child as illustrated in Fig. 9.1.

Investigations at first presentation

- Urine dipstick analysis (protein, blood).
- Early morning Upr:Ucr or Ua:Ucr to quantify proteinuria.
- Urinary sodium concentration (➔ see 'Fluid balance, hypovolaemia, and hypervolaemia in nephrotic syndrome') particularly if there are symptoms and signs of intravascular depletion (hypo- or hypertension,

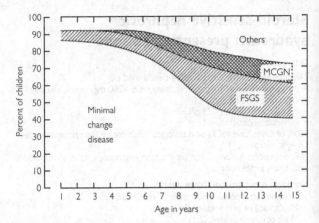

Fig. 9.1 'Smoothed' representation of the distribution of major causes of childhood nephrotic syndrome by age. Based on pooled data from the ISKDC and patients investigated at Guy's Hospital, London (n = 566). MCGN, mesangiocapillary glomerulonephritis (previously known as membranoproliferative glomerulonephritis, and now known as C3 glomerulopathy and immune complex-mediated glomerulonephritis).

Reproduced with permission from Webb, N.J.A. and Postlethwaite, R.J. (eds) (1994) *Clinical Paediatric Nephrology*, 2nd Ed. Oxford, UK: OUP. Copyright © 1994 OUP.

abdominal pain, decreased capillary refill, increased core–periphery temperature gap by >2°C).
• Plasma albumin, creatinine, and electrolytes.
• FBC.
• Complement C3 and C4 levels.
• VZV serology (IgG) to determine immune status in case of exposure to varicella while receiving high-dose steroids.
• Hepatitis B and C serology.
• ASO titre, anti-DNAase B, and lupus antibody serology (antinuclear antibody (ANA), extractable nuclear antibody (ENA), and ds-DNA) in older children, and those with atypical presenting features.

Indication for renal biopsy at disease presentation

• As >90% of children with MCD and an additional 20% of those with FSGS will respond to steroid therapy, the large majority of children with no atypical presenting features are given an empirical course of prednisolone or prednisone without a renal biopsy being performed.
• Children with atypical presenting features should be referred for specialist paediatric nephrology assessment, including, in most cases, a renal biopsy. These features include:
  • age <12 months or >12 years
  • persistent hypertension or impaired renal function
  • gross haematuria
  • low plasma C3
  • hepatitis B or C positivity.

Up to 25% of children with MCD may have microscopic haematuria or transient hypertension (which may be paradoxically related to intravascular volume depletion resulting in peripheral vasoconstriction) at presentation: neither should be a contraindication to empirical steroid therapy, but hypertension should prompt clinical assessment of intravascular volume status.

Management

The large majority of children presenting for the first time with nephrotic syndrome should be admitted to hospital to ensure adequate monitoring of their clinical status, and to allow the parents to undergo an education programme about the disease and its treatment, and the importance and practicalities of home urine monitoring.

Steroids

- *ISKDC regimen*: prednisolone 60 mg/m^2 (maximum dose 80 mg) once daily for 28 days, followed by 40 mg/m^2 (maximum dose 60 mg) given on alternate days for a further 28 days.
- *Prednisolone, the active drug, is the agent of first choice in the UK, whereas in France, Germany, and much of the USA prednisone is used. Dosing is the same for both agents. No head-to-head study has compared their efficacy and safety in childhood nephrotic syndrome.*
- In Germany, France, and other nations, a more intensive course of initial therapy has traditionally been used, with daily prednisone 60 mg/m^2 for 6 weeks followed by alternate-day prednisone 40 mg/m^2 for 6 weeks. In some centres, this has been followed by a progressively reducing course of alternate-day therapy resulting in a total course duration of up to 6 months. This strategy is based upon the results of early studies and a subsequent Cochrane review which showed that a longer-duration course of steroid therapy (12 weeks or more) at first presentation reduced the subsequent rate of relapse. Standard regimens in Germany and France incorporate 12 weeks or more of initial steroid therapy. More recent, high-quality placebo-controlled studies have not confirmed this observation and the most recent Cochrane review (2015) concluded that there was no benefit to increasing the duration of prednisone beyond 2 or 3 months in the initial episode of SSNS. The PREDNOS study, a 237-patient UK study comparing standard with prolonged prednisolone therapy in UK children, has also shown no clinical benefit in extending prednisolone therapy beyond the 2-month ISKDC regimen.
- A response to steroid therapy is indicated by the resolution of proteinuria, urinary remission being defined as three consecutive days of zero or trace proteinuria on Albustix®. It takes a number of additional days following the resolution of proteinuria for the plasma albumin to return to normal.
- Of those children who respond to steroids, ~80% will have entered remission within 14 days using this protocol.
- A clinical diagnosis of SSNS is used in children who enter remission during the first 28 days of therapy and such steroid sensitivity is associated with a good long-term prognosis in the very large majority.
  - The large majority of children therefore never undergo renal biopsy and the diagnostic title of SSNS is used in place of a histological diagnosis of MCD. The two are sometimes used interchangeably;

however, this is strictly incorrect as there will be a small number of children with MCD who do not respond to steroids and similarly a number of children with SSNS who have a histology other than MCD, e.g. those with FSGS.
* IgM nephropathy is a controversial clinicopathological entity characterized by IgM diffuse deposits in the mesangium on immunofluorescence with minimal changes on light microscopy. Some consider this a variant of MCD and others a distinct entity; no good follow-up/outcome data are available.
* Conversely, those who fail to respond to steroid treatment have a poorer long-term prognosis and require further investigations to guide further therapy. These include genetic testing and/or a renal biopsy to obtain a histological diagnosis. This is discussed elsewhere (➔ see 'Steroid-resistant nephrotic syndrome').

Infection
* Children are at increased risk of bacterial infection because of urinary losses of immunoglobulins and complement components alongside other factors.
* Peritonitis, septicaemia, and cellulitis are significant causes of morbidity and mortality.
* *Streptococcus pneumoniae* and Gram-negative organisms are the commonest infective pathogens. Broad-spectrum antibiotics should always be used in suspected infection until the results of bacterial cultures are available.
* While there is little good evidence to support this practice, prophylactic phenoxymethylpenicillin 12.5 mg/kg twice daily (against *Streptococcus pneumoniae*) may be given while the child is oedematous and there should be a low threshold for investigating and adequately treating infection should this be suspected.
* Children with no previous exposure to VZV should receive varicella zoster immunoglobulin if exposed to the virus. All patients with SSNS should have their VZV antibody status documented (anti-VZV IgG).
* If varicella infection occurs, this should be treated aggressively with IV aciclovir if the child is immunosuppressed at the time.
* Children should be immunized against VZV when off immunosuppressive therapy. A number of countries have now adopted universal VZV immunization, though uptake rates have generally been poor.
* Children with nephrotic syndrome should receive all of the routine childhood immunizations. Live vaccines should only be administered when the child is off all immunosuppressive therapy, remembering that immunosuppression may continue for some time after drug discontinuation; a period of 3 months following discontinuation of steroids or ciclosporin and 6 months following discontinuation of cyclophosphamide is likely to be safe. Children should additionally receive pneumococcal vaccine (this is now part of the routine infant vaccination schedule in most countries) and an annual influenza vaccine.

Fluid balance, hypovolaemia, and hypervolaemia
➔ See 'Fluid balance, hypovolaemia, and hypervolaemia in nephrotic syndrome'.

Diet

- No evidence exists to support any alteration in dietary protein content in children with SSNS.
- A no-added-salt diet is a sensible measure in view of the generalized oedema (salt and water overload) and the use of steroids.

Hypercoagulability

- Children will become hypercoagulable while nephrotic (➔ see 'Steroid-resistant nephrotic syndrome'):
  - Given that the presenting episode is generally short-lived, systemic anticoagulation is not indicated.
  - Patient mobility should be encouraged.

Information

- Families should be provided with written information about nephrotic syndrome:
  - A range of written and online information is available in a variety of European and other languages, e.g. ℘ http://www.infokid.org.uk/nephrotic-syndrome, http://www.ipna-online.org/patient-education.
  - Families need to be taught urinalysis to allow home urine testing and the early detection of relapses prior to the development of oedema.
- Many centres provide families with a diary in which to enter results of urine tests and medications given. This should be brought to all clinic appointments.

Steroid-sensitive nephrotic syndrome: relapsing disease

>70% of children with SSNS will develop disease relapses necessitating further courses of immunosuppressive therapy and ~50% of these will develop frequently relapsing or steroid-dependent disease. A suggested outline to the management of relapsing disease is shown in Fig. 9.2.

Management of initial relapses

- Relapses (⦿ see 'Nephrotic syndromes: definitions') are generally detected through routine home first morning urinalysis, allowing the early commencement of treatment without hospital admission prior to the development of generalized oedema with its attendant complications.
- It is not uncommon to have such a degree of proteinuria during an intercurrent infection, and there may be a case for observing the child for a little longer prior to commencing steroids provided that the child is otherwise well and that there is no evidence of peripheral oedema.

Relapse

Prednisolone 60 mg/m^2/24 h (maximum 80 mg/kg/24 h) until remission followed by prednisolone 40 mg/m^2/48 h for 28 days

↓

Frequent relapses

Following treatment of relapse, commence maintenance prednisolone 0.1–0.5 mg/kg/48 h for 6 months, then taper

↓

Relapses on prednisolone

Consider addition of levamisole 2.5 mg/kg/alternate-days for 6–12 months and/or the use of a marginally higher alternate daily steroid dose if this is well tolerated. Thereafter prednisolone can be tapered and levamisole could be continued for 2–3 years.

↓

Relapses on levamisole/prednisolone or prednisolone alone at >0.5 mg/kg/48 h or the presence of steroid side effects

Cyclophosphamide 3 mg/kg/day for 8 weeks

↓

Post-cyclophosphamide relapses

As 1 and 2 above

↓

Relapse on prednisolone >0.5 mg/kg/alternate-day

Ciclosporin 6 mg/kg/day in two doses for 1–3 years +/– alternate-day steroids

↓

Relapse on ciclospsorin +/– alternate-day prednisolone

↓

Individual treatment

Options include the use of a higher alternate-day prednisolone dose in conjunction with ciclosporin, a second course of cyclophosphamide or a course of chlorambucil or the use of tacrolimus, mycophenolate mofetil, or rituximab.

Fig. 9.2 Treatment of relapsing steroid-sensitive nephrotic syndrome.

- Systematic review of three small RCTs performed in Sri Lankan and Indian children receiving alternate-day steroid therapy has shown that changing from alternate-day to daily steroid therapy at the same dose (e.g. 10 mg alternate days to 10 mg daily) at the time of a febrile URTI significantly reduces the rate of subsequent relapse. A further larger study (PREDNOS 2) is currently ongoing to address whether this strategy is effective and safe in UK children.
- *ISKDC relapse regimen*: prednisolone 60 mg/m^2 (maximum dose 80 mg) daily until urinary remission (3 days of zero or trace proteinuria), followed by 40 mg/m^2 (maximum dose 60 mg) on alternate days for 14 doses over a 28-day period.
  - Recent clinical trials and systematic review have shown that intensification of the relapse regimen has not been shown to be of long-term clinical benefit. No good quality clinical trials have investigated a less intensive regimen.

Infrequently relapsing disease

- Children experiencing less than three relapses per year can be managed with repeated courses of the ISKDC relapse regimen, provided that they continue to grow well and that there are no other adverse effects of steroid therapy.
- Should side effects of steroids develop, then alternative therapeutic strategies should be considered.

Management of frequently relapsing and steroid-dependent SSNS

(➔ See 'Nephrotic syndromes: definitions'.)
- More than two relapses in the first 6 months after initial steroid response predicts a high risk of frequently relapsing nephrotic syndrome or SDNS.
- These patients should generally be managed by, or in consultation with, a paediatric nephrologist.

Notes on drug therapy

Long-term, low-dose maintenance steroid therapy

- The side effects of steroids are reduced by the use of the drug in a single alternate daily morning dose at a level that prevents disease relapse.
- Prednisolone dose is gradually tapered from treatment dose, aiming for a maintenance dose in the range of 0.1–0.5 mg/kg on alternate days.
- After around 6 months of therapy, the dose should be tapered so that the smallest dose possible that maintains remission is used.
- Those with steroid dependency generally require higher maintenance doses than those with frequently relapsing disease.
- Where relapses occur, the subsequent maintenance dose should be targeted just above the dose at which relapse occurred.
- Close monitoring for the well-known adverse effects of steroids is mandatory:
  - posterior subcapsular cataract is reported to occur in up to one-third of children. It is at present unclear whether there is a link between total dose of steroid administered and risk of cataract.

- Normal growth has been reported in prepubertal children on long-term alternate-day steroids, though it appears to fall off after 10 years of age, particularly in boys, in whom there is also some evidence of pubertal delay.
- Bone mineral density may be reduced by prolonged steroid therapy, though the majority of the evidence suggests that the bone effects of long-term alternate-day steroids are minimal in this population.
- If the child cannot be maintained in stable remission on an acceptably low dose of alternate-day steroids, particularly where steroid side effects have developed, the use of alternative agents should be considered.
- Despite the widespread use of alternate-day steroid regimens in SSNS over many decades, there have been very few studies reporting the outcomes of this strategy.

Levamisole
- Immunomodulatory properties not completely understood.
- Dose 2.5 mg/kg on alternate days. Available in UK in dispersible tablet to assist with accurate dose administration.
- Allows the tapering and possible discontinuation of concomitant alternate-day steroids. Significantly more effective than prednisolone alone.
- Efficacy of levamisole is dependent upon its continuous administration.
- If remission can be successfully maintained, levamisole is typically continued for a period of up to 2–3 years, though many children have safely received in excess of 5 years of treatment.
- Very low incidence of adverse effects: neutropenia (reversible upon drug discontinuation), GI upset, abnormality of LFTs, and rash.
- Blood count should be performed regularly (6–8-weekly initially then up to 4-monthly after 6 months) and if neutropenia develops, drug should be discontinued.

Alkylating agents: cyclophosphamide and chlorambucil
- The alkylating agents bind to purine bases and impair normal DNA transcription.
- Cyclophosphamide is the most widely used agent, though chlorambucil may also be used. Both significantly reduce the risk of relapse compared with prednisolone alone at up to 24 months.
- Both agents have been shown to induce a period of steroid-free remission, 2-year relapse-free rates following cyclophosphamide therapy being ~70% in frequently relapsing nephrotic syndrome and 25% in SDNS. In general, those with heavier levels of steroid dependence have shorter durations of steroid-free remission.
- Cyclophosphamide dose is 3 mg/kg for a total of 8 weeks (total dose 168 mg/kg).
- No benefit has been shown by prolongation of this course at the same daily dose to 12 weeks and shorter courses have been shown to be less efficacious. 12-month outcome is no better with IV rather than oral therapy.
- Chlorambucil dose 0.2 mg/kg daily for 8 weeks.
- Prednisolone dose is tapered (e.g. 40 mg/m² for the first 4 weeks of therapy, then 20 mg/m² for the second 4 weeks with further subsequent taper) so that steroids are discontinued shortly after completion of cyclophosphamide/chlorambucil.

Table 9.3 Short-term adverse effects of cyclophosphamide and their incidence

Adverse event	Cyclophosphamide (%)	Chlorambucil (%)
Infection	11	4
Serious infection	5	4
Leucopenia	18	18
Leucopenia necessitating medication cessation	7	6
Thrombocytopenia	6	9
Hair loss	17	4
Cystitis	4	0

Source: data from Pravitsitthikul, N. et al. Non-corticosteroid treatment for nephrotic syndrome in children. *Cochrane Database of Systematic Reviews.* 2013, 10 Art. No.:CD002290. Copyright © 2013 Cochrane.

- Short-term adverse effects and their incidence (where available) are shown in Table 9.3.
- Blood count should be performed weekly throughout therapy and if neutropenia develops, the dose should be halved (neutrophil count $1.0–1.5 \times 10^9/L$) or discontinued ($<1 \times 10^9/L$): cyclophosphamide or chlorambucil can be recommenced at a lower dose once the neutrophil count recovers, with prolongation of the course so that a total dose of 168 mg/kg (cyclophosphamide) or 11.2 mg/kg (chlorambucil) is administered (Fig. 9.3).
- Prompt medical advice should be sought if febrile illness develops.
- *Longer-term adverse effects:*
  - Risk of azoospermia with multiple courses of therapy, though a single 8-week course is not thought to have a significant effect. Fig. 9.3 shows the relationship between the cumulative dose of cyclophosphamide received and the sperm count.
  - The ovary is more resistant than the testis to effects of these drugs.
  - The theoretical risk of malignancy remains unproven; however, it is widely acknowledged that, as witnessed in the transplant population, the long-term administration of all immunosuppressive therapies is associated with an increased risk of malignancy.
- While this practice occurs less frequently now than in previous decades, a second course may be administered during childhood. There is little point in pursuing this strategy if the first course of treatment was unsuccessful. Long-term adverse effect risk increases with the cumulative dose administered.

Ciclosporin
- Modifies T-cell function, inhibiting IL-2 production by activated T cells (Table 9.4).
- Response to ciclosporin depends upon its continuous administration, with a high rate of relapse occurring upon its discontinuation.

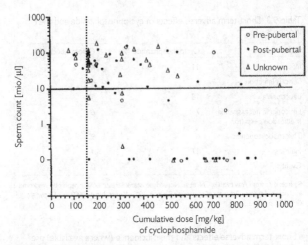

Fig. 9.3 Relationship between cumulative dose of cyclophosphamide and sperm count in adult life. Vertical dotted line indicates total dose administered during an 8-week course of cyclophosphamide at 3 mg/kg/day.

Adapted with permission from Latta, K. et al. A meta-analysis of cytotoxic treatment for frequently relapsing nephrotic syndrome in children. *Pediatric Nephrology.* 16(3), 271–82. Copyright © IPNA—International Pediatric Nephrology Association New York, USA 2001.

Table 9.4 Short-term adverse effects of ciclosporin and their incidence

Adverse effect	Incidence (%)
Gingival overgrowth	23
Hypertrichosis	27
Hypertension	13
Renal dysfunction	10

Source: data from Pravitsitthikul, N. et al. Non-corticosteroid treatment for nephrotic syndrome in children. *Cochrane Database of Systematic Reviews.* 2013, 10 Art. No.:CD002290. Copyright © 2013 Cochrane.

- Often used after a previous course of cyclophosphamide, although it may be used earlier in preference to cyclophosphamide, e.g. in peripubertal boys possibly at increased risk of cyclophosphamide-related gonadal toxicity.
- Dose 6 mg/kg/day divided into two doses.
- While monitoring of trough ciclosporin levels is recommended to ensure compliance and to avoid toxicity, there is no evidence to support any specific target range. Most centres will aim for trough blood levels of 50–125 micrograms/L, but successful management with lower doses

or once-daily dosing has been reported. Thus, if remission is stably maintained on ciclosporin, dosage may be tapered to minimize adverse effects.
- Alternate-day steroid therapy may be tapered or discontinued once stable remission achieved.

Longer-term adverse effects
- *Chronic ciclosporin-induced nephrotoxicity*:
  - Check for microalbuminuria (Ua:Ucr) on an early morning urine at each clinic visit.
  - It is widely accepted practice to perform a renal biopsy after 18–24 months of therapy or if there is microalbuminuria.
  - Ciclosporin may be continued beyond 2 years in those patients with no histological evidence of chronic nephrotoxicity, though an annual biopsy is recommended.

Other agents
- *Tacrolimus* has a similar mode of action to ciclosporin and there are an increasing number of reports of efficacy in patients who relapse on ciclosporin therapy.
  - Dose 0.2–0.3 mg/kg in two divided doses. Advice for monitoring trough levels as with ciclosporin—suggested levels 3–5 micrograms/L.
  - Two small case series have reported tacrolimus to be at least as effective as ciclosporin.
  - Preferred by some because of absence of cosmetic adverse effects.
  - However, the literature contains a number of reports of permanent diabetes developing in children with SSNS following a switch from ciclosporin to tacrolimus.
- *MMF* has similarly been shown to be efficacious. Dose 600–1200 mg/m^2/day divided into two doses. Blood count monitoring is mandatory as with renal transplant patients. No evidence to support the monitoring of mycophenolic acid (the active drug) levels:
  - The initial open-label study of MMF in SSNS reported that 24 of 32 patients (predominantly SSNS without SDNS) remained in remission during the 6-month study period.
  - In one small study, ciclosporin significantly reduced the relapse rate compared with MMF and limited data from a German cross-over study suggested that ciclosporin was more effective than MMF in maintaining remission, despite being potentially more nephrotoxic. However, when a comparison was made with MMF recipients where there had been higher MPA exposure (mean MPA-AUC 74.0 micrograms/h/mL), outcomes were comparable.
- *Rituximab*:
  - The use of this chimeric anti-CD20 monoclonal antibody has risen significantly in recent years.
  - A number of case reports and RCTs, including at least two well-conducted placebo-controlled RCTs, have now shown the use of rituximab to be effective, allowing the reduction of other immunosuppressive agents.
  - A recent meta-analysis showed that compared with other immunotherapies, rituximab significantly improved relapse-free survival.

- A dose of 375–750 mg/m^2 has been used, though precisely which dose and the number of doses required (one to four) remains uncertain. This controversy is highlighted in the RCTs which have been performed; in one, patients received 375 mg/m^2 weekly for 4 weeks, while in the other, a single dose of 375 mg/m^2 was used.
- It is standard practice to monitor CD19 counts post administration, principally to confirm that the B-cell population has been depleted. Some authorities have recommended that re-dosing should take place once there is evidence of B-cell repopulation, i.e. a rise in CD19 count. This has not, however, been shown in prospective studies to reduce the overall relapse rate and others will simply await the development of breakthrough relapses prior to re-dosing.
- Commonly reported adverse effects include infusion reactions, hypoproteinaemia, lymphocytopenia, and neutropenia. Other adverse effects include rash, bronchospasm, abdominal pain, and vomiting.
- Fatal pulmonary interstitial fibrosis has been reported, as has progressive multifocal leucoencephalopathy in patients with lupus. There is at least one report of agammaglobulinaemia subsequently requiring bone marrow transplantation. However, all of these patients were treated with multiple other immunosuppressants at the same time, making the establishment of a direct causal relationship with rituximab (or indeed any other agent) difficult.
- There are no data regarding the long-term safety of this agent in children with renal disease.
- The efficacy of vaccinations following the administration of rituximab remains unclear.

Secondary steroid resistance

- Up to 4.5% of SSNS patients will develop a steroid-resistant pattern of illness in a subsequent relapse.
- The majority will regain corticosteroid responsiveness following further immunosuppressive therapy.
- A small percentage will remain corticosteroid resistant and develop progressive CKD leading to dialysis and transplantation. These children almost invariably have FSGS on histological examination. It is likely that these children have a circulating factor causing their disease (in comparison to children with recognized genetic abnormalities), and are at high risk of disease recurrence post transplant.

Further reading

Larkins N, Kim S, Craig J, et al. Steroid-sensitive nephrotic syndrome: an evidence-based update of immunosuppressive treatment in children. *Arch Dis Child* 2016;101:404–408.

Lombel RM, Gipson DS, Hodson EM, et al. Treatment of steroid-sensitive nephrotic syndrome: new guidelines from KDIGO. *Pediatr Nephrol* 2013;28:415–426.

Steroid-resistant nephrotic syndrome

Primary steroid-resistant nephrotic syndrome

Introduction

- Definition: failure of proteinuria to resolve following at least 28 days of prednisolone at a dose of 60 mg/m^2/day.
- ~10% of children presenting with idiopathic nephrotic syndrome will fail to respond to an initial course of corticosteroids and receive the diagnostic label of SRNS.
- Around two-thirds of SRNS patients present in the first 5 years of life.
- There is some heterogeneity in the definition of SRNS; the ISKDC defined non-responders as those children who failed to achieve remission following 8 weeks of the standard ISKDC oral prednisone regimen (60 mg/m^2 daily for 4 weeks followed by 40 mg/m^2 on alternate days for 4 weeks). Other reported definitions include failure to achieve remission following 4 weeks of daily oral prednisone at a dose of 60 mg/m^2 and 4 weeks of daily oral prednisone at a dose of 60 mg/m^2 followed by three doses of IV methylprednisolone.
- Renal biopsy should be considered mandatory, as histology may alter the treatment options: rarer causes of nephrotic syndrome require a very different approach to therapy.
- Genetic analysis should also be considered to be mandatory, as the results may influence the intensity of subsequent treatment. Identification of an underlying genetic cause may sometimes obviate the need for renal biopsy, e.g. in affected first-degree relatives of an index case. Furthermore, identification of mutations allows appropriate genetic counselling to take place.
- Differential diagnosis:
  - FSGS (58%).
  - MCD (22%).
  - C3G (➔ see 'C3 glomerulopathy') (13%).
  - Diffuse mesangial proliferation (2%).
  - MN (➔ see 'Membranous nephropathy').
  - Causes of congenital and infantile nephrotic syndromes (➔ see 'Congenital and infantile nephrotic syndrome'): these are forms of SRNS, though in practice, therapeutic trials of steroids are rarely given.

Histology

- The majority of cases of SRNS will have either FSGS or MCD on biopsy.
- There is increasing evidence that significant differences exist and that children with a histological diagnosis of FSGS have a wide range of diseases which may or may not have a genetic aetiology (see below).
- Repeat biopsy may show apparent 'transformation' from MCD to FSGS. It is unclear whether such FSGS lesions were missed on the initial biopsy, or have developed with time.
- US data shows that FSGS accounts for 30% of all black patients >13 years of age in the NAPRTCS database, in part related to the high prevalence of FSGS in black patients who possess the high risk APOL1 genotype linked to rapid disease progression.

Genetics
(● See 'Overview of inherited glomerular diseases'.)
* PodoNet registry data (℗ www.podonet.org) report that 24% of SRNS patients have a genetic mutation. This figure is similar to those found in other cohorts in the UK and USA; however, these registries suffer from strong bias by referrals from consanguineous families. In most Western centres, the mutation rate is probably closer to 10%.
* Mutations in the *NPHS2* (podocin) gene are the most commonly detected genetic mutations in SRNS.
* Other more commonly reported causative genes include *WT1*, *NPHS1*, *PLCE1*, and *TRPC6*.
* The identification of genetic mutations in SRNS is of great importance for therapeutic decisions and genetic counselling; those with mutations generally respond less well to immunosuppressive therapy and have a high risk of ESKD. However, following transplantation, the risk of disease recurrence is significantly lower where a genetic mutation has been identified (● see Chapter 21).
* Patients with mutations in genes affecting the coenzyme Q pathway may respond to supplementation with coenzyme Q

Outcomes
* Overall, 52% of children with SRNS will develop ESKD by 15 years post diagnosis.
* Renal survival is greatest in those who achieve a full response to treatment in the first year (10-year renal survival 94%).
* Of those who achieve partial remission and those with multidrug resistance (failure to respond to treatment), the corresponding 10-year CKD stage 5-free survivals are 72% and 43%, respectively.
* The presence of a genetic mutation markedly worsens prognosis; in one study, 15-year CKD stage 5-free survival rates were 17% in those with a genetic diagnosis and 48% in those with sporadic multidrug-resistant disease.
* Notably among patients with familial disease, families without an identified genetic mutation have better renal survival than those with one.
* Children with MCD have better 10-year CKD stage 5-free survival compared with FSGS (79% vs 52%).

Treatment
* The evidence to support most therapies for SRNS is poor and few large, high-quality randomized trials have been performed.
* Of those trials that have been performed, none have stratified patients according to genetic mutation status; this is potentially important given the significant influence of the presence of such mutations on both response to therapy and long-term outcomes.
* Therapy is justified on the grounds that patients with persistent nephrotic syndrome have a poor prognosis with a high rate of decline into CKD stage 5.
* It should, however, be remembered that continued heavy immunosuppressive therapy in the persistently non-responsive patient may place the patient at significant risk of morbidity or mortality and in these instances, abandoning 'active' treatment should be considered.

- Given the increasing evidence that children with *NPHS2* and other genetic mutations have a very low rate of response to immunosuppressive therapy, the abandonment of therapy should be considered at an earlier point than in those with no known mutation.
  - There are an increasing number of experts who believe that children with mutation-positive SRNS should not be treated with immunosuppressive therapy.
- Retrospective analysis of the PodoNet registry has shown that there is no good evidence of efficacy for any single agent or regimen. Overall, independent of mutation status, complete remission was achieved in 24.5% and partial remission in 16.5%.
  - Ciclosporin appeared to have the greatest efficacy with a complete remission rate of 29.8%. Complete remission rates for other agents were cyclophosphamide 9.2%, MMF 8.3%, CNI + MMF 11.8%, and pulsed cyclophosphamide plus other agents 12.5%.

Immunosuppression

- Corticosteroids:
  - Many recommend the use of IV methylprednisolone (500–1000 mg/m^2/dose, maximum dose 1 g, daily for 3–5 days) prior to the renal biopsy as this may induce remission in a small proportion.
    - This depends upon the definition used of SRNS (see earlier in this topic).
    - A response to such therapy may indicate the presence of steroid-sensitive disease, which has been effectively 'undertreated' because of poor absorption of oral prednisolone over the preceding 28 days or non-compliance.
    - It is unclear as to whether responders should be classified as having steroid-sensitive disease, though most will treat them as such.
    - An ISKDC study showed that the use of a prolonged course of alternate-day steroid therapy (40 mg/m^2 for 12 months) resulted in complete resolution of proteinuria in 28%.
  - Some other small, uncontrolled series have reported success with the use of IV methylprednisolone alone.
- Ciclosporin:
  - In addition to the PodoNet registry data, Cochrane meta-analysis of controlled studies comparing ciclosporin with placebo or no treatment showed that this agent increased the number of children with SRNS who achieved complete remission. However, this was based on only eight children who achieved remission with ciclosporin compared with no children who achieved remission with placebo/no treatment (three studies, 49 children: relative risk (RR) 7.66, 95% confidence interval (CI) 1.06–55.34). Ciclosporin also significantly increased the number with complete or partial remission compared with IV cyclophosphamide (two studies, 156 children: RR 31.98, 95% CI 1.25–3.13)
  - No difference was detected in the response to ciclosporin between patients with MCD and FSGS.
  - One study showed no difference in the number who achieved complete remission with tacrolimus vs ciclosporin (41 children: RR 0.86, 95% CI 0.61–1.87).
  - This evidence probably warrants ciclosporin being favoured as the agent of first choice in SRNS.

- *Alkylating agents*:
  - Meta-analysis of controlled studies of children with SRNS showed no significant difference in the number of children who achieved complete remission between oral cyclophosphamide with prednisone vs prednisone alone (two studies, 91 children: RR 1.06, 95% CI 0.61–1.87), IV vs oral cyclophosphamide, or IV cyclophosphamide vs oral cyclophosphamide with IV dexamethasone (one study each).
- *MMF*:
  - A non-randomized Brazilian study has shown the use of 6 months of MMF to be of benefit in children with SRNS. Of 34 children previously treated with ciclosporin, 21% achieved complete remission and 39% partial remission and of 18 treated with MMF *de novo* (no prior ciclosporin), 28% achieved complete remission and 33% partial remission.
- A study comparing ciclosporin vs MMF and dexamethasone showed no difference in the proportion achieving complete remission (138 children: RR 2.14, 95% CI 0.87–5.24).
- *Rituximab*:
  - There are many single case reports and small series of the use of this chimeric anti-CD20 monoclonal antibody in both SDNS and SRNS.
  - Appears to be less efficacious in SRNS than in SDNS.
  - A dose of 375–750 mg/m^2 has been used, though the number of doses required (one to four) remains uncertain.
  - Fatal pulmonary interstitial fibrosis has been reported, as has progressive multifocal leucoencephalopathy in patients with lupus.
  - Appropriately powered RCTs of the use of this agent are urgently required; a small number are currently ongoing.
- *Other agents*:
  - There are reports of SRNS being successfully treated with tacrolimus, sirolimus, and vincristine.

Non-immunosuppressive treatment
- *Antiproteinuric agents*:
  - ACE inhibitors and/or ARBs may be used to reduce proteinuria either alone or in conjunction with immunosuppressive therapy. While these will not eliminate proteinuria, they may make urinary protein losses more easily manageable.
  - The use of these agents may be associated with deterioration in renal function, particularly where intravascular volume depletion is present. It is therefore of great importance that these agents are temporarily discontinued during episodes of acute illness (ACE inhibitor/ARB holidays).
  - Sparsentan, a dual endothelin A and angiotensin II receptor antagonist, has shown promising results in early phase studies and is currently undergoing further evaluation in a multicentre study in the USA.
- *Antihypertensive agents*:
  - Therapy is needed where significant hypertension is present.
  - ACE inhibitors and ARBs are a logical choice in light of their additional proteinuria-reducing properties.
  - BP should be maintained below the 50th percentile for age and height (European Society of Hypertension paediatric guideline recommendation).

- *Diuretics*:
  - May be of benefit in children with symptomatic oedema. Furosemide is most commonly used, often in combination with spironolactone.
  - Need to be used with caution, as contraction of intravascular volume may already be present, and diuretic therapy may worsen this.
  - Plasma electrolytes require regular monitoring.
- Anti-infection strategies.
- Persistently nephrotic children are at increased risk of infection, predominantly from *Streptococcus pneumoniae* peritonitis and septicaemia.
- Despite the importance of *Streptococcus pneumoniae*, many infections are caused by other Gram-positive and -negative organisms and broad-spectrum antibiotic therapy should be used until culture results become available.
- Classical signs of infection may be masked in the immunosuppressed child and there should be a low threshold for treating suspected infection.
- While there is no evidence to support such an approach, prophylactic phenoxymethylpenicillin (12.5 mg/kg twice daily) can be considered to be given to children while nephrotic in conjunction with pneumococcal vaccination.
- Varicella is a major threat to nephrotic children and their varicella immunity status should be known.
  - Seronegative children should be immunized when off immunosuppressive therapy.
  - Varicella zoster immunoglobulin or possibly aciclovir should be given following proven exposure in the non-immune child.
  - Where varicella develops, this should be treated with high-dose IV or oral aciclovir (➔ see Chapter 21).
- *Hyperlipidaemia*:
  - Children with persistent heavy proteinuria may develop significant dyslipidaemia including hypercholesterolaemia.
  - There are no data regarding long-term cardiovascular outcomes in this group though most authorities would recommend dietary modification and possibly the use of a statin where cholesterol levels are very high.
- *Thrombosis*:
  - The nephrotic state confers an increased risk of both arterial and venous thrombosis.
  - Proven episodes should be treated with formal anticoagulation with heparin or thrombolytic therapy where thrombosis is extensive or involves major organ systems (bilateral renal vein/IVC, massive pulmonary embolism, etc.). This should be followed by 3–6 months of warfarin therapy.
  - To prevent the development of thrombosis, hypovolaemia should be avoided by ensuring adequate hydration, ACE inhibitor/ARB 'holidays' during periods of acute illness, etc.
  - There is no consensus about the use of prophylactic LMWH or antiplatelet agents such as aspirin or dipyridamole in persistently nephrotic children, though there may be a reasonable case for their use in those with a prior history of thrombotic complications.

- *Nutrition*:
  - The urinary albumin losses and poor appetite seen in SRNS may result in the development of malnutrition.
  - Expert paediatric renal dietetic advice is required to ensure an adequate intake of protein, carbohydrate, and essential vitamins. Enteral feeding may prove necessary in some. Sodium is a major driver of oedema formation and should be restricted in nephrotic children.
- Fluid balance, hypovolaemia, and hypervolaemia (➲ see 'Fluid balance, hypovolaemia, and hypervolaemia in nephrotic syndrome')
- Thyroid function: children may need thyroxine as levels may be low due to losses of thyroid-binding globulin in the urine.

Secondary steroid-resistant nephrotic syndrome

- This refers to the development of steroid resistance in a child with previous steroid-sensitive disease.
- May develop in up to 5% of patients with previous SSNS.
- Biopsy has been recommended prior to the commencement of further immunosuppressive therapy (generally with alkylating agents); however, there is some evidence that previously steroid-sensitive patients are likely to respond to further treatment, regaining their steroid sensitivity and that biopsy should be reserved for those who remain unresponsive.
  - Where there is unresponsiveness, this is very often associated with the development of FSGS on renal biopsy.

Further reading

Hodson EM, Wong SC, Willis NS, et al. Interventions for idiopathic steroid-resistant nephrotic syndrome in children. *Cochrane Database Syst Rev* 2016;10:CD003594.

Trautman A, Schnaidt S, Lipska-Ziętkiewicz BS, et al. Long-term outcome of steroid resistant nephrotic syndrome in children. *J Am Soc Nephrol* 2017;28:3055–3065.

Fluid balance, hypovolaemia, and hypervolaemia in nephrotic syndrome

- A low-salt diet is crucial to control thirst and minimize oedema. This will reduce thirst and spontaneous fluid intake. Salt restriction is considerably more efficacious as a measure to control fluid intake than simple fluid restriction alone.
- Where this measure alone is unsuccessful, the subsequent addition of diuretics (furosemide plus/minus K-sparing diuretic or metolazone) will help resolve oedema.
- It must be stressed that the child with overt nephrotic syndrome who is being salt restricted with or without additional diuretic therapy should be kept under very close review to ensure that hypovolaemia (intravascular volume depletion) is avoided. Hypovolaemia the risk of AKI, thrombosis, and other complications.
- Generalized abdominal pain is a common presenting feature of hypovolaemia. Risk factors for the development of hypovolaemia include diarrhoea, vomiting, sepsis, and the injudicious use of diuretic therapy.
- The child should undergo regular clinical assessment of peripheral temperature and capillary refill time, JVP, BP, pulse, and weight during the presenting illness.

Clinical assessment of the intravascular compartment of the oedematous child is difficult:

- *Hypovolaemia*:
  - Increased capillary refill time (>3°C core–periphery temperature gap).
  - JVP not raised (may be difficult to see in the oedematous child).
  - Normal BP usually, although the BP may be increased due to the vasoconstriction and/or prednisolone.
- *Hypervolaemia*:
  - Normal capillary refill time.
  - BP normal or high.
  - JVP high.
- Urinary sodium must be interpreted with caution in nephrotic states as urinary sodium levels may be low (<10 mmol/L) in both hypo- and hypervolaemia:
  - In *hypovolaemia*, levels will be low due to avid salt and water retention by the kidney.
  - In *hypervolaemia*, however, levels may also be low. There is good evidence for primary sodium retention in nephrotic syndrome due to pathologically filtered proteases, such as plasmin, activating ENaCs.
  - Moreover, nephrotic syndrome is associated with a deficiency in certain proteases, such as corin, needed to activate natriuretic peptides.
- Urinary sodium levels are uninterpretable when loop diuretics, e.g. furosemide, have been administered.
- An elevated haemoglobin level is suggestive of haemoconcentration, i.e. hypovolaemia.
- Hypovolaemia should be promptly corrected with the use of 10–20 mL/kg of 4.5% albumin solution or another colloid and diuretics should be stopped or avoided in this setting.

- The increased risk of vascular thrombosis in this condition is further enhanced by hypovolaemia.
- 20% (salt-poor) albumin can be used in combination with diuretics to relieve symptomatic oedema refractory to diuretics and fluid restriction, particularly where skin is compromised:
  - Up to 1 g/kg (up to 5 mL/kg 20% albumin) should be infused slowly over 2–4 h with furosemide 1–2 mg/kg being given IV during the second half of the infusion.
  - There are a number of reports of intravascular volume overload with the development of pulmonary oedema associated with such therapy, particularly when large doses of albumin are delivered or where the rate of delivery is rapid. The dose of albumin should not exceed 1 g/kg and the infusion time should not be shorter than 4 h to avoid this occurring—strict monitoring of vital signs should take place, and treatment should be given during routine hours where possible.
  - There is no indication to use 20% albumin to correct asymptomatic hypoalbuminaemia alone; treat the patient, not the plasma albumin result.
- Remission is heralded by an increase in urine output: this should prompt cessation of diuretic therapy.

C3 glomerulopathy and immune complex-mediated glomerulonephritis

Patients present with proteinuria, haematuria, hypertension ± CKD and low C3, although C3 can be normal. The severity is variable. The old term of membranoproliferative glomerulonephritis has now been abandoned and reclassified into two diseases based on the underlying pathological mechanism rather than histology:

- C3G: loss of alternative pathway regulation results in glomerular C3 deposition. C3G is further divided into:
  - C3 glomerulonephritis (C3GN)
  - dense deposit disease (DDD).
- ICGN: immune complex GN with IgG deposition.

Complement proteins and/or Ig immune complexes are deposited in the mesangium and/or capillary walls resulting in the appearance of 'double contouring'.

C3 glomerulopathy

- Mutations or autoantibodies affecting the alternative pathway of complement are present in 80% of patients. They act via C3 convertase to increase C3 consumption:
  - Autoantibodies stabilize the decay of the alternative pathway C3 convertase (C3NeF).
  - Complement factor H (CFH) mutations or CFH antibodies impair regulation of the decay of C3 convertase.
  - C3 and complement factor B mutations make C3 convertase resistant to decay.
- C3G is a proliferative nephropathy with predominant C3 deposition.
- It is divided by electron microscopy into:
  - C3GN: discrete C3 deposits in mesangium and capillary wall
  - DDD: deposits are denser and in mesangium and GBM.
- There may be a preceding partial lipodystrophy, particularly affecting the face and upper body, and/or ocular deposits (Drusen).
  - Thrombotic microangiopathy may rarely occur either pre or post transplant.
  - Spontaneous recovery may occur.
  - 50% progress to ESKD.
  - Japanese children undergo screening for haematuria results in a larger number of mild cases (e.g. children with isolated haematuria) being detected.

Differentiation of C3GN from PIGN

- Persistent low C3 after 6 months with C3GN.
- On biopsy C4d is present in C3GN but not PIGN.
- The deposits in PIGN have IgG deposition and mesangial subepithelial and subendothelial humps.

Treatment of C3G

There are no controlled trials to guide management.
* Immunosuppression:
  * Studies of the use of steroids, MMF, and CNIs in C3G are few with small numbers and use the old classification. Outcomes are variable.
  * Rituximab and MMF have been used when C3NeF is present, with some success.
  * There are no reports showing any benefit from immunosuppression in DDD.
* Complement targeted therapy:
  * There are case reports of the use of plasma exchange or eculizumab, with variable outcomes.

Non-evidence-based suggestions for treatment

Treatment will depend on the severity of presentation:
* Reduction of proteinuria with ACE inhibitors or ARBs is suggested for all patients.
* If renal function is normal with no nephrotic syndrome, no other treatment and wait for potential recovery.
* If C3NeF is present, consider MMF or rituximab.
* If abnormal renal function and/or nephrotic syndrome, consider plasma exchange or eculizumab if available.
* Continue with treatment for 6 months then reassess whether there has been a benefit.

Renal transplantation

* Disease recurrence rate is 50–60%.
* Graft loss after recurrence is 50% overall but nearer 70% for DDD.
* Transplant survival is currently just >50% at 10 years.
* Whether complement-targeted therapies will improve outcome is not yet known.

Immune complex-mediated glomerulonephritis (ICGN)

IgG deposition results from a specific cause such as infection, autoimmune disease, and malignancy.
Complement activation is by the classical pathway.

Treatment of ICGN

* Treatment is of the primary cause.
* Prednisolone or other immunosuppression may benefit those with nephrotic-range proteinuria and/or abnormal renal function.

Reference

Riedl M, Thorner P, Licht C. C3 glomerulopathy. *Pediatr Nephrol* 2017;32:43–57.

Membranous nephropathy

Introduction

In contrast to nephrotic syndrome affecting adults, this is a rare disorder in children, accounting for ~1–5% of cases of idiopathic childhood nephrotic syndrome.

- Estimated incidence 1 per million childhood population.
- Boys and girls equally affected.
- MN may additionally be diagnosed in children being investigated for asymptomatic non-nephrotic proportion proteinuria.
- There are no clear aetiological factors in the majority of children (idiopathic MN).
- Two podocyte proteins have been identified as autoantigens:
  - The M-type phospholipase A2 receptor (PLA2R), a transmembrane receptor that is highly expressed in glomerular podocytes, has been identified as a major antigen in idiopathic MN, circulating autoantibodies to PLA2R being identified in up to 80% of adults with idiopathic MN. PLA2R antibody levels appear to be associated with disease activity. There are a small number of reports of PLA2R antibody positivity in children with idiopathic MN.
  - Antibodies to thrombospondin 1 domain 7A are much rarer.
- Measurement of antibody levels may be used to follow the course of the disease and the effect of treatment. Higher levels predict a lower rate of remission, either spontaneous or with treatment. A fall in levels precedes clinical remission.
- Up to 43% of cases (a higher proportion than in adult MN) are secondary to:
  - infection (including hepatitis B and C, HIV, malaria (*Plasmodium malariae*), congenital and secondary syphilis, leprosy, and schistosomiasis)
  - multisystem disease (SLE is the commonest cause, though MN has been reported secondary to rheumatoid disease, dermatomyositis, diabetes mellitus, inflammatory bowel disease, and sarcoidosis)
  - drugs (including penicillamine, captopril, gold, NSAIDs, COX-2 inhibitors, lithium, and clopidogrel)
  - malignancy (including Wilms tumour, lymphomas, leukaemia, melanoma, and multiple carcinomas).
- The incidence of secondary MN is higher in areas where hepatitis B is endemic.
- A small number of cases may be familial.
- *De novo* MN may develop in the transplanted kidney in a previously unaffected individual (incidence 1–2%) and may also recur post transplantation where CKD stage 5 has occurred secondary to MN (➔ see 'Recurrent and de novo renal disease following renal transplantation').
- Neonatal MN is very rare and occurs secondary to fetomaternal alloimmunization: mothers are deficient for a gene encoding a protein expressed in placenta and glomerulus. If the child expresses the protein on the placenta, the mother produces antibodies which cross the placenta and bind to the antigen in the glomerulus. One such recognized antigen is neutral endopeptidase. The disease improves with degeneration of the maternal antibodies over time.

Presenting clinical features

- Nephrotic syndrome (70%).
- Asymptomatic proteinuria (30%).
- Macroscopic haematuria (2%).
- Microscopic haematuria (70%).
- Hypertension (20%).
- Renal impairment at presentation (<5%).

Diagnosis

- C3 and C4 levels are normal in idiopathic MN but depressed in MN secondary to SLE or hepatitis B.
- Diagnosis is histological:
  - Renal biopsy shows uniform thickening of the capillary wall within the glomerulus secondary to deposition of subepithelial immune aggregates (between the basement membrane and the podocyte (➔) see Fig. 1.11, p. 31). There is no inflammatory cell infiltrate or proliferative change (➔ see Fig. 1.11, p. 31). Advanced cases show glomerular sclerosis with tubular atrophy and interstitial fibrosis.
  - Immunofluorescence shows finely granular IgG deposits. Positive staining for IgA or IgM indicates the presence of secondary disease, e.g. SLE.
  - Electron microscopy shows the presence of subepithelial immune deposits.
- Where the diagnosis is made, a search should be made for aetiological factors (causes of secondary MN), particularly where the C3 and C4 levels are low.

Treatment

Secondary MN

- Where possible, causes of secondary MN (e.g. infection, malignancy) should receive specific treatment.
- This often results in resolution of the proteinuria without the need for immunosuppressive therapy.
- Hepatitis B-associated MN has a high rate of spontaneous remission, but in those with persistent disease there is a good response to interferon A.

Idiopathic MN

- There is no evidence base for the management of idiopathic childhood MN.
- Recommendations have to be made on the basis of uncontrolled reports in children and controlled trials performed in adults.
- ~20% of children will develop CKD stage 5. This is more common in those with heavy proteinuria and hypertension at presentation. CKD stage 5 does not appear to develop in those with asymptomatic, low-level proteinuria; proteinuria in this group may resolve within 12–18 months.
- Children with nephrotic syndrome due to idiopathic MN should generally receive immunosuppressive therapy, this being more intensive where there is evidence of renal impairment or hypertension at presentation.

- About 30–35% of adults with idiopathic MN will undergo spontaneous resolution of nephrotic syndrome, therefore it is reasonable to delay specific therapy for at least 6 months, utilizing supportive therapy, including RAS blockade, unless the patient has an unexplained rapid deterioration in kidney function or there are complications related to uncontrolled nephrotic syndrome (KDIGO 2012 recommendation).

Alkylating agents

- Controlled studies in adults have shown alkylating agents in combination with steroids to significantly increase the rate of disease remission. KDIGO guidelines (2012) recommended that first-line therapy for adults is a 6-month course of alternating monthly cycles of oral and IV steroids and oral alkylating agents. Cyclophosphamide is preferred to chlorambucil as initial therapy.
- Ponticelli regimen: three consecutive doses of IV methylprednisolone (1 g in adults), then oral prednisolone at 0.5 mg/kg for 27 days, then chlorambucil 0.2 mg/kg/day or oral cyclophosphamide 2.0 mg/kg/day for 1 month, then alternating the prednisolone and chlorambucil monthly regimens for a total of 6 months.

Calcineurin inhibitors (the authors' personal preference)

- KDIGO 2012 guidelines suggestion as an alternative to alkylating agents.
- Adult controlled studies have also shown the use of ciclosporin and tacrolimus for 6–12 months to reduce proteinuria and the incidence of declining renal function. The choice of ciclosporin vs tacrolimus should be one of physician and patient preference, considering adverse effect profiles etc.
- If treatment is going to be effective, children will generally have entered remission by 6 months. If no response by 6 months then treatment should be discontinued and an alternative considered.

Corticosteroid monotherapy

- Has produced conflicting results in controlled adult studies.
- There are reports of successful outcomes in uncontrolled studies performed in children.
- Many will have received at least 4 weeks of daily steroids prior to diagnosis as empiric treatment for childhood nephrotic syndrome.
- One recommended schedule is prednisolone 2 mg/kg/day (maximum 60 mg) for 4–8 weeks followed by a similar dose on alternate days with a gradual taper of this dose to a dose of 10–30 mg on alternate days over 6 months to 5 years depending on clinical response.
- Most children who respond do so within 2–3 months.

Other immunosuppressive treatments

- There is increasing experience with rituximab, particularly in adults with relapsing disease. Experience in children is limited.
- A small number of adult studies have shown some benefits of treatment with both MMF and ACTH.
- Ongoing studies are investigating anti-PLA2R antibody immunoadsorption.

Non-immunosuppressive therapy

* Hypertension should be well controlled (below the 50th centile for age, sex, and height), ACE inhibitors or ARBs being the logical agents of first choice as they also reduce proteinuria.
  * Proteinuria should be minimized with the use of an ACE inhibitor or ARB.
* Dyslipidaemia should be managed with dietary modification and/or the use of statins where this is local practice in children with persistent nephrotic syndrome.
* Antithrombotic prophylaxis (e.g. aspirin) where this is local practice in children with persistent nephrotic syndrome.
* Children with nephrotic syndrome should receive pneumococcal vaccine or phenoxymethylpenicillin prophylaxis.
* Monitor thyroid function. Some may need thyroxine replacement therapy due to loss of binding protein in the urine. TSH (not free T4) is the best guide to monitor thyroid function in nephrotic syndrome.

Children with asymptomatic proteinuria alone (i.e. no hypertension, renal impairment, or nephrotic syndrome)

* Have a very low rate of progression to CKD and may enter spontaneous remission.
* Should be treated with an ACE inhibitor or ARB to reduce proteinuria.
* The adverse effects of immunosuppressive therapy probably outweigh the benefits.

References

KDIGO. Idiopathic membranous nephropathy. In: KDIGO clinical practice guideline for glomerulo-nephritis. *Kidney Int Suppl* 2012;2:186–187.

Menon S, Valentini RP. Membranous nephropathy in children: clinical presentation and therapeutic approach. *Pediatr Nephrol* 2010;25:1419–1428.

Systemic disease affecting the kidney

Systemic lupus erythematosus: background, clinical evaluation, and investigation

Background

- Systemic lupus erythematosus (SLE) is an episodic, multisystem, autoimmune disease with polyclonal B-cell activation and widespread production of autoantibodies.
- Both genetic factors and environmental triggers (ultraviolet light, medications) have been implicated in the pathogenesis.
- Genome-wide association studies have identified various SLE susceptibility genes associated with antigen processing and presentation, clearance of apoptotic debris, leucocyte cell surface receptors, and cell signalling and transcription molecules.
- Circulating self-reactive antibodies deposit in tissues leading to a widespread inflammatory response in blood vessels and connective tissue.
- Gene expression profiling of blood in lupus patients consistently reveals an alpha-interferon signature and upregulation of granulopoiesis suggesting the importance of innate immunity in the perpetuation of the disease.
- Paediatric-onset lupus represents 10–20% of all SLE cases with an incidence in the paediatric population between 0.3 and 0.9 per 100,000, and most cases presenting in the teenage years.
- More common in females (5–10:1) and in the non-white population.
- Haematological and renal disease is more severe in patients with childhood-onset lupus than in those with adult-onset disease.
- Renal involvement occurs in 20–80% of paediatric patients. In prospective studies of childhood-onset lupus, the prognosis is most closely related to the severity of renal disease.
- The classification of lupus nephritis, initially developed by the World Health Organization (WHO), has been modified (⊃ see 'Systemic lupus erythematosus: classification and treatment of lupus nephritis').
- SLE is associated with significant morbidity and mortality, although this appears to be improving:
  - A retrospective, serial, cross-sectional analysis of a large paediatric hospital database in the USA for the years 2000, 2003, 2006, and 2009 identified 26,903 paediatric SLE hospitalizations.
  - Mean length of stay was 5.9 days and was constant across time.
  - There was a significant downward trend in mortality across time from 1% to 0.6% ($p = 0.04$).
  - The rate of dialysis, blood transfusions, and vascular catheterization procedures increased with time.
  - Patients with SLE nephritis and non-white race were at risk for increased healthcare utilization and death.
- Causes of death in paediatric lupus have remained unchanged and are due primarily to infections and renal involvement.

• As survival increases in SLE patients, focus has shifted to long-term morbidities particularly premature atherosclerosis which is now the leading cause of death in adults with lupus. In one study, the increased risk of death from cardiovascular disease (CVD) was 16 times that of the general population. Attention to minimizing cumulative steroid dose is also important in ameliorating a host of other morbidities such as osteoporosis, growth failure, cataracts, and diabetes.

The American College of Rheumatology (ACR) classification criteria of systemic lupus erythematosus

Four of the following 11 criteria are required for the classification) of SLE. It should be noted that in children, the features may present sequentially with different manifestations of lupus evolving over time. Diagnosis of lupus does not require meeting these criteria. Nevertheless, these criteria are an excellent guide. Several studies have demonstrated that most children who prove in time to have SLE meet or exceed the minimum of four of these criteria at presentation.

1 *Malar rash*: fixed erythema, flat or raised, over the malar eminences, tending to spare the nasolabial folds.
2 *Discoid rash*: erythematous raised patches with adherent keratotic scaling and follicular plugging; atrophic scarring may occur in older lesions.
3 *Photosensitivity*: skin rash as a result of unusual reaction to sunlight, by patient history or physician observation.
4 *Oral or nasopharyngeal ulceration*: usually painless, observed by a physician.
5 *Arthritis*: non-erosive arthritis involving two or more peripheral joints, characterized by tenderness, swelling, or effusion.
6 *Serositis*:
   • Pleuritis (convincing history of pleuritic pain, or rub heard by a physician, or evidence of effusion), *or*
   • Pericarditis (documented by ECG or rub or evidence of pericardial effusion).
7 *Renal disorder*:
   • Persistent proteinuria >0.5 g/day or >+++ on dipstick analysis, *or*
   • Cellular casts (may be red cell, haemoglobin, granular, tubular, or mixed).
8 *Neurological disorder*: seizures or psychosis in the absence of offending drugs or known metabolic derangements, such as uraemia, ketoacidosis, or electrolyte imbalance.
9 *Haematological disorder*:
   • Haemolytic anaemia with reticulocytosis, *or*
   • Leucopenia (<4 × 10⁹/L on two or more occasions), *or*
   • Lymphopenia (<1.5 × 10⁹/L on two or more occasions), *or*
   • Thrombocytopenia (<150 × 10⁹/L in the absence of offending drugs).
10 *Immunological disorder*:
   • *Anti-DNA*—antibody to native DNA in abnormal titre, *or*
   • *Anti-Sm (Smith antibody)*—presence of antibody to Sm nuclear antigen, *or*
   • *Positive finding of antiphospholipid antibodies* based on—abnormal serum level of IgG or IgM anticardiolipin antibodies; positive test result for lupus anticoagulant; or false-positive serological test for syphilis.

11 *Antinuclear antibodies (ANAs)*: abnormal titre of ANAs by
immunofluorescence or an equivalent assay at any point in time, and in
the absence of any drugs known to be associated with 'drug-induced
lupus' syndromes.

The Systemic Lupus International Collaborating Clinics (SLICC) published
a classification system for SLE in 2012. Validation of these criteria in paediatric lupus patients demonstrated that in comparison to the ACR criteria
they are more sensitive (98.7% vs 76.6%) but less specific (85.3% vs 93.4%).
Further studies on larger populations are needed to confirm these results.

Systemic lupus erythematosus syndromes in the paediatric population

* There are different clinical presentations of lupus disease, including
drug-induced lupus, neonatal lupus, discoid lupus, systemic lupus
erythematosus, and atypical lupus.
* It is important to note that a diagnosis of SLE can be made in a patient
who has negative anti-double-stranded (ds) DNA antibodies—
'seronegative' lupus. This is observed in 3–5% of cases at presentation
and that, in children, clinical features of SLE may evolve slowly
over time.

It is also important to note that a patient with an isolated positive ANA
lacking other classification criteria is unlikely to evolve into SLE.

Clinical evaluation of systemic lupus erythematosus

General points in the history
* Pyrexia and weight loss.
* Fatigue, malaise, and lethargy.
* Anorexia, nausea, and vomiting.
* Poor school attendance.
* Drug, past medical, and family history.

Mucocutaneous
* Maculopapular eruption and discoid lesions.
* Alopecia, malar erythema, and swollen fingers.
* Mucosal ulceration.

Neurological
* Headache and/or migraines.
* Confusion, delirium, or psychosis.
* Deteriorating level of consciousness.
* Seizures, stroke, ataxia, or chorea.

Musculoskeletal
* Myalgia and arthralgia.

Cardiorespiratory
* Dyspnoea and pleuropericardial pain.
* Intermittent chest pain.
* Major cutaneous vasculitis (e.g. ulcers).
* Recurrent thromboembolism.

Renal

- Proteinuria, haematuria, oedema, or hypertension,

Examination findings

The important clinical parameters on examination should include the following:

General

- Weight, height centiles, and changes over time.
- Systolic and diastolic BP and centiles.
- Lymphadenopathy and hepatosplenomegaly.

Mucocutaneous

- Maculopapular eruption and discoid lesions.
- Alopecia.
- Swollen fingers.
- Angio-oedema and panniculitis.
- Telangiectasia, malar, and periungual erythema.
- Mucosal ulceration especially of the hard palate.

Neurological

- Confusion, delirium, or psychosis.
- Deteriorating level of consciousness.
- Seizures, stroke, ataxia, or chorea.
- Peripheral or cranial neuropathy.
- Transverse myelitis.

Musculoskeletal

- Myositis, tendonitis, and arthritis.
- Contractures, fixed deformities, and aseptic bone necrosis.

Cardiorespiratory

- Cardiac failure, friction rub.
- Pericardial or pleural rub.

Vasculitis

- Raynaud's phenomenon.
- Purpura, urticaria, nail fold, and digital vasculitis.
- Livedo reticularis.
- Superficial phlebitis.

Renal

- Oedema (nephrotic syndrome).

Blood tests in systemic lupus erythematosus (first presentation)

Haematology

- FBC and blood film.
- ESR.
- Coagulation screen and international normalized ratio.
- Direct Coombs test.
- Reticulocyte count.
- Ferritin.
- Lupus anticoagulant.

Biochemistry
- Plasma U&Es, CO_2, Cl, urate, and creatinine.
- CRP (relatively normal compared to ESR in active SLE, but may rise in infection).
- Glucose.
- Liver function, albumin, creatine kinase (CK), LDH, and bone profile (Ca, Mg, PO_4, and ALP).
- Ionized Ca and intact PTH.
- Thyroid function tests.
- Amylase and lipase (for pancreatitis).
- Haptoglobins (if suspicion of haemolytic anaemia).

Immunology
- ANA.
- Anti-dsDNA.
- Rheumatoid factor.
- ANCA.
- ENA (Ro, La, Smith[Sm], RNP, Jo1, and other).
- *Complement*: C3 and C4, mannose binding lectin (if available).
- Anticardiolipin IgG and IgM antibodies.
- Anti-liver kidney microsomal (LKM) antibodies if hepatic dysfunction.
- Immunoglobulins G, A, M (can get hypogammaglobulinaemia, mimicking common variable immunodeficiency).
- Organ specific autoantibodies if indicated
- Varicella IgG to check immunity prior to immunosuppression.

Urine investigations in systemic lupus erythematosus

- Dip test.
- MC&S.
- Ua:Ucr.
- Tubular reabsorption of inorganic phosphate (TRP), urine *N*-acetyl glucosaminidase (Unag):Ucr, and Urbp:Ucr if tubulopathy suspected.

Other investigations in systemic lupus erythematosus

The following investigations need to be considered where appropriate:
- Renal US.
- ECG.
- Chest X-ray.
- Echocardiography.
- Pulmonary function tests.
- Bronchoalveolar lavage if opportunistic lung infection suspected.
- Bone marrow aspirate and trephine (exclude malignancy, macrophage activation syndrome).
- Lumbar puncture: microscopy and culture; viral polymerase chain reaction (PCR) (HSV, CMV, *Enterovirus*, VZV); protein; glucose; oligoclonal bands (present in cerebral lupus).
- MRI brain ± spinal cord (for central nervous system (CNS) lupus).
- Electroencephaloogram (EEG).
- GFR.
- Tissue biopsy: skin, lung, intestinal, lymph node (Kikuchi–Fujimoto's disease: necrotizing lymphadenitis, sometimes complicating SLE);

lymphoma—increased risk with SLE, as intrinsic aspect of disease, and/or complicating therapy.
- Renal biopsy if there is:
  - significant proteinuria (reproducible proteinuria ≥0.5 g/24 h) especially with glomerular haematuria (>5 RBCs per high power field) and/or cellular casts
  - deteriorating renal function.

Generally, renal biopsy is reserved for children with clinical or laboratory evidence of renal involvement with glomerular dysfunction, aiming to identify diffuse proliferative lupus nephritis (DPLN), which is the most severe subtype. DPLN adversely affects the prognosis and may influence patient management by requiring an increase in immunotherapy. However, extensive glomerular abnormalities have been identified on biopsies of patients who have no clinical evidence of renal disease. Renal biopsy can differentiate whether proteinuria is caused by renal scarring or active disease.

Follow-up investigations

At every follow-up visit (at least every third month) the child should have:
- a full clinical evaluation including height and weight
- BP
- urine dipstick and Ua:Ucr on first morning urine
- blood tests including:
  - FBC, ESR, and CRP
  - U&Es
  - LFTs
  - serum albumin.
- dsDNA, C3 and C4, anticardiolipin antibody (ACL). NB: ANA is insensitive as a biomarker and to measure it repetitively is counter to current recommendations.
- coagulation screen and direct Coombs test if low Hb.

Once yearly, the following evaluations should be done:
- Bone density measurement (dual-energy X-ray absorptiometry (DXA) scan) for osteoporosis.
- Fasting blood lipids: cholesterol, triglycerides, high-density lipoprotein (HDL), and very low density lipoprotein (VLDL).
- Pubertal status (self-reported using validated self-reporting tool is acceptable).

Further reading

Banchereau R, Hong S, Cantarel B, et al. Personalized immunomonitoring uncovers molecular networks that stratify lupus patients. Cell 2016;165:551–565. Erratum in: Cell 2016;165:1548–1550. Erratum in: Cell 2016;165:1548–1550.
Petri M, Orbai AM, Alarcón GS, et al. Derivation and validation of Systemic Lupus International Collaborating Clinics classification criteria for systemic lupus erythematosus. Arthritis Rheum 2012;64:2677–2686.

Systemic lupus erythematosus: treatment of non-renal systemic lupus erythematosus

In an attempt to reduce the burden of short- and long-term therapy-related morbidity and mortality, recent paradigm shifts to the approach to therapy of SLE (renal and non-renal) include the following:
* Increasing use of mycophenolate mofetil (MMF) in place of IV cyclophosphamide (IVCYC) for induction of remission.
* Attempts to minimize corticosteroid exposure where possible.
* Increasing use of rituximab or other B-cell depletion strategy for those who fail standard therapy or where cumulative IVCYC toxicity is a concern.
* Where cyclophosphamide is used, this is given IV, rather than orally because of a better therapeutic index, i.e. lower cumulative IV dose required to induce remission.

The phases of treatment of systemic lupus erythematous

One approach to therapy is to consider the treatment of SLE in three phases:
* Induction of remission.
* Maintenance of remission.
* Maintenance withdrawal.

This approach provides a useful framework for the clinical management of patients, and informs the design of most clinical studies relating to SLE treatment.

Induction of remission

To rapidly reduce inflammation and gain control of disease activity, and limit organ damage or death:
* Typically with high dose of corticosteroids, with subsequent taper; immunosuppressant agents (MMF, IVCYC, azathioprine, or methotrexate (MTX)); rarely plasma exchange. Plasma exchange is generally less helpful in lupus than in ANCA-associated vasculitides but is essential in the setting of thrombotic thrombocytopenic purpura (TTP) or catastrophic antiphospholipid syndrome (CAPS).
* Depending on severity, this phase typically lasts 3–6 months.

Maintenance therapy

To maintain remission of disease activity while minimizing therapy-related toxicity:
* Low-dose daily or alternate-day corticosteroids (e.g. prednisolone 0.1–0.3 mg/kg daily, sometimes alternate days).
* *Plus* least toxic immunosuppressant, e.g. hydroxychloroquine (HCQ), azathioprine, MMF, MTX.
* *Duration*: months to years (or indefinitely).

Maintenance therapy withdrawal phase

Attempts can be made to withdraw corticosteroids and immunosuppressants, e.g. after 2–3 years of remission on maintenance therapy:

- There is little or no evidence to guide this decision and relapse and disease progression is a major concern even after many years of disease quiescence.
- Thus, most patients with SLE require lifelong treatment in one form or another. There are active trials in progress, which in the future will guide long-term management.

General therapeutic considerations

Sun protection

All children with SLE and especially those with active skin disease should always use appropriate sunscreen and protect themselves from the sun, since ultraviolet light exposure can precipitate cutaneous and systemic disease relapse.

Immunizations

- Children with SLE and treated with immunosuppressive treatment should avoid immunizations with live vaccines.
- Routine vaccination with killed vaccines is advised.
- Seasonal influenza vaccine should be given annually.
- Pneumococcal vaccination is now being recommended by the UK Department of Health for all patients likely to be on steroids for more than a month and all patients with renal disease.

Management of infection

Children on immunosuppressive treatment are more susceptible to severe infections then other children.

- It should be emphasized to the parents and the children that they need to seek medical advice early in the case of symptoms suggestive of an infection.
- Intercurrent infection can often precipitate flares of SLE so infection and active SLE often coexist: increased corticosteroids under broad-spectrum antibiotic cover may be required. Consider infection (rather than assume disease flare) if CRP elevated.

Management of specific non-renal organ systems

Skin and joint disease

- *NSAIDs*: e.g. naproxen 10–20 mg/kg/day divided into two doses, maximum 500 mg twice daily. Monitor renal function carefully when administering scheduled NSAIDs in SLE.
- *HCQ*: 5–6.5 mg/kg/day—beneficial for skin and joint disease, may reduce fatigue, and is good for long-term cardiovascular protection:
  - the risk of HCQ retinal toxicity is rare, but appears to be related to cumulative dose. Screening is important since objective changes on retinal exam typically precede complaints of visual loss. In the UK, the Royal College of Ophthalmologists recommends baseline assessment of renal and liver function, inquiry about visual symptoms, and recording of near-visual acuity at each visit and measurement of visual acuity annually. A yearly sight test including colour vision (local optician) is recommended. Use of HCQ in children <7 years may be complicated by the difficulty of obtaining satisfactory visual testing.

- *Topical tacrolimus*: in resistant cutaneous lesions, 0.1% topical tacrolimus may be useful.
- Thalidomide (50 mg orally on alternate days to 100 mg orally daily) can be used to treat severe recalcitrant cutaneous lupus that does not respond to more conventional therapy: thalidomide is associated with risk of peripheral neuropathy and teratogenicity—seek expert advice if considering this approach (refer also to the relevant guideline in the
  → *Oxford Handbook of Paediatric Rheumatology*).
- MTX (10–15 mg/m², orally or SC, once a week) can be used for those with more severe arthritis if renal function is stable.

Moderate multisystemic disease (including haematological involvement)
- HCQ at dose 5–6.5 mg/kg/day to a maximum of 400 mg/day orally with guidelines as shown in → 'Skin and joint disease':
  - HCQ is usually given in addition to other immunosuppressants if these latter agents are required (other immunosuppressants are dealt with in the sections that follow).
- Oral prednisolone at 2 mg/kg once daily, *or*
- Pulsed IV methylprednisolone (IVMP) 30 mg/kg/dose for 3 days followed by oral prednisolone.
- Azathioprine 2–3 mg/kg/once a day: many advocate checking red cell thiopurine transmethyltransfersase (TPMT) levels or genotyping prior to starting—individuals with both intermediate and absent TPMT activity have an increased risk of developing thiopurine-induced myelosuppression, compared with individuals with normal activity.

The following serves only as a guide, and remember that those with normal TPMT levels can also develop myelosuppression thus everyone should have standard azathioprine monitoring (→ see 'The standard treatment of child-hood vasculitis'. Units quoted here are pmol/h/mg haemoglobin, but this may vary between laboratories:
- Normal TPMT 26–50: azathioprine starting dose 2 mg/kg once daily.
- Intermediate TPMT (carriers of mutant allele) 10–25 mL—starting dose 1 mg/kg once daily, then work up while monitoring FBC.
- Deficiency (homozygotes, 1:300 of the population) of TPMT <10: 0.5 mg/kg/ once daily (or less) and monitor closely for myelosuppression; or consider another agent.
- Oral MMF 1200–1800 mg/m²/day in two or three divided doses:
  - Evidence in adults now suggests that MMF also improves non-renal SLE.
  - The dose is slowly increased over 2–3 weeks from a starting dose of ~300 mg/m² twice daily to a target dose of 600–900 mg/m² twice daily (maximum 3 g/day, but approximately 2 g/day is tolerated by most).
  - This approach is to avoid the main side effects of gastric upset, diarrhoea, and leucopenia.
  - If GI side effects are a continuing problem the daily dose may be divided up and given three or four times a day or mycophenolate sodium can be prescribed.

For severe life-threatening multisystemic SLE, Box 10.1 describes one suggested approach.

Box 10.1 One approach to induction therapy for life-threatening multisystemic SLE ± HLH

- IV methylprednisolone 30 mg/kg (maximum 1 g) for three daily doses (may need to be repeated 5–7 days later) followed by:
- Oral prednisolone 2 mg/kg/day, weaning to 0.5 mg/kg once daily by 2 months.
- IVCYC 250–1000 mg/m^2 (maximum 1.2 g with 2-mercaptoethanesulfonic acid sodium salt (mesna) cover):
  - Reduce dose to lower end of range if renal, hepatic, or cardiac failure present.
  - If able to take oral medication MMF could be considered as an alternative to IVCYC, but experience in critically ill patients is limited.
- Consider plasma exchange (5–10 daily sessions) for TTP or CAPS.
- Consider IV ciclosporin 1 mg/kg twice daily if secondary *haemophagocytic lymphohistiocytosis* (HLH) is suspected clinically or confirmed on bone marrow aspirate, and has not responded to the measures given here. Suspect HLH in a clinically deteriorating patient if one or more of:
  - haemophagocytosis observed on bone marrow aspirate (not always present)
  - progressive cytopenia observed (low Hb, falling white cell count, falling platelets)
  - ferritin >5000 micrograms/mL
  - high aspartate aminotransferase (AST), alanine transaminase (ALT), gamma-glutamyltransferase, LDH
  - falling or low fibrinogen or other progressive unexplained coagulopathy
  - falling ESR, but patient getting worse clinically (hepatosplenomegaly, unremitting fever, encephalopathy, purpuric rash or other haemorrhage)
  - high fasting triglycerides
  - low serum sodium.

Central nervous system involvement
- IV methylprednisolone followed by oral prednisolone (see Box 10.1).
- Pulsed IV cyclophosphamide: 250–1000 mg/m^2 (maximum 1.2 g) monthly for 6 months; then 3-monthly for 6–18 months *or* consider switching to azathioprine or MMF.
- MMF may be a reasonable alternative to IVCYC for induction of remission of CNS disease, although there are limited data to support this.
- Consider rituximab or other B-cell depletion therapy (currently limited data in children—see plasma exchange if CNS dysfunction secondary to TTP or CAPS as Box 10.1 (and ➲ see 'Plasmapheresis and immunoadsorption', p. 575)).
- Anticonvulsants if seizures (cerebral lupus).

Antiphospholipid syndrome (thrombosis plus presence of lupus anticoagulant and/or anticardiolipin antibodies)

Standard treatment of SLE as appropriate *plus*:
* aspirin, *and*
* warfarin: lifelong treatment if one major thrombotic episode has occurred (such as pulmonary or femoral arterial thrombus). NB: initial warfarinization *must* be covered with full heparinization to prevent 'paradoxical' thrombosis, which can occur at international normalized ratio levels <2
* consider IV immunoglobulin, plasma exchange, and/or rituximab in addition for CAPS:
  * CAPS is a rapidly progressive life-threatening disease causing multiple organ thromboses and dysfunction in the presence of antiphospholipid antibodies.
  * Despite treatment, mortality is still 48%.

Alternative induction therapies (limited formal trial data available to support use)

IV immunoglobulin: can be useful particularly in haematological disease. Dose 2 g/kg IV over 12 h, maximum 70 g.

Further reading

Ginzler EM, Wofsy D, Isenberg D, et al. Non-renal disease activity following mycophenolate mofetil or intravenous cyclophosphamide as induction treatment for lupus nephritis. *Arthrit Rheumat* 2010;62:211–221.

Marmor MF, Kellner U, Lai TY, et al. Recommendations on screening for chloroquine and hydroxychloroquine retinopathy (2016 revision). *Ophthalmology* 2016;123:1386–1394.

Systemic lupus erythematosus: classification and treatment of lupus nephritis

This section should be read in conjunction with ➔ 'Systemic lupus erythematosus: treatment of non-renal systemic lupus erythematosus'.

Clinical features of lupus nephritis in children

- Renal involvement occurs in 20–80% of paediatric patients. In adults, the widely quoted frequency of renal involvement is 60%.
- Children may have earlier and more severe presentation of renal involvement than adults.
- Renal SLE presents (in variable combination) with proteinuria, nephrotic syndrome, microscopic haematuria, hypertension, and renal dysfunction, and is confirmed by renal biopsy. The indication for first renal biopsy is any sign of renal involvement, in particular proteinuria >0.5 g/24 h. especially with glomerular haematuria and/or cellular casts.
  - Tubulointerstitial nephritis (TIN) with or without glomerulonephritis is also observed. The severity of tubulointerstitial inflammation is predictive of renal survival.
  - Renal impairment ± haematuria and hypertension can occur from small vessel thrombosis in the kidneys due to antiphospholipid syndrome (APS).
  - Renal impairment should be distinguished from glomerulonephritis and will (in most cases) be detected by renal biopsy.
  - Treatment of renal impairment requires full anticoagulation (➔ see 'Systemic lupus erythematosus: treatment of non-renal systemic lupus erythematosus').
- In prospective studies of childhood-onset lupus, the prognosis is most closely related to the severity of renal disease:
  - Advances in treatment have led to an improved prognosis for renal SLE.
  - Despite this, SLE is still associated with significant morbidity and mortality (➔ see 'Systemic lupus erythematosus; background, evaluation and investigation').

Histological classification of lupus nephritis

- The classification of lupus nephritis is critical to patient care and for the comparison of outcome results from therapeutic trials. This classification provides useful information to assist in how aggressively to treat patients.
- Consensus concerning the definition of the different classes of SLE nephritis is therefore imperative.
- A group of renal pathologists, nephrologists, and rheumatologists have updated the classification of lupus nephritis (see Table 10.1).

Table 10.1 Abbreviated International Society of Nephrology/Renal Pathology Society (ISN/RPS) classification of lupus nephritis (2003)

Class I	Minimal mesangial lupus nephritis
Class II	Mesangial proliferative lupus nephritis
Class III	Focal lupus nephritis[a]
Class IV	Diffuse segmental (IV-S) or global (IV-G) lupus nephritis[b]
Class V	Membranous lupus nephritis[c]
Class VI	Advanced sclerosing lupus nephritis

Indicate and grade (mild, moderate, severe) tubular atrophy, interstitial inflammation and fibrosis, severity of arteriosclerosis, or other vascular lesions.

[a] Indicates the proportion of glomeruli with active and with sclerotic lesions.

[b] Indicates the proportion of glomeruli with fibrinoid necrosis and cellular crescents.

[c] Class V may occur in combination with class III or IV, in which case both will be diagnosed.

Treatment

(➔ See also 'Systemic lupus erythematosus: treatment of non-renal systemic lupus erythematosus'.) ACE inhibitors or ARBs should be prescribed for proteinuria and hypertension.

Guidelines for the treatment of lupus nephritis have been published as joint European League Against Rheumatism and European Renal Association-European Dialysis and Transplant Association (EULAR/ERA-EDTA) recommendations for the treatment of adult and paediatric lupus nephritis. The American College of Rheumatology (ACR) has published very similar guidelines for the treatment of adult lupus nephritis. The Childhood Arthritis and Rheumatology Research Alliance, a consortium of the majority of academic paediatric rheumatologists in North America have also published consensus treatment plans for the treatment of juvenile SLE-associated proliferative nephritis.

WHO class I and II

* No specific therapy: same treatment as mild to moderate non-renal disease if present (➔ see 'Systemic lupus erythematosus: treatment of non-renal systemic lupus erythematosus', p. 266).

WHO class III, IV, and V lupus nephritis: evidence for MMF

* WHO class III nephritis is typically grouped with class IV in treatment protocols. Class III/V and class IV/V overlaps also follow these same treatment regimens. Pure class V has less of an evidence base but is treated initially with MMF and corticosteroids.
* Most nephrologists (paediatric and adult) now advocate MMF in place of IVCYC as first-line 'standard of care' for severe lupus nephritis based on the results of RCTs in adults:
  * Initial trials suggested superior efficacy and fewer adverse events for MMF versus IVCYC.
  * More recent trial data (the Aspreva Lupus Management Study (ALMS) trial described here) suggest that MMF is equally efficacious to IVCYC, and that short-term adverse events are comparable.

- MMF is associated with more diarrhoea, whereas IVCYC is associated more nausea and vomiting.
- There is still a belief that MMF spares patients from late toxic side effects of IVCYC such as infertility and bladder cancer, but this remains unproven.
- The main practical concern regarding the use of MMF is adherence to therapy, a major issue particularly in adolescent patients.
- The biggest MMF trial was recently published by the ALMS group:
  - 370 adult patients with classes III–V lupus nephritis were randomly assigned to MMF (target dose 3 g per day) or IVCYC 0.5–1 g/m²/ month in a 24-week induction study.
  - Both groups received an identical weaning prednisolone regimen.
  - The primary endpoint was a prespecified decrease in Up:Ucr and stabilization or improvement in serum creatinine.
  - There was no difference in response rate between the two groups— 56.2% responded to MMF compared with 53% in the IVCYC group.
  - There were no significant differences with regard to rates of adverse events, including infections.
  - There were nine deaths in MMF group and five in IVCYC group;

Suggested induction treatment protocol using MMF and corticosteroids (see also published guidelines and consensus treatment plans as cited earlier):
- Oral prednisolone 2 mg/kg/day to a maximum of 60–80 mg/day, *or*
- IVMP 30 mg/kg (maximum 1 g) for three consecutive days followed by oral prednisolone.
- In severe cases, IVMP may be repeated 1 week later.
- To minimize corticosteroid side effects, aim to wean the prednisolone over the following 6–8 weeks to a dose of 0.5 mg/kg/day. Further weaning to 0.2 mg/kg/day over the subsequent 2–3 months is dependent upon individual response.
- MMF is slowly increased over 2–3 weeks from a starting dose of ~300 mg/m² twice daily to a target dose of 600–900 mg/m² twice daily (maximum 3 g/day, but ~2 g/day is tolerated by most):
  - This approach is to avoid the main side effect of gastric upset and diarrhoea.
  - If GI side effects are a continuing problem, the daily dose may be divided up and given three or four times a day or mycophenolate sodium can be prescribed.
- If patients are too critically ill to take MMF, or if there are concerns about adherence to oral medication or other clinical reason, then IVCYC is still an option:
  - IVCYC 250–1000 mg/m² monthly for 6 months (induction) then switch to a steroid-sparing agent (MMF or azathioprine).
  - Mesna prophylaxis is recommended to reduce risk of haemorrhagic cystitis and late bladder cancer, always document cumulative doses of CYC treatment (cumulative doses of 500 mg/kg can cause azoospermia in males).
  - Always start with a low dose (such as 250–500 mg/m²) with renal impairment (beware cardiotoxicity and other side effects).

Influence of ethnicity on choice of therapy

- The ALMS group report in post hoc analysis that black and Hispanic patients responded better to MMF than IVCYC.
- More data are required before making any firm recommendations.

WHO class V lupus nephritis: alternative therapy

- Recent evidence from the ALMS group and others suggests that MMF and IVCYC are similar as induction therapies for class V lupus nephritis.
- Alternative agents used with corticosteroids as already described for induction of remission of class V lupus nephritis include:
  - IVCYC as shown in ➔ 'Treatment', or
  - oral ciclosporin at 5 mg/kg/day (in two divided doses): aim for levels between 90 and 110 micrograms/L. Check levels

Crescentic nephritis

(As per ➔ 'WHO class III, IV, and V lupus nephritis: evidence for MMF.') Although most paediatric nephrologists would still consider plasma exchange for severe lupus nephritis or other life-threatening complications, such as pulmonary haemorrhage or severe cerebral lupus, based on favourable retrospective clinical experience, a meta-analysis in adult patients with severe lupus nephritis did not confirm any benefits from adding plasma exchange to the standard treatment of IVMP and IVCYC.

Refractory disease

Evidence to guide the treatment of refractory lupus nephritis is scant. Patients failing to respond to either MMF or IVCYC can be switched to the alternative agent. Rituximab or other anti-B-cell therapy can be given as an add-on or alternative therapy for severe renal (± extrarenal) disease or for disease resistant to standard therapy.

The use of rituximab in paediatric systemic lupus erythematosus

- Although B cells have critical roles in the pathogenesis of SLE, including cytokine production, presentation of self-antigen, T-cell activation, and (indirectly via plasma cells) autoantibody production, trials of B-cell therapy in lupus have been disappointing.
- Both rituximab trials (EXPLORER and LUNAR) reported negative results.
- More recently tested B-cell therapies (ocrelizumab, epratuzumab, and atacicept) have failed to reach primary endpoints and/or had significant safety concerns.
- Both belimumab trials reported positive results, however, patients with severe renal disease were excluded and benefit appeared modest.

The reasons for these trial failures is unclear, but is in distinct contrast to the success of B-cell depletion in the treatment of ANCA-positive vasculitis. A recent publication which tracked longitudinal gene expression profiles in a large cohort of paediatric lupus patients demonstrates that there is molecular heterogeneity of these patients with different biological pathways dysregulated in individual patients; in some lupus patients, B cells do not play a prominent role. In the future, it may be possible to individualize therapy for lupus patients, selecting those patients most likely to respond to a specific therapy.

Given the negative recent trial data for rituximab in adults with SLE, albeit with positive retrospective clinical experience with this therapy in children with SLE resistant to standard therapy, rituximab should only be given upon expert advice.

- In rare circumstances, rituximab can be considered for primary induction of remission—suggest under expert advice only.

Patient selection criteria

- Severe active lupus previously treated with standard lupus treatment either IVCYC or MMF for a minimum of 6 months, *or*
- As add-on to standard induction therapy for those with severe life-threatening disease—little available evidence of its efficacy in this context.
- No known severe reaction to humanized chimeric antibodies.

Exclusion criteria

- Chronic active infection.
- Recent severe infection (screen for hepatitis B virus).
- Pregnancy or planned pregnancy.
- Hypogammaglobulinaemia (these patients should be considered with caution).

Rituximab treatment protocol

Rituximab may be given in addition to CYC, except where cumulative CYC toxicity, side effects, or other clinical contraindication preclude this.

Suggested protocol

- Day 1 and day 15: rituximab infusion 750 mg/m² (rounded up to the nearest 100 mg); max dose—1 g.
- Premedicate with chlorphenamine (5–10 mg) and paracetamol (15 mg/kg) 1 h prior to the rituximab infusion.
- In addition, a dose of methylprednisolone IV 100 mg (absolute dose, not per kg) is given 30 min prior to the rituximab infusion.

Administration of rituximab: practical aspects

- Dilute the required dose with sodium chloride 0.9% or glucose 5% to a final concentration of 1–4 mg/mL.
- The initial infusion rate is 50 mg/h, which can be increased by increments of 50 mg/h every 30 min up to a maximum of 400 mg/h as tolerated.

Rituximab: side effects

- *Serum sickness*: fevers and rigors, which usually present within the first 2 h. Other reported symptoms include pruritus and rashes, dyspnoea, bronchospasm, angio-oedema, and transient hypotension:
  - In the event of an infusion-related adverse event, stop the infusion, and assess the patient. Mild to moderate infusion reactions may require slowing of infusion, additional antihistamines, paracetamol, bronchodilators, or glucocorticoids. Severe reactions requiring discontinuation of drug are rare. NB: of fatal infusion reactions within 24 h of rituximab infusion, 80% occurred with first infusions.
  - Premedication with chlorphenamine, paracetamol, and methylprednisolone will reduce the incidence of adverse effects.

- *Infections*:
  - Herpes zoster infection described in children.
  - Progressive multifocal leucoencephalopathy caused by JC virus (a polyoma virus).
- *Rituximab-associated neutropenia*: occurring usually several months following the administration of rituximab:
  - Usually not clinically significant and is self-limited but should be differentiated with neutropenia from other cause such as active SLE.
  - Mechanism remains largely speculative.

Follow-up post rituximab

Follow up carefully with:
- clinical status
- FBC including differential, ESR, CRP, U&Es, and LFTs; Ua:Ucr (minimum of fortnightly FBC for 6 weeks then monthly)
- dsDNA, C3, C4
- screen for B-cell response and agammaglobulinaemia (see Table 10.2). The use of replacement immunoglobulins in deficient patients is not standard practice at this stage, but will be continually monitored. The decision to commence IV immunoglobulin replacement will be decided on an individual basis and will depend on the findings of hypogammaglobulinaemia, and/or the occurrence and nature of infections

Repeat rituximab dosing

Repeated doses of rituximab are only recommended for those with evidence of return of disease activity after return of peripheral blood lymphocytes (Table 10.2).

Further reading

Bertsias G, Tektonidou M, Amoura Z, et al. Joint European League Against Rheumatism and European Renal Association-European Dialysis and Transplant Association (EULAR/ERA-EDTA) recommendations for the management of adult and paediatric lupus nephritis. *Ann Rheum Dis* 2012;71:1771–1782.

Weening JJ, D'Agati VD, Schwartz MM, et al. The classification of glomerulonephritis in systemic lupus erythematosus revisited. *Kidney Int* 2004;65:521–530.

Table 10.2 Monitoring rituximab treatment in patients with SLE

Test	Timing (after first dose)	Notes
Lymphocyte subsets	Day 7–10 Monthly from 4 months after first dose until B cells normal	Measures T, B (CD19) and NK cells. Must do FBC same day
Immunoglobulins GAM	Day 7–10 2 months after first dose. Monthly from 4 months after first dose until B cells normal.	

Note: B cells express CD19 and CD20, and it is routine to measure CD19 as a B-cell marker. Rarely (normally in the context of malignancy) B cells may not express CD20 and will not therefore be eliminated by rituximab. If there is concern that B cells are not eradicated after 7–10 days, routine B-cell measurement should be repeated and direct measurement of CD20 may be helpful. This will rarely be required.

Diabetes and metabolic syndrome

Type 1 diabetes

Background

- Diabetic nephropathy is the commonest cause of CKD stage 5 in adults in the USA and accounts for 22% of new patients requiring dialysis in the UK, this figure rises to 30% in areas of ethnic diversity.
- Microalbuminuria can occur within 5 years of the onset of type 1 diabetes mellitus and is therefore seen in the paediatric population, as well as in adults.
- The natural history includes progression in several stages over 10–15 years, starting with apparent normality in the first few years after diagnosis, followed by incipient nephropathy characterized by the presence of small amounts of albumin in the urine (undetectable on dipstick), known as microalbuminuria, terminating in overt proteinuria and nephropathy.
- 20–30% of patients develop subclinical microalbuminuria, which is potentially reversible with tight glucose control.
- Once overt proteinuria has developed, it is irreversible and heralds the onset of CKD.
- 25–45% of patients develop overt clinical nephropathy (the minimal criterion for which is a persistently positive urine dipstick for protein).
- Patients with nephropathy will almost invariably have other signs of diabetic microvascular disease, such as neuropathy or retinopathy.
- There is no specific therapy for diabetic nephropathy, and patient management should generally be targeted at preventing the onset of CKD, and slowing its progress once detected.
- Sodium–glucose co-transporter 2 inhibitors reduce glycaemia as well as weight, BP, and albuminuria in adults with diabetes and have recently been shown to reduce the incidence of cardiovascular complications of the disease.

Pathology

The three major histological changes in the glomeruli in diabetic nephropathy are:

- mesangial expansion
- glomerular basement membrane thickening
- glomerular sclerosis which may have a nodular appearance: the Kimmelstiel–Wilson lesion.

There may be associated hyaline deposits in the glomerular arterioles. Renal biopsy in diabetics with microalbuminuria only may reveal normal histology or evidence of glomerulosclerosis or other changes of diabetic nephropathy. Normal histology is more likely where the level of albumin excretion is low and there is no hypertension or impairment of GFR.

Microalbuminuria

- Microalbuminuria refers to levels of albuminuria that are too low to be detected by conventional dipstick analysis and require the use of sensitive laboratory techniques.
- Microalbuminuria is defined as an excretion of 30–300 mg/day (20–200 micrograms/min) of albumin in an adult. In comparison,

dipstick-positive albuminuria typically reflects values >300 mg/day (200 micrograms/min).
* It is common practice to use early morning spot Ua:Ucr for the detection of microalbuminuria in children: Ua:Ucr >2.5 mg/mmol would define microalbuminuria.
* The renal excretion of albumin can be elevated by vigorous exercise, acute illness, fever, severe cardiac disease, UTI, menstrual bleeding, severe hypertension, poor glycaemic control, and ketoacidosis. Sample collection should therefore be avoided when such intercurrent problems are present, and vigorous exercise avoided for 24 h prior to testing. Three serial early morning urine samples should be checked to rule out problems such as these.

Management of the child with microalbuminuria

The presence of overt diabetic nephropathy in childhood is rare, so:
* management should concentrate on the prevention of the development of and screening for the presence of microalbuminuria
* microalbuminuria screening should be annual. NICE guidelines (2016) state that this should commence at 12 years of age. As in all monitoring for albuminuria/proteinuria, this should be performed on a first morning specimen of urine. Where an initial Ua:Ucr is >3 mg/mmol but below 30 mg/mmol then the test should be repeated on two further first morning specimens
* when persistent microalbuminuria is detected, treatment strategies should be introduced to reduce the degree of albumin excretion with the aim of postponing the progression to overt nephropathy
* optimal management should address all possible risk factors: hyperglycaemia, hypertension, microalbuminuria and dyslipidaemia.

Glycaemic control

A number of studies in adult patients have shown that strict control of the plasma glucose through the use of intensive insulin therapy results in a reduction in the cumulative incidence of microalbuminuria, and can also halt the progression to overt diabetic nephropathy in those with existing microalbuminuria.

ACE inhibition

A Cochrane systematic review of adult studies confirms that ACE inhibition results in a significant reduction in albumin excretion and a lowering of systemic BP. These drugs were shown to prevent the new onset of kidney disease and reduce the number of deaths in adults with diabetes and normal plasma albumin levels compared with placebo or calcium channel inhibitors. However, no effect of ARBs was seen on either development of CKD stage 5 or death.

Management of hypertension

The presence of hypertension is a known adverse risk factor for the progression of microalbuminuria to overt nephropathy:
* NICE guidelines (2015) recommend that BP is measured annually in children with type 1 diabetes.
* As ACE inhibitors reduce albumin excretion in addition to BP, they are the logical drug of first choice where hypertension is detected.

- It is fairly well established that the use of antihypertensive agents in diabetic patients is beneficial (when compared with no treatment), in terms of maintaining renal function and protein excretion.
- Lifestyle: avoidance of obesity and smoking, and increased physical activity.

Type 2 diabetes

Background
- The incidence of type 2 diabetes and the ratio of type 2:type 1 diabetes in children is rising in the USA and Europe. This is strongly linked to the rising incidence of obesity, which is a major risk factor for insulin resistance, glucose intolerance, and type 2 diabetes.
- Microalbuminuria is more common in type 2 than type 1 diabetes in children.
- Children with type 2 diabetes have a fivefold increased risk of CKD stage 5 over patients with adult onset:
  - There is the possibility that diabetes may reflect genetic kidney disease, e.g. HNF1B mutations.

Management
- As for type 1 diabetes, though there should be a major focus on weight reduction strategies including increased physical activity.
- The use of metformin is now recommended from diagnosis.
- NICE guidelines (2015) state that children and young adults with type 2 diabetes should undergo annual monitoring for:
  - hypertension starting at diagnosis
  - dyslipidaemia starting at diagnosis
  - retinopathy starting at diagnosis
  - microalbuminuria starting at diagnosis (recommendations as for type 1 diabetes).

Other causes of proteinuria in children and young adults with diabetes
It is important to remember that albuminuria may occasionally be due to an alternative glomerular disease. Clues pointing to a non-diabetic nephropathy include:
- the early onset of proteinuria (within 5 years of diagnosis)
- acute onset of proteinuria
- the presence of an active urinary sediment (red cells and casts)
- the absence of diabetic retinopathy or neuropathy.

Diabetic nephropathy is generally not confirmed histologically in adult patients, with biopsy being reserved for those with such atypical presenting features where an alternative pathology is suspected. This is also sensible practice in children.

Obesity and the metabolic syndrome
- 18.5% of children in the USA are obese (body mass index ≥95th percentile). Similar figures are developing in Europe.
- Childhood obesity tends to track into adulthood: 85% of obese toddlers become obese adults.
- Childhood obesity is associated with many significant health issues. While children do not generally develop cardiovascular events such as myocardial infarction, evidence of atherogenesis can be detected in those with obesity.

- Obesity is harmful to the kidney; fat is metabolically active and leads to insulin resistance, increased inflammatory cytokines, sympathetic activity, oxidative stress and leptin, and reduced adiponectin. Increased activity of the renin–angiotensin system results in hypertension, hyperfiltration, and CKD.
- The metabolic syndrome comprises a cluster of cardiovascular risk factors including hypertension, altered glucose metabolism, dyslipidaemia, and abdominal obesity. >25% of the adult population of the USA is affected. In addition to CVD and type 2 diabetes, the metabolic syndrome is associated with chronic low-grade inflammation, hyperuricaemia, hyperandrogenism, polycystic ovary syndrome, hepatic steatosis, obstructive sleep apnoea, hypogonadism, vascular dementia, Alzheimer disease, and certain malignancies.
- Many attempts have been made to define metabolic syndrome in children, though to date no consensus definition exists.

Further reading

NICE. *Diabetes (Type 1 and Type 2) in Children and Young People: Diagnosis and Management*. NICE guideline NG18. London: NICE, 2015 (updated November 2016).

Weiss R, Bremer AA, Lustig RH. What is metabolic syndrome and why are children getting it? *Ann NY Acad Sci* 2013;1281:123–140

Sickle cell disease

Haematuria is very common. In early adulthood, up to 40% have microalbuminuria, 30% proteinuria, and 18% ESKD. Mortality on RRT is high due to co-morbidities.

Haematuria

Haematuria may occur in sickle cell disease due to sickling of RBCs in the renal medulla. This occurs because:

- the PaO_2 in the renal medulla is below the threshold for sickling
- the osmolality of the medulla is high
- the medulla is relatively acidic.

Characteristics of renal problems in sickle cell disease

- Haematuria may occur with HbSS or HbAS.
- Renal involvement causing haematuria may be unilateral and associated with discomfort in the loin of the affected side.
- Haematuria may be severe and prolonged.
- The medullary pyramids are echo bright on US.
- Papillary necrosis may occur (see later in topic).
- FSGS may develop.

Treatment of macroscopic haematuria

- 0.45% saline at 4 L/1.73 m²/day.
- Furosemide to increase urine flow.
- Alkalinization with oral sodium bicarbonate.

Papillary necrosis

- May develop even without obvious haematuria and even in young children.
- May be identified by CT scan, where clubbed calyces and an irregular medullary cavity are seen.
- Causes a urine-concentrating defect so patients with sickle cell disease should be encouraged to maintain a high fluid intake. This develops early in life and can be associated with enuresis.

Other renal pathology

- Repeated vaso-occlusive episodes in the vasa recta lead to ischaemia–hyperperfusion injury, early glomerular enlargement, then FSGS, the most common cause of CKD in sickle cell disease.
- The ischaemia–hyperperfusion generates a chronic inflammatory response which leads to tubulointerstitial changes, loss of nephrons, and eventual sclerosis.
- Proteinuria is the most common clinical manifestation of these changes and may progress to nephrotic syndrome.
- In the distal nephron, the loss of the vasa recta results in impaired concentrating ability.

Further reading

Becker AM. Sickle cell nephropathy: challenging the conventional wisdom. *Pediatr Nephrol* 2011;26:2099–2109.

Renal involvement in cystic fibrosis

* As the prognosis improves for patients with cystic fibrosis (CF), renal complications of the illness are more frequently seen.
* There are several possible mechanisms of renal injury in CF, including complications arising from chronic infection, immunological dysregulation (perhaps as a result of chronic infection or inflammation), and drug therapy.
* Even though the CF transmembrane regulator gene (*CFTR*) is widely expressed in the kidney, there is no evidence for a primary renal involvement.

Nephrocalcinosis and nephrolithiasis

CF is associated with an increased risk of nephrocalcinosis and nephrolithiasis for various reasons:
* Prolonged periods of immobilization.
* Use of lithogenic drugs (e.g. corticosteroids or furosemide).
* *Secondary alimentary hyperoxaluria*: calcium usually complexes with oxalate in the gut, preventing oxalate absorption (i.e. calcium is an 'oxalate binder', as well as a phosphate binder, as used in CKD). In fat malabsorption, as can occur in CF due to exocrine pancreatic dysfunction, fatty acids compete with oxalate for calcium binding, thereby increasing oxalate absorption.

Nephrotoxic drugs

* A number of potentially nephrotoxic drugs are routinely used in the management of children with CF including aminoglycoside antibiotics, cephalosporins, loop diuretics, and NSAIDs. Nephrotoxic acute tubular necrosis (ATN) is a recognized complication of certain drug therapy (e.g. aminoglycosides) and differs clinically from ischaemic ATN in that the former is more likely to be associated with a non-oliguric presentation and gradual onset of renal failure.
* The drug most commonly associated with AKI in CF is gentamicin, which should therefore be avoided. Tobramycin appears to have less nephrotoxicity. As much as possible, antibiotics should be given nebulized, rather than systemically. The risk for AKI can be further minimized by once-daily dosing and close attention to drug levels.
* NSAIDs are used in CF for the management of CF-related arthropathy, and may be associated with renal vasoconstriction and acute renal dysfunction, especially in the context of the chronic salt depletion associated with CF.

Tubulointerstitial nephritis

* TIN may complicate CF as a result of an allergic reaction to antibiotics or infection. Polyuria/polydipsia is common and systemic signs of allergy, such as rash and non-specific symptoms, such as malaise, fever, and vomiting may be present.
* Laboratory investigations demonstrate elevation of plasma urea and creatinine, occasionally accompanied by hypokalaemia and hypophosphataemia (due to the proximal tubular dysfunction), and sometimes a peripheral blood and/or urinary eosinophilia (request Wright stain on urine sample).

- Urinary examination may reveal haematuria, proteinuria (positive dipstick for protein, but little urinary albumin implying tubular rather than glomerular protein leak), and glycosuria.
- US usually demonstrates large, echo-bright kidneys.
- Renal biopsy demonstrates an interstitial infiltrate with frequent eosinophils, sometimes with tubular dilatation and areas of TIN fibrosis (→ see 'Tubulointerstitial nephritis', p. 197).

IgA nephropathy

IgA nephropathy (IgAN) is a rare complication and coexistence may be co-incidental, but there may be a real association due to recurrent respiratory tract infections, with increased circulating IgA with glomerular deposition.

Other renal manifestations of cystic fibrosis

- Amyloidosis may complicate CF due to the chronic inflammatory nature of the disease. The prognosis is generally poor.
- Systemic vasculitis occasionally complicates CF, the cause of which is unknown, but presumably reflects an aberrant immune response to chronic infection or drug therapy, or both. The vasculitis is predominantly cutaneous, but occasionally is more widespread with both cerebral and renal involvement (renal failure and focal glomerular sclerosis and capsular adhesions) reported.
- CF may be complicated by diabetes mellitus, and reports of diabetic nephropathy in this context have been documented.

Sarcoidosis

Background

- A spectrum of idiopathic, multisystemic inflammatory diseases characterized by the formation of non-caseating granulomata in affected tissues.
- Two distinct forms of the disease exist in children. Older children usually have disease similar to adult manifestations with pulmonary involvement and lymphadenopathy. Early-onset sarcoidosis (EOS), with onset of disease before the age of 5 years, is a very different disease from later presentations, and will be discussed separately.

Pathogenesis

- The cause is unknown:
  - An exaggerated immune host response (under genetic control) to so far unidentified antigens remains the main hypothesis.
  - Candidate genes may reside in loci that influence regulation of the immune response.
- Epidemiology:
  - Incidence and prevalence vary worldwide by age, sex, ethnic origin, and geographic location: primarily a disease of 20–40-year-olds.
- The disease is more common in Japanese children and black children, although this racial distribution varies with geographic location. Sarcoid is seen more commonly in developed than underdeveloped areas.
- True incidence and prevalence in children is unknown.
- In Denmark, where the disease has a high prevalence, the incidence in children younger than 15 years is 0.22–0.27 per 100,000/year; 0.06 per 100,000 children under the age of 4 years; and increases gradually with age to 1.02 per 100,000 in children aged 14–15 years.

Genetics of sarcoidosis

- There is an increased incidence of sarcoidosis in certain families.
- In the USA, familial clusters are observed in African Americans in 19%, compared to 5% in white families.
- Monozygotic twins are two to four times more concordant for disease than dizygotic twins.
- Sarcoidosis is associated with a genetic risk profile comprised of many variant genes:
  - HLA-DRB1*03 predisposes to disease with spontaneous resolution
  - HLA-DRB1*14 or HLA-DRB1*15 predispose a chronic course.
- Recent studies suggest a unique candidate gene BTNL2 in the MHC II region on chromosome 6 that may function as a costimulatory molecule.

Clinical features

This is a multisystem disease so presentation can vary greatly:
- Multisystemic presentation: older children usually present in a similar manner as adults with lymphadenopathy, pulmonary involvement, and systemic symptoms (fever, malaise, fatigue, and weight loss).
- Renal and biochemical findings:

- Renal involvement is rare in children and adults, and may be asymptomatic; renal involvement is usually secondary to hypercalcaemia and/or hypercalciuria (occurring in ~30% of paediatric sarcoid cases), rather than renal infiltration with granulomata.
- Polyuria, enuresis (secondary nephrogenic diabetes insipidus (NDI) from hypercalcaemia).
- Hypercalcaemia ± hypercalciuria.
- Hypercalciuria in the absence of hypercalcaemia.
- Nephrocalcinosis and nephrolithiasis (only if hypercalciuria).
- Bilateral enlargement of the kidneys.
- TIN.
- Rarely, glomerular lesions: classically membranous glomerulonephritis, but crescentic nephritis has also been reported.
- Pulmonary disease—is the most commonly involved organ:
  - Chronic cough with or without dyspnoea.
  - Bilateral hilar lymphadenopathy with or without parenchymal involvement is the most common radiographic finding.
  - The hilar lymphadenopathy is usually symmetrical.
  - Parenchymal disease, pleural effusions, and atelectasis occur less commonly in children than in adults (25% of affected adults are affected with these).
  - Nearly half of all children with sarcoidosis demonstrate restrictive lung disease on pulmonary function tests.
  - An obstructive pattern secondary to intrabronchial granuloma or mediastinal lymph node airway compression may occasionally be observed.
- Lymphadenopathy and hepatosplenomegaly: lymphadenopathy, including retroperitoneal lymphadenopathy, is commonly observed, and can occur with or without hepatosplenomegaly.
- Skin disease—24–40%:
  - Sarcoid should be considered in the differential diagnosis of unusual skin lesions in children.
  - Most common is a cutaneous eruption with soft, yellowish-brown flat topped papules found most frequently on the face.
  - Larger violatious plaque-like lesions may be found on the trunk and extremities.
  - Erythema nodosum is reported in 31%.
  - Other lesions include nodules and subcutaneous tumours, hyper- or hypo-pigmented lesions, and ulcers.
- Eye disease: it should be remembered that young children may be asymptomatic, although blind in one eye at presentation. All of the following are described in sarcoid:
  - Uveitis: general term used to describe inflammation of the uvea, comprising the iris, ciliary body and choroid.
  - Iridocyclitis (inflammation of the iris and ciliary body).
  - Posterior uveitis: predominantly choroid but not iridocyclitis.
  - Lacrimal gland swelling.
  - Conjunctival granulomata.
  - Vitritis.
  - Chorioretinitis.

- Optic neuritis.
- Proptosis.
- Interstitial keratitis.
- Musculoskeletal disease—affects 15–58% of affected children:
  - Arthralgia.
  - Arthritis, usually affecting multiple joints: boggy tenosynovitis with relatively painless effusion and little or no overlying erythema of skin; erosive changes on X-ray usually absent.
  - Bone cysts (especially small bones of hand and foot).
  - Muscle involvement can occur, but is unusual.
- Neurological—neurosarcoidosis is rare in children, but is described, and includes:
  - encephalopathy and seizures
  - cranial nerve involvement
  - cerebral mass lesion (rare in posterior fossa)
  - spinal cord involvement
  - aseptic meningitis
  - obstructive hydrocephalus.
- Other:
  - Parotid enlargement (with uveitis sometimes called 'uveo-parotid fever').
  - Rectal prolapse.
  - Sicca syndrome.
  - Testicular mass.
  - Pericardial effusion.
  - Myocardial involvement.
  - Granulomatous large and medium-size vessel vasculitis.

Differential diagnosis

- Infection causing granulomatous inflammation, including:
  - *Mycobacterium tuberculosis*
  - leprosy
  - histoplasmosis
  - blastomycosis.
- Chronic granulomatous disease (exclude with nitroblue tetrazolium test; ➔ see 'Laboratory findings and investigations').
- Blau syndrome (➔ see 'Early-onset sarcoidosis and Blau syndrome').
- Systemic juvenile idiopathic arthritis.
- Granulomatous small vessel vasculitis including granulomatosis with polyangiitis (formerly known as Wegener's granulomatosis), and eosinophilic granulomatosis with polyangiitis (formerly known as Churg–Strauss syndrome).
- Crohn's disease may rarely be confused with sarcoidosis.
- Lymphoma.
- Berylliosis: inhalation of beryllium has been associated with a granulomatous lung disease known as chronic beryllium disease.

Laboratory findings and investigations

No single test is diagnostic of sarcoid. Ultimately, tissue diagnosis and the exclusion of other diseases that can mimic sarcoid are required. The historical Kveim–Siltzbach test, whereby intradermal injection of a splenic extract from a known sarcoid patient resulted in sarcoid granulomata in a suspected case, is antiquated, and the standard test reagent no longer available. Observed laboratory findings include the following:

- Leucopenia, thrombocytosis, and eosinophilia relatively common.
- High ESR and CRP.
- Hypercalcaemia: varies from 2% to 60% of cases. The mechanism of this appears to be that abnormal pulmonary macrophages synthesize $1,25(OH)_2$ vitamin D from 25-hydroxy vitamin D, and are relatively insensitive to feedback by hypercalcaemia.
- Abnormal liver function.
- Raised Ua:Ucr.
- Tubular function abnormalities (➔ see 'Tubulointerstitial nephritis').
- Serum angiotensin-converting enzyme (sACE), produced by epithelial cells in the granulomas may be elevated. ACE levels are influenced by ACE gene polymorphisms and physiological values vary according to age with children having a higher normal range. The value of sACE in the diagnosis and management of sarcoidosis remains unclear.
- Mantoux test or QuantiFERON® (interferon-gamma release assay) to exclude TB. NB: sarcoid patients commonly demonstrate anergy (no response) to purified protein derivatives of *Mycobacterium tuberculosis* even if previously exposed.
- Nitroblue tetrazolium (NBT) test (alternatively a flow cytometric test of neutrophil oxidative metabolism using dihydrorhodamine) to exclude chronic granulomatous disease.
- Eye screen for uveitis.
- X-rays of affected bones and joints.
- Chest X-ray: standard screen for pulmonary sarcoid.
- Increased sensitivity of detection of pulmonary involvement with high-resolution CT of chest.
- Pulmonary function tests including transfer factor (diffusing capacity, DLCO).
- MRI of brain for suspected neurosarcoidosis.
- Tissue biopsy: skin, lung, salivary glands. Occasionally renal biopsy.
- ECG and echocardiogram for suspected cardiac involvement. Cardiac MRI may also have a role in this context.

Treatment

- Acute transient disease requires rest and NSAIDs.
- Chronic and/or severe multisystemic disease requires corticosteroid therapy, e.g. 0.5–2 mg/kg daily prednisolone, tapering over 2–3 months.
- An additional immunosuppressant agent may be required for persistent progressive sarcoidosis: MTX, or azathioprine: a RCT of MTX in 24 adults with sarcoid demonstrated steroid-sparing efficacy.
- Occasionally cyclophosphamide or ciclosporin has been used for more aggressive disease.
- Ocular involvement usually responds to corticosteroid administered locally or systemically.
- Although evidence-based data are scant for the treatment of paediatric sarcoidosis, the recognition of the toxicity of long-term steroids, even in lower doses, has encouraged the use of MTX 10–15 mg/m^2 once weekly as a steroid-sparing strategy. Biological therapy especially anti-tumour necrosis factor (TNF) alpha has been increasingly used in severe and refractory cases with moderate success.

Early-onset sarcoidosis and Blau syndrome

- EOS refers to young children with disease onset in the first 5 years of life. These children differ from those with sarcoidosis of later presentation:
  - EOS typically presents with the classic triad of rash, arthritis, and uveitis (in that order), but without apparent pulmonary involvement or hilar lymphadenopathy.
  - EOS typically presents in the first year of life.
  - Uveitis, which occurs in more than half of the children with EOS, is relatively less common in patients with later-onset disease. This ocular disease can be difficult to control despite aggressive therapy. Significant visual loss occurs in 20–30% of affected children.
- Blau syndrome is an AD granulomatous disease that occurs in families and has the same classic triad of rash, arthritis, and uveitis, i.e. an identical clinical phenotype to EOS.
- Recent data suggest that EOS and Blau syndrome represent the sporadic and familial forms of the same disease since both share genetic mutations in the nucleotide-binding oligomerization domain 2 gene (NOD2, also referred to as the CARD15 gene).
- The NOD2 gene probably has no major effect on sarcoidosis susceptibility in older patients, however.

Renal disease is very rare in EOS but the following have been described:
- Renal granulomata.
- TIN.
- Renal insufficiency.
- Renal clear cell carcinoma in a 14-year-old.

Prognosis

- Guarded prognosis for young children with EOS: nearly all develop long-term morbidity from uveitis, polyarthritis, or other organ involvement.
- An international Blau registry with 31 patients after a median disease duration of 12.8 years found:
  - joint damage leading to mild impairment in 31%, and severe impairment in 28%
  - moderate to severe visual loss in 33%
  - expanded manifestations beyond classic triad (visceral, vasculitis) in 52%.
- Older children have a variable prognosis, dependent on organ involvement, geography, sex, and race:
  - Long-term follow-up of 46 Caucasian Danish children reported 78% complete recovery.
  - 11% still had chronic active disease with multiorgan involvement.
  - 7% died.
  - 4% were recovered, but with residual organ damage including unilateral loss of vision and abnormal chest radiography.
  - The presence of erythema nodosum was associated with a good prognosis, and CNS sarcoidosis was associated with a poor prognosis.
- In another series of 29 children from a French national registry followed up for a mean of 4–5 years:

- In the patients >10 years old, 47% of patients had experienced relapses, with current steroid treatment in all but one. Seven of this group were also on additional immunosuppressive medications.
- Relapse occurrence was significantly associated with systemic disease extension, evaluated by number of involved organs ($p = 0.004$).

Further reading

Rosé CD, Pans S, Casteels I, et al. Blau syndrome: cross-sectional data from a multicentre study of clinical, radiological and functional outcomes. *Rheumatology* 2015;54:1008–1016.
Valeyre D, Prasse A, Nunes H, et al. Sarcoidosis. *Lancet* 2014;383:1155–1167.

Mitochondrial cytopathies

Basic principles

- Mitochondria are intracellular organelles involved in ATP generation (cellular 'power plants'). They are derived from symbiotic bacteria that were eventually incorporated into the cell. Consequently, they carry their own circular DNA—the mitochondrial DNA.
- Because mitochondrial DNA (which also encodes ribosomal RNA) is derived from bacteria, mitochondria are particularly susceptible to antibiotics that target prokaryotic protein synthesis, such as aminoglycosides, chloramphenicol, and tetracyclines. This is the basis for the human toxicity of these antibiotics—an acquired mitochondrial cytopathy.
- Mitochondria derive from the oocyte only. Thus, mitochondrial DNA is inherited from the mother.
- The oocyte contains multiple mitochondria. A mutation may not be present in all of them. The passing on of mitochondria to daughter cells occurs randomly, thus some cells may contain more mutated mitochondrial DNA than others. This is referred to as 'heteroplasmy' and explains why some tissues may be affected more than others in a given patient. Similarly, if a mother carries a mitochondrial mutation, some oocytes may receive a higher proportion of the mitochondria carrying the mutation than others, resulting in phenotypic variability.
- The mitochondrial genome is incomplete for the functioning of mitochondria as it encodes only 37 genes. A mitochondrion hosts about 3000 proteins and the genes encoding all the other proteins are localized in the nuclear DNA. Consequently, mitochondrial diseases can be inherited maternally (if the mutation is localized in the mitochondrial DNA) or AR (if the mutation is in the nuclear DNA).
- Because mitochondria are responsible for ATP and thus cellular energy generation, the symptoms can be extremely variable. Several defined syndromes exist, but there is considerable overlap and variability.

Clinical manifestations of mitochondrial disease

- *Bone marrow*: pancytopenia.
- *Brain*:
  - Ataxia.
  - Stroke.
  - Seizures.
  - Dementia.
  - Migraine.
- *Eye*:
  - External ophthalmoplegia.
  - Optic neuropathy.
  - Pigmentary retinal degeneration.
  - Cataract.
  - Corneal dystrophy.
  - Ptosis.

- *Heart*:
  - Cardiomyopathy.
  - Conduction blocks.
  - Wolff–Parkinson–White syndrome.
- *Inner ear*: sensorineural deafness.
- *Intestine*: malabsorption.
- *Kidney*:
  - Tubulopathy.
  - Nephrocalcinosis.
  - Glomerulopathy/FSGS.
  - CKD.
- *Liver*: hepatopathy.
- *Pancreas*:
  - Diabetes mellitus.
  - Exocrine dysfunction.
- *Skeletal muscle*:
  - Myopathy.
  - Fatigue.
  - Weakness.
- *Other*:
  - Short stature.
  - Episodic nausea and vomiting.
  - Hypoparathyroidism.
  - Adrenal insufficiency.
  - Lactic acidosis.
  - Elevated cerebrospinal fluid protein.
  - Peripheral neuropathy.
  - Myoclonus.

Classical syndromes associated with mitochondrial cytopathy

- *MERRF*: myoclonic epilepsy with ragged red fibres.
- *NARP*: neuropathy, ataxia, and retinitis pigmentosa.
- *MELAS*: mitochondrial encephalopathy, lactic acidosis, and stroke-like episodes.
- *Leigh syndrome*: maternally inherited Leigh syndrome (somnolence, blindness, deafness, peripheral neuropathy, degeneration of brainstem).
- *Pearson syndrome*: pancytopenia, exocrine pancreatic deficiency, and hepatic dysfunction.
- *Kearns–Sayre syndrome*: ophthalmoplegia, pigmentary retinopathy, heart block, and ataxia.
- *Alper syndrome*: intractable epilepsy, liver disease, and neuronal degeneration.

The kidney and mitochondrial cytopathy

- The most common renal manifestation associated with mitochondrial cytopathies in childhood is renal Fanconi syndrome, although a few patients have FSGS. Some may have nephrocalcinosis.
- Renal manifestations rarely occur alone and are usually associated with other symptoms, mainly neurological disease. Most patients present in the first months of life. The prognosis is guarded for infants with severe neurological and renal disease associated with mitochondrial cytopathy.

- The most prevalent pathogenic mutation in mitochondrial disease is the m.3243A>G point mutation in the tRNA^{Leu(UUR)} (*MTTL1*) gene, which has an estimated frequency of ~1:400. It is associated with a whole spectrum of severity both for renal and extrarenal manifestation, ranging from no apparent symptoms to multiorgan involvement. Glomerular dysfunction with CKD is more common in older mutation carriers.
- Recessive mutations in *ADCK4* are a cause of steroid-resistant nephrotic syndrome, associated with FSGS on biopsy and rapid progression to ESKD. *ADCK4* is involved in CoQ10 synthesis and isolated reports suggest that the disease can be halted by CoQ10 (ubiquinone) supplementation, highlighting the importance of early diagnosis and screening of family members at risk.
- There is increasing recognition of the importance of mitochondrial function in AKI, because of their essential role in providing cellular energy.

Investigations to be considered in suspected mitochondrial disease

- FBC, U&Es, creatinine, bicarbonate, albumin, bone and liver function, and fasting glucose.
- Formal GFR or cystatin C-based methods may be helpful as, due to poor muscle mass, creatinine may be deceptively low and therefore underestimate GFR.
- Thyroid function.
- PTH.
- Plasma cortisol (24 h profile).
- Synacthen® test.
- Plasma lactate, pyruvate, ketone bodies (acetoacetate and beta-hydroxybutyrate) and lactate: pyruvate molar ratio.
- Cerebrospinal fluid lactate:pyruvate ratio.
- Bone marrow aspirate/trephine if there is evidence of marrow failure as other causes of this, e.g. leukaemia, must be excluded.
- ECG (24 h monitor), chest X-ray, and echocardiogram.
- Ophthalmological review.
- EEG, EMG, nerve conduction.
- MRI brain.
- Audiometry or other age-specific hearing test.
- Muscle biopsy (quadriceps): to include standard histological stains, electron microscopy, and respiratory chain assays.
- Skin biopsy for fibroblast culture.
- Blood for nuclear and mitochondrial DNA analysis.
- Urine for tubular function tests: amino acids, pH, tubular proteins, TRP.
- Ua:Ucr.
- Urine organic acids to exclude other inborn error of metabolism associated with acidosis.
- Renal and abdominal US.
- Renal biopsy.

Treatment

There is no cure although some forms can be dramatically improved, e.g. by coenzyme Q supplementation in patients with mutations in *COQ2*, *PDSS2*, or *ADCK4*, who cannot synthesize coenzyme Q themselves (➜ see 'Overview of inherited glomerular diseases', p. 214). Expert advice is imperative in suspected mitochondrial disease in order not to miss such a therapeutic opportunity. Therapy is divided into general supportive and specific pharmacological attempts to improve the respiratory chain defect.

General

- Treat tubulopathy: adequate hydration, correction of acidosis, potassium, sodium, phosphate supplementation. Alfacalcidol for rickets and hypocalcaemia.
- Treat underlying endocrinopathy/exocrinopathy (diabetes, exocrine pancreas insufficiency, adrenocortical insufficiency, hypoparathyroidism, hypothyroidism).
- Treat seizures.
- Cochlear implants for deafness (NB: there can be no more MRI scans after insertion of cochlear implants since they contain metal, unless patients receive an implant with a removable magnet).
- Eyelid (ptosis) and cataract surgery.
- Cardiac pacing.
- Gastrostomy.
- Speech and physiotherapy.
- Renal transplantation (and cardiac/hepatic transplantation) has been performed in children with mitochondrial disease. The indication for this needs to be considered in the context of the potential extra renal disease.

Specific: seek expert advice (systematic studies lacking)

- Ubiquinone (coenzyme Q10).
- Vitamins C, E, and K.
- Carnitine.
- Vitamins B1 and B2.
- Avoid drugs known to interfere with respiratory chain: valproate, barbiturates.
- Avoid drugs that inhibit mitochondrial protein synthesis: aminoglycosides, tetracyclines, chloramphenicol.
- Ketogenic diet.
- Genetic counselling.

Further reading

Emma F, Montini G, Parikh SM, et al. Mitochondrial dysfunction in inherited renal disease and acute kidney injury. *Nat Rev Nephrol* 2016;12:267–280.

Fabry disease

Background

* An X-linked, recessive lysosomal storage disorder caused by mutations of the gene *GLA* encoding the lysosomal hydrolase, alpha-galactosidase A, resulting in systemic accumulation of globotriaosylceramide (Gb3).
* Usually presents in young adults but may present in childhood in hemizygous males and some heterozygous females, but the diagnosis is often unrecognized due to its variable presentations and low incidence.
* Classical presenting symptoms are neuropathic pain (principally in the hands and feet), angiokeratomas (purple vascular lesions anywhere on the body), and hypohidrosis.
* A swirling pattern in the cornea seen on slit lamp is often present early in life.
* Later there is cardiac, cerebral, and renal involvement, leading to multiorgan dysfunction and death.
* A family history is present in up to one-half of patients and this often is how the diagnosis is made.

Renal involvement

* Presenting symptoms can include NDI, proteinuria, haematuria, and/or CKD, although this is rare in childhood.
* Gb3 is deposited in glomeruli, particularly the podocytes, leading to proteinuria. Nephrotic-range proteinuria is uncommon.
* Gb3 is also deposited in the tubules, so proteinuria may also be tubular in origin. The distal tubules are affected first, leading to decreased urinary concentrating capacity, so polyuria and polydipsia may be the earliest symptoms. Eventually the proximal tubules become affected, occasionally producing renal Fanconi syndrome.
* Urine sediment contains oval fat bodies (degenerating tubular epithelial cells).
* Urinary excretion of Gb3 may be increased.

Diagnosis

* Diagnosis is confirmed by measurement of alpha-galactosidase A activity in leucocytes, plasma, or cultured skin fibroblasts. Enzyme activity is not reliable in females due to potentially distinct X-inactivation in the various organs.
* Genetic diagnosis is most accurate, especially if a mutation has been identified in the family.

Treatment

* Enzyme replacement therapy decreases neuropathic pain and Gb3 deposition (seek expert advice).
* Early institution of this therapy may be able to prevent irreversible tissue damage.
* ACE inhibitor/ARB use to reduce proteinuria may be challenging, since low BP is common.

Further reading

Najafian B, Mauer M, Hopkin RJ, et al. Renal complications of Fabry disease in children. *Pediatr Nephrol* 2013;28:679–687.

Amyloidosis

Background

- Amyloidosis refers to a heterogeneous group of diseases characterized by normally soluble proteins deposited extracellularly in an abnormally folded, insoluble fibrillar form.
- The type of amyloid protein that is misfolded and the organ or tissue in which the misfolded proteins are deposited determines the clinical manifestations.
- Can lead to organ impairment including CKD and premature death.
- Is now rarely seen largely since inflammatory diseases leading to secondary (reactive) amyloidosis are now better controlled with newer drugs.
- Similarly, dialysis-related amyloidosis is rare in the young, principally due to their shorter waiting times for renal transplantation.
- Genetic autoinflammatory diseases (also referred to as periodic fever syndromes) are now emerging as the leading cause of reactive systemic amyloidosis affecting children and adults.

Amyloid

- Amyloid represents a heterogeneous group of proteins. Present in most forms of amyloid, however, is a carbohydrate moiety in the form of glycosaminoglycans and proteoglycans. Most forms of amyloid also contain the protein amyloid-P. This can be exploited diagnostically (⊃ see 'Investigation of suspected amyloidosis', p. 296).
- At least 30 different amyloid proteins are described. The two most clinically important are amyloid-A (AA) and amyloid-L (AL).
- AL comprises monoclonal immunoglobulin light chains and occurs in patients with myeloma-associated amyloidosis. Hence it is usually seen in adults, although some genetic forms of amyloidosis contain AL.
- Protein AA (derived from serum amyloid A—SAA) is an acute phase reactant, and is associated with the amyloidosis of chronic inflammation such as that seen in poorly controlled juvenile idiopathic arthritis, and familial Mediterranean fever (⊃ see 'Familial Mediterranean fever', p. 297).
- The remainder of this section will deal with this type of reactive AA amyloidosis, since it is the commonest type seen in children.

Causes of reactive amyloid-A amyloidosis

Poorly-controlled inflammatory disease of any cause, including:

Juvenile idiopathic arthritis

- Particularly systemic juvenile idiopathic arthritis (SJIA; previously called Still's disease).
- Adolescent-onset rheumatoid arthritis.
- Other forms of arthritis in children including enthesitis (inflammation at tendinous insertions into bones) and related arthritis (including juvenile ankylosing spondylitis and its variants).

Autoinflammatory diseases
- Familial Mediterranean fever (FMF) associated with mutation of the *MEFV* gene.
- Cryopyrin-associated periodic fever syndromes (CAPS) associated with mutation in the *NLRP3* gene, which include:
  - chronic infantile neurological cutaneous and articular (CINCA) syndrome, also referred to as neonatal onset multisystemic inflammatory disease (NOMID)
  - Muckle–Wells syndrome
  - familial cold autoinflammatory syndrome.
- TNF-alpha receptor-associated periodic fever syndrome (TRAPS, previously known as 'familial Hibernian fever') associated with mutation in the *TNFRSF1A* gene.
- Hyper IgD syndrome ('Dutch fever') associated with mutations in the *MVK* gene.

Apart from FMF, these are beyond the scope of this chapter.
- Worthy of note is that SLE and systemic sclerosis are rarely associated with amyloidosis.

Clinical features of reactive AA amyloidosis

The spleen, liver, and kidneys are often involved first in reactive AA amyloidosis. Symptoms and signs develop insidiously, usually on the background of a chronic inflammatory disorder, and the clinician must remain vigilant to the possibility of amyloidosis. Symptoms and signs include the following:
- Weakness.
- Fatigue.
- Weight loss.
- Proteinuria and nephrotic syndrome with CKD—the major cause of death in AA amyloidosis.
- Malabsorption, bowel obstruction, diarrhoea, and hepatosplenomegaly.
- Other manifestations relate mainly to AL amyloidosis, although may occur in AA amyloidosis, and include:
  - cardiac conduction defects
  - restrictive cardiomyopathy and cardiac failure
  - lung involvement
  - skin papules
  - neuropathy—particularly carpal tunnel syndrome
  - arthropathy
  - macroglossia
  - vasculopathy
  - autonomic dysfunction.

Investigation of suspected amyloidosis

- Diagnosis and staging of amyloidosis involves confirmation of amyloid deposition, identification of fibril type, assessment of the underlying amyloidogenic disorder, and extent and severity of amyloidotic organ involvement.
- *Tissue biopsy*: rectal, renal, skin, or SC fat. Stain with Congo red, which reveals apple green birefringence when examined under polarized microscopy. This birefringence remains the histological gold standard for confirming the presence of amyloid in tissue samples.
- Immunohistochemistry remains the most widely used method for fibril typing and its diagnostic value is very high in AA amyloidosis.

- Genetic studies to determine underlying cause if chronic inflammatory disease not apparent or undiagnosed—seek expert advice:
  - Suspected autoinflammatory diseases.
  - Other genetic tests for the many primary genetic types of amyloidosis—all rare in children but occasionally seen.
- SAA will be chronically elevated.
- Renal function.
- Ua:Ucr.
- Radiolabelled serum amyloid-P scintigraphy ('SAP scan'), available in specialized centres only. Helps localize the amyloid, and helpful in monitoring response to therapy. SAP scans are relatively poor at detecting cardiac amyloidosis. Cardiac MRI is increasingly used in this context.

Treatment and prognosis of reactive AA amyloidosis

- Depends on cause.
- If not detected and treated early will ultimately progress leading to CKD and death since no definitive cure available. Thus, prevention is of prime importance.
- Historically, in chronic inflammatory diseases, cytotoxic therapy with chlorambucil and melphalan in combination with corticosteroids has been used to treat amyloidosis in JIA and rheumatoid arthritis (RA) patients. Increasingly, novel biological agents, such as anakinra (IL-1 receptor antagonist) or tocilizumab (IL-6 blocker) are being used to treat amyloidosis with some anecdotal success describing regression of amyloid.
- Colchicine plays an important role in the prevention of amyloidosis in FMF, and may also improve the prognosis for established amyloidosis in this context. Specifically it slows the progression of CKD and reduces proteinuria. Colchicine acts by inhibiting leucocyte chemotaxis through a direct effect on their microtubules. May also down-regulate cell adhesion molecule expression on leucocytes and endothelial cells.

Familial Mediterranean fever

- FMF is common in eastern Mediterranean countries, and is the commonest periodic fever syndrome with propensity to develop reactive AA amyloidosis.
- Inheritance is AD with a gene dosage effect. The MEFV mutations, exons 2, 10 (chromosome 16) result in abnormalities of the protein pyrin, an important regulator of inflammation.
- Duration of fever attacks: 1–4 days. Other features include:
  - serositis: abdominal pain, chest pain, pericarditis, scrotal pain
  - splenomegaly
  - erysipelas-like rash on lower limbs
  - HSP/PAN-like presentation in some patients
  - propensity to reactive (AA) amyloidosis.

Treatment

Colchicine 500–2000 micrograms/day. This will ameliorate fever attacks, lower SAA, and protect against the onset of reactive AA amyloidosis. It will also slow the progression of established AA amyloidosis. Concerns regarding long-term toxicity have not been borne out, and thus colchicine therapy in this context is for life. Colchicine is usually started at a low dose (e.g. 250 micrograms/day) and increased over a few weeks in order to limit GI side effects, which are usually transient.

Corticosteroids are usually ineffective for the treatment of FMF.

Prognosis

With continuous colchicine therapy, most FMF patients are free from inflammatory attacks, and will not develop amyloidosis.

Amyloidosis can also recur in transplanted kidneys, so colchicine needs to be continued after renal transplantation for amyloidosis in FMF patients.

Dialysis-related amyloidosis

* A specific form of beta-2-microglobulin amyloidosis related to long-term dialysis. Affects virtually all patients dialysed for >20 years.
* Symptomatic amyloid is rare in children, but beta-2-microglobulin may be raised.
* A prospective postmortem study found deposition of amyloid in joints in 21% of patients haemodialysed for 2 years, 50% after 7 years, and 100% after 13 years.
* Dialysis amyloidosis occurs because of the inability of conventional HD membranes and time schedules or PD to remove the relatively large molecule beta-2-microglobulin, the primary component of amyloid deposits. New high flux membranes offer better removal of beta-2-microglobulin for HD patients as do haemodiafiltration and longer times on dialysis.
* Since there is limited beta-2-microglobulin clearance by PD, those patients undergoing long-term PD are at risk.
* Histological demonstration of amyloid deposits in synovial, fat or tissue biopsy is diagnostic. Beta-2-microglobulin has a high affinity for collagen, which may explain the predominance of joint and bone disease in patients with dialysis-related amyloidosis. Synovial biopsy, aspiration, and joint fluid and radiographic features are especially important diagnostically.
* Diagnosis is supported by the finding of grossly elevated plasma beta-2-microglobulin levels of the order of 30–50 mg/mL (normal 0.8–3).

Clinical features appear after 10–15 years on dialysis and include:
* carpal tunnel syndrome
* arthropathy
* chronic tenosynovitis of finger flexor tendons
* subcutaneous and glossal lumps
* destructive spondyloarthropathy of cervical spine
* cord compression from amyloidosis in the dural space
* pathological bone fracture
* cardiac amyloid causing arrhythmias and/or cardiac failure from myocardial and conductive system involvement, valvular dysfunction, and restrictive pericarditis
* genitourinary deposition with renal, ureteric, and bladder deposits causing urinary obstruction.

Further reading

Kastner DL, Aksentijevich I, Goldbach-Mansky R. Auto-inflammatory disease reloaded: a clinical perspective. *Cell* 2010;140:784–790.
Wechalekar AD, Gillmore JD, Hawkins PN. Systemic amyloidosis. *Lancet* 2016;387:2641–2654.

Emergency renal management of inborn errors of metabolism

Background

Inborn errors of metabolism (IEMs) may first present in the neonatal/early infancy periods with hyperammonaemic encephalopathy, acidosis, and hypoglycaemia. Neonatal hyperammonaemia is a medical emergency, as brain damage ensues. These patients should only be treated in a centre with experience in neonatal dialysis and metabolic diseases. In addition, metabolic decompensation may occur at any age in patients with IEM during intercurrent illness.

The following is a guideline for the acute renal management of neonates/ infants who present with metabolic crises when the diagnosis is not established, and for those who present with metabolic decompensation in the context of an established diagnosis. This section does not provide a comprehensive review of the many and varied metabolic diseases.

Important general points of note

- The key to success for the management of hyperammonaemia is rapid removal of ammonia from the body. Unlike the rapid removal of urea, this is not associated with a disequilibrium syndrome.
- Children with IEMs may be significantly malnourished; therefore plasma creatinine may provide a poor estimate of GFR. If a more accurate estimate of GFR is needed, cystatin C or similar methods may be advisable (→ see Chapter 18).
- Renal replacement therapy (RRT) (HD, PD, continuous venovenous haemofiltration (CVVH), plus dialysis (CVVHD), exchange transfusion) are rarely required for the management of metabolic crises, for which diet and emergency metabolic regimens form the mainstay of treatment.

Acute severe encephalopathy (including hyperammonaemia and aminoacidopathies)

Hyperammonaemia (>170 µmol/L) strongly suggests metabolic disease. Lower levels may be a non-specific consequence of illness. Children with IEMs may develop permanent brain damage as a result of the accumulation of ammonia and other toxic low-molecular-weight molecules. Those with ammonia levels >1000 µmol/L rarely escape without neurological handicap.

Possible causes include:

- urea cycle disorders (e.g. ornithine transcarbamylase deficiency, arginosuccinic acid synthetase deficiency (ammonia levels typically >400 µmol/L with respiratory alkalosis))
- maple syrup urine disease (NB: ammonia normal in most cases)
- organic acidaemias (methylmalonic acidaemia (MMA), propionic acidaemia (ammonia levels typically 200–500 µmol/L and ketones in urine are characteristic findings).

Investigations

Diagnostic investigations

Seek expert advice from a metabolic disease specialist about likely diagnosis and consequent investigations. Typical investigations include:

* plasma amino acids
* urine organic and amino acids including orotic acid
* acyl carnitines (Guthrie card).

To monitor response to treatment:

* Ammonia, U&Es, creatinine, LFTs (6-hourly).
* Clotting.
* Glucose.
* Plasma amino acids.
* Blood gas.
* Plasma lactate.

Emergency treatment

* Hyperammonaemia: the goals of treatment are to decrease ammonia production and increase ammonia removal rate. Blood purification should be performed in any child with a plasma ammonia >400 µmol/L, although prognosis and neurodevelopmental outcome needs to be considered, if plasma ammonia >1000 µmol/L and/or persistent for >3 days. The most commonly used modality is CVVHD, as it is better tolerated and can be continued for prolonged periods of time.
* Provide adequate calories, fluid, and electrolytes IV (10% glucose).
* Hyperammonaemia causes vasomotor instability, and boluses of colloid may be required.
* Metabolic (no blood purification) treatment of hyperammonaemia typically includes ammonium scavengers (sodium benzoate, sodium phenylacetate or sodium phenylbutyrate). Seek expert advice regarding dosing for individual cases and consider the sodium load from these drugs in the fluid prescription.

Management of severe metabolic acidosis in organic acidaemias, and severe lactic acidosis

* Calculate the anion gap (AG): (Na) − (HCO$_3$ + Cl) (normal range 8–12 mmol/L; ➔ see Chapter 6). In organic acidaemias and lactic acidosis (e.g. MMA, propionic acidaemia (PA)) the AG is increased, whereas in renal tubular acidosis, the AG is normal or decreased. Ensure that hypovolaemia and sepsis are adequately treated, if present.
* Consider correcting acidosis using a 'half correction' based on the formulae:

Pre-term: $(0.6 \times \text{weight}(kg) \times \text{base excess})/2$

Term neonate / children : $(0.3 \times weight(kg) \times \text{base excess}) / 2$
$= mL \text{ of } 8.4\% IV \text{ NaHCO}_3$

This is hyperosmolar and should be administered diluted (in normal saline or 5% albumin) by at least 50%, i.e. give as 4.2%).

- Multiple corrections may be required. Beware hypernatraemia/carbia—
  consider tris(hydroxymethyl)aminomethane (THAM) if this occurs
  (1 mL of 7.2% THAM = 1 mmol of sodium bicarbonate); however, the
  use of THAM involves the administration of a significant volume of fluid
  and should only be administered in an intensive care unit: beware fluid
  overload and secondary hypokalaemia (due to shift into cells).
- If there is considerable encephalopathy, acidosis, or large amounts of
  bicarbonate have been required, consider CVVHD or HD. If vascular
  access is not feasible, consider PD using a bicarbonate-containing
  solution such as Physioneal®.

Methylmalonic acidaemia

With early diagnosis and treatment, the more severe cases of MMA are
surviving longer. There are four important renal considerations in MMA:
- Prerenal AKI during metabolic decompensation, with acute tubular
  dysfunction resulting in severe tubular sodium leak.
- CKD possibly secondary to urate nephropathy or chronic interstitial
  nephritis, particularly in non-vitamin B12 responders.
- Renal tubular dysfunction, impaired urinary concentrating ability.
- Hypertension.

It is important to appreciate that children with MMA may have pre-existing
renal impairment since this will contribute to the acidosis and dehydration, which occur during episodes of acute decompensation. The severity
of AKI may be masked by a relatively low plasma creatinine because of
small muscle bulk and a low-protein diet. Consider HD in severe metabolic
decompensation.

   Successful management of CKD stage 5 in MMA with dialysis, and isolated kidney or combined liver–kidney transplant has been achieved.

Further reading

Häberle J, Boddaert N, Burlina A, et al. Suggested guidelines for the diagnosis and management of
   urea cycle disorders. *Orphanet J Rare Dis* 2012;7:32.

Cystinosis

Background

Nephropathic cystinosis is an AR lysosomal storage disorder leading to cystine accumulation within all cells. Deposition of cystine in the kidney leads first to failure of the proximal tubule and renal Fanconi syndrome. Cystinosis is the commonest cause of the renal Fanconi syndromes in children (➜ see 'Disorders presenting with hypokalaemic acidosis: proximal tubule', p. 166). The estimated incidence is 1 in 100–200,000 live births. Three broad types of cystinosis are described:

* Nephropathic (classic renal and systemic disease with infantile presentation).
* Intermediate (a late-onset variant of nephropathic cystinosis).
* Non-nephropathic (clinically affecting only the cornea).

Genetics

* Mutations in the gene *CTNS* cause all three forms of cystinosis. The gene product, cystinosin, is a lysosomal transport molecule. Loss of function results in intracellular cystine accumulation, which if left untreated, ultimately leads to a variety of organ failures.
* For pregnancies at risk for nephropathic cystinosis, prenatal diagnosis is available through molecular genetic testing.

Nephropathic cystinosis

* Infants appear normal at birth, but develop failure to thrive and manifest renal tubular Fanconi syndrome, with its concomitant metabolic (normal AG) acidosis and volume depletion, electrolyte imbalances, growth retardation, and hypophosphataemic rickets by 6–12 months of age.
* All racial groups are affected, so the typically described appearance of blond hair and fair complexion can be misleading.
* Later, photophobia reflects progressive corneal crystal accumulation. Crystals appear early in the disease (>16 months) and ophthalmological review should be part of the assessment of any child presenting with renal Fanconi syndrome.
* In the natural history of untreated cystinosis, CKD stage 5 develops by 10 years of age.
* Later in the untreated patient, extrarenal complications occur with varying frequencies. These include:
  * distal vacuolar myopathy (with wasting of the small muscles of the hand in particular)
  * swallowing abnormalities
  * retinal blindness
  * hepatosplenomegaly, sometimes with hypersplenism
  * hypothyroidism
  * hypogonadism, with pubertal delay (particularly males)
  * diabetes mellitus
  * pancreatic exocrine insufficiency
  * decreased pulmonary function due to muscle involvement
  * neurological deterioration
  * male infertility.

Diagnosis

- Early diagnosis is critical to instigate treatment and thus delay the onset of complications. Diagnosis relies upon the findings of failure to thrive and renal Fanconi syndrome. Cystinosis remains the most common, and the most treatable, identifiable cause of renal Fanconi syndrome in children. Diagnosis before 1 year of age is feasible, if clinicians consider the diagnosis in patients with failure to thrive and polyuria. A dipstick examination can be helpful, if positive for protein and/or blood. However, false negatives are possible as the dipstick do not recognize low-molecular-weight proteins and the glucose concentration may be <5 mM (the threshold for the dipstick) due to the diluted urine. Thus, dipstick should be accompanied by sending the urine for low-molecular-weight proteins and by a blood electrolyte panel.
- Definitive diagnosis is reached by genetics or biochemically by an elevated leucocyte cystine level in *specialized* labs, generally 3–20 nmol half-cystine/mg protein, at any age. However, normal values are <0.2 nmol half-cystine/mg protein, and values higher than this should raise suspicion sufficient to warrant discussion of the case with an expert in cystinosis.
- In addition to elevated leucocyte cystine levels, the finding of corneal crystals on slit lamp examination by an experienced ophthalmologist can also make the diagnosis, but some patients do not have crystals until 1–2 years of age.

Treatment

- Treatment should involve a team approach, including a paediatric nephrologist, a metabolic disease expert, a genetic counsellor, ophthalmologist, endocrinologist, and a local paediatrician or family practitioner, and dietician.
- Principle therapeutic issues include:
  - oral cysteamine (also called mercaptamine, brand name Cystagon®) therapy should be initiated within days of diagnosis (⊃ see 'Oral cysteamine (Cystagon® or Procysbi®) therapy', p. 304 for dosage);
- Cysteamine treatment is not a cure, but significantly delays the onset of complications. Retrospective cohort analysis suggests that each year of adequate treatment delays the onset of ESKD by 0.9 years. This highlights the need for early diagnosis and adequate cystine depletion (⊃ see 'Oral cysteamine (Cystagon® or Procysbi®) therapy'):
  - Ready access to water and sodium (2–6 mmol/kg/day).
  - Provision of supplemental phosphate salts (⊃ see 'Rickets', p. 193).
  - Oral repletion with potassium (2–6 mmol/kg/day) and alkalinizing agents (e.g. K-citrate or bicarbonate 2–15 mmol/kg/day).
  - Vitamin D preparations (alfacalcidol or calcitriol at 0.2–1 micrograms/day) may be needed to increase intestinal absorption of calcium and decrease urinary losses of phosphate, and for the healing of rickets which may have developed in some.
  - Blood chemistry should be monitored frequently at the initiation of therapy, perhaps every other week for the first month, and then monthly for 6 months.

- For unclear reasons, patients often deteriorate after initiation of treatment with respect to fluid and electrolyte homeostasis, before eventually stabilizing and they need to be monitored closely during this time period.
- Stabilization of blood chemistry should be complete within several weeks and healing of rickets within 3–6 months.
- Ophthalmic examination should be performed approximately every year to monitor corneal deposits and to rule out idiopathic intracranial hypertension (flat optic discs).
- Neurological progress should be monitored on a regular basis to assess the presence of coordination problems and learning difficulties in childhood, and for myopathic changes and cognitive deterioration in adults.
- Linear growth should be evaluated every 6 months and typically improves after 6–12 months of initiation of cysteamine with optimal control of blood chemistry and nutrition. In some patients, the use of recombinant human growth hormone (rhGH) has been reported.
- Poor appetite/poor adherence with medication and nutrition may require NG tube or gastrostomy.
- Thyroxine and testosterone (males >14 years) replacement may be required. Insulin may be required for diabetes mellitus, particularly following renal transplantation.
- Renal transplantation is the treatment of choice for CKD stage 5 in cystinosis, and is curative for the renal Fanconi syndrome, although some children may continue to need supplementation of water and electrolytes because of ongoing losses from their native kidneys.
- A glucose tolerance test prior to transplantation may help to assess the risk for diabetes with consequent consideration for altered immunosuppression (steroid and tacrolimus minimization/avoidance).
- Steroid minimization or avoidance after transplantation can also help maximize growth potential. The use of carnitine for improvement in muscle function remains controversial, but may be used in selected circumstances.

Oral cysteamine (Cystagon® or Procysbi®) therapy

- Oral mercaptamine therapy provides the mainstay of cystinosis treatment and should be started as soon as possible. The main limitation of this therapy from the patient's point of view is that it is highly unpalatable and leaves a sulfuric body odour and halitosis. This can negatively affect their interactions with their peers and negatively affects adherence.
- Initial dosing is incremental (over ~2–4 weeks) to achieve a dose of 60 mg/kg per day. Further dose increases, to between 60 and 90 mg/kg per day (or between 1.3 and 1.95 g/m² per day), should be implemented to optimize cystine depletion.
- Cystine depletion can be assessed by determining the leucocyte cystine level. This should be performed in an experienced laboratory. Treatment target is a level <1.0 nmol half-cystine/mg protein. Yet, since a level of <0.2 nmol half-cystine/mg protein is normal, consideration should be given to administering doses that achieve leucocyte cystine

values approaching this level (e.g. doses >60 mg/kg per day can be prescribed to lower the leucocyte cystine value from 0.9 half-cystine/mg protein closer to the normal level of <0.2). The dose should never exceed 90 mg/kg per day of cysteamine. The dose recommended for adults is 2000 mg every day, but higher doses may be required in adolescents to achieve satisfactory cystine depletion.
- With doses >90 mg/kg/day (or >1.95 g/m^2/day), rare side effects in the form of vascular, neurologic, muscular, or bone lesions have been described, which improve with reduction in the cysteamine dose
- Cystagon® is available in capsules of 50 and 150 mg. It can be given with food or drink, but must be taken in bolus form (i.e. within 5 min), rather than dissolved and sipped over time. It needs to be given every 6 h to achieve sustained cystine depletion.
- A sustained-release form of cysteamine is marketed under the trade name of Procysbi®. It can be administered every 12 h, thus simplifying the life of patient and family and potentially improving adherence. Side effects of body odour and halitosis remain the same, as these relate to the active compound cystamine. Availability has been impaired by the dramatically increased cost of this formulation compared to Cystagon®. In the USA in 2013, treatment with a daily dose of 2000 mg costs was ~$10,000 per year with Cystagon®, compared to $250,000 for Procysbi®.
- Leucocyte cystine levels should be monitored every 3 months to help monitor therapy. Because the effect of the drug wears off within hours, the levels should be obtained immediately before the next dose (4–6 h after the last dose with Cystagon® (or 10–12 h with Procysbi®) to assess at the time of presumably highest cystine level.
- For patients with gastric acid-related symptoms, proton pump inhibitors may prove helpful.
- Cystine depletion therapy delays the onset of all complications of cystinosis and thus must be continued also after kidney transplant to help preserve other organs.

Mercaptamine eye drops
- Oral therapy does not influence corneal cystine deposition. Thus, in addition to oral therapy, mercaptamine eye drops are required. These can dissolve corneal crystals within months and relieve photophobia within weeks. Mercaptamine eye drops are given ideally up to 10–12 times per day as a 0.55% solution in normal saline with a preservative, although in practical terms most only manage up to six times a day. Adherence is often driven by the symptoms of corneal irritation and photophobia.
- A gel formulation of topical cysteamine is now available, requiring application only four times per day and thus simplifying the life of patients and their families. Unfortunately, as with the extended-release oral formulation, availability is impaired by a steep increase in price. In the UK, weekly treatment with the gel formulation is £865 per week, compared to £48.85 for the regular cysteamine drops.

Transfer to adult care

Transitioning of care from paediatric to adult services remains an important area of concern. Patients should be transferred to adult centres with experience in this condition. Renal transplantation has improved the prognosis for nephropathic cystinosis, but this does not correct the accumulation of cystine in extrarenal tissues, and multisystemic involvement may still occur, even with optimal mercaptamine treatment.

Further reading

Langman CB, Barshop BA, Deschênes G, et al. Controversies and research agenda in nephropathic cystinosis: conclusions from a 'Kidney Disease: Improving Global Outcomes' (KDIGO) Controversies Conference. *Kidney Int* 2016;89:1192–1203.

Nesterova G, Williams C, Bernardini I, et al. Cystinosis: renal glomerular and renal tubular function in relation to compliance with cystine-depleting therapy. *Pediatr Nephrol* 2015;30:945–951.

Vasculitis

The classification of paediatric vasculitis

Background to classification criteria

- Classification criteria (see Table 11.1) are often described for diseases where the pathogenesis and/or molecular mechanisms are poorly understood.
- They are used to facilitate clinical trials and improve epidemiological descriptions by providing a set of agreed criteria that can be used by investigators anywhere in the world.
- Classification criteria for vasculitis are designed to differentiate one form of vasculitis from another once the diagnosis of vasculitis has been secured. They are not the same as diagnostic criteria (such as those described for Kawasaki disease), but are often misused as such.
- Thus, classification criteria aim to:
  - identify a set of clinical findings (criteria) that recognize a high proportion of patients with the particular disease (sensitivity)
  - exclude a high proportion of patients with other diseases (specificity).
- Classification criteria typically include manifestations that are characteristics of the disease in question that occur with less frequency or are absent in other conditions.
- Symptoms or findings that might be typical or common, but may also be present in other diseases tend to be excluded.
- An important limitation to these criteria is that they are not based on a robust understanding of the pathogenesis and as such are relatively crude tools that are likely to be modified as scientific understanding of these diseases progresses.

Paediatric vasculitis classification 2010

- New paediatric classification criteria are now described, and validated in >1300 cases worldwide.
- These criteria do not include Kawasaki disease (➔ see 'Kawasaki disease', p. 326); nor do they include definitions for microscopic polyangiitis (too few cases included in dataset).
- Since these classification criteria were devised, the proper terminology for Wegener granulomatosis has changed to granulomatosis with polyangiitis (GPA).
- For Takayasu arteritis, care must be taken to exclude fibromuscular dysplasia (or other cause of non-inflammatory large and medium vessel arteriopathy) since undoubtedly there could be scope for overlap in the clinical presentation between these two entities, although the pathogenesis and treatment are clearly distinct.

General scheme for the classification of paediatric vasculitides

- This is based on the size of the vessel predominantly involved in the vasculitic syndrome and is summarized in Box 11.1.
- It should be noted, however, that most vasculitides exhibit a significant degree of 'polyangiitis overlap': e.g. GPA can affect the aorta and its major branches, and small vessel vasculitis can occur in polyarteritis nodosa.

Table 11.1 Classification criteria for specific vasculitic syndromes[1]

Vasculitis	Classification criteria	Sensitivity[a]	Specificity[a]
HSP	Purpura, predominantly lower limb *or* diffuse* (mandatory) *plus* 1 out of: abdominal pain IgA on biopsy haematuria/proteinuria arthritis/arthralgia * If diffuse (i.e. atypical distribution) then IgA deposition on biopsy required	100%	87%
GPA	At least 3 out of 6 of the following: histopathology upper airway involvement laryngo-tracheobronchial stenoses pulmonary involvement ANCA positivity renal involvement	93%	99%
PAN	Histopathology or angiographic abnormalities (mandatory) plus 1 out of 5 of the following criteria: skin involvement myalgia/muscle tenderness hypertension peripheral neuropathy renal involvement	89%	99%
TA	Angiographic abnormalities of the aorta or its main branches (also pulmonary arteries) showing aneurysm/dilatation (mandatory criterion), plus 1 out of 5 of the following criteria: pulse deficit or claudication four-limb blood pressure discrepancy bruits hypertension acute phase response	100%	99%

GPA, granulomatosis with polyangiitis; HSP, Henoch–Schönlein purpura; PAN, polyarteritis nodosa; TA, Takayasu arteritis.

[a] Based on 1347 children with miscellaneous vasculitides.[2]

[1] Ozen S, Pistorio A, Iusan SM, et al. for the Paediatric Rheumatology International Trials Organisation (PRINTO) (2010). EULAR/PRINTO/PRES criteria for Henoch-Schönlein purpura, childhood polyarteritis nodosa, childhood Wegener granulomatosis and childhood Takayasu arteritis: Ankara 2008. Part II: Final classification criteria. *Ann Rheum Dis* 69:798–806.

[2] Ruperto N, Ozen S, Pistorio A, et al. for the Paediatric Rheumatology International Trials Organisation (PRINTO) (2010). EULAR/PRINTO/PRES criteria for Henoch-Schönlein purpura, childhood polyarteritis nodosa, childhood Wegener granulomatosis and childhood Takayasu arteritis: Ankara 2008. Part I: Overall methodology and clinical characterisation. *Ann Rheum Dis* 69:790–797.

Box 11.1 Classification of paediatric vasculitides by size of vessel involved

Predominantly large vessel vasculitis

- Takayasu arteritis (TA).

Predominantly medium-sized vessel vasculitis

- Childhood polyarteritis nodosa (PAN).
- Cutaneous polyarteritis.
- Kawasaki disease (KD).

Predominantly small vessel vasculitis

- Granulomatous:
  - Granulomatosis with polyangiitis (GPA; formerly known as Wegener granulomatosis).
  - Eosinophilic granulomatosis with polyangiitis (EGPA; formerly known as Churg–Strauss syndrome).
- Non-granulomatous:
  - Microscopic polyangiitis (MPA).
  - Henoch–Schönlein purpura (HSP).
  - Isolated cutaneous leucocytoclastic vasculitis.
  - Hypocomplementaemic urticarial vasculitis.

Other vasculitides

- Behçet disease.
- Vasculitis secondary to infection (including hepatitis B-associated PAN), malignancies, and drugs, including hypersensitivity vasculitis.
- Vasculitis associated with other connective tissue diseases.
- Isolated vasculitis of the central nervous system (CNS; childhood primary angiitis of the central nervous system: cPACNS).
- Cogan syndrome.
- Unclassified.

Investigation of primary systemic vasculitis

Background

Clinical features that suggest a vasculitic syndrome are:

- Pyrexia of unknown origin.
- Palpable purpura, urticaria, dermal necrosis.
- Mononeuritis multiplex.
- Unexplained arthritis, myositis, serositis.
- Unexplained pulmonary, cardiovascular, or renal disease *plus* one or more of:
  - leucocytosis
  - eosinophilia
  - hypocomplementaemia
  - cryoglobulinaemia
  - circulating immune complexes
  - raised ESR or CRP, thrombocytosis.

Characteristic features of individual vasculitides

(→ see also 'The classification of paediatric vasculitis', p. 308)

- *PAN*—either:
  - biopsy evidence of necrotizing vasculitis of small or medium sized arteries, or
  - suggestive visceral angiography in a child who is systemically unwell (antineutrophil cytoplasmic antibody (ANCA) usually negative).
- *Microscopic polyangiitis*: small vessel vasculitis with focal segmental pauci-immune glomerulonephritis, but without granulomatous disease of the respiratory tract. Clinically, it can be difficult to distinguish from GPA and often presents with rapidly progressive glomerulonephritis (RPGN). Typically associated with perinuclear antineutrophil cytoplasmic antibody (p-ANCA), especially myeloperoxidase (MPO)-ANCA
- *Renal-limited form of microscopic polyangiitis*: manifestation solely in the kidneys with crescentic nephritis (± p-ANCA positivity).
- *GPA*: combination of sinus, lung, and kidney disease with biopsy evidence of granuloma or necrotizing vasculitis. Typically associated with cytoplasmic (c)-ANCA especially proteinase 3 (PR3)-ANCA, occasionally p-ANCA or ANCA-negative in the young.
- *Takayasu arteritis*: symptoms or signs of large vessel disease; systemically unwell; characteristic angiography. May present with severe hypertension and pulse deficits ('pulseless disease').
- *Other vasculitides*:
  - There are many other vasculitic syndromes (→ see 'Kawasaki disease', p. 326, and 'Henoch–Schönlein purpura', p. 320). Goodpasture syndrome is characterized by crescentic nephritis (linear staining on immunofluorescence) and pulmonary haemorrhage, associated with anti-glomerular basement membrane (anti-GBM) antibodies.

Level 1 investigations

To be performed in the following cases:

Haematology and acute phase reactants

FBC, ESR, CRP, clotting, prothrombotic screen (if patchy ischaemia of digits or skin), blood film.

Basic biochemistry

Renal and liver function, creatine phosphokinase, thyroid function, LDH, amylase/lipase, urine dip, and Ua:Ucr.

Infectious disease screen

- Blood cultures and urine MC&S.
- ASOT and anti-DNase B.
- *Mycoplasma pneumoniae* serology.

Immunological tests

- ANAs, dsDNA antibodies, ENAs, ANCA, rheumatoid factor (RF).
- Anti-GBM antibodies.
- Tissue transglutaminase (TTG) antibodies (coeliac disease screen).
- Immunoglobulins IgGAM and E.
- Anticardiolipin antibodies, lupus anticoagulant.
- C3/C4, mannose binding lectin, CH100.
- VZV antibody status (prior to starting immunosuppressive therapy).
- Serum ACE.

Radiological

Chest X-ray, abdominal and renal US.

Other

ECG, echocardiography, digital clinical photography of lesions.

Level 2 investigations

To be considered on an individual basis.

- *Tissue biopsy*: skin, nasal or sinus, kidney, sural nerve, lung, liver, gut, temporal artery, muscle, brain, other.
- Selective contrast visceral angiography.
- MRI/MRA of brain (for suspected cerebral vasculitis).
- Cerebral contrast angiography (for suspected cerebral vasculitis).
- Sinus X-ray (for GPA).
- CT abdomen, thorax, brain.
- Four-limb BP.
- Doppler US of peripheral arteries.
- Ophthalmology review.
- Cryoglobulins (if there is a history of cold sensitivity/vasculitis mainly present in exposed areas of the body).
- Ventilation/perfusion (V/Q) scan.
- Nerve conduction studies (PAN, GPA, Behçet's—before starting thalidomide).
- Formal GFR.
- 24 h ambulatory BP monitoring.
- X-ray of bones and joints.
- Labelled white cell scan (for extent and location of inflammation).

- DMSA scan.
- Bone marrow analysis and/or lymph node excision biopsy (for suspected malignancy).
- Urinary catecholamines (consider plasma catecholamines as well), and urine vanillylmandelic acid (VMA), homovanillic acid (HVA) (for phaeochromocytoma, or neuroblastoma).
- Positron emission tomography (PET)–CT: for differential of malignancy or Castleman disease.
- Nitroblue tetrazolium test if granulomatous inflammation found on biopsy.
- DNA analysis for periodic fever syndromes that can mimic vasculitis: *MEFV* (familial Mediterranean fever (FMF)) gene, *TNFRSF1A* (tumour necrosis factor (TNF) alpha receptor-associated periodic fever syndrome (TRAPS)), mevalonate kinase (*MVK*; hyper IgD syndrome (HIDS)), NLRP3 (cryopyrin-associated periodic syndrome), and *NOD2* (Crohn disease/Blau syndrome/juvenile sarcoid mutations).
- IgD.
- Serum amyloid A (SAA).
- Mitochondrial DNA mutations.
- Mantoux 1:1000, and/or QuantiFERON®.
- Viral serology for:
  - HBV, HCV
  - parvovirus B19.
- PCR for CMV, EBV, enterovirus, adenovirus, VZV, hepatitis B and C viruses.
- Serology for HIV, rickettsiae, *Borrelia burgdorferi*.
- Thermography and nail-fold capillaroscopy.
- Organ specific autoantibodies.
- Beta-2-glycoprotein 1 antibodies.
- Basic lymphocyte panel and CD19 count if monitoring post rituximab.

The standard treatment of childhood vasculitis

Standard vasculitis therapy (*excluding* crescentic glomerulonephritis)

See Fig. 11.1.

Prior to using this approach, there should be:
* a well-established diagnosis
* severe, potentially life-threatening disease
* inadequate response to less toxic therapy—milder cases of vasculitis (e.g. isolated cutaneous forms) may respond to less toxic agents, such as colchicine. So therapy should always be tailored for each individual
* no known infection or neoplasm
* no pregnancy or possibility thereof
* informed consent obtained and documented in notes

(➜ See Table 11.2 for guidelines for the use of cytotoxic drugs in non-malignant disease.)

Other points of note

* Therapy for all types of paediatric chronic vasculitis, as adapted from adult studies, consists of remission induction followed by remission maintenance with specific treatments in each phase dependent on disease type and severity.
* Although the use of oral cyclophosphamide is highlighted in Fig. 11.1, increasingly IV cyclophosphamide is favoured over the oral route in children and adults because of reduced side effects and lower cumulative dose, but comparable efficacy as suggested by a number of studies in adults with ANCA vasculitis (e.g. the 'CYCLOPS' trial).
* IV cyclophosphamide has the added advantage of ensuring adherence to therapy, of particular relevance in adolescents with vasculitis.

Use of biological therapy in systemic vasculitis of the young

* While the therapeutic approach and drugs used as suggested in Figs. 11.1 and 11.2 undoubtedly have improved survival and long-term outlook for children with severe vasculitis, concerns relating to toxicity, particularly with cyclophosphamide, and relapses despite this conventional therapeutic approach have led to the increasing use of biological therapy, such as rituximab, anti-TNF alpha, or other biological therapy.
* Evidence to support the use of rituximab as a primary induction agent in place of cyclophosphamide for the treatment of ANCA-associated vasculitis is now available for adults with this group of diseases (RITUXVAS and RAVE trials).
* Evidence to support this approach in children remains anecdotal, but undoubtedly rituximab is being increasingly used for children with

ANCA vasculitis that is not adequately controlled using the conventional cyclophosphamide followed by azathioprine therapeutic regimen outlined in Fig. 11.1.
• Evidence for the use of anti-TNF alpha or other biological agents, such as anakinra, remains anecdotal for children and adults with vasculitis.
• While there is not enough evidence to recommend specific biological therapy for specific vasculitic syndromes, a general approach favoured by the authors is given in Table 11.3.

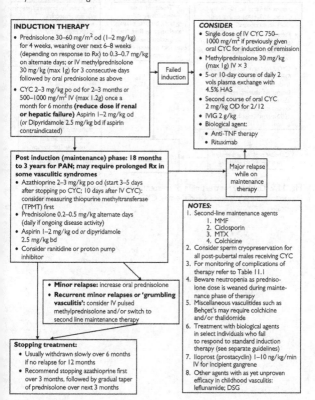

INDUCTION THERAPY
• Prednisolone 30–60 mg/m² od (1–2 mg/kg) for 4 weeks, weaning over next 6–8 weeks (depending on response to Rx) to 0.3–0.7 mg/kg on alternate days; or IV methylprednisolone 30 mg/kg (max 1g) for 3 consecutive days followed by oral prednisolone as above
• CYC 2–3 mg/kg po od for 2–3 months *or* 500–1000 mg/m² IV (max 1.2g) once a month for 6 months **(reduce dose if renal or hepatic failure)** Aspirin 1–2 mg/kg od (*or* Dipyridamole 2.5 mg/kg bd if aspirin contraindicated)

Failed induction →

CONSIDER
• Single dose of IV CYC 750–1000 mg/m² if previously given oral CYC for induction of remission
• Methylprednisolone 30 mg/kg (max 1g) IV × 3
• 5-or 10-day course of daily 2 vols plasma exchange with 4.5% HAS
• Second course of oral CYC 2 mg/kg OD for 2/12
• IVIG 2 g/kg
• Biological agent:
  • Anti-TNF therapy
  • Rituximab

Post induction (maintenance) phase: 18 months to 3 years for PAN; may require prolonged Rx in some vasculitic syndromes
• Azathioprine 2–3 mg/kg po od (start 3–5 days after stopping po CYC; 10 days after IV CYC): consider measuring thiopurine methyltransferase (TPMT) first
• Prednisolone 0.2–0.5 mg/kg alternate days (daily if ongoing disease activity)
• Aspirin 1–2 mg/kg od *or* dipyridamole 2.5 mg/kg bd
• Consider ranitidine or proton pump inhibitor

Major relapse while on maintenance therapy →

NOTES:
1. Second-line maintenance agents
   1. MMF
   2. Ciclosporin
   3. MTX
   4. Colchicine
2. Consider sperm cryopreservation for all post-pubertal males receiving CYC
3. For monitoring of complications of therapy refer to Table 11.1
4. Beware neutropenia as prednisolone dose is weaned during maintenance phase of therapy
5. Miscellaneous vasculitides such as Behçet's may require colchicine and/or thalidomide
6. Treatment with biological agents in select individuals who fail to respond to standard induction therapy (see separate guidelines)
7. Iloprost (prostacyclin) 1–10 ng/kg/min IV for incipient gangrene
8. Other agents with as yet unproven efficacy in childhood vasculitis: leflunamide; DSG

• **Minor relapse:** increase oral prednisolone
• **Recurrent minor relapses or 'grumbling vasculitis':** consider IV pulsed methylprednisolone and/or switch to second line maintenance therapy

Stopping treatment:
• Usually withdrawn slowly over 6 months if no relapse for 12 months
• Recommend stopping azathioprine first over 3 months, followed by gradual taper of prednisolone over next 3 months

Fig. 11.1 Standard vasculitis therapy (excluding crescentic glomerulonephritis). CYC, cyclophosphamide; DSG, gusperimus; od, once daily; po, orally.

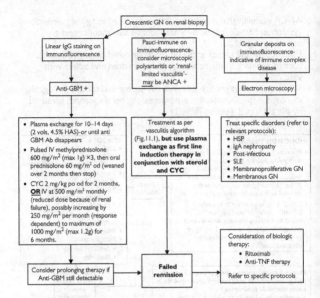

Fig. 11.2 Guideline for treatment of crescentic glomerulonephritis. Of major importance is early diagnosis and therapy. CYC, cyclophosphamide; od, once daily; po, orally.

Table 11.2 Doses, side effects, and clinical monitoring of commonly used immunosuppressant and cytotoxic immunosuppressant drugs used for the treatment of vasculitis

	Cyclophosphamide (CYC)	Azathioprine	Mycophenolate mofetil (MMF)	Ciclosporin	Methotrexate (MTX)
Dose	2–3 mg/kg once daily orally 2–3 months; 0.5–1.0 g/m² IV monthly with mesna to prevent cystitis ⊕ see 'Appendix', p. 681, for mesna dose and IV CYC administration protocol).	0.5–2.5 mg/kg once daily orally for 1 year or more	600 mg/m² twice daily	3–5 mg/kg /day orally in 2 divided doses	10–15 mg/m²/week orally or SC (single dose)
Side effects	Leucopenia; haemorrhagic cystitis; reversible alopecia; infertility; leukaemia; lymphoma, transitional cell carcinoma of bladder	GI toxicity; hepatotoxicity; rash; leucopenia; teratogenicity; no increase in malignancy in adults with rheumatoid arthritis; no conclusive data for cancer risk in children	Bone marrow suppression; severe diarrhoea; pulmonary fibrosis	Renal impairment, hypertension, hepatotoxicity, tremor; gingival hyperplasia, hypertrichosis, lymphoma	Bone marrow suppression and interstitial pneumonitis (decreased risk with folic acid), reversible elevation of transaminases, hepatic fibrosis
Cumulative toxic dose	Not described for malignancy; 500 mg/kg for azoospermia	Not described	Not described	Not described	Not described

(Continued)

Table 11.2 (Contd.)

	Cyclophosphamide (CYC)	Azathioprine	Mycophenolate mofetil (MMF)	Ciclosporin	Methotrexate (MTX)
Clinical monitoring	Weekly FBC for duration of therapy (usually 2–3 months); baseline and monthly renal and liver function. Temporarily discontinue and/or reduce dose if neutropenia <1.5 × 10⁹/L, platelets <150 × 10⁹/L, or haematuria. Day 10 FBC if IV. Reduce dose if renal or hepatic failure e.g. to 250–300 mg/m²	Weekly FBC for 1 month, then 3 monthly. Temporarily discontinue and/or reduce dose if neutropenia <1.5 × 10⁹/L, platelets <150 × 10⁹/L, and check TPMT enzyme—patients deficient in TPMT require reduced doses (or may not tolerate) azathioprine because of increased marrow toxicity	Fortnightly FBC for 2 months, then monthly for 2 months, 3-monthly when stable. Baseline monthly renal and liver function until stable. Discontinue temporarily and/or reduce dose if neutropenia <1.5 × 10⁹/L, platelets <150 × 10⁹/L, or significant GI side effects	Weekly measurement of BP; baseline then monthly renal and liver function; maintain 12 h trough level at 50–100 ng/ml. 6–12-monthly GFR. Consider renal biopsy every 2 years	Baseline chest X-ray, FBC, and LFTs, then FBC and LFTs fortnightly until dose stable, then monthly to every 6 weeks (after 6 months). Reduce or discontinue if hepatic enzymes >3 × upper limit of normal, neutropenia <1.5× 10⁹/L, new or worsening cough, severe nausea, vomiting, or diarrhoea, platelets <150 × 10⁹/L or falling rapidly

TPMT, thiopurine transmethyltransfersase.

Table 11.3 Recommendations for indication and choice of biological therapy for primary systemic vasculitis of the young based on published experience.

Vasculitis type	Indication for biological agent	Proposed first choice of biological agent
ANCA-associated vasculitis	Critical organ or life-threatening disease, which has failed to respond to standard vasculitis therapy or concerns regarding cumulative CYC dose	Rituximab or other B-cell depleting monoclonal antibody
Takayasu arteritis	Failed therapy with standard agents	Anti-TNF or tocilizumab
Polyarteritis nodosa	Failed therapy with standard agents or concern regarding cumulative CYC dose	Anti-TNF alpha or rituximab
Behçet's disease	Recalcitrant and severe disease; alternative to thalidomide	Anti-TNFA (infliximab, adalimumab)

CYC, cyclophosphamide.

Reproduced with permission from Eleftheriou D, Melo M, Marks SD, et al. Biologic therapy in primary systemic vasculitis of the young. *Rheumatology*. 48(8), 978–86. Copyright © 2009 OUP.

Further reading

Eleftheriou D, Brogan P. Therapeutic advances in the treatment of vasculitis. *Pediatr Rheumatol* 2016;14:26

Henoch–Schönlein purpura

Epidemiology

* HSP (anaphylactoid purpura) is a multisystem small vessel systemic vasculitis.
* It is the commonest vasculitis in the paediatric population.
* The annual incidence is estimated at 20.4 per 100,000 children in the UK, with greater incidence in children from the Indian subcontinent (24 per 100,000) compared with white Caucasians (17.8 per 100,000) and black populations, predominantly Afro-Caribbean (6.2 per 100,000).
* North American series also report a higher incidence of HSP in white compared with black children.
* Other epidemiological studies from Holland and the Czech Republic place the incidence between 6.1 and 10.2 per 100,000 children respectively, possibly reflecting differences in ethnicities and/or methodological differences in data collection.
* Younger children are most frequently affected, the peak incidence occurring at around 4–5 years of age and the disease is more prevalent in boys. The disease appears to follow a seasonal pattern, with a higher incidence during winter and the early spring.

Pathogenesis

* Remains largely unknown.
* Probable polygenic contribution.
* The most commonly accepted theory of HSP nephritis pathogenesis is that polymeric galactose-deficient IgA (formed under genetic control) is produced in response to infection or immunization in some individuals, resulting in pathological formation of immune complexes with naturally occurring anti-glycan IgG or IgA1, with subsequent glomerular deposition, and activation of mesangial cells and initiation of glomerulonephritis.

Clinical features of Henoch–Schönlein purpura

HSP is defined as a vasculitis with IgA-dominant immune deposits affecting small vessels and typically involving skin, gut and glomeruli and associated with arthralgias or arthritis. The classification criteria are:
* Purpura, commonly palpable and predominantly lower limb or diffuse (if diffuse, i.e. atypical distribution, then IgA deposition on biopsy is required (mandatory)) plus one out of four of:
  * abdominal pain
  * IgA on biopsy
  * haematuria/proteinuria
  * arthritis/arthralgia.

Mainly affects skin, GI tract, joints, and kidneys:
* *Skin*: purpura generally symmetrical, affecting the lower limbs and buttocks in the majority of cases, the upper extremities being involved less frequently; abdomen, chest, and face are generally unaffected. New crops of purpura may develop for several months after the disease onset, though generally fade with time. Lesions can be induced by mild trauma. Angio-oedema and urticaria can also occur.

- *Joints*: around two-thirds of children have joint manifestations at presentation. The knees and ankles are most frequently involved. Pain, swelling, and decreased range of movement tend to be fleeting and resolve without the development of permanent damage.
- *GI tract*: three-quarters of children develop abdominal symptoms ranging from mild colic to severe pain with ileus and vomiting. Haematemesis and melaena are sometimes observed. Other complications include intestinal perforation and intussusception. The latter may be difficult to distinguish from abdominal colic, and the incidence of intussusception is significant enough to warrant exclusion by US when suspected.
- *Acute pancreatitis*: rare complication.
- One complication worth emphasizing for paediatric nephrologists is the rare, but well-recognized complication of ureteric obstruction.
- Other organs less frequently involved include the CNS (cerebral vasculitis), gonads (orchitis may be confused with torsion of the testis), and the lungs (pulmonary haemorrhage).
- Many cases follow an upper respiratory tract infection and the onset of the disorder may be accompanied by systemic symptoms, including malaise and mild pyrexia.
- Multiple organ involvement may be present from the outset of the disease, or alternatively an evolving pattern may develop, with different organs becoming involved at different time points over the course of several days to several weeks.
- Around one-third of children have symptoms for <14 days, one-third 2–4 weeks, and one-third >4 weeks.
- Recurrence of symptoms occurs in around one-third of cases, generally within 4 months of resolution of the original symptoms. Recurrences are more frequent in those with renal involvement.

Henoch–Schönlein purpura nephritis

- Incidence reported between 20% and 61% of HSP patients, depending on criteria for definition of nephritis.
- Renal involvement is normally manifest between a few days and a few weeks after clinical presentation, but can occur up to 2 months or (rarely) more from presentation.
- There appears to be an increased risk of renal disease in those with bloody stools.
- May present with isolated microscopic haematuria, proteinuria with microscopic or macroscopic haematuria, acute nephritic syndrome (haematuria with at least two of hypertension, raised plasma creatinine and oliguria), nephrotic syndrome (usually with microscopic haematuria), or a mixed nephritic–nephrotic picture.

Pathological findings in Henoch–Schönlein purpura

- The skin lesion of HSP is that of a leucocytoclastic vasculitis with perivascular accumulation of neutrophils and mononuclear cells. Immunofluorescence studies reveal vascular deposition of IgA and C3 in affected skin, although similar changes may be observed in skin unaffected by the rash. An important caveat is that if biopsies are taken from the centre of a necrotic skin lesion then IgA may be falsely

negative because it is cleaved by proteolytic enzymes involved in the inflammatory vasculitic process.
* The renal lesion of HSP nephritis is characteristically a focal and segmental proliferative glomerulonephritis.

Investigation of Henoch–Schönlein purpura

* No single laboratory test has been shown to be helpful.
* Immunological investigations including complement levels and ANAs are normal.
* Serum IgA is elevated in around one-half of children and a small number exhibit ANCA positivity.
* Coagulation studies are normal and platelet numbers are normal or occasionally increased. Factor XIII may be low.
* Where significant nephritis is present at presentation, renal function and electrolytes may be correspondingly abnormal.

Differential diagnosis

* Sepsis.
* Other systemic vasculitides (SLE, PAN, GPA, microscopic polyangiitis, and hypersensitivity vasculitis), all of which can present with similar clinical features.
* FMF can also mimic HSP.

Who needs a renal biopsy?

* Nephritic/nephrotic presentation (urgent).
* Raised creatinine, hypertension, or oliguria (urgent).
* Heavy proteinuria (Ua:Ucr persistently >100 mg/mmol) on an early morning urine sample at 4 weeks. Serum albumin not necessarily in the nephrotic range.
* Persistent proteinuria (not declining) after 4 weeks.
* Consider biopsy for persistent impaired renal function (GFR <80 mL/min/1.73^2).

General treatment of Henoch–Schönlein purpura

* The large majority of cases of HSP are mild and immunosuppressive treatment is usually not justified; children should receive symptomatic treatment only.
* The skin lesion usually requires no treatment (except where there is severe haemorrhagic oedema affecting the face or scrotum, where systemic corticosteroid therapy may be indicated).
* Arthropathy should be treated with rest and simple analgesia (paracetamol or NSAIDs).
* While never subjected to a controlled clinical trial, there is some evidence to suggest that the more severe GI symptoms, particularly abdominal pain and GI bleeding, respond well to corticosteroid therapy, which has also been used for the treatment of testicular involvement and pulmonary haemorrhage.

Treatment of Henoch–Schönlein purpura nephritis

Currently prescribed treatments for HSP nephritis are not adequately guided by evidence obtained in robust RCTs.

*Treatment with oral prednisolone to prevent development
of Henoch–Schönlein purpura nephritis*
- Meta-analysis of four RCTs, which evaluated prednisone therapy at presentation of HSP, showed that there was no significant difference in the risk of development or persistence of renal involvement at 1, 3, 6, and 12 months with prednisone, compared with placebo or no specific treatment.
- Thus, prophylactic corticosteroid does not prevent the onset of HSP nephritis.
- There could still be a role for early use of corticosteroids in patients with severe extrarenal symptoms and in those with renal involvement, however.

Rapidly progressive glomerulonephritis
- There are good data indicating that crescents in >50% of glomeruli and nephrotic range proteinuria carry an unfavourable prognosis.
- Unfortunately, to date, there is only one RCT evaluating the benefit of treatment, which showed no difference in outcome using cyclophosphamide vs supportive therapy alone. This study did not examine combined therapy, i.e. cyclophosphamide and steroid, however, a regimen used in most other severe small vessel vasculitides.
- For patients with RPGN with crescentic change on biopsy, uncontrolled data suggest that treatment may comprise aggressive therapy with corticosteroid, cyclophosphamide, and possibly plasma exchange, as for other causes of crescentic nephritis (➔ see 'The standard treatment of childhood vasculitis', p. 314).
- Other therapies, such as ciclosporin, azathioprine, and cyclophosphamide have been reported by some authors to be effective.
- As HSP is probably the commonest cause of RPGN in childhood, more aggressive therapeutic approaches have been employed in some cases including 14 children with severe HSP nephritis treated successfully with plasma exchange alone these treatment options, while potentially important in select cases, are not yet supported by randomized controlled trials.

*Treatment of Henoch–Schönlein purpura nephritis that is
not rapidly progressive*
Patients may include the following features: <50% crescents on renal biopsy, suboptimal GFR; heavy proteinuria that is not necessarily nephrotic range:
- Three daily doses of IV methylprednisolone 30 mg/kg (maximum 1 g per dose).
- Followed by 4 weeks of 2 mg/kg oral prednisolone for 4 weeks.
- At 4-week assessment, if there is no improvement the prednisolone will be rapidly weaned and stopped.
- If there is improvement, oral prednisolone could be continued for up to 6 months in total.
- Some advocate the use of steroids and cyclophosphamide in HSP nephritis with biopsy showing diffuse proliferative lesions or sclerosis, but with <50% crescentic change, who have ongoing heavy proteinuria. A typical regimen would comprise 8 weeks of oral cyclophosphamide (2 mg/kg/day) with daily prednisolone, converting to alternate-day prednisolone and azathioprine for a total of 12 months.

- The published evidence for the efficacy of this approach is lacking, but this may be a reasonable option bearing in mind the adverse prognosis of children with HSP who have a nephritic/nephrotic phenotype.
- Fish-oil treatment has been reported in analogy to IgA nephropathy, but no good evidence exists.

Use of ACE inhibitors in Henoch–Schönlein purpura nephritis

In patients with >6 months duration of proteinuria an ACE inhibitor may be indicated to limit secondary glomerular injury.

Long-term outcome of Henoch–Schönlein purpura

The majority of children with HSP make a full and uneventful recovery with no evidence of ongoing significant renal disease.

- Renal involvement is the most serious long-term complication of HSP:
  - A single study of long-term outcome of 78 subjects who had had HSP nephritis during childhood (mean of 23.4 years after onset) demonstrated overall that initial findings on renal biopsy correlated well with outcome, but had poor predictive value in individual patients.
  - 44% of patients who had nephritic, nephrotic, or nephritic/nephrotic syndromes at onset had hypertension or impaired renal function, whereas 82% of those who presented with haematuria (with or without proteinuria) were normal.
  - 7 patients deteriorated clinically years after apparent complete clinical recovery.
  - 16 of 44 full-term pregnancies were complicated by proteinuria and/or hypertension, even in the absence of active renal disease.
- A recent systematic review of all published literature with regards to long-term renal impairment in children with HSP has been performed:
  - 12 studies with 1133 children were reviewed.
  - Renal involvement occurred in 34% of children; 80% had isolated haematuria and/or proteinuria while 20% had acute nephritis or nephrotic syndrome.
  - Renal complications, if they did occur, developed early—by 4 weeks in 85% and by 6 months in nearly all children.
  - Persistent renal involvement (hypertension, reduced renal function, nephrotic or nephritic syndrome) occurred in 1.8% of children overall, but the incidence varied with the severity of the kidney disease at presentation, occurring in 5% of children with isolated haematuria and/or proteinuria, but in 20% who had acute nephritis and/or nephrotic syndrome in the acute phase.
  - Children with significant renal impairment at presentation, and/or persistent proteinuria should undergo regular assessment of their GFR, e.g. at 1, 3, and 5 years after the acute episode of HSP.
  - Some instances of hypertension have been reported many years after normalization of renal function and urinalysis.
  - An increased incidence of pre-eclampsia has also been reported.
  - Interestingly, in children who underwent repeat renal biopsies the majority of children with HSP still had IgA deposition years later, which could explain in part late the renal morbidity sometimes described.

Recurrence of Henoch–Schönlein purpura in renal allografts

- It is recognized that HSP can occur in renal allografts.
- True recurrence should, however, be differentiated from IgA deposits, which are sometimes seen in renal transplants in patients who did not have HSP or IgA nephropathy.
- One worrying suggestion is that recurrence rates may be higher for living donor transplants, although data are limited.

Further reading

Narchi H. Risk of long term renal impairment and duration of follow up recommended for Henoch–Schönlein purpura with normal or minimal urinary findings: a systematic review. *Arch Dis Child* 2005;90:916–920.

Zaffanello M, Fanos V. Treatment-based literature of Henoch–Schönlein purpura nephritis in childhood. *Pediatr Nephrol* 2009;24:1901–1911.

Kawasaki disease

Kawasaki disease (KD) is an acute, self-limiting vasculitic syndrome that targets the coronary arteries. It occurs predominantly in infants and young children. KD is the second commonest vasculitic illness of childhood (after HSP) and is the leading cause of childhood acquired heart disease in developed countries.

Pathogenesis and epidemiology

* Pronounced seasonality and clustering of KD cases have led to the hunt for infectious agents as a cause. So far, no single agent has been identified.
* The aetiology of KD remains unknown, but it is currently felt that one or more widely distributed infectious agents evoke an abnormal immunological response in genetically susceptible individuals, leading to the characteristic clinical presentation of the disease.
* KD has a worldwide distribution with a male preponderance, an ethnic bias towards Asian children, seasonality, and occasional epidemics.
* Incidence of KD continues to increase in North-East Asian countries such as Japan, Korea, and Taiwan. The incidence in North America, Europe, and Australia increased until the last decade when it seems to have largely plateaued. The current incidence in England is 8.4/100,000 children <5 years old.

Diagnostic criteria

Fever persisting for 5 days (4 days if treatment with intravenous immunoglobulin (IVIG) eradicates fever) or more plus at least four of the following clinical signs not explained by another disease process:
* Peripheral extremity changes (reddening of the palms and soles, indurative oedema, and subsequent desquamation) (80%).
* A polymorphous exanthema, primarily truncal; non-vesicular (>90%).
* Bilateral non-exudative conjunctival injection/congestion (80–90%).
* Lips and oral cavity changes (reddening/cracking of lips, strawberry tongue, oral, and pharyngeal injection) (80–90%).
* Acute non-purulent cervical lymphadenopathy with at least one node >1.5 cm in diameter (50%).
* Patients with fewer than four out of five principal features can be diagnosed with KD when coronary aneurysm or dilatation is recognized by two-dimensional echocardiography or coronary angiography.

Numbers in parentheses indicate the approximate percentage of children with KD who demonstrate the criterion.
Note: at least 10% of children who develop aneurysms never meet criteria for KD. Children <6 months of age are more likely to have atypical features and to develop aneurysms.

Clinical features

The cardiovascular features are the most important manifestations of the condition with widespread vasculitis affecting predominantly medium size muscular arteries, especially the coronary arteries. Coronary artery involvement occurs in 15–25% of untreated cases with additional cardiac features in a significant proportion of these including pericardial effusion, electrocardiographic abnormalities, pericarditis, myocarditis, valvular incompetence, cardiac failure, and myocardial infarction. It is important to involve a paediatric cardiologist early if this diagnosis is suspected.

Fever is the hallmark of KD and the diagnosis must be suspect in the absence of fever. Typically the fever is persistent, minimally responsive to antipyretics and often remains >38.5°C throughout the illness.

- Of note, irritability is an important sign, which is virtually universally present although not included in the diagnostic criteria.
- Another clinical sign that may be relatively specific to KD is the development of erythema and induration at sites of BCG inoculations. The mechanism of this sign is thought to be cross-reactivity of T cells in KD between specific epitopes of mycobacterial and human heat shock proteins.
- An important point is that the principal symptoms and signs may present sequentially, such that the full set of criteria may not be present at any one time. Awareness of other non-principal signs (such as BCG scar reactivation) may improve the diagnostic pick-up rate of KD.
- Most children are photophobic and as many as two-thirds develop anterior uveitis. Slit lamp examination may be useful in diagnostically ambiguous cases.
- Other clinical features include arthritis, aseptic meningitis, pneumonitis, uveitis, gastroenteritis, meatitis and dysuria, and otitis.
- Relatively uncommon abnormalities include hydrops of the gallbladder, GI ischaemia, jaundice, petechial rash, febrile convulsions, and encephalopathy or ataxia, macrophage activation syndrome, and syndrome of inappropriate antidiuretic hormone secretion (SIADH).

Differential diagnosis

Conditions that can cause similar symptoms to KD and must be considered in the differential diagnosis include:

Infections

- Adenovirus, enterovirus, EBV, CMV, parvovirus, influenza virus infection.
- Measles.
- Scarlet fever.
- Rheumatic fever.
- Streptococcal or staphylococcal toxic shock syndrome.
- Staphylococcal scalded skin syndrome.
- Rickettsiae infection.
- Leptospirosis.
- *Mycoplasma pneumoniae* infection.

Drug reactions

- Stevens-Johnson syndrome
- Mercury toxicity (acrodynia)

Rheumatic diseases

- Systemic juvenile idiopathic arthritis.
- Infantile polyarteritis nodosa.
- SLE.

Malignancy

- Lymphoma—particularly for IVIG-resistant cases.

Investigations

Systemic inflammation is most characteristic with elevated CRP, ESR, leucocytosis with neutrophilia, a normocytic anaemia, and by the second week of illness a thrombocytosis which may reach $1,000,000/mm^3$. Patients frequently have a sterile pyuria.

In cases of suspected KD, the following investigations should be considered:

• FBC and blood film.
• ESR.
• CRP.
• Urine MC&S.
• Dip test of urine for blood and protein.
• Renal and liver function tests.
• Coagulation screen.
• Chest X-ray.
• ECG.
• Two-dimensional echocardiography to identify coronary artery involvement acutely and monitoring long-term changes.
• Coronary arteriography has an important role for delineating detailed anatomical injury, particularly for children with giant coronary artery aneurysms (>8 mm), where stenoses adjacent to the inlet/outlet of the aneurysms are a concern. Note that the procedure may need to be delayed until at least 6 months after disease onset since there could be a risk of myocardial infarction if performed in children with ongoing severe coronary artery inflammation.

Investigations for differential diagnosis

• Blood cultures.
• CSF culture, cell count, chemistries.
• ASOT and anti-DNase B.
• Serology (IgG and IgM) for *Mycoplasma pneumoniae*, enterovirus, adenovirus, measles, parvovirus, EBV, CMV.
• Nose and throat swab, and stool sample for culture (superantigen toxin typing if *Staphylococcus aureus* and/or beta-haemolytic streptococci detected).
• Consider serology for rickettsiae and leptospirosis if history suggestive.
• Autoantibody profile (ANA, ENA, ANCA).

Treatment

The goal of therapy is to reduce inflammation as rapidly as possible and to prevent the formation of coronary artery aneurysms. For this reason, patients should be treated as soon as a diagnosis of KD is established.

The treatment of KD (➲ see Fig. 11.3) comprises of:

• IVIG at a dose of 2 g/kg as a single infusion over 12 h (consider splitting the dose over 2–4 days in infants with cardiac failure)
• IVIG should be started early preferably within the first 10 days of the illness. However, clinicians should not hesitate to give IVIG to patients who present after 10 days if there are signs of persisting inflammation.

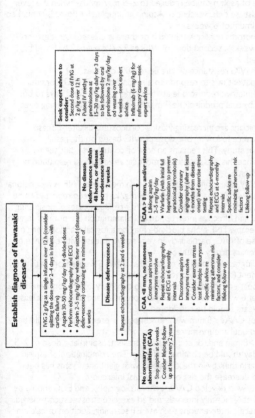

Establish diagnosis of Kawasaki disease*

- IVIG 2 g/kg as a single infusion over 12 h (consider splitting the dose over 2–4 days in infants with cardiac failure)
- Aspirin 30–50 mg/kg/day in 4 divided doses
- Perform echocardiography and ECG
- Aspirin 2–5 mg/kg/day when fever settled (disease deferrescence) continuing for a minimum of 6 weeks

No disease deferrescence within 48 hours, or disease recrudescence within 2 weeks

Seek expert advice to consider:
- Second dose of IVIG at
  - 2 g/kg over 12 h
- Pulsed IV methyl prednisolone at 15–30 mg/kg daily for 3 days to be followed by oral prednisolone 2 mg/kg/day od weaning over 6 weeks—seek expert advice
- Infliximab (6 mg/kg) for refractory cases—seek expert advice

Disease deferrescence

Repeat echocardiography at 2 and 6 weeks†

No coronary artery abnormalities (CAA)
- Stop aspirin at 6 weeks
- Consider lifelong follow up for at least every 2 years

CAA <8 mm, no stenoses
- Continue aspirin until aneurysms resolve
- Repeat echocardiography and ECG at 6-monthly intervals
- Discontinue aspirin if aneurysms resolve
- Consider exercise stress test if multiple aneurysms
- Specific advice re minimizing atheroma risk factors, and consider lifelong follow-up

‡CAA > 8 mm, and/or stenoses
- Lifelong aspirin
- Clopidogrel 1 mg/kg/day
- Warfarin (with initial full heparinization to prevent paradoxical thrombosis)
- Consider coronary angiography (after at least 6 months from disease onset) and exercise stress testing
- Repeat echocardiography and ECG at 6-monthly intervals
- Specific advice re minimizing atheroma risk factors
- Lifelong follow-up

Fig. 11.3 Guideline for the management of Kawasaki disease.

* Treatment can be commenced before a full 5 days of fever if sepsis has been excluded. Treatment should also be given if the presentation is 10 days from fever onset.

† Refer to paediatric cardiologist.

‡ Other specific interventions, such as PET scanning, addition of calcium channel blocker therapy, and coronary angioplasty at the discretion of paediatric cardiologist.

Recent evidence suggests that steroids combined with IVIG as initial treatment reduces the overall risk of coronary artery disease in severe KD. However, it is not known what dose, duration, and route of corticosteroids should be used or whether all children would benefit from initial treatment with steroids. In severely ill KD patients, expert consultation should be obtained.

* Aspirin 30–50 mg/kg/day in four divided doses.
* The dose of aspirin can be reduced to 2–5 mg/kg/day when the fever settles (disease defervescence). Aspirin at antiplatelet doses is continued for a minimum of 6 weeks.
* If the symptoms persist within 48 h or there is disease recrudescence within 2 weeks a second dose of IVIG at 2 g/kg over 12 h should be considered.
* However, IVIG resistance occurs up to 20% of cases.
* When a patient fails to respond to a second dose of IVIG, consider IV pulsed methylprednisolone at 15–30 mg/kg daily for 3 days to be followed by oral prednisolone 2 mg/kg/day once daily weaning over 6 weeks.
* Some clinicians are increasingly using corticosteroids after disease recrudescence following one dose of IVIG based on the results of a recent study. This remains an area of controversy, but seems rational since this is associated in most cases with rapid resolution of inflammation.
* In refractory cases, infliximab, a human chimeric anti-TNF-A monoclonal antibody, given IV at a single dose of 6 mg/kg has been reported to be effective, and is increasingly used for IVIG-resistant cases. Considering that rapid and effective interruption of inflammation is a primary target of KD therapy, TNF-alpha blockade may be a logical step following one failed dose of IVIG, particularly in very active disease with evidence of early coronary artery dilatation.
* Echocardiography should be repeated at 2 and 6 weeks from initiation of treatment (refer to paediatric cardiology).
* If the repeat echocardiogram shows no coronary artery abnormalities (CAAs) at 6 weeks, aspirin can be discontinued and follow-up at least every 2 years should be considered.
* In cases of CAAs <8 mm with no stenoses present, aspirin should be continued until aneurysms resolve.
* If CAAs >8 mm and/or stenoses are present, aspirin at a dose of 2–5 mg/kg/day should be continued lifelong. The combination of aspirin and warfarin therapy in these patients with giant aneurysms has been shown to decrease the risk of myocardial infarction.
* In patients who develop CAAs, echocardiography, and ECG should be repeated at 6-monthly intervals and an exercise stress test considered.
* Other specific interventions such as PET scanning, addition of calcium channel blocker therapy, and coronary angioplasty should be organized at the discretion of the paediatric cardiologist.

Outcome

* Treatment with IVIG and aspirin reduces CAAs from 25% for untreated cases to 4–9%.
* IVIG resistance occurs in ~20%, and is associated with a higher risk of CAA.

- The overall outlook of children with KD is good, with the acute mortality rate due to myocardial infarction having been reduced to <1% by increased alertness of the clinicians to the diagnosis and prompt treatment.
- Nonetheless, the disease may contribute to the burden of adult CVD and cause premature atherosclerosis, an area of active ongoing research.

Polyarteritis nodosa

Background

- PAN is a necrotizing vasculitis associated with aneurysmal nodules along the walls of medium-sized muscular arteries.
- Despite some overlap with smaller-vessel disease, PAN appears to be a distinct entity and, in adults in Europe and the United States, appears to have an estimated annual incidence of 2.0–9.0/million.
- Although comparatively rare in childhood, it is the most common form of systemic vasculitis after HSP and KD.
- Peak age of onset in childhood is 7–11 years, often with a male preponderance.
- Classification criteria for PAN are not diagnostic criteria, and meeting classification criteria is not equivalent to making a diagnosis in an individual patient—see elsewhere in this section and ➜ 'The classification of paediatric vasculitis').

Aetiology

- *Unknown*: possible interaction between infection and aberrant host response.
- There may be genetic factors that may make individuals vulnerable to PAN and other vasculitides. There are reports of PAN occurring in siblings that add weight to this hypothesis. Mutations in the gene encoding adenosine deaminase 2 (*ADA2*) resulting in a syndrome of livedoid rash, intermittent fevers, early-onset lacunar strokes, and a systemic PAN-like vasculopathy have been described by two independent groups.
- There is a well-recognized association of PAN and FMF in parts of the world where this is common.
- There are data to support roles for hepatitis B and reports of a higher frequency of exposure to parvovirus B19 and cytomegalovirus in PAN patients compared with control populations.
- HIV has also been implicated, and PAN-like illnesses have been reported in association with cancers and haematological malignancies. However, in childhood, associations between PAN and these infections or other conditions are rare.
- Streptococcal infection and bacterial superantigens may play a role in some cases, particularly cutaneous limited forms of PAN.
- Occasional reports suggest immunization as a cause, but this is not proven.

Clinical features

A diagnosis is made by considering all clinical features in a patient, only some of which may be classification criteria. Clinical manifestations (and investigation findings) can be very confusing, especially in the early phase of the disease with absence of conclusive diagnostic evidence. There is an entity that involves the skin only (cutaneous PAN).

- The main systemic clinical features of PAN are malaise, fever, weight loss, skin rash, myalgia, abdominal pain, and arthropathy.

- Skin lesions are variable, and may masquerade as those of HSP or multiform erythema. The cutaneous features described in a recent international classification exercise for PAN in children occurred commonly and were defined as follows:
  - *Livedo reticularis*—purplish reticular pattern usually irregularly distributed around SC fat lobules, often more prominent with cooling.
  - *Skin nodules*—tender SC nodules.
  - *Superficial skin infarctions*—superficial skin ulcers (involving skin and superficial SC tissue) or other minor ischaemic changes (nail-bed infarctions, splinter haemorrhages, digital pulp necrosis).
  - *Deep skin infarctions*—deep skin ulcers (involving deep SC tissue and underlying structures), digital phalanx or other peripheral tissue (nose and ear tips) necrosis/gangrene.
- Renal manifestations such as haematuria, proteinuria, and hypertension.
- GI features and abdominal pain are relatively common and include:
  - *indeterminate intestinal inflammation*—intestinal inflammation without characteristic histological features of either ulcerative colitis or Crohn's disease. *NB*: routine mucosal gut biopsies rarely detect overt vasculitis, since the small- and medium-sized arteries lie below the mucosa
  - GI haemorrhage (upper and lower)
  - intestinal perforation
  - pancreatitis.
- Neurological features such as focal defects, hemiplegia, visual loss, mononeuritis multiplex, and organic psychosis may be present.
- Other important clinical features include ischaemic heart and testicular pain. Rupture of arterial aneurysms can cause retroperitoneal and peritoneal bleeding, with perirenal haematomata being a recognized manifestation of this phenomenon, although this is rare.
- In contrast to ANCA-associated vasculitis, involvement of lung is rare in PAN.

Differential diagnosis

- *Other primary vasculitides*: HSP, GPA, microscopic polyangiitis (MPA), KD. ➐ See 'Henoch–Schönlein purpura', p. 320 and ➐ 'Kawasaki disease', p. 326.
- Autoimmune or autoinflammatory diseases:
  - Juvenile idiopathic arthritis (JIA)—particularly the systemic form.
  - Juvenile dermatomyositis (JDM).
  - SLE.
  - Undifferentiated connective tissue disease.
  - Sarcoidosis.
  - Behçet's disease.
- *Infections*:
  - *Bacterial*: particularly streptococcal infections, and sub-acute bacterial endocarditis.
  - *Viral (many)*: specifically look for hepatitis B and C, CMV, EBV, parvovirus B19, and consider HIV.
- *Malignancy*: lymphoma, leukaemia, and other malignancies can mimic PAN.

Diagnostic laboratory and radiological investigation

Blood tests
- Anaemia, polymorphonuclear leucocytosis, thrombocytosis, increased ESR, and CRP.
- Platelets are hyperaggregable.
- Circulating immune complexes, or cryoglobulins may be present.
- Evidence of antecedent streptococcal infection may be present particularly in cutaneous PAN.
- Positive hepatitis B serology in children is unusual in association with PAN, but can occur.
- ANCA is not thought to play a major part in the causality of PAN, but there are reports demonstrating their presence in some adults and children with PAN:
  - The presence of c-ANCA with antibodies to PR3 in a patient suspected of having PAN makes it mandatory to eliminate GPA as a diagnosis.
  - Likewise, a significant titre of p-ANCA with antibodies to MPO would necessitate steps to eliminate MPA as the diagnosis.

Tissue biopsy
Biopsy material is diagnostically important, especially skin or muscle, although tissue biopsy has overall low diagnostic sensitivity, since the disease is patchy and vasculitis can be easily missed.
- The characteristic histopathological changes of PAN are fibrinoid necrosis of the walls of medium or small arteries, with a marked inflammatory response within or surrounding the vessel.
- However, absence of such changes would not exclude the diagnosis, as the vasculitic features are variable and affected tissue may not have been sampled.
- Renal biopsy is usually not helpful and carries a greater risk than usual of bleeding and the formation of arteriovenous fistulae.

Radiological tests
- The most valuable investigative procedure is catheter-selective visceral digital subtraction arteriography to include flush aortogram, and selective renal, hepatic, and mesenteric arteriography. This should be performed and interpreted only by those with expertise in this test in paediatric patients:
  - Arteriography findings include aneurysms, segmental narrowing and variations in the calibre of arteries, together with pruning of the peripheral renal vascular tree (Fig. 11.4).
  - Treatment with prior corticosteroids will alter the arteriography and can result in false negatives.
  - Non-invasive arteriography, such as CT or MRA, are *not* as sensitive as catheter arteriography for the detection of medium-sized vessel vasculitis such as PAN.
  - Consider formal cerebral arteriography if clinical and MRI features suggest cerebral vasculitis.
- Indirect evidence of the presence of medium-size artery vasculitis affecting renal arteries may be obtained by demonstrating patchy areas within the renal parenchyma of decreased isotope uptake on Tc-99m dimercaptosuccinic acid (DMSA) scanning of the kidneys.

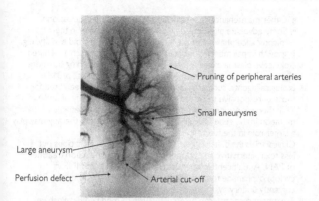

Pruning of peripheral arteries

Small aneurysms

Large aneurysm

Perfusion defect

Arterial cut-off

Fig. 11.4 PAN: renal arteriogram.

- MRA usually fails to detect aneurysms of small- and medium-sized muscular arteries, although it may demonstrate large intra- and extrarenal aneurysms and stenoses/occlusions of the main renal arteries, and areas of ischaemia and infarction. A caveat is that MRA may overestimate vascular stenotic lesions.
- Computed tomography angiography (CTA) may also reveal larger aneurysms and arterial occlusive lesions, and demonstrate areas of renal cortical ischaemia and infarction, but:
  - at the expense of high ionizing radiation exposure
  - with less sensitivity than catheter arteriography.
- Echocardiography can be useful for the identification of pericarditis, valve insufficiency, myocarditis, or coronary artery abnormalities.

Treatment

(See Table 11.2.)
- In most patients, it is appropriate to treat aggressively to induce remission (typically 3–6 months), followed by less aggressive therapy to maintain remission (typically 18–24 months).
- In those presenting with mild predominantly cutaneous disease, corticosteroid alone may be appropriate, with careful monitoring of clinical and laboratory parameters as this is weaned.
- *Induction therapy*: high-dose corticosteroid with an additional cytotoxic agent such as cyclophosphamide:
  - Cyclophosphamide is usually given as pulsed monthly IV injections for up to 6 months or for shorter periods in children if remission is achieved.
  - Oral cyclophosphamide 2 mg/kg per day for 2–3 months is an alternative, although for other vasculitides the IV regimen has been shown to have a more favourable therapeutic index.
- Aspirin 1–5 mg/kg/day as an antiplatelet agent may be considered.
- *Maintenance therapy*: once remission is achieved, therapy with daily low-dose prednisolone and oral azathioprine is frequently used for up to 18–24 months:

- Other maintenance agents include MTX, MMF, and ciclosporin.
- Some advocate alternate-day low-dose prednisolone in the maintenance phase with the intention of limiting steroid toxicity, e.g. growth impairment), but data to support this approach are limited.
- Adjunctive plasma exchange can be used in life-threatening situations (➔ see 'The standard treatment of childhood vasculitis', p. 314).
- Biological agents, such as infliximab or rituximab have been used for those unresponsive to conventional therapy. The efficacy of anti-TNF therapy including etanercept in the treatment of patients with a mutation in the gene encoding ADA2 suggests that this therapy may play a larger role in the future.
- Clinical trials in adults suggest that MMF may be an efficacious but less toxic alternative to cyclophosphamide in the induction treatment of PAN. A multicentre, open-label RCT (MYPAN) of MMF vs cyclophosphamide for the induction of remission of childhood PAN is currently underway.
- Treatment response can be assessed using a modified Birmingham Vasculitis Activity Score (BVAS) or the paediatric version of BVAS, 'PVAS', which has been recently validated and by monitoring of conventional acute phase reactants, urinary sediment, BP, and growth.

Outcome

- PAN, unlike some other vasculitides, such as GPA, appears to be a condition in which permanent remission can be achieved.
- However, relapses can occur. Two recent studies indicated relapse rates between 35% and 75%. Relapses occurred more frequently in those with severe GI involvement. An increased cumulative dose of cyclophosphamide was associated with a lower relapse rate. Long-term data from the French Vasculitis study group registry indicate increased rates of relapse for childhood onset PAN after the age of 18 years.
- However, if treatment is delayed or inadequate, life-threatening complications can occur due to the vasculitic process.
- Severe complications, especially infections, can occur from immunosuppressive treatment.
- In comparison with the almost 100% mortality rate in the pre-steroid era, mortality rates as low as 1.1% were reported in a recent retrospective multicentre analysis. However, this may not truly reflect mortality in circumstances of severe disease because 30% of patients in that series were considered to have predominantly cutaneous PAN.
- A mortality rate of 10% was recently recorded from a major tertiary referral centre seeing predominantly children with aggressive advanced disease.
- Late morbidity can occur years after childhood PAN from chronic vascular injury, possibly resulting in premature atherosclerosis. This remains a cause for concern and an area of ongoing research.

Further reading

Eleftheriou D, Batu E, Ozen S, et al. Vasculitis in children. *Nephrol Dial Transplant* 2014;30:i94–i103.
Ozen S, Anton J, Arisoy N, et al. Juvenile polyarteritis: results of a multicenter survey of 110 children. *J Pediatr* 2004;145:517–522.

The antineutrophil cytoplasmic antibody-associated vasculitides

Background

- ANCA-associated vasculitides (AAVs) are:
  - granulomatosis with polyangiitis (GPA) formerly known as Wegener granulomatosis
  - microscopic polyangiitis (MPA)
  - eosinophilic granulomatosis with polyangiitis (EGPA) formerly known as Churg–Strauss syndrome (CSS)
  - renal limited vasculitis (previously referred to as idiopathic crescentic glomerulonephritis).
- Although rare, the AAVs do occur in childhood.

Definitions of antineutrophil cytoplasmic antibody-associated vasculitides

Definitions for each of the AAVs describing the salient major clinical and laboratory features are given here. These are not the same as classification criteria, which (for GPA) are provided in ➔ 'The classification of paediatric vasculitis', p. 308.

- GPA: granulomatous inflammation involving the respiratory tract and necrotizing vasculitis affecting small- to medium-sized vessels often associated with a cytoplasmic ANCA (c-ANCA, PR3-ANCA) positivity.
- MPA:
  - Necrotizing vasculitis, with few or no immune deposits, affecting small vessels.
  - Necrotizing arteritis involving small- and medium-sized arteries may be present.
  - Pulmonary capillaritis often occurs—clinically, it often presents with rapidly progressive pauci-immune glomerulonephritis, in association with p-ANCA (MPO-ANCA) positivity.
- EGPA: an eosinophil-rich and granulomatous inflammation involving the respiratory tract and necrotizing vasculitis affecting small- to medium-sized vessels; there is an association with asthma and eosinophilia.
- Renal limited: RPGN, often with ANCA positivity (usually MPO-ANCA), but without other organ involvement.

Pathogenesis

- It is not known why patients develop ANCA in the first instance:
  - The pathogenicity of the ANCA antibody especially in MPA is suggested by a mouse model in which the injection of anti-MPO IgG is able to recapitulate human disease with resultant necrotizing and crescentic glomerulonephritis and vasculitis including haemorrhagic pulmonary capillaritis. Additionally, two cases of transplacental transfer of MPO-ANCA inducing neonatal MPA have been reported.

- When ANCAs are present, the most accepted current model of pathogenesis proposes that ANCA activates cytokine-primed neutrophils, leading to bystander damage of endothelial cells and an escalation of inflammation with recruitment of mononuclear cells.
  - However, other concomitant exogenous factors and genetic susceptibility appear to be necessary for disease expression since ANCA can be present in asymptomatic individuals.

Clinical features of granulomatosis with polyangiitis

From a clinical perspective, GPA may be broadly considered as having two forms, which may coexist or present sequentially in individual patients:
- A predominantly granulomatous form with mainly localized disease. Localized disease appears to be less common in childhood.
- A florid, acute small vessel vasculitic form characterized by severe pulmonary haemorrhage, and/or rapidly progressive vasculitis or other severe vasculitic manifestations.

At disease onset, the most common features are constitutional symptoms such as malaise, fever, weight loss, or growth failure

Organ-specific involvement
Includes the following:
- *Upper respiratory tract*:
  - Epistaxis.
  - Otalgia, and hearing loss (conductive and/or sensorineural); chronic otitis media; mastoiditis.
  - Nasal septal involvement with cartilaginous collapse results in the characteristic saddle nose deformity.
  - Chronic sinusitis.
  - Glottic and subglottic polyps and/or large and medium-sized airway stenosis. Note that airway stenosis is a classification criterion due to this finding's specificity for GPA.
- *Lower respiratory tract manifestations*—include (singly or in combination):
  - granulomatous pulmonary nodules with or without central cavitation
  - pulmonary haemorrhage with respiratory distress, frank haemoptysis, and/or evanescent pulmonary shadows on chest X-ray
  - interstitial pneumonitis.
- *Renal involvement*: typically a focal segmental necrotizing glomerulonephritis, with pauci-immune crescentic glomerular changes. The clinical manifestations associated with this lesion are:
  - hypertension
  - proteinuria
  - nephritic and nephrotic syndrome
  - other protean manifestations of renal failure.
- *Ophthalmological disease*: retinal vasculitis, conjunctivitis, episcleritis, uveitis, optic neuritis. Unilateral or bilateral proptosis may be caused by granulomatous inflammation affecting the orbit (pseudotumour).
- Arthralgia and arthritis.
- *Other manifestations*: include peripheral gangrene with tissue loss, and vasculitis of the skin, gut (including appendicitis), heart, CNS and/or peripheral nerves (mononeuritis multiplex), salivary glands, gonads, and breast.

Investigations

(➔ See 'Investigation of primary systemic vasculitis', p. 311.)

The diagnosis of GPA is based on a combination of typical clinical features, the presence of serologic markers, and characteristic histopathology. If GPA is suspected, a careful assessment of the upper and lower airway as well as the kidneys must be performed to assess extent and severity of the disease.

* GPA is commonly associated with a cytoplasmic staining pattern of ANCA by indirect immunofluorescence, and enzyme-linked immunosorbent assay (ELISA) reveals specificity against proteinase 3 (PR3; PR3-ANCA).
* MPA and renal limited AAV are typically associated with p-ANCA by indirect immunofluorescence and with MPO-ANCA specificity on ELISA. Note that p-ANCA can also be seen ulcerative colitis and primary sclerosing cholangitis.
* ANCA-negative forms of GPA, MPA, renal limited vasculitis, and EGPA are well described in children.
* While the diagnostic value of ANCA is without question important, the value of ANCA for the longitudinal monitoring of disease activity is probably unreliable in many patients with GPA.
* Tissue diagnosis, in particular renal biopsy, but also biopsy of skin, nasal septum, or other tissue, can be important diagnostically for diagnosing all of the AAVs, and can help stage the disease for therapeutic decision-making.
* Other commonly observed non-specific findings include:
  * a mild normochromic normocytic anaemia together with a leucocytosis and thrombocytosis
  * elevated ESR and CRP
  * raised immunoglobulins (polyclonal IgG).
* Laboratory manifestations relating to renal involvement include:
  * dipstick haematuria and proteinuria positive
  * raised Upr:Ucr
  * raised serum creatinine and other associated laboratory features of renal failure
* Assessments of airway.
* Chest X-ray may be abnormal but high-resolution CT chest has better sensitivity for demonstrating pulmonary infiltrates or discrete nodular and/or cavitating lesions.
* Plain X-ray or CT sinuses for sinusitis.

Pulmonary function tests are frequently abnormal. A decrease in the diffusing capacity of carbon monoxide (DLCO) may be an early sign of pulmonary haemorrhage.

Treatment of antineutrophil cytoplasmic antibody-associated vasculitides

(➔ see 'The standard treatment of childhood vasculitis', p. 314.)

When considering therapy, it is useful to remember that most evidence for treatment is derived from adult trials. It is also useful to consider the different phases of the therapeutic journey for AAVs:

* The pre-diagnostic phase: occasionally lasting years. Significant organ damage can accrue in this phase, or even death.

- Induction of remission phase: typically 3–6 months.
- Maintenance of remission phase: usually 18–24 months.
- Therapy withdrawal phase: not all patients achieve this.

The following general points are worthy of note:
- Key to successful treatment is early diagnosis to limit organ damage.
- Treatment for paediatric AAV is broadly similar to the approach used in adults, and involves corticosteroids, cyclophosphamide, and in some individuals plasma exchange (particularly for pulmonary capillaritis and/or RPGN 'pulmonary–renal syndrome') to induce remission; followed by low dose corticosteroids and azathioprine to maintain remission.
- Antiplatelet doses of aspirin can also be considered empirically on the basis of the increased risk of thrombosis associated with the disease process.
- MTX in combination with corticosteroids may have a role for inducing remission in patients with limited GPA.
- Co-trimoxazole is commonly added to therapeutic programmes for the treatment of GPA, particularly in those with upper respiratory tract involvement, serving both as prophylaxis against opportunistic infection and as a possible disease-modifying agent.
- Newer immunosuppressive agents and immunomodulatory strategies such as MMF and rituximab (see the 'RAVE' and 'RITUXVAS' trials in adults) have been reported to be effective at inducing or maintaining remission in adults with AAVs and are increasingly used in children for recalcitrant disease. Some now advocate the use of rituximab for initial therapy in younger patients in whom the need to preserve fertility is an important consideration.
- Although anti-TNF therapy has been used anecdotally with some success in select patients, it failed to prevent relapse during maintenance therapy in a randomized controlled trial.

Outcome of antineutrophil cytoplasmic antibody-associated vasculitides

- The AAVs still carry considerable disease-related morbidity and mortality, particularly due to progressive CKD or aggressive respiratory involvement, and therapy-related complications, such as sepsis.
- The mortality for GPA from one recent paediatric series was 12% over a 17-year period of study inclusion. The largest paediatric series of patients with GPA reported 40% of cases with CKD at 33 months of follow-up despite therapy.
- Mortality in paediatric patients with MPA during follow-up has been reported to be between 0% and 14%.
- For EGPA in children, the most recent series quotes a related mortality of 18%.

Further reading

Moroshita K, Brown K, Cabral D. Pediatric vasculitis. *Curr Opin Rheumatol* 2015;27:493–499.

Takayasu arteritis

Background

- Takayasu arteritis (TA) is an idiopathic, chronic granulomatous vasculitis affecting the aorta and its major branches.
- Other names include 'pulseless disease', aortic arch syndrome, or idiopathic aortoarteritis.
- Classification criteria are provided in ➔ 'The classification of paediatric vasculitis', p. 308.

Epidemiology

- TA is more prevalent in Southeast Asia, Central and South America, and Africa. It is rarer in Europe and North America.
- Most studies report an incidence of 1–3 per million/year in Caucasian populations. In Japan, the estimated incidence is up to 100 times higher: 1 per 3000/year.
- In adult studies there is a 9:1 female predominance. In children, however, sex ratios vary amongst different studies. A recent study from Southeast Asia and Africa report a female to male ratio of 2:1.
- TA is a rare vasculitis in children:
  - Age of onset may range from infancy to middle age.
  - The peak period of onset is in the second and third decade of life.

Aetiopathogenesis

- The cause remains unknown.
- Genetic factors may play a role, and there are several reports of familial TA including in identical twins:
  - HLA associations include HLA-A10, HLA-B5, HLA-Bw52, HLA-DR2, and HLADR4 in Japan and Korea; HLA B22 association has been described in the USA population.
  - The presence of HLA Bw52 has been associated with coronary artery and myocardial involvement, and worse prognosis.
- TA is described in association with rheumatoid arthritis, ulcerative colitis, and other autoimmune diseases suggesting an autoimmune mechanism for the pathogenesis of the disease.
- Circulating anti-aortic endothelial cell antibodies in patients with TA have been reported; their exact role, however, is yet to be determined.

Histopathology

TA is characterized by granulomatous inflammation of all layers of the arterial vessels (panarteritis):

- Inflammation progresses in a patchy fashion from the adventitia to the intima. The initial finding is neutrophil infiltration of the adventitia and cuffing of the vasa vasorum with proliferation and penetration of the latter within the tunica intima.
- Destruction of tunica elastica and muscularis cause dilatation and aneurysms.
- Inflammation of the tunica intima is followed by intimal hyperplasia leading to stenoses or occlusions.
- Endothelial cell damage leads to a prothrombotic tendency.
- Various mixed chronic inflammatory cells including T cells contribute to granuloma formation in the tunica media and adventitia mediated by the release of interferon-gamma and TNF-alpha.

• Later, the adventitia and media are replaced by fibrous sclerotic tissue and the intima undergoes acellular thickening, thus narrowing the vessel's lumen and contributing to ischaemia.

In paediatric series:
• Occlusions and stenoses were present in 98% of the patients, while aneurysms were only seen in 15.6% of the patients.
• Post-stenotic dilatations were present in 34% of cases.
• Lesions are most commonly seen in the subclavian arteries (90%), the common carotids (60%), the abdominal aorta (45%), the aortic arch (35%), and the renal arteries (35%). Pulmonary arteries are involved in 25% of the cases.

Clinical features

Acute phase
Non-specific features of systemic inflammation (systemic, pre-stenotic phase). In children, up to 65% of cases of TA present abruptly with systemic features:
• Pyrexia, malaise, weight loss, headache, arthralgias and/or myalgias.
• Rash (erythema nodosum, pyoderma gangrenosum).
• Arthritis.
• Myocarditis causing congestive heart failure (± hypertension) or valvular involvement (aortic valve most commonly affected followed by mitral valve).
• Myocardial infarction.
• Hypertension occurs in 65–100% of paediatric patients and may be the only clinical finding.
• Hypercoagulable state: thrombotic tendency.

Chronic phase
Features and signs secondary to vessel occlusion and ischaemia (stenotic phase):
• *Asymmetric or absent pulses*: a measured difference of >10 mmHg on four-limb BP monitoring is likely to indicate arterial occlusion.
• *Systemic hypertension*: commonest finding.
• Arterial bruits.
• Congestive heart failure secondary to hypertension and/or aortic regurgitation when the valve is affected.
• *Angiodynia*: localized tenderness on palpation of the affected arteries.
• Claudication.
• Coronary angina.
• Mesenteric angina presenting with abdominal pain and diarrhoea from malabsorption.
• Recurrent chest pain from chronic dissection of the thoracic aorta or pulmonary arteritis.
• Pulmonary hypertension.
• *CNS involvement*: may be attributed to ischaemia ± hypertension. Dizziness or headache; seizures; transient ischaemic attacks, stroke.

Eye involvement
Diplopia, blurry vision, amaurosis, visual field defect. Fundoscopy findings include:
• retinal haemorrhage

- micro aneurysms of the peripheral retina
- optic atrophy.

Renal involvement
- Renal hypertension secondary to renal artery stenosis with secondary glomerular damage.
- CKD.
- Secondary amyloidosis.
- Glomerulonephritis (GN) has been described in association with TA: IgA nephropathy; membranoproliferative GN; crescentic GN; mesangioproliferative GN.

Differential diagnoses

- *Other vasculitides including medium and small vessel vasculitis:*
  - KD; PAN. GPA is a recognized cause of aortitis.
- *Other rheumatic diseases:*
  - Behçet disease, sarcoidosis, SLE, and spondyloarthritis.

Infectious causes
- Bacterial endocarditis.
- Septicaemia without true endocarditis.
- TB.
- Syphilis.
- HIV.
- Borreliosis (Lyme disease).
- Brucellosis (very rare).
- Non-inflammatory large vessel vasculopathy of congenital cause. Treatment with immunosuppression will be ineffective or may worsen the disease:
  - Fibromuscular dysplasia.
  - Williams syndrome.
  - Congenital coarctation of the aorta.
  - Congenital mid-aortic syndrome.
  - Ehler–Danlos type IV.
  - Marfan syndrome.
  - NF1.
- *Other:* post-radiation therapy.

Laboratory investigations

(➜ See also 'Investigation of primary systemic vasculitis', p. 311.)
There are no specific laboratory tests for TA. During the acute stage of disease, the most common laboratory abnormalities reflect systemic inflammation.
- Normochromic normocytic anaemia, leucocytosis, thrombocytosis; raised ESR, raised CRP— these signs of inflammation may not be present in chronic (stenotic) phase of illness.
- Elevated transaminases and hypoalbuminaemia.
- Deranged renal function tests in cases of renal involvement.
- Polyclonal hyperglobulinaemia. (Elevated globulin in the blood due to inflammation. If this comes from a single B-cell population (monoclonal), it is associated with myeloma. Polyclonal is likely normal and associated with inflammation.)

- Further tests required to exclude other causes mimicking TA or for disease monitoring.
- Regular four-limb BP measurement (preferably with a manual manometer).
- In cases of significant peripheral artery stenosis, central BP measurements may be required.
- Renal function tests, urinalysis.
- Autoimmune screen.
- Baseline immunology tests including lymphocyte subsets, nitroblue tetrazolium (NBT) test.
- Blood cultures (acute phase).
- Mantoux test or interferon gamma-releasing assays (IGRAs).
- Syphilis serology.
- Tissue biopsy, rarely performed, but should include microbiological culture, and 16S and 18S ribosomal PCR if available to exclude bacterial and fungal infection, respectively.

Imaging

- Imaging of the aorta and its branches are fundamental for the diagnosis and monitoring of TA.
- An echocardiogram (and ECG) and chest X-ray are simple first-line imaging tests and should be performed in all cases where TA is suspected.
- Conventional digital subtraction catheter arteriography is the method used routinely for obtaining a generalized arterial survey when TA is suspected, but essentially only provides 'lumenography' with no imaging of arterial wall pathology.
- MRI and MRA, and CTA, or a combination of these may help accurately diagnose TA and monitor disease activity, and (for MRA and CTA) provide cross-sectional aortic wall images allowing detection of arterial wall thickness and intramural inflammation.
- MRI and MRA are gradually replacing conventional angiography in most centres and are useful for diagnosis and follow up; however, they lack sensitivity in evaluation of the distal aortic branches, and may overestimate the degree of arterial stenosis, especially in small children; cardiac MRI is increasing employed to look for valvular involvement and/or myocarditis.
- Angiographic findings form the basis of one classification for TA (Takayasu Conference, 1994; see Box 11.2).
- Doppler US scan:
  - High-resolution duplex US technology is a valuable tool in evaluation and follow-up of TA.
  - This modality offers high-resolution imaging of the vascular wall and can be useful for the detection of increased wall thickness.
  - 18F-FDG-PET co-registered with CTA can be a powerful technique combining information relating to the metabolic activity of the arterial wall (18F-FDG uptake detected using PET) with detailed lumenography (CTA) thus providing information on disease activity and anatomy. This technique is not available in all centres, and carries a high radiation exposure limiting its use for routine follow-up of disease activity.

Box 11.2 Classification of Takayasu arteritis

* *Type I*: classic pulseless type that affects blood vessels of aortic arch involving the brachiocephalic trunk, carotid, and subclavian arteries.
* *Type II*: affects middle aorta (thoracic and abdominal aorta).
* *Type III*: affects aortic arch and abdominal aorta.
* *Type IV*: affects pulmonary artery in addition to any of types I–III.
* *Type V*: includes patients with involvement of the coronary arteries.

Diagnosis

The diagnosis of TA is based on clinical and laboratory findings of systemic inflammation and/or of large vessel ischaemia and angiographic demonstration of lesions in the aorta or its major branches, with exclusion of other causes listed in the differential diagnosis.

Treatment

(➔ See 'The standard treatment of childhood vasculitis', p. 314.)

Early diagnosis and aggressive treatment is fundamental for the outcome of the disease, although new lesions can continue to develop even in the presence of clinical remission in 60% of cases.

* Vascular damage already established in some patients will usually not respond to medical treatment.
* Medical management of TA includes high-dose corticosteroids, usually in combination with MTX or cyclophosphamide for induction of remission. Maintenance agents include MTX , azathioprine, or more recently MMF.
* Corticosteroids constitute the first line of treatment for active large vessel vasculitis. IV pulsed methylprednisolone 30 mg/kg/day (maximum 1 g) for 3 days followed by a second course a week later and subsequent oral prednisolone 2 mg/kg/day. Although 60% of patients respond there is a 50% risk of relapse while corticosteroids are tapered. Moreover, better and more rapid remission may be achieved with additional immunosuppressive treatment added early.
* MTX (15 mg/m²/week orally or SC) improves the remission rate in steroid-dependent TA. Half of the cases will achieve complete and sustained remission on MTX for a follow up period of 5 years. It is the authors' personal preference to use the SC route for TA.
* *Cyclophosphamide*: a recent study showed promising results for oral cyclophosphamide for the induction of remission.
* *Azathioprine*: recently published data in adults advocate the use of azathioprine in combination with prednisolone as a safe and effective drug accomplishing both clinical remission and prevention of further vascular damage.
* *MMF*: in patients with TA who did not respond to steroid treatment the use of MMF has shown clinical improvement along with reduction of inflammatory markers. It may work as a safe alternative in cases where other immunosuppressants have failed.
* *Anti-TNF alpha*: case series of children and adults with TA treated with anti-TNF alpha such as infliximab suggest efficacy, although no data from RCTs exist yet to support this approach.

Hypertension

* At least 40% of TA patients are hypertensive.
* Optimal control of hypertension is essential in the longer term since it is a major contributor to long-term morbidity.
* Medical treatment of hypertension in TA may be challenging since renovascular hypertension may not respond to medical therapy alone.
* Revascularization procedures may be required
  (→ see 'Revascularization and other surgical procedures').

Revascularization and other surgical procedures

Techniques

* Angioplasty (including percutaneous transluminal angioplasty; or patch angioplasty).
* Arterial bypass procedures.
* Endarterectomy.
* Arterial stenting.
* Cardiac valve repair/replacement.
* Surgery during the acute phase of the disease carries significant risk of re-occlusion and procedural complication, so should be deferred until the acute phase is treated.
* These techniques should only be undertaken in centres with expertise.

Indications for revascularization

* Hypertension from stenotic coarctation of the aorta or renovascular disease.
* End organ ischaemia or peripheral limb ischaemia.
* Cerebral ischaemia.
* Aortic or other arterial aneurysms, or aortic regurgitation.

Prognosis

* There is usually a significant time lag (~18 months, occasionally much longer) between initial presentation and diagnosis of TA in children. Arterial damage accrues during this pre-diagnostic phase, and influences prognosis.
* The course of the disease is variable, but most patients experience new lesions over time. Typically, vascular inflammation persists even in patients thought to be clinically in remission.
* Aortic valve insufficiency and congestive heart failure are reported in 25%.
* Vascular claudication limiting activities occurs in up to 40%.
* Long-term mortality ranges from 10% to 30%: the main causes of death include congestive cardiac failure, myocardial infarction, aneurysm rupture, or renal failure.
* After commencement of treatment ~60% will respond to corticosteroids, while 40% will relapse when these are tapered off.
* Poor prognostic factors are severe aortic regurgitation, severe hypertension, cardiac failure, and aneurysms.

Further reading

Gulati A, Bagga A. Large vessel vasculitis. *Paediat Nephrol* 2010;25:1037–1048.

Szugye H, Zeft A, Spalding S. Takayasu arteritis in the pediatric population: a contemporary United States-based single center cohort. *Pediatr Rheumatol* 2014;12:21.

Infections and the kidney

Introduction

Any infection causing septicaemia can cause AKI, the commonest being meningococcal septicaemia. Acute postinfectious glomerulonephritis and UTI are described in ➔ Chapter 9 and ➔ Chapter 4, respectively. This chapter describes infections that can specifically affect the kidneys.

The general principle in all infection-associated renal complications is that treatment should be aimed at the underlying infection. Eradicating or suppressing the underlying infection is usually the best treatment for the associated renal disease.

Hepatitis B

* Can cause secondary membranous nephropathy (➔ see 'Membranous nephropathy') but has been associated with other glomerulonephritides.
* Most have active hepatitis B infection (hepatitis B surface antigen (HBsAg) and e antigen (HBeAg) positive) without antibodies, although core antibody may be present.
* Remission occurs with disappearance of the HBeAg and development of hepatitis B surface antibodies.
* No kidney-specific treatment is of proven benefit.
* HBsAg-positive children being considered for renal transplantation require assessment by a paediatric hepatologist. Untreated active viral replication, chronic active hepatitis, and cirrhosis have a poor prognosis post transplant.

Hepatitis C

* Has been associated with glomerulonephritis of various types. The commonest is membranoproliferative histology associated with cryoglobulinaemia. Hepatitis C virus (HCV) leads to chronic overstimulation of B lymphocytes and production of mixed cryoglobulins which are deposited in the mesangium and glomerular capillaries.
* Antiviral therapy includes interferon alfa and ribavirin (seek expert advice). Long-term prognosis depends on sustained HCV RNA clearance from serum at least 6 months after cessation of therapy, but no treatment is of proven benefit to the kidney outcome.
* Hepatitis C-positive children being considered for renal transplant require assessment by a paediatric hepatologist. Survival post transplant is increased compared to remaining on dialysis.

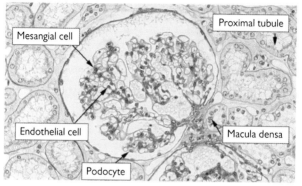

Mesangial cell

Proximal tubule

Endothelial cell

Macula densa

Podocyte

Plate 1 Normal renal biopsy.

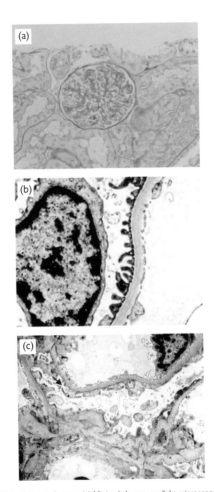

Plate 2 Minimal change disease. (a) Minimal changes on light microscopy. (b) Electron microscopy (EM) of normal foot processes. (c) Minimal change disease with effacement of podocyte foot processes.

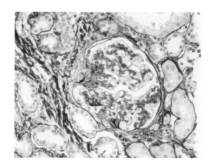

Plate 3 Focal and segmental glomerulosclerosis: sclerosis of part of a glomerulus, not all glomeruli affected (silver stain). A capsular adhesion is present. There is a propensity for FSGS to affect predominantly the deep, juxta-medullary glomeruli, so cortical glomeruli may not demonstrate the lesion (false-negative renal biopsy).

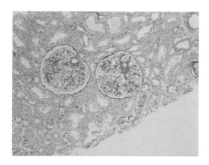

Plate 4 Mesangial proliferative glomerulonephritis. Increase in mesangial cells and matrix (>4 cells/mesangial area), but without peripheral capillary loop involvement (PAS). This pattern is most characteristic of Henoch–Schönlein nephritis, IgA nephropathy, IgM nephropathy, and SLE, but may be present in many other conditions.

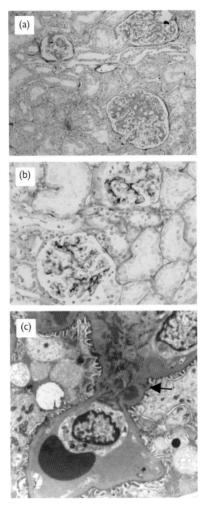

Plate 5 IgA nephropathy. (a) Mesangial proliferation (PAS). (b) Granular immune complexes containing predominantly IgA in the mesangium of most or all glomeruli (immunohistochemistry). (c) EM showing electron-dense deposits in the mesangium.

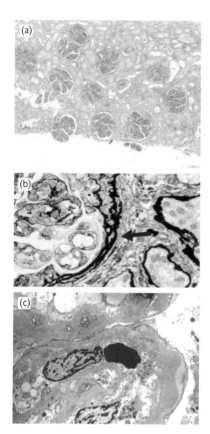

Plate 6 Membranoproliferative glomerulonephritis type 1. (a) Diffuse increase in glomerular cellularity with mesangial cell proliferation and lobulation of the glomerular tufts (PAS). (b) Thickening of the capillary wall caused by circumferential interposition of mesangial cells and matrix between the endothelium GBM, resulting in capillary luminal narrowing and 'double-contour' formation on silver staining (silver). (c) EM revealing separation of the endothelial cells from the GBM by interposed mesangial cell cytoplasm and subendothelial deposits, resulting in narrowing of the capillary lumen.

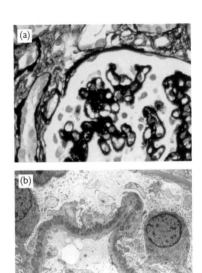

Plate 7 Membranous glomerulonephritis. (a) Light microscopy demonstrating thickening of the GBMs with 'spike' formation (silver). (b) EM of membranous glomerulonephritis with thickened GBM and numerous, regular subepithelial electron-dense deposits.

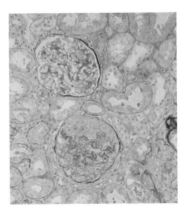

Plate 8 Crescentic nephritis. Cellular crescent impinging on glomerulus (PAS). Immunohistochemistry was 'pauci-immune' compatible with antineutrophil cytoplasmic antibody (ANCA) vasculitis (in this case granulomatosis with polyangiitis).

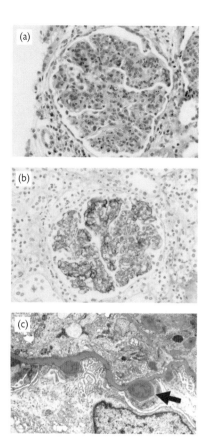

Plate 9 Post-infectious glomerulonephritis (acute diffuse proliferative glomerulonephritis). (a) Glomeruli show hypercellularity. There is obliteration of the capillary lumens (endocapillary proliferation). Some polymorphonuclear leucocytes can be seen (PAS). (b) Coarse granular pattern of staining with IgG in the GBM ('lumpy bumpy' pattern), typical of post-infectious glomerulonephritis (IHC). (c) EM showing large subepithelial deposits (humps) in the GBM (arrows).

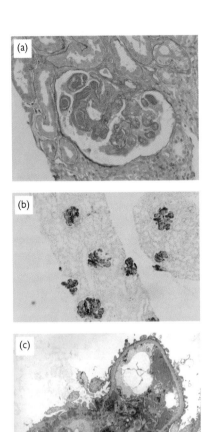

Plate 10 Systemic lupus erythematosus. (a) Diffuse proliferative (World Health Organization (WHO) class 4) lupus nephritis with endocapillary cellular proliferation and massive subendothelial deposit forming 'wire-loop' and 'hyaline-drop' lesions. (b) Immunostaining in such cases often shows a 'full-house' pattern with deposition of IgG, IgM, IgA, and complement. (c) Large electron-dense deposits are seen in the subendothelial region of the GBM (arrow). See also Plate 10.

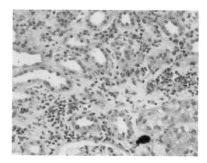

Plate 11 Tubulointerstitial nephritis. Extensive interstitial infiltration of mononuclear inflammatory cells and eosinophils with tubular damage.

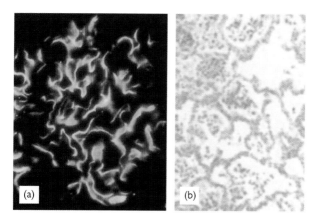

Plate 12 Goodpasture disease. (a) Linear staining of immunoglobulin deposited in the glomerulus. In Goodpasture disease, the autoantibody is directed against an antigen in the GBM deposited in a linear fashion, in contrast to immune complex-mediated disease. (b) Lung of a patient with evidence of intra-alveolar haemorrhage.

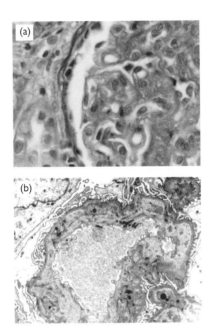

Plate 13 Haemolytic uraemic syndrome. (a) A glomerulus affected by thrombotic microangiopathy with luminal reduction and double-contour formation (silver). (b) Electron micrograph demonstrating subendothelial widening containing fibrin-like material.

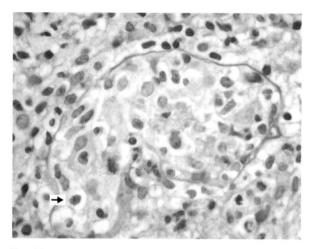

Plate 14 Tubulitis. Lymphocyte nuclei seen within tubular epithelium inside tubular basement membrane.

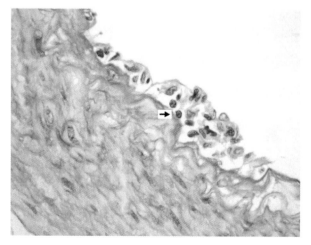

Plate 15 Endothelialitis. Lymphocytes seen within intima of artery—a histological change suggestive of acute ABMR.

Human immunodeficiency virus

- HIV-associated nephropathy (HIVAN) is defined by the presence of proteinuria associated with mesangial hyperplasia and/or global focal segmental glomerulosclerosis, in combination with microcystic transformation of renal tubules. Glomerular capillary collapse associated with hyperplasia of podocytes (collapsing glomerulopathy) may also occur.
- Alternatively, there may be mesangial proliferative lesions secondary to immune complex deposits and lupus-like changes.
- African Americans show a unique susceptibility to develop HIVAN.
- Children may present with nephrotic syndrome and CKD.
- Treatment is with antiretroviral therapy.
- Renal transplantation has been successful, provided there is stable maintenance of antiretroviral therapy, the HIV viral load is undetectable for at least 6 months, and the CD4 cell count is >200 cells/mm^3.

Malaria

- *Plasmodium falciparum* can cause AKI as malarial parasites in RBCs affect their circulation in the renal microvasculature.
- Plasmodium malaria infections can be associated with nephrotic syndrome, also called quartan malaria nephropathy; however, a direct causal link has not been demonstrated, and neither antimalarial therapy nor steroid therapy is effective.

Leptospirosis

- Infection is through skin contact with the urine of infected animals.
- Presentation is with fever, muscle pain, conjunctivitis, and, in severe cases, renal and liver failure.
- Organisms invade the renal tubules and can be found in the urine.
- Treatment is with penicillin and tetracyclines. Occasionally, steroids are required to treat severe late immunological sequelae (caused by immune complex disease) such as pulmonary haemorrhage after the acute infection is treated.

Schistosomiasis

- Occurs in Asia, Africa, and South America.
- Renal disease is associated with *Schistosoma mansoni* infection.
- May present with dysuria and terminal haematuria as the worms lay their eggs in the venous plexuses surrounding the bladder and ureters.
- Fibrosis and obstruction may develop in the long term, as can bladder carcinoma.

Tuberculosis

TB of the kidney and urinary tract is more common in developing countries and is up to 70 times more common in immunosuppressed populations. TB may be due to reactivation of latent infection or to new infection, including from a donor at the time of transplantation.

Presentation

- Asymptomatic or non-specific symptoms.
- LUT symptoms.
- Haematuria and pyuria.
- Mild hyponatremia due to SIADH from pulmonary involvement.

Pathology

- Direct infection of the kidney with granuloma formation, glomerulonephritis, tubulointerstitial nephritis, fibrosis, and abscess formation.
- Direct invasion of the LUT with fibrosis and stenosis leading to obstructive uropathy.
- Secondary amyloidosis.

Screening for latent TB

- Is recommended in any patient due to start immunosuppression who is at risk for TB.
- Can be by:
  - Mantoux test, but this may give a positive result in the first one to two decades after immunization and can be falsely negative in children on dialysis
  - interferon-γ release assays (e.g. QuantiFERON®-TB Gold) can detect latent TB and can distinguish between latent infection and a positive response to a Mantoux test due to previous vaccination.
- Prednisolone can cause false-negative results so it is important to assess immune status and look for latent TB in high-risk children before immunosuppression.

Diagnosis of renal TB

- At least three first-morning midstream urine specimens for microscopy for acid-fast bacilli (AFBs) and culture.
- PCR on potentially infected tissue.
- Radiology may show both upper and lower urinary tract involvement, calcifications, calyceal blunting and erosion, narrowing of infundibula, papillary necrosis, parenchymal scarring, ureteric strictures, and/or bladder involvement.

Treatment

- Ensure the patient does not have concurrent HIV.
- Prevention is with BCG pre transplant in non-immune children but BCG cannot be given to anyone who is immunosuppressed. Effectiveness decreases with age and is ~80% if administered before 15 years of age. BCG is not available in some areas.
- If latent TB is suspected, obtain an infectious disease consultation. Usual treatment is with isoniazid 10–15 mg/kg (maximum dose 300 mg) initially for 6 months and oral pyridoxine 25–50 mg daily.
- Also consider isoniazid as prophylaxis in unvaccinated patients on or starting immunosuppression in those who have a history of TB or who are going to endemic areas.
- In confirmed TB, antituberculous drugs for 6 months. Some drugs are nephrotoxic and interfere with CNI levels. Consider longer treatment if immunosuppressed.
- Progressive fibrosis of infected areas may continue during treatment.

Renal cystic diseases and ciliopathies

Renal cystic diseases: basic principles

- Typically we separate multicystic from polycystic kidney disease:
  - 'Multicystic' is a term usually used in the context of renal cystic dysplasia, including the MCDK (➲ see 'Renal dysplasia').
  - 'Polycystic' refers to defined genetic diseases, mainly autosomal dominant (ADPKD) and recessive polycystic kidney disease (ARPKD), including the contiguous gene syndrome with tuberous sclerosis (TS; see Table 13.1).
- Cysts can be microscopically small (microcysts) and thus not be identifiable as discrete cysts on US, but instead lead to an appearance of increased echogenicity.
- Glomerulocystic kidney disease is a histological diagnosis. It is typically seen in the renal cysts and diabetes syndrome (Table 13.1)
- Investigations into the causes of cystic kidney diseases identified dysfunction of primary cilia or the centrosome, an intracellular structure closely associated with ciliary function, as a unifying aetiology. Cilia are hair-like appendages, which can be motile or non-motile. They are important sensory organelles involved in cell polarity and proliferation. Cilia are found on many epithelial cells explaining the wide spectrum of associated symptoms.
- In ADPKD, cysts develop on the basis of a germline mutation and a 'second hit', i.e. an acquired mutation in the second allele. This has been shown by genetic testing of individual cysts—each cyst has an individual mutation on one allele in addition to the inherited mutation on the other allele. This may explain some of the phenotypic variability within families, as 'second hits' occur essentially at random.
- 'Second-hit' somatic mutations are also the disease mechanism in TS.
- In ADPKD, cysts can arise anywhere in the nephron; in ARPKD, they are exclusively in the collecting duct.
- Nephronophthisis and cystic dysplasia probably form a spectrum of the manifestations of ciliopathies, as both forms can be associated with typical ciliopathies, such as Bardet–Biedl, Jeune, Joubert, and Ivemark syndromes.

Table 13.1 shows the inheritance, affected gene, age at onset, renal imaging, and symptoms of the inherited cystic renal diseases. Genetic testing for these genes is becoming increasingly available. However, US and associated clinical features can usually establish a clinical diagnosis.

Particular issues relevant to all cystic diseases

- A careful family history (including for diabetes) and US of the parents' kidneys may help in the diagnosis.
- Examination of the child for associated symptoms, such as hepatosplenomegaly, retinal changes, signs of TS (also in the parents), and Bardet–Biedl syndrome (BBS) may help in the diagnosis.
- Screening of other family members or antenatal diagnosis can be offered (➲ see 'Genetic testing and antenatal diagnosis', p. 39).
- Long-term follow-up is essential.
- Recurrence after transplantation has not been described for cystic diseases.

Table 13.1 The inherited cystic kidney diseases

Inherited cystic disease	Inheritance, genes and incidence	Age cysts noted	Imaging	Other manifestations
Autosomal dominant polycystic kidney disease (ADPKD)	Mutations of PKD1 (80–90%) and PKD2, which is associated with slower progression. Phenotype varies even within families. Affects 1:1000	May be detected antenatally, incidentally, or on screening. Cannot be excluded until the fourth decade of life	Cysts may be isolated at presentation and progressively increase in number and size. May be asymmetrical. Kidneys are large	Cysts in liver and pancreas. Cerebral aneurysms Mitral valve prolapse
Tuberous sclerosis (TS) Contiguous gene syndrome (TSC2 and PKD1)	AD, mutations of TSC1 and TSC2 Disruption of TSC2 and the adjacent PKD1 gene (2% of TS patients)	Childhood Early childhood	75% of patients with TS develop angiomyolipomata and 35% develop cysts Large, polycystic kidneys	Adenoma sebaceum, intracerebral tubers, ungual fibromas, cardiac rhabdomyomas, hypopigmented patches and shagreen patches, developmental delay
Autosomal dominant tubulointerstitial kidney disease: UMOD and MUC1	AD, mutations in MUC1 or UMOD	Early adulthood, rarely CKD in childhood	Kidneys may be normal or reduced in size. Mostly medullary cysts	May be associated with hyperuricaemia
Autosomal dominant tubulointerstitial kidney disease: HNF1B	AD, mutations of HNF1β	Any age, including antenatally (bright kidneys)	Variable renal size, cysts, dysplasia	Maturity-onset diabetes, genital abnormalities in females, gout, deafness, hypomagnesaemia

(Continued)

Table 13.1 (Contd.)

Inherited cystic disease	Inheritance, genes and incidence	Age cysts noted	Imaging	Other manifestations
Autosomal recessive polycystic kidney disease (ARPKD)	AR, mutations of *PKHD1*. Affects 1:20,000	May present antenatally with large bright kidneys, and oligohydramnios if severe with respiratory distress at birth; or with palpable kidneys in infancy or later childhood	Kidneys are large with poor corticomedullary differentiation and scattered small cysts, usually 1–2 mm	Ductal plate malformation, hepatic fibrosis
Hyperinsulinism and polycystic kidney disease (HIPKD)	AR, mutations in *PMM2*, including a promoter mutation in at least one allele	Antenatal to childhood	Enlarged kidneys with macro- and microcysts,	Hyperinsulinaemic hypoglycaemia, liver cysts, and ductal plate malformation
Nephronophthisis	AR, mutations in >15 genes Most commonly in *NPHP1* (25%). Affects 1:50,000	Infancy, childhood and adolescence	Normal sized kidneys with poor corticomedullary differentiation, increased echogenicity, cysts at the corticomedullary junction	May be associated with retinitis pigmentosa (Senior–Loken syndrome), oculomotor apraxia, cone-shaped epiphyses, developmental delay and hypoplasia of the cerebellar vermis (Joubert syndrome), situs inversus
Bardet–Biedl syndrome	AR, mutations in >12 *BBS* genes; 1:135,000	Antenatal	Fetal lobulation, increased echogenicity, cystic dysplasia, calyceal abnormalities	Polydactyly, obesity, developmental delay, retinal dystrophy, hypogenitalism

Autosomal dominant polycystic kidney disease

Background

- Most common inherited renal disease, incidence estimated at 1:500–1000.
- Due to mutations in either *PKD1* (16p13) or *PKD2* (4q21–23).
- ~10% of cases are due to spontaneous mutations (no family history).

Presentation and prognosis

- Wide spectrum of clinical severity: from intrauterine death with Potter sequence to mild CKD well into late adulthood.
- The phenotype may be variable even within families.
- Approximately half of patients reach end-stage kidney disease by 60 years of age.
- Once progression begins, the mean decline in GFR is ~4–6 mL/min/1.73 m^2 per year.
- Extrarenal manifestations include polycystic liver disease, pancreatic cysts, and intracranial aneurysms (rarely seen in childhood).
- CKD stage 5 is extremely rare in childhood. The median onset of CKD stage 5 is in the sixth decade of life with *PKD1* and eighth decade with *PKD2* mutations.
- Complications of ADPKD do occur in childhood—hypertension incidence is 15–30%, and proteinuria 30–40%; CKD stage ≥2 is seen in up to 40% of teenagers.

Diagnosis

- Diagnostic screening of at-risk children is controversial—establishing the diagnosis may not provide a benefit, yet impose a burden of psychological stress, and may impair the child's ability to obtain health or life insurance or a mortgage later in life.
- Conversely, failing to rule out the diagnosis in at-risk children may unnecessarily relegate unaffected children to annual follow-up and continuing worries about being affected.
- These issues of diagnostic screening need to be discussed with the family. Many may want to delay diagnostic testing until the at-risk child is old enough to make a fully informed decision.
- The potential introduction of medical treatment (➔ see 'tolvaptan' in the following 'Management' section) may change the risk:benefit ratio of screening.
- Currently, the most common modality for diagnostic screening is a renal US. However, the first cysts may not appear until the fourth decade of life, so ADPKD cannot be excluded until then. The presence of any cyst in an at-risk child is highly suggestive of the disease; the presence of two or more cysts is considered diagnostic. Genetic testing is the definitive screening tool, if a family mutation can be identified.
- Diagnostic screening of all children at risk will become standard of care, once a proven treatment slowing disease progression is available.

Management

- Annual review of BP and early morning urine for protein is recommended for affected children and those at risk (with family history of ADPKD). Treatment with ACE inhibitors has demonstrated efficacy with respect to target-organ damage (cardiac hypertrophy). Long-term studies to assess the effect of ACE inhibitors on progression of CKD are ongoing.
- US is used for diagnostic purposes (➜ see 'Diagnosis', p. 357), but has no bearing on clinical management, once the diagnosis is established.
- Initial tests in those with an established diagnosis should include blood and urine tests. The frequency of subsequent blood tests depends on kidney function.
- Routine screening for intracranial aneurysms is not recommended unless there is a strong family history of cerebrovascular accidents. MRA can detect all but the smallest aneurysms.
- A phase III trial (TEMPO) in adult ADPKD patients of tolvaptan has demonstrated slowing in the increases in kidney and/or liver volume and the drug has been approved for the treatment of ADPKD in several jurisdictions. A trial of tolvaptan in paediatric ADPKD patients commenced in 2016.
  - Tolvaptan is a vasopressin receptor type 2 (AVPR2) antagonist, initially developed for the treatment of euvolaemic hyponatraemia (➜ see 'Disorders of renal water handling presenting with hyponatraemia'). It thus induces a pharmacologically induced form of nephrogenic diabetes insipidus. By blocking AVPR2, it inhibits formation of cAMP in the collecting duct, which is considered a key driver of cyst formation. Polyuria, the intended effect in the original indication of hyponatraemia, is thus a marked side effect when used in the treatment of ADPKD.

Further reading

Ong AC, Devuyst O, Knebelmann B, et al. Autosomal dominant polycystic kidney disease: the changing face of clinical management. *Lancet* 2015;385:1993–2002.

Renal structural abnormalities in tuberous sclerosis

Introduction

- TS is an autosomal dominant disorder caused by mutations in the *TSC1* (9q34) and *TSC2* (16p13.3) genes. The incidence is 1:6500 to 1:10,000.
- *TSC2* lies adjacent to *PKD1*, the gene responsible for ADPKD, suggesting a role for *PKD1* in the aetiology of renal cystic disease in TS. A high proportion of TS patients with renal cystic disease have contiguous deletions of *TSC2* and *PKD1*.
- Neurological features predominate, although there are a number of significant renal manifestations.
- A severe form of angiodysplasia affecting any part of the arterial tree is also described in TS.

Renal disease in tuberous sclerosis

Angiomyolipomata (AML)

- Benign hamartomas.
- Present in 80% of TS patients and may be detected in early childhood.
- Major complications include bleeding and rarely mechanical obstruction—most lesions that bleed are >3.5 cm in diameter. Bleeding lesions are treated by arterial embolization.
- Treatment with mammalian target of rapamycin (mTOR) inhibitors (see guidelines mentioned later in this topic) is recommended as first-line treatment of non-bleeding AML.

Cystic disease (simple cysts and polycystic disease)

- 20% develop simple cysts.
- Polycystic kidney disease develops in <5%, and may result in CKD stage 5 in children and adults.

Renal cell carcinoma

- This develops in <1% and appears to follow a less aggressive course than in unaffected individuals.
- Suspicion should be raised where apparent angiomyolipomata appear to have a low fat content on US.

Guidelines for the management of patients with tuberous sclerosis

International guidelines for the management of TS were published in 2012 (as recommendations of the 2012 International Tuberous Sclerosis Complex Consensus Conference). For the renal aspects, these include the following:

- Annual measurement of BP and renal function.
- Initial MRI of the abdomen to assess for the presence of angiomyolipomas and renal cysts. MRI was specifically recommended over US due to better sensitivity. Follow-up thereafter with US or MR annually.
- Refer for a specialist opinion if macroscopic haematuria develops.
- Refer to a specialist unit if treatment of a renal lesion is contemplated.

- Clinical trials (EXIST) have shown a reduction in AML with mTOR inhibitors, with an overall response rate of ~50%.
- Everolimus is licensed for adults with TS for the following indications:
  - Growing AML >3 cm.
  - Aneurysms within AML.
  - Multiple or bilateral lesions.

Use of everolimus
- The starting dose is 5–10 mg daily in adults, scaled down for children and if liver involvement, and titrated against side effects and response.
- Check trough levels within 2 weeks of starting, aiming for 3–15 ng/mL.
- Enzyme-inducing agents will decrease levels (e.g. carbamazepine).

Indications to stop everolimus: reassess after 6 months
- Intolerable side effects (stomatitis, nasopharyngitis, acne, headaches, cough, hypercholesterolaemia).
- No response of AML despite blood levels in target range (i.e. new enlarging lesions >30 mm or a >25% increase in size in existing lesions).
- Progressive decline in GFR to <30 mL/min/1.73 m^2.
- Proteinuria >3 g/L.
- Bleeding lesions necessitating embolization/surgery.

Transplantation
- Native nephrectomies pre transplant due to technical reasons and nephromegaly, and risk of ongoing renal lesions.
- Consider an mTOR inhibitor as part of the immunosuppressive regimen.

References

Kingswood JC, Bissler JJ, Budde K, et al. Review of the tuberous sclerosis renal guidelines from the 2012 Consensus Conference: current data and future study. Nephron 2016;134:51–58.

Krueger DA, Northrup H, International Tuberous Sclerosis Complex Consensus Group. Tuberous sclerosis complex surveillance and management: recommendations of the 2012 International Tuberous Sclerosis Complex Consensus Conference. Pediatr Neurol 2013;49:255–265.

Autosomal recessive polycystic kidney disease

Background

- Due to recessive mutations in *PKHD1* (6p21–12).
- Incidence of ~1:20,000 live births.
- Other ciliopathies, e.g. due to mutations in *TMEM67* or *NPHP1* or biallelic mutation in *PKD1/2* and even a specific form of a congenital disorder of glycosylation ("Hyperinsulinism and PKD" due to a promoter mutation in *PMM2*) can mimic ("phenocopy") the clinical symptoms of ARPKD.

Presentation and prognosis

- *Clinical variability*: from severe renal disease with fetal or neonatal death with Potter sequence and pulmonary hypoplasia to exclusive liver disease (congenital hepatic fibrosis).
- *Some genotype–phenotype correlation*: two truncating mutations in *PKHD1* appear incompatible with life, although individual survivors have been reported. Most patients surviving the neonatal period have at least one missense mutation. However, no specific mutation profile is seen for patients with predominant liver disease.
- Those surviving the neonatal period have reported survival rates of 80–90% at 10 years of age.

Renal manifestations

- *Enlargement of the kidneys*: >90% have kidneys ≥2 SD for age. In severe cases, enlargement is massive with consequent pulmonary hypoplasia and abdominal protuberance. These kidneys are easily palpable as firm masses. Severe abdominal distension can cause problems with feeding and respiration to the extent that unilateral nephrectomy may be considered.
- Hyponatraemia is often seen in early infancy, presumably due to impaired urinary dilution.
- Hypertension is a common complication (up to 80% of patients).
- Over 50% of patients will have developed CKD stage 5 by age 20 years.

Extrarenal manifestations

Mainly restricted to the liver:

- All patients have some degree of congenital hepatic fibrosis (Caroli disease).
- US may show dilated biliary ducts.
- A hepatobiliary imino-diacetic acid (HIDA) scan may show abnormal biliary drainage, but may be normal before the age of 1 year.
- A biopsy is not routinely recommended, but if performed shows ductal plate malformation.
- Assessment for hepatosplenomegaly should be part of routine clinical examinations.
- Hypersplenism may present as a falling platelet and white cell count.

- Oesophageal varices may develop and screening with US is necessary, particularly prior to transplant.
- Cholangitis may present with recurrent septicaemia with enteric organisms (especially *Klebsiella*, *Escherichia coli* and *Enterobacter*) without the classical features of 'Charcot's triad' (fever, hepatic pain, and jaundice).
- Occasionally, pancreatic cysts are seen.

Diagnosis

- Usually a clinical diagnosis based on US appearance of the kidneys with nephromegaly and liver involvement.
- *Ultrasound appearance:*
  - Antenatal screening typically shows bright and/or enlarged kidneys; however, antenatal bright kidneys can be seen in other conditions, too, especially with HNF1B disease.
  - Cysts are usually too small to resolve by US (microcysts), but lead to increased echogenicity.
  - Larger cysts (macrocysts) may also be seen, which can be difficult to distinguish from ADPKD.
- Genetic testing can confirm the diagnosis in ~80% of cases with clinically suspected ARPKD. Genetic testing can be especially helpful in cases with unclear clinical diagnosis and for genetic counselling.

Management

- Dependent on CKD stage (➔ see Chapter 18).
- Hypertension typically responds well to ACE inhibitors (➔ see Chapter 16).
- Hyponatraemia is usually self-limited. Concentration of feeds to decrease fluid intake may help. Salt supplementation will worsen hypertension, consistent with the hyponatraemia being due to water retention. Aquaretics (AVPR2 blockers like tolvaptan) may be beneficial based on anecdotal evidence.
- Cholangitis needs treatment with appropriate IV antibiotics; subsequent prophylactic antibiotics should be considered, such as:
  - *cefalexin*—12.5 mg/kg (maximum 500 mg) once a day
  - *amoxicillin*—25 mg/kg (maximum 1 g) once a day
  - *trimethoprim*—2 mg/kg (maximum 50 mg) once a day.
- These can also be used in a rotating fashion, e.g. changing antibiotics every 12 weeks.
- Nephrectomies may need to be performed prior to transplantation because of nephromegaly. It may also be necessary prior to initiation of peritoneal dialysis (PD).
- Patients should be assessed for potential combined kidney-liver transplant when approaching CKD stage 5.

Further reading

Bergmann C. ARPKD and early manifestations of ADPKD: the original polycystic kidney disease and phenocopies. *Pediatr Nephrol* 2015;30:15–30.

Nephronophthisis

Background

- The commonest inherited aetiology in a newly presenting child with CKD stage 5.
- There are usually few preceding symptoms, other than long-standing polydipsia and polyuria.
- More than 20 genes have been identified so far, which account for approximately one-third of cases. Thus, more genes still await identification.
- The most common mutation (accounting for ~20% of cases) is a homozygous deletion of *NPHP1*.

Presentation and prognosis

Progression to CKD stage 5 is virtually universal. However, age at onset and extrarenal manifestations vary according to the underlying gene, but also individually.

Extrarenal manifestations
- *Eye*:
  - Retinal dysplasia/retinitis pigmentosa (Senior–Løken syndrome, Leber amaurosis).
  - Oculomotor apraxia (Cogan syndrome).
- *Skeleton*:
  - Thoracic deformity (Jeune asphyxiating thoracic dystrophy).
  - Cone-shaped epiphysis (Mainzer–Saldino syndrome).
  - Skeletal dysplasia (Ellis van Crefeld syndrome).
- *Heart*:
  - Situs inversus (infantile nephronophthisis, Ivemark syndrome).
  - Cardiac malformations.
- *Brain*:
  - Cerebellar vermis aplasia (Joubert syndrome).
  - Encephalocoele (Mekkel–Gruber syndrome).
- *Liver*: ductal plate malformation.

Diagnosis

- On US, kidneys typically are of normal size, but echo-bright and may contain cysts.
- Anaemia is often severe because of the tubulointerstitial fibrosis affecting the peritubular erythropoietin-producing cells.
- The most important differential diagnostic consideration is tubulointerstitial nephritis (TIN), which can present with similar symptoms. Chronicity of symptoms, as assessed by history, degree of anaemia, and parathyroid hormone (PTH) elevation will argue for nephronophthisis (NPHP). Renal biopsy can help distinguish between the two diagnoses: histology in NPHP is characterized by the triad of renal tubular (and glomerular) cysts, tubular membrane disruption, and tubulointerstitial cell infiltrates with interstitial fibrosis. Conversely, TIN is characterized by an eosinophilic infiltrate.

Management

- No specific therapy is available but standard CKD management applies (➔ see Chapter 18).
- All should have ophthalmological and cardiac reviews in view of the known extrarenal manifestations.
- Post-transplant recurrence of the disease has not been reported.

Further reading

Wolf MT. Nephronophthisis and related syndromes. *Curr Opin Pediatr* 2015;27:201–211.

Bardet–Biedl syndrome

BBs is characterized by the primary manifestations of:
- rod-cone dystrophy
- truncal obesity
- postaxial polydactyly
- cognitive impairment
- male hypogonadotropic hypogonadism, complex female genitourinary malformations
- renal abnormalities.

Secondary features include:
- speech delay/disorder
- developmental delay
- behavioural abnormalities
- eye abnormalities: strabismus, cataracts, and astigmatism
- brachydactyly/syndactyly
- ataxia/poor coordination/imbalance
- mild hypertonia (especially lower limbs)
- diabetes mellitus
- orodental abnormalities: dental crowding, hypodontia, small dental roots, and high-arched palate
- cardiovascular anomalies: valvular stenoses and atrial/ventricular septal defects, patent ductus arteriosus and unspecified cardiomyopathy
- hepatic involvement: perilobular fibrosis, periportal fibrosis with small bile ducts, bile duct proliferation with cystic dilatation, biliary cirrhosis, portal hypertension, and congenital cystic dilations of both the intrahepatic and extrahepatic biliary tract
- craniofacial dysmorphism
- Hirschsprung disease
- anosmia.

Diagnosis

- The presence of four primary features or three primary plus two secondary features is considered diagnostic.
- The diagnosis can be confirmed by genetic testing. Mutations in >15 genes have been associated with BBS.

Renal involvement

- Renal involvement is seen in ~30–50% of children with BBS.
- It is predominantly diagnosed antenatally or in infancy.
- A child with no evidence of renal disease at the age of 5 years is highly unlikely to develop significant renal disease during childhood.
- Most common manifestation is cystic renal dysplasia and structural renal abnormalities (horseshoe, duplex, and ectopic kidney).
- Urinary concentrating defect and bladder dysfunction (detrusor instability) can also occur.
- A second peak of renal disease occurs during adulthood and is likely related to longstanding obesity and diabetes.
- Severe renal disease is most likely with *BBS10* mutations (20% of patients progress to CKD stage 5, compared to <5% with *BBS1*), as well as *BBS2* and *BBS12*.

Management

- Patients with BBS should be assessed for renal involvement by measuring BP, urine protein excretion, and a renal US.
- If there is no evidence of renal involvement by the age of 5 years, routine follow-up with a GP or infrequent (every few years) specialist follow-up may be sufficient.
- For those with CKD, the usual management (➜ see Chapter 18) applies.
- In BBS patients undergoing renal transplantation, steroid avoidance or minimization should be considered given the risk/presence of diabetes and obesity.

Further reading

Forsythe E, Sparks K, Best S, et al. Risk factors for severe renal disease in Bardet-Biedl syndrome. J Am Soc Nephrol 2017;28:963–970.

Renal cysts and diabetes syndrome (HNF1B disease)

Background

- Mutations in the transcription factor hepatocyte nuclear factor-1-beta gene (*HNF1B*) can cause a variety of manifestation, chiefly renal cysts and diabetes; ~50% are due to microdeletions at chromosome 17q12, which includes 14 other genes.
- The most commonly found genetic abnormality is antenatal bright kidneys (~30%).

Presentation and prognosis

- Renal manifestations are highly variable and include MCDK; hypo-, a-, and dysplasia; cysts, including glomerular cysts; malformations such as horseshoe kidney; and occasionally LUT abnormalities.
- Progression to CKD stage 5 in childhood is seen in ~10–20% of patients.

Associated features may include

- *pancreas*:
  - type 2 diabetes mellitus (maturity onset diabetes of the young type 5 (MODY5), onset usually in adulthood, but can occur earlier)
  - there may be an increased risk for new-onset diabetes mellitus after transplantation (NODAT)
  - pancreatic exocrine dysfunction and agenesis of pancreatic body and tail
- *kidney*:
  - hypouricosuria with hyperuricaemic gout
  - hypomagnesaemia with renal magnesium wasting and hypochloraemic hypokalaemic metabolic alkalosis (Gitelman-like tubulopathy; ➔ see Chapter 7)
- *genitalia*:
  - abnormalities of the female genitalia, including bicornuate uterus, rudimentary uterus, uterus didelphys, hemiuterus, and vaginal aplasia
  - abnormalities of the male genitalia, including epididymal cysts atresia of vas deferens, hypospadias, and cryptorchidism
- *liver*:
  - elevated liver enzymes
  - neonatal cholestasis
- *other*:
  - in addition, autism, schizophrenia, developmental delay, epilepsy, and eye abnormalities (coloboma and cataract) have been reported in patients with 17q12 microdeletions; these additional manifestations likely represent a contiguous gene syndrome, and may not be directly related to the loss of *HNF1B*, but of other genes contained within the deletion
  - lipodystrophy
  - biallelic mutations in *HNF1B* are associated with renal chromophobe cancer.

Diagnosis

* *HNF1B* gene mutations should be considered in any child with a combination of these symptoms (➔ 'Presentation and prognosis', p. 367), especially if there is a family history of renal disease, early-onset diabetes, or gout.
* Genetic testing provides a definitive diagnosis. Because of the high proportion of deletions, gene dosage assays (such as multiplexed ligation-dependent probe amplification (MPLA) or array comparative genomic hybridization (aCGH) (➔ see 'Genetic testing and antenatal diagnosis', p. 39) need to be performed if sequencing is normal.

Management

* The large number of potential extrarenal manifestations suggests that patients with *HNF1B* mutations should be carefully screened for the presence of these.
* If hyperuricaemia is present, treatment with allopurinol should be considered (➔ see Chapter 18).
* Hypomagnesaemia can be ameliorated with magnesium supplementation.
* Modification of post-transplant immunosuppression (avoidance/minimization of tacrolimus) because of a potential increased risk of NODAT should be considered, but needs to be balanced against risks of other immunosuppressants. Currently, there is insufficient experience to warrant specific recommendations.

Further reading

Bockenhauer D, Jaureguiberry G. HNF1B-associated clinical phenotypes: the kidney and beyond. *Pediatr Nephrol* 2016;31:707–714.

Solitary renal cysts

- With increasing use of abdominal imaging, occasionally an incidental solitary renal cyst is identified.
- The Bosniak classification (see Table 13.2) was developed in adults to assess for potential malignancy, but has been used also in children.
- Incidentally noted cysts in children are typically stage 1 or 'simple' cysts.
- Solitary simple cysts, in the absence of a family history of renal disease are rare in children: in one US study of ~30,000 babies, the incidence was 0.007%. The incidence increases with age to ~2% in young adults (<40 years of age).
- An incidentally noted solitary simple cyst is most likely of no clinical relevance, but if there is a family history of ADPKD, it is suggestive of the patient being affected.
- A parental US may help to assess for undiagnosed familial cystic kidney disease.
- Follow-up for a solitary simple cyst is probably not indicated, but a repeat US after a few years to assess for cyst growth and cyst number may help relieve anxiety. Since ~10% of ADPKD cases arise from *de novo* mutations (➔ see 'Autosomal dominant polycystic kidney disease'), there is a very small risk that the solitary cyst may reflect ADPKD even with no family history.
- Complicated and/or symptomatic cysts require consultation with a paediatric urologist.

Table 13.2 The Bosniak renal cyst classification

Stage	Cyst wall	Septa	Calcification
I	Hairline thin	No	No
II	Minimal regular thickening	Few, hairline thin	Smooth, hairline thin
IIF[a]	Minimal regular thickening	Multiple, minimal smooth thickening	Thick, nodular
III[b]	Irregular thickening	Measurably thick, irregular	Thick, nodular, irregular
IV	Gross, irregular thickening	Irregular gross thickening	Thick, nodular, irregular

[a] IIF F denotes follow-up. Cyst size of diameter of 3 cm is also an indication for follow-up.

[b] III: indeterminate stage III should be managed as IIF, while definitive stage III should be managed surgically.

Renal dysplasia and other manifestations in syndromic diseases

Background

- The most common cause of CKD in childhood.
- May occur in association with other congenital abnormalities of the urinary tract (➔ see Chapter 3).
- The kidneys are usually small with increased echogenicity on US and may or may not contain cysts that, if present, are usually cortical.
- There is a familial incidence, with a recurrence risk of up to 10%.
- Renal dysplasia can occur in a variety of genetic disorders.
- With the introduction of antenatal screening, which detects these lesions before potential infections, the diagnosis of reflux nephropathy has become rare. Presumably, many of the children previously diagnosed with reflux nephropathy actually had primary renal dysplasia.
- No imaging modality can distinguish between primary renal dysplasia and acquired renal scarring/reflux nephropathy.

Presentation and prognosis

- The majority of children are diagnosed antenatally.
- Renal dysplasia typically affects tubular salt handling, so polyuria and acidosis are common.
- Severity is variable, with some presenting at birth with severe CKD and others presenting later in childhood or even early adult life.
- CKD progression is slow. Infants and young children may even show an improvement in renal function in the first few years of life and then function can remain relatively stable or with a very slow decline throughout childhood with an increase in CKD progression at puberty.

Management

➔ See Chapter 18, sections on 'Management', pp. 460–494.
- Because of the obligatory tubular salt and water losses, children need free access to water and some may need sodium supplementation. Hypertension is therefore unusual before CKD stage 5.
- Large doses of sodiumbicarbonate may be necessary due to renal wasting.
- Because urine output usually continues into CKD stage 5, children can be managed with very low GFRs without dialysis with good dietary care.

Overview of genetics and renal abnormalities in inherited syndromes

Mendelian disorders

See Table 14.1.

Table 14.1 Mendelian disorders

Syndrome	OMIM	Gene(s)	Mode	Type of RM	Features other than RM
Alagille	118450 610205	JAG1 NOTCH2	AD	Dysplasia	Cholestasis, cardiac disease, skeletal abnormalities, ocular abnormalities, characteristic facies
Apert	101200	FGFR2	AD	Hydronephrosis	Craniosynostosis, midface hypoplasia, syndactyly
Bardet–Biedl	209900	BBS1-15	AR	Abnormal calyces (on IVP) Cystic dysplasia, NPHP	Retinal dystrophy, polydactyly, mental retardation and obesity
Beckwith–Wiedemann	130650	P57 CDKN1 CH19 LIT1	AD GI	Dysplasia	Exomphalos, macroglossia, gigantism, hypoglycaemia
Branchio-oto-renal	113650	EYA1 SIX1	AD	Agenesis, dysplasia	Pre-auricular pits, branchial fistulae, deafness
Campomelic dysplasia	114290	SOX9	AD	Dysplasia	Skeletal defects, abnormal genitalia

(Continued)

Table 14.1 (Contd.)

Syndrome	OMIM	Gene(s)	Mode	Type of RM	Features other than RM
CHARGE	214800	CHD7 SEMA3E	AD	Dysplasia	Coloboma, heart defects, atresia (choanal), retarded growth and development, genital and ear anomalies
Duane–radial ray	607323	SALL4	AD	Agenesis, migration defect	Upper limb anomalies, ocular anomalies
Fraser	219000	FRAS1 FREM2	AR	Agenesis	Cryptophthalmos, syndactyly, abnormal genitalia, laryngeal malformations, anal stenosis
Jeune (asphyxiating thoracic dystrophy)	208500 611263 613091 603297 61177	ATD1 ATD2 ATD3 DYNC 2H1 IFT80	AR	Cystic dysplasia, NPHP	Severely constricted thoracic cage and respiratory insufficiency, cysts in the liver and pancreas, retinal degeneration, short limbs, abnormal pelvis
Joubert	613037 613277 608629 607100 610142 609884 610937 608922 612013 300804	INPP5E TMEM216 AHI9 NPHP1 CEP290 TMEM67 RPGRIP1L ARL13B CC2D2A OFD1	AR	Cystic dysplasia, NPHP	Cerebellar vermis hypoplasia, dysregulation of breathing pattern and eye movement, developmental delay, retinal dystrophy

Condition	OMIM	Gene	Inheritance	Renal phenotype	Other features
Kallman	308700	KAL1	XR	Agenesis, dysplasia	Hypogonadotropic hypogonadism, anosmia
	147950	FGFR1	AD		
	244200	PROK2	AD		
	610628	PROK2R	AD+AR		
	612370	CHD7	AD		
	612702	FGF8	AD+AR		
Meckel–Gruber	249000	MKS1	AR	Cystic dysplasia, NPHP	Encephalocoele, hepatic ductal dysplasia and cysts and polydactyly
	603194	TMEM216			
	607361	TMEM67			
	611134	CEP290			
	611561	RPGRIP1L			
Nail–patella	161200	LMX1B	AD	Congenital NS or glomerulonephritis	Ungual dysplasia, absent or hypoplastic patellae, elbow and other skeletal abnormalities
Neurofibromatosis type I	162200	NF1	AD	Arterial stenosis and hypertension	Neurofibromas, pigmented patches
Pallister–Hall	146510	GLI3	AD	Dysplasia	Hypothalamic hamartoma, pituitary dysfunction, central polydactyly, and visceral malformations
Renal coloboma	120330	PAX2	AD	Hypo-/dysplasia, VUR	Optic disc coloboma
Renal cysts and diabetes	137920	HNF1B	AD	Hypo-/dysplasia	Diabetes, gout, hypomagnesaemia, uterus malformation

(Continued)

Table 14.1 (Contd.)

Syndrome	OMIM	Gene(s)	Mode	Type of RM	Features other than RM
Renal tubular dysgenesis	179820 106150 106180 106165	REN AGT ACE AGTR1	AR	Tubular agenesis	Potter sequence with fetal death
Senior–Loken	266900 606995 606996 609254 610189 613615	NPHP1 NPHP3 NPHP4 IQCB1 NPHP6 SDCCAG8	AR	NPHP	Retinitis pigmentosa, retinal a-/dysplasia (Leber's amaurosis)
Simpson–Golabi–Behmel	312870 300209	GPC3 CXORF5	XR	Dysplasia	Polydactyly, macrosomia, cleft palate
Townes–Brocks	107480	SALL1	AD	Hypo-/dysplasia	Imperforate anus, hand, foot and ear abnormalities, deafness
Zellweger	214100	PEX1, 2, 3, 5, 6, 12, 14, 26	AR	Dysplasia	Craniofacial abnormalities, hepatomegaly

AD, autosomal dominant; AR, autosomal recessive; GI, genomic imprinting; NPHP, nephronophthisis; OMIM, Online Mendelian Inheritance in Man; RM, renal manifestation; XR, X-linked recessive.

In AD diseases, parents may not show symptoms due to incomplete penetrance or spontaneous mutation in the child. Renal involvement is not obligate in many of the disorders. Dysplasia often includes cysts.

Associations and chromosomal abnormalities

See Table 14.2.

Table 14.2 Associations and chromosomal abnormalities

	OMIM	RM	Clinical findings
Association			
VATER and VACTERL	192350	40% unilateral agenesis, others varied	Vertebral defects, anal atresia, tracheoesophageal fistula with oesophageal atresia, and radial dysplasia (VATER) with cardiac malformations and limb anomalies (VACTERL)
COACH (variant of Joubert)	216360	Cystic dysplasia	Cerebellar vermis hypo/aplasia, oligophrenia, ataxia, coloboma, and hepatic fibrosis
Chromosomal abnormalities			
Trisomies and deletions (➲ see 'Down syndrome', p. 378)		Variable and common	Variable
Turner (45,X)		Variable structural anomalies	Short stature, webbed neck, heart defects
Williams (microdeletion chromosome 7)	194050	Infantile hypercalcaemia with nephrocalcinosis, renal agenesis, pelvic kidney, renal artery stenosis, hypertension	Supravalvular aortic stenosis, multiple peripheral pulmonary arterial stenosis, elfin face, mental and statural deficiency, characteristic dental malformation
DiGeorge (microdeletion chromosome 22)	188400	Unilateral renal agenesis, dysplasia, hydronephrosis	Hypocalcaemia arising from parathyroid hypoplasia, thymic hypoplasia, and outflow tract defects of the heart

OMIM, Online Mendelian Inheritance in Man; RM, renal manifestation.

Down syndrome

Introduction

Down syndrome (trisomy 21) is the commonest chromosomal abnormality in live-born infants with an incidence of ~1:800. Current guidelines from the American Academy of Pediatrics (℘ http://pediatrics.aappublications. org/content/107/2/442) and the UK Down Syndrome Medical Interest Group (℘ http://www.dsmig.org.uk/publications/guidelines.html) do not recommend screening for renal or urological problems, although some small studies suggest an increased incidence of these.

Renal structural abnormalities in Down syndrome

- A variety of urological abnormalities have been reported in children with Down syndrome including:
  - vesicoureteric reflux (VUR) and vesicoureteric junction (VUJ) obstruction
  - renal hypoplasia and dysplasia
  - obstructive uropathy
  - posterior urethral valves.
- There also appears to be an increased rate of glomerular microcyst formation, the significance of which is uncertain.
- As large population studies have not been performed, it is not possible to determine whether any of these abnormalities occur with any greater frequency in Down syndrome than in the general population.
- Autopsy studies have reported that the rate of renal abnormalities such as hypoplasia, dysplasia, and obstruction may be as high as 21%.
- Some have recommended that all children with Down syndrome undergo US assessment of the urinary tract to screen for abnormalities, with further investigations being performed when US abnormalities are detected.

Renal functional abnormalities in Down syndrome

- A number of cases of CKD, including stage 5, have been reported in children with Down syndrome, several of whom underwent successful renal transplantation.
- Down syndrome per se is not a contraindication to dialysis and transplantation, although significant co-morbid features need to be considered as in all patients being assessed for suitability for CKD stage 5 active management.

Further reading

Mercer ES, Broecker B, Smith EA, et al. Urological manifestations of Down syndrome. J Urol 2004;171:1250–1253.

Williams syndrome

Background

AD disorder which in the full-blown form includes:

* supravalvular aortic stenosis classically, but any arterial stenosis can occur, including renal artery stenosis and multiple peripheral pulmonary arterial stenoses
* characteristic facial features with full lips and retroussé nose
* stellate iris pattern due to stromal hypoplasia
* short stature
* small, wide-spaced primary dentition
* idiopathic infantile hypercalcaemia
* learning difficulties with uneven profile of abilities
* characteristic behavioural phenotype.

Caused by a microdeletion on the long arm of chromosome 7, usually containing 25–27 genes including the elastin gene.

Urinary tract disease in Williams syndrome

* Structural renal abnormalities (agenesis, duplex, pelvic kidney).
* Nephrocalcinosis secondary to hypercalcaemia and hypercalciuria.
* Unilateral or bilateral renal artery stenoses.
* *Voiding issues*: frequency, urgency, enuresis, detrusor instability.
* Bladder diverticulae (50%).
* *Hypertension*:
  * More prevalent in adult life (50%).
  * May be associated with renal artery stenosis, generalized arterial stiffening, or increased sympathetic drive.
  * The *NCF1* gene can be included in the chromosome 7 deletion. Loss of this gene is associated with a lower risk of hypertension.

Hypercalcaemia and hypercalciuria

* Aetiology unknown.
* Symptomatic hypercalcaemia usually resolves during childhood.
* Lifelong abnormalities of calcium and vitamin D metabolism which are poorly understood.
* Hypercalciuria is common and may predispose to nephrocalcinosis.
* Some infants with Williams syndrome require a feed with a low-calcium content, e.g. Locasol®.

Recommended renal investigations in Williams syndrome

(Full 2010 management guidelines are available at ℘ https://kr.ihc.com/ ext/Dcmnt?ncid=521096048&tfrm=default—the guidelines provide much useful information including Williams syndrome growth charts.)

* US of the urinary tract including Doppler studies of the renal arteries.
* Echocardiogram (annual cardiac examination until 4 years of age).
* Urinalysis for presence of microscopic haematuria.
* Uca:Ucr.
* Plasma biochemistry including calcium.
* Measurement of BP annually.

Where nephrocalcinosis is detected, refer to nephrologist for 6-monthly screening. Where a structural abnormality is detected, management or referral as necessary. Where renal artery stenosis is detected, refer to nephrologist.

Further reading

Martin NDT, Smith WR, Cole TJ, et al. New height, weight and head circumference charts for British children with Williams syndrome. *Arch Dis Child* 2007;92:598–601.

DiGeorge syndrome

Background

- Also called CATCH22 to denote the affected chromosome (22) and the clinical manifestations:
  - CArdiac malformations.
  - T-call deficit due to hypo- or aplasia of the thymic gland.
  - Cleft palate.
  - Hypocalcaemia, due to parathyroid hypoplasia.
- Microdeletion syndrome, associated with heterozygous deletion on chromosome 22q11.2. The deletions are of various sizes, containing various numbers of genes, potentially explaining some of the heterogeneity in the phenotype.
- The main manifestations appear to be related to deficiency in a gene called *TBX1*.
- Renal involvement, if present, is in the form of CAKUT (➔ see Chapter 3), typically renal hypodysplasia or aplasia, but also ureteric abnormalities.
- Renal involvement appears to be restricted to patients in whom the deletion includes the genes *SNAP29, AIFM3,* and *CRKL*.

Further reading

Lopez-Rivera E, Liu YP, Verbitsky M, et al. Genetic drivers of kidney defects in the DiGeorge syndrome. *N Engl J Med* 2017;376:742–754.

DiGeorge syndrome

Renal tumours

Wilms tumour

Introduction

* Incidence is 8.1 cases per million Caucasian children <15 years of age.
* Usually presents before 5 years of age. Median age at diagnosis is 3–4 years of age.
* Nephrogenic rests (clusters of blastemal cells, tubules, and stromal cells found at the periphery of the renal lobe) are thought to be precursor lesions. The term nephroblastomatosis indicates the presence of multifocal or diffuse nephrogenic rests in one or both kidneys, and has a distinctive radiological appearance compared with Wilms tumour.
* In 10–15% of individuals, the cause is considered to be a germline pathogenic variant or an epigenetic alteration (an alteration that changes gene expression, without a change in DNA sequence) occurring during early embryogenesis. The most commonly reported germline mutations involve the WT1 gene and the 11p15.5 locus (which harbours a number of imprinted genes involved in growth regulation), but a growing number of variants in other genes have been reported.
* A number of different syndromes are associated with genetic abnormalities linked to the development of Wilms tumour, most commonly in the WT1 gene located on chromosome 11:
  * Denys–Drash syndrome (cryptorchidism, diffuse mesangial sclerosis causing heavy proteinuria). The majority have a heterozygous germline mutation in WT1. Reported risk of Wilms tumour is up to 74%.
  * WAGR syndrome (Wilms tumour, Aniridia, Genitourinary malformations, mental Retardation). Heterozygous contiguous gene deletion at 11p13 that includes both WT1 and PAX6 is causative. Risk of Wilms tumour estimated to be 45–60%.
  * Frasier syndrome (undermasculinized external genitalia ranging from ambiguous to normal-looking female in an individual with a 46,XY karyotype, FSGS, and gonadoblastoma. Heterozygous single nucleotide variants in WT1 intron 9. Risk for Wilms tumour considered low.
  * Beckwith–Wiedemann syndrome (macrosomia, macroglossia, hemihypertrophy, visceromegaly, embryonal tumours (Wilms tumour, hepatoblastoma, neuroblastoma, and rhabdomyosarcoma), omphalocoele, neonatal hypoglycaemia, ear creases/pits, adrenocortical cytomegaly, and renal anomalies. Abnormal gene transcription regulation in chromosome 11p15.5. Risk of Wilms tumour 7%.
  * Less common causes of Wilms tumour predisposition include Bloom syndrome, Fanconi anaemia, mosaic variegated aneuploidy, Perlman syndrome, Simpson–Golabi–Behmel syndrome, and Li–Fraumeni syndrome.

Presenting features of Wilms tumour

* Abdominal mass or swelling (commonest).
* Abdominal discomfort.
* Gross or microscopic haematuria.

- Pyrexia.
- Hypertension: may be associated with hyperreninaemia, often due to distortion of the renal arteries, and responds to therapy with ACE inhibitors or angiotensin II receptor blockade.
- US abnormality detected during the screening of at-risk individuals.

Diagnosis

Radiology
- Abdominal US and MRI or CT to determine the extent of spread of tumour into adjacent structures, e.g. liver and IVC, with tumour, and radiological abnormalities of the opposite kidney.
- Chest CT to exclude pulmonary metastases.

Histology
- Needle biopsy performed by an experienced operator is recommended in the UK and does not change the tumour stage.
- Following pre-nephrectomy chemotherapy, nephrectomy is performed to confirm histology of excised renal tissue, and lymph nodes and local abdominal staging.
- Diffuse or focal anaplastic histological change, which is present in ~5% of cases, is associated with a poorer prognosis and is an indication for more aggressive therapy. Focal anaplasia does not have the same high risk and puts the patients into an intermediate risk group.

Staging

Depends on the involvement of sampled regional lymph nodes and direct examination of the contralateral kidney by the surgeon. The presence/ absence of metastases is evaluated at presentation on the basis of imaging studies (see Box 15.1).

Treatment

- Combination of surgery, chemotherapy, and radiotherapy, which is dependent on the stage and histology of the tumour.
- Most centres in the USA advocate primary surgery followed by chemotherapy or radiotherapy: cited advantages include avoidance of possible modification of tumour histology and staging, and the administration of chemotherapy to children with non-Wilms malignancies or benign lesions.
- In the UK and Europe, most patients receive pre-nephrectomy chemotherapy: vincristine/dactinomycin for localized disease and vincristine, dactinomycin, and doxorubicin for metastatic disease. Post-nephrectomy chemotherapy depends on abdominal stage and response to preoperative chemotherapy. Cited advantages include a lower tumour rupture rate at operation and the identification of good prognostic subgroups based on tumour response.
- The tumour is radiosensitive, although radiotherapy is reserved for localized, high-risk Wilms tumours stage II and III, and all abdominal stage III. Radiotherapy may be indicated in lung and brain metastases.
- In children with bilateral disease, consideration is given to renal-sparing surgery.

- Treatment of nephroblastomatosis is somewhat different. As part of the recommendations in the current SIOP (Societe Internationale D'oncologie Pediatrique) Wilms tumour protocol, chemotherapy should be tried first as long as the lesions respond, and surgery is reserved for lesions which progress or become radiologically suggestive of a Wilms tumour. This should be renal sparing as feasible.

Box 15.1 Staging of Wilms tumours

Stage I

- The tumour is limited to kidney or surrounded with a fibrous pseudocapsule if outside of the normal contours of the kidney. The renal capsule or pseudocapsule may be infiltrated with the tumour, but it does not reach the outer surface, and it is completely resected (resection margins 'clear').
- The tumour may be protruding ('bulging') into the pelvic system and 'dipping' into the ureter (but is not infiltrating their walls).
- The vessels of the renal sinus are not involved.
- Intrarenal vessel involvement may be present.

Stage II

- The tumour extends beyond kidney or penetrates through the renal capsule and/or fibrous pseudocapsule into perirenal fat, but is completely resected (resection margins 'clear').
- Tumour infiltrates the renal sinus and/or invades blood, and lymphatic vessels outside the renal parenchyma, but is completely resected.
- Tumour infiltrates adjacent organs or vena cava, but is completely resected.

Stage III

- Incomplete excision of tumour which extends beyond resection margins (gross or microscopical tumour remains postoperatively).
- Any abdominal lymph nodes are involved.
- Tumour rupture before or intraoperatively (irrespective of other criteria for staging).
- The tumour has penetrated through the peritoneal surface.
- Tumour implants are found on the peritoneal surface.
- The tumour thrombi present at resection margins of vessels or ureter; transected or removed piecemeal by surgeon.
- The tumour has been surgically biopsied (wedge biopsy) prior to preoperative chemotherapy or surgery.

Stage IV

Haematogenous metastases (lung, liver, bone, brain, etc.) or lymph node metastases outside the abdominopelvic region.

Stage V

Bilateral renal tumours at diagnosis. Each side should be substaged according to above classifications.

Prognosis

- Overall survival rates of ~90% have been reported.
- For children with relapsed Wilms tumour, high-dose chemotherapy with carboplatin, etoposide, and melphalan has been reported to confer a prolonged disease-free survival in ~50% of cases.
- ~1% of children with unilateral Wilms tumour develop disease in the contralateral kidney, and as for children with bilateral Wilms tumour at presentation, consideration is given to renal-sparing surgery.
- If bilateral disease results in CKD stage 5, it is arbitrarily suggested that transplantation be delayed until 2 years following completion of all therapy provided that post-therapy assessment has shown no evidence of recurrent disease.
- For the child with remnant renal tissue post surgery who subsequently progresses to CKD stage 5, it is wise to remove the remnant tissue prior to transplantation as there is a risk of recurrent tumour developing in it following commencement of immunosuppression.

Surveillance for Wilms tumour in at-risk individuals

UK Wilms Tumour Surveillance Working Group recommendations

- Surveillance should be offered to children at >5% risk of Wilms tumour.
- Surveillance should only be offered after review by a clinical geneticist.
- Surveillance should be by renal US every 3–4 months.
- Surveillance should continue until 5 years of age in all conditions except Beckwith–Wiedemann syndrome, Simpson–Golabi–Behmel syndrome, and some familial Wilms tumour pedigrees, when it should continue until 7 years.
- Surveillance can be undertaken in a local centre, but should be performed by someone with experience of paediatric ultrasonography.
- Screen-detected lesions should be managed at a specialist centre.

Clear cell sarcoma

- Primary renal tumour, very rare.
- More common in boys.
- Presents at a median age of 1.5 years.
- Significantly higher relapse and mortality rate than favourable histology Wilms tumour.
- Metastasizes most frequently to the lungs, and has a tendency to metastasize to bone and brain.
- Overall survival for clear cell sarcoma is 69%, with stage I patients having a 98% survival rate.

Malignant rhabdoid tumour

- Highly aggressive, rare renal tumour, which is often lethal.
- Most are diagnosed in the first year of life, typically with metastatic disease.
- All tumours have a deletion of the *SMARCB1* gene.
- May be associated with concomitant primary tumour in the brain.
- Overall survival rate is <50%, with stage IV patients <25%.

Hypertension

Basic concepts of blood pressure and defining hypertension in children

The concept of blood pressure

- The force exerted by the blood against any unit area of the vessel wall (see Fig. 16.1a).
- Physiologists (and intensivists) traditionally use end-on pressure obtained by placing catheters into vessels and measuring the pressure 'in line' with the vessel: this may not be the same as the lateral wall pressure of palpation, auscultation, or oscillation (see Fig. 16.1b).

(a)   (b)

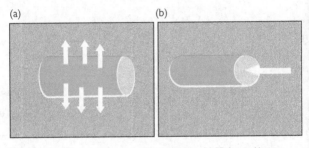

Fig. 16.1 (a) BP detected by auscultation or palpation. (b) BP detected by intra-arterial catheter.

- BP can be affected by changes in vessel size (vasoconstriction/ vasodilatation) and the volume of blood pumped through the arterial system. The latter is affected by cardiac output, as well as fluid volume itself, which is regulated by the kidney.
- Short-term changes in BP are mostly mediated by the heart and blood vessels (key hormones are catecholamines).
- Long-term BP is mediated by the kidney through regulation of salt reabsorption (key hormone is aldosterone).
- All forms of hypertension with a defined aetiology are related (directly or indirectly) to altered renal salt handling, establishing the central role of the kidney in BP regulation.

Example of phaeochromocytoma: the direct mediator of hypertension is the increased catecholamine level which leads to vasoconstriction and increased cardiac output. However, this could be easily counteracted by the kidneys by adapting the arterial filling volume via excretion of salt and water. Yet aldosterone levels are typically increased! The reason for this is the fact that the renal arteries are exquisitely sensitive to catecholamines. The resultant constriction leads to decreased renal perfusion with up-regulation of aldosterone and distal salt reabsorption, thus sustaining the hypertension.

Defining hypertension in children

- *In adults*—epidemiological definition based on risk of adverse event (e.g. stroke): >140/90 mmHg.
- *In children*—statistical definition: stage 1, BP >95th, but <99th percentile for sex, height, and age, plus 5 mmHg; stage 2, BP >99th percentile for sex, height, and age, plus 5 mmHg.
- Thus, a fundamental difference in children as compared with adults is that, in children, hypertension is defined statistically, whereas in adults, definitions are based on the risk of an adverse event.
- Recent guidelines suggest to use the adult definition in children >16 years.

The importance of recognizing hypertension in the young

- Despite the relatively arbitrary definitions of hypertension, severe untreated hypertension carries a high risk of morbidity and mortality.
- Signs of target organ damage are:
  - blood vessel changes (visible in the retina)
  - cardiac hypertrophy
  - microalbuminuria.

Measurement of blood pressure in infants and children

Important points

- Measuring BP in young children can be difficult.
- BP measurements using different techniques give different results.
- Check unexpected values, especially when obtained by oscillometry (e.g. Dinamap® device). Check that the cuff size and circumstances of measurement are correct.

Techniques used to measure blood pressure in children

- Direct, which requires an intra-arterial catheter.
- Auscultatory, using either mercury or aneroid devices or an Accoson Greenlight® sphygmomanometer.
- Doppler US (the technique of choice in young children because Korotkoff sounds are not consistent under the age of 5 years).
- Oscillometry.
- Ambulatory BP measurement (Ⓢ see 'Ambulatory blood pressure measurement in children').
- Newer methods estimate the central aortic systolic pressure by pulse wave analysis of peripheral arteries. It is thought that the central pressure better correlates with vascular disease and outcomes than the peripheral BP, but evidence in children is lacking.

Selecting the right cuff size

- Too small a cuff will give an overestimation of BP.
- Underestimation of BP due to too large a cuff is more of a theoretical concern than a real clinical problem.
- The widest cuff that can be applied to the arm should be used. The length of the inflation bladder should be at least 70%, preferably 90–100% of the circumference of the arm.
- To cover ages 0–14 years, a minimum of three cuff sizes are required:
  - 4 × 13 cm (infant).
  - 8 × 18 cm (child).
  - 12 × 35 cm (adult).
- An 'alternative adult' and thigh cuff (to use on the arm) are needed for obese patients.

Circumstances of measurement

- Child resting for at least 3 min in a warm room.
- Measurements taken if the child is crying may be spuriously high.
- Brachial artery at level of heart, with arm supported.

Korotkoff phases

Inflate cuff until palpable pulse disappears:
- K1: corresponds to systolic BP.
- K2: tapping disappears—'auscultatory gap'.
- K3: tapping returns.

- K4: tapping muffled—paediatric diastolic BP until age 13 years.
- K5: tapping disappears—diastolic BP after age 13 years.

Comments
- K1 typically appears 10–12 mmHg higher than the palpated pulse.
- K1 is, on average, 3 mmHg below direct systolic BP (i.e. systolic measured using an intra-arterial catheter).
- K5 disappears on average 9 mmHg above direct diastolic BP (K4 is even more unreliable).

Doppler ultrasound technique

Recommended for children <5 years:
- The technique of choice for children <5 years of age.
- A Doppler probe held over the pulse is used to magnify the sound so that it is audible without a stethoscope.
- Preferable because phases of K may not be heard reliably by stethoscope in sick children, those under the age of 1 year, and some healthy children <5 years.
- Using the mercury-Doppler technique ('Hg-D'), the first sound heard represents the systolic pressure. However, Hg-D may be 5 mmHg higher than K1 since the Doppler flow signal is likely to be detected before the K1 by auscultation.

Alternatives to mercury sphygmomanometers

There has been a gradual disappearance of mercury sphygmomanometers from hospitals in the UK because of concerns regarding mercury toxicity. There are a number of alternatives:

Aneroid manometers
- Register pressure through a bellows and lever system.
- Accurate initially, but very sensitive to jolts and bumps; with time, they usually underestimate BP, and require regular calibration and maintenance.
- 58% of aneroid manometers have errors >4 mmHg; 33% of these have errors >7 mmHg.

Accoson Greenlight®
Validated as comparable with the mercury manometer. Self-calibrating each time the apparatus is switched on, less maintenance required.

Oscillometry
- Pulsatile blood flow through a vessel produces arterial wall oscillation that is transmitted to a cuff encircling the extremity.
- Systolic BP is recorded at the point where a rapid increase in the oscillation amplitude occurs (approximates to K1).
- Diastolic BP is recorded where there is a sudden decrease in the oscillation amplitude (approximates to K5).
- Oscillometric devices measure the mean arterial BP and then calculate the systolic and diastolic values using proprietary algorithms.
- Some devices overestimate BP in young children and very few devices have been validated in hypertensive children <5 years old.
- Normative data for casual BP recordings is available (➔ see 'Appendix').

Other important points in the clinical evaluation

* In the absence of any significant symptoms, an elevated BP should be measured three times on three separate occasions before starting medications.
* If available, ambulatory BP monitoring (ABPM) should be considered to confirm hypertension in children old enough to tolerate it (usually >5 years old).

Family history
* Essential hypertension, other familial hypertension.
* Sudden death, renal failure, heart attacks, or stroke.

Patient history
* *Symptoms of renal disease*: e.g. polyuria, dysuria, and enuresis; or of phaeochromocytoma, e.g. palpitations, flushing.
* *Symptoms of high BP*: failure to thrive, lethargy, visual disturbance, headache, nausea, and vomiting.
* *Drugs*: amphetamines, ecstasy, and oral contraceptives.

Physical examination
* *Femoral delay and BP discrepancy between the arm and leg*: coarctation of the aorta or Takayasu disease.
* *Café au lait spots, axillary freckles*: neurofibromatosis type 1 (NF1).
* *Abdominal bruit*: renovascular diseases (also check for orbital and cranial bruit).
* *Signs associated with CKD*: short stature, bone disease, anaemia, and deafness.
* *Ambiguous genitalia*: adrenogenital syndromes.
* *Fundi and cardiovascular system*: assess end-organ damage.
* Check urine for protein and blood.

Investigation of hypertension in the young

The aims of investigation are to:
- assess the presence and severity of target organ damage
- define aetiology.

See Table 16.1 for causes of severe hypertension.

First-line investigations to be considered in all cases of paediatric hypertension

- FBC.
- U&Es, creatinine, albumin, bicarbonate, Ca, PO_4, and LFTs; ± urine electrolytes, urine creatinine.
- Fasting lipids.
- Plasma renin (activity).
- Plasma aldosterone.
- Plasma catecholamines (adrenaline and noradrenaline).
- Dip test of urine.
- Spot Ua:Ucr.
- Urine microscopy (to check for red cell casts).
- Urine for catecholamines (adrenaline, noradrenaline/metadrenaline, and dopamine) to creatinine ratio. Ideally 24 h urine, due to pulsatile nature of catecholamine excretion in phaeochromocytoma, which can be missed with spot urine.
- Echocardiography.
- Fundoscopy.
- Renal US with Doppler flow studies of the renal vessels.

Table 16.1 The causes of severe hypertension in the young, presentation by age

Age	Cause of hypertension
Neonatal period to 1 year	Renal artery stenosis (fibromuscular dysplasia; thrombus of renal artery secondary to umbilical arterial catheterization)
	ARPKD
	Infantile nephronophthisis
	Renal venous thrombosis
	Drugs (corticosteroids)
	Neuroblastoma
	Raised intracranial pressure
	Coarctation of the aorta
	Wilms tumour

(Continued)

Table 16.1 (Contd.)

Age	Cause of hypertension
1–5 years	Renal artery stenosis
	Middle aortic syndrome
	Glomerulonephritis
	Renal venous thrombosis
	Phaeochromocytoma
	Neuroblastoma
	Cystic kidney disease/infantile nephronophthisis
	Corticosteroids
	Monogenic hypertension (e.g. Liddle syndrome)
	Wilms' tumour
5–10 years	Renal scarring
	Glomerulonephritis
	Cystic renal disease
	Renal artery stenosis
	Middle aortic syndrome
	Endocrine tumours: Cushing syndrome and disease, Conn syndrome, phaeochromocytoma, neuroblastoma
	Wilms tumour
	Other parenchymal renal disease (e.g. glomerulocystic disease, nephronophthisis)
	Essential hypertension
	Obesity
10–20 years	Obesity
	Essential hypertension
	Reflux nephropathy
	Glomerulonephritis
	Renal artery stenosis
	Endocrine tumours
	Monogenic hypertension
	Pregnancy
	Drugs: oral contraceptive pill, corticosteroids, alcohol, amphetamines, ecstasy

This serves as a guide and is not an exhaustive list. There may be some overlap in causality at different ages. CKD or AKI (from any cause) should be considered at all ages. In addition, pain and raised intracranial pressure should be excluded as a potential cause.

Second-line investigations

See Table 16.2.

Table 16.2 Second-line investigations to be performed in selected cases only, and usually only in specialist centres

Suspected aetiology	Investigations
Glomerulonephritis	➔ See Chapter 9
Reflux nephropathy/ renal scarring	Cystogram (direct/indirect)
Obstructive uropathy	MAG3
Renal scarring	DMSA scan
Phaeochromocytoma	Meta-iodobenzylguanidine scintigraphy
	Adrenal/abdominal US scan
	MRI abdomen or PET scan
	DNA for genetic testing: up to 70% of children with phaeochromocytoma have an identifiable genetic basis. Recognized disease genes include *VHL* (von Hippel–Lindau syndrome), *RET* (multiple endocrine neoplasia type 2), *SDHD* (paraganglioma syndrome type 1), *SDHC* (paraganglioma syndrome type 3), *SDHB* (paraganglioma syndrome type 4) and *NF1* (neurofibromatosis type 1), *SDHA*, *SDHAF2*, *KIF1B*, *GDNF*, *MAX*, and *TMEM127*
	Genetic identification is important to assess risk for associated morbidities, including cancer
Monogenic hypertension	Monogenic forms of hypertension all affect renal Na reabsorption and are thus discussed in ➔ 'Tubulopathies: basic principles'
Miscellaneous	Genetics when appropriate; urine toxicology screen (amphetamines, ecstasy)

Further reading

Lurbe E, Agabiti-Rosei E, Cruickshank JK, et al. 2016 European Society of Hypertension guidelines for the management of high blood pressure in children and adolescents. *J Hypertens* 2016;34:1887–1920.

Renovascular hypertension

* Renovascular disease (renal arterial stenosis being the commonest cause) is the cause of 5–10% of all cases of hypertension in children.
* Presents at all ages.
* After coarctation of the aorta it is the commonest surgically remediable form of hypertension.

Causes of renovascular disease

* Fibromuscular dysplasia.
* NF1.
* Williams syndrome.
* Following vasculitis, in particular Takayasu disease.
* Following trauma or renal artery thrombosis associated with umbilical artery catheterization.
* Following abdominal radiotherapy.
* External compression of renal arteries by hilar lymph nodes or tumour (including Wilms tumour).
* Post-renal transplantation (5% of renal transplants).
* Idiopathic

Presenting symptoms

* Incidental.
* Congestive heart failure.
* Cerebral symptoms including:
  * cerebrovascular incident
  * acute hypertensive encephalopathy
  * headache
  * facial palsy.
* Failure to thrive.
* Screening of children with syndromes (➔ see 'Causes of renovascular disease').

When to suspect renovascular disease

* Very high BP. Not uncommonly systolic BP of 200 mmHg or more.
* Secondary symptoms of high BP including cerebral symptoms, cardiac failure, and facial palsy.
* Difficult-to-treat hypertension that is not well controlled on full doses of at least two antihypertensive drugs.
* Hypokalaemic, hypochloraemic metabolic alkalosis (the biochemical 'fingerprint' of aldosterone).
* Diagnosis of a syndrome with a higher risk of vascular disease (e.g. NF1 or Williams syndrome).
* Signs of vasculitis.
* Known or suspected previous vascular insult.
* Transplanted kidneys (with deteriorating function in the absence of rejection).
* Bruit heard over the artery/ies.
* Elevated peripheral plasma renin/aldosterone.

Investigations

- Renal US and Doppler studies.
- DMSA.
- CT and/or MRA has poor sensitivity in children.
- Selective renal arteriography. Note that all other imaging modalities have at least 10–20% false-negative and false-positive results.
- Renal vein renin studies can in some cases be used to define the kidney or the area of the kidney driving the hypertension.
- MRI of the brain including both parenchyma and blood vessels.
- Peripheral plasma renin (➔ see also 'Investigation of hypertension in the young').

Involvement of vascular beds

- Bilateral renal artery disease is more common than unilateral.
- Intrarenal artery disease is seen in many patients and is not amenable to interventional treatment.
- A quarter of the children have middle aortic syndrome, i.e. narrowing of their aorta.
- A third of the patients have associated stenosis of one or several of their intestinal arteries. This is often asymptomatic and mostly does not need treatment.
- At least one-fifth of the patients have cerebrovascular disease. The extent of this can affect the target BP.

Treatment

- The goals of the treatment are twofold:
  - Improvement of BP.
  - Improvement or preservation of kidney function.
- Medical treatment in most cases is not sufficient.
- Interventional treatment includes:
  - angioplasty with or without stenting; in many centres this is now the most commonly used treatment modality
  - surgery: due to the fact that vessels need to grow in children, surgical treatment (especially with fixed-sized grafts) is used only in cases not amenable to angioplasty.
- Treatment should be individualized after discussions in teams including a nephrologist, interventional radiologist, and vascular surgeon.
- Note that kidneys with seemingly no function, i.e. no DMSA uptake, can recover some or all of their function after revascularization. Thus, a conservative approach to nephrectomy is advised unless the kidney looks severely shrunken or dysmorphic on US.

Further reading

Tullus K, Brennan E, Hamilton G, et al. Renovascular hypertension in children. *Lancet* 2008;371:1453–1463.

Treatment

Treatment of hypertensive emergency

* Children and adolescents with severe elevation of BP are at increased risk of hypertensive encephalopathy, seizures, and congestive heart failure. Severe, symptomatic hypertension with decompensation is a medical emergency and should be treated with IV antihypertensive drugs.
* If the crisis is of known short duration (<72 h), e.g. a dialysis patient who consumed a high-salt diet, the BP can be brought down more quickly than in children who have long-standing hypertension (➔ see 'Long-term treatment in children and adolescents').
* If the patient is on dialysis, the treatment is immediate fluid removal by emergency dialysis.
* Conditions that may mimic hypertensive emergency, e.g. intracranial pathology, seizures, and dysautonomia, must be excluded.
* In a new presentation of hypertension, the duration is unlikely to be known so the BP must be brought down slowly. The first one-third of total targeted BP reduction should be aimed for over the first 12 h, the next one-third over 12 h, and the final one-third over 24 h.
* The preferred drug for hypertensive encephalopathy is labetalol by infusion. If there are contraindications, such as asthma and heart failure, a sodium nitroprusside infusion can be used.
* Hydralazine as a slow IV injection or as an IV infusion may be given to stabilize the patient. The patient must have two large-bore IV cannulae inserted so that IV NaCl 0.9% can be given if the BP is reduced too quickly.

It is preferable to use drugs with a short duration of action in the first instance so that if there is a sudden potentially harmful drop in BP this can be reversed more readily. Conversion to once-daily agents can be made subsequently. Sublingual nifedipine may cause a precipitous drop in BP so should be avoided, particularly in those with long-standing (or uncertain duration) hypertension. It can be an option if IV access cannot be secured. See Fig. 16.2 for a general scheme for the management of paediatric hypertension.

Hypertensive crisis

See Boxes 16.1 and 16.2.

Initiation of treatment of acute severe (>99th percentile) hypertension (non-hypertensive crisis)

Acute treatment of hypertension is as an in-patient. Preferred first-line drugs are oral nifedipine and IV hydralazine, or if fluid overloaded, oral or IV furosemide (see Table 16.3).

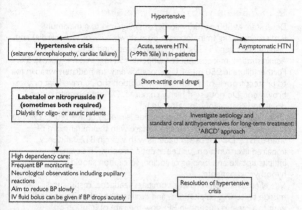

Fig. 16.2 General scheme for the management of paediatric hypertension (HTN).

Box 16.1 Labetalol infusion (combined alpha and beta blocker)

- *Dose*: start at 500 micrograms (0.5 mg)/kg/h to maximum 3 mg/kg/h.
- *Administration*: dilute to 1 mg in 1 mL (maximum 2 mg in 1 mL) in glucose 5% or glucose 4%/NaCl 0.18% *or* can be given neat (5 mg in 1 mL)—protect neat solution from light. Do not use NaCl 0.9% or mix with other drugs.
- *Contraindications*: second- or third-degree heart block. Low cardiac output. Caution in asthmatics (control with salbutamol).
- *Side effects*: nasal congestion, rash, pruritus, nausea, and vomiting. Severe hepatocellular damage has been reported after both short- and long-term treatment. Check for hepatic dysfunction.

Box 16.2 Sodium nitroprusside infusion

* *Dose*: start at 500 ng (0.5 micrograms)/kg/min to a maximum 8 micrograms/kg/min. Increase dose slowly (risk of tachycardia) and discontinue over 15–30 min to prevent rebound effect.
* *Administration*: mix contents of ampoule (50 mg) in 2 mL glucose 5%. Further dilute in 250 mL–1 L glucose 5% *only*. Immediately wrap in foil to protect from light. Fresh infusion solution should have faint orange-brown tint. Do not use if highly coloured. Do not mix with other drugs and change infusion after 24 h.
* *Contraindications*: sodium nitroprusside is rapidly converted to cyanide and to thiocyanate, which may interfere with the metabolism of vitamin B12. Do not use in patients with vitamin B12 deficiency, impaired liver function, or Leber optic atrophy. Thiocyanate inhibits uptake and binding of iodine, so caution should be used in hypothyroid patients.
* *Side effects*: nausea, retching, vomiting, headache, restlessness, muscle twitching, palpitations, and dizziness are often associated with too rapid reduction in BP: slow the rate of infusion or temporarily stop. Cyanide inhibits cellular oxidative metabolism. Excessive concentrations of cyanide can cause tachycardia, sweating, hyperventilation, cardiac arrhythmias, and metabolic acidosis. The infusion may be continued for several days but the blood cyanide concentration must not exceed 100 micrograms/100 mL and the serum cyanide concentration must not exceed 8 micrograms/100 mL. If administering over >3 days, blood thiocyanate concentration should be checked.

Table 16.3 Drugs used in the treatment of acute severe (>99th percentile) hypertension

Drug	Route	Normal starting dose	Normal dose range (to maximum)	Divided doses/day	Preparations
Furosemide (if fluid overloaded)	IV	500 micrograms/kg/dose	0.5–4 mg/kg/day	2–4	Injection 10 mg in 1 mL
	Oral	500 micrograms/kg/dose	1–4 mg/kg/day (maximum 12 mg/kg/day)	1–4	Tablets 20 mg, 40 mg
					Syrup 50 mg in 5 mL
Nifedipine SR	Oral	250 micrograms/kg/dose	1–2 mg/kg/day (maximum 3 mg/kg/day up to 120 mg/day)	2–4	Drops 20 mg in 1 mL (not licensed—short-acting)
				2 (older children)	SR tablets 10 mg, 20 mg, preferably cut SR tablets with tablet cutter; when crushed and dispersed in water, long-acting effect reduced
Hydralazine	IV	100–500 micrograms/kg/dose or 10–50 micrograms/kg/h	Maximum 4-hourly (maximum 3 mg/kg in 24 h)	Slow IV or infusion if required	Injection 20 mg

SR, slow release.

Long-term treatment in children and adolescents

The focus here is to use drugs that preferably can be used once daily, maximizing treatment dosage before adding a further drug. The agent(s) used will come from the following 'ABCD' groups:

* ACE inhibitor and ARBs.
* Beta blocker.
* Calcium channel blocker.
* Diuretic.

The British Hypertension Society (BHS) launched this ABCD algorithm to provide more didactic advice on the sequencing of drugs for the treatment of hypertension in adults, but the principles also apply to the paediatric population (see Table 16.4):

* Children generally respond better to drugs that block the RAS. These include 'A' drugs (ACE inhibitors and ARBs) and 'B' drugs (beta blockers).
* If combination treatment is necessary, it is recommended to combine A or B with C or D.
* The third step would involve triple therapy with either A+C+D or B+C+D.
* The clinical situation, including the presence of any proteinuria (for which ACE inhibition or angiotensin II blockade would be recommended), will determine which group you should start with. When the GFR is <10 mL/min/1.73 m^2, always start with the lowest dose, although careful assessment of fluid status is required as the cause in the majority will be fluid overload and dialysis is likely the best treatment.
* *For infants (<1 year old)*: use shorter-acting agents for flexibility of dosage—propranolol instead of atenolol; captopril instead of enalapril. Once stable, the patient may be changed to the longer-acting antihypertensives.
* While approaches such as the ABCD algorithm are useful, in some cases it is possible to predict which drugs might be most efficacious depending on the cause of the hypertension (Table 16.5).

Table 16.4 Drugs commonly used in the ABCD algorithm

Drug	Route	Normal starting dose	Normal dose range (to maximum)	Divided doses/day	Preparations and comments
Amlodipine	Oral	100–200 micrograms/kg/dose	6–15 kg: 1.25 mg 15–25 kg: 2.5 mg >25 kg: 5 mg (maximum 10 mg/day)	1	Tablets 5 mg, 10 mg Tablets may be dispersed in water and still maintain long-acting effect
Atenolol[a]	Oral	1 mg/kg/dose	1–2 mg/kg/day (maximum 100 mg/day or 50 mg/day when GFR <10)	1	Tablets 25 mg, 50 mg, 100 mg Syrup 25 mg in 5 mL Caution in asthma although cardioselective
Enalapril	Oral	100 micrograms/kg/dose	200–500 micrograms/kg/day (maximum 600 micrograms/kg/day up to 40 mg/day)	1	Tablets 2.5 mg, 5 mg, 10 mg Contraindicated commencing treatment in pregnancy and hyperkalaemia Caution in renal artery stenosis and when GFR <30

(Continued)

Table 16.4 (Contd.)

Drug	Route	Normal starting dose	Normal dose range (to maximum)	Divided doses/day	Preparations and comments
Irbesartan	Oral	2 mg/kg/dose	*6–12 years:* 75–150 mg/day *>13 years:* 150–300 mg/day	1	Tablets 75 mg, 150 mg May be useful to add in presence of persistent proteinuria Contraindicated in pregnancy and caution in renal artery stenosis
Bendroflumethiazide	Oral	Maximum 400 micrograms/kg once a day initially then reduce to maintenance	Up to 12 months: 1.25 mg 1–4 years: 1.25–2.5 mg 5–12 years: 2.5 mg >12 years: 2.5–5 mg	1	Tablets 2.5 mg, 5 mg May exacerbate SLE
Furosemide	Oral	500 micrograms/kg/dose	1–4 mg/kg/day	1–4	Tablets 20 mg, 40 mg Syrup 50 mg in 5 mL

[a] Recent studies in adults (*Lancet*, systematic review and ASCOT data) have suggested that atenolol should not be used alone as first-line therapy.

Table 16.5 Treatment of choice for select causes of hypertension

Suspected aetiology	Treatment of choice
Obesity	Weight reduction
Acute glomerulonephritis	Diuretics
	Standard oral antihypertensives
Reflux nephropathy/obstructive uropathy	Relieve obstruction if present
	Standard oral antihypertensives
	ACE inhibitor
Renovascular disease	Standard oral antihypertensives
	(ACE inhibitor), risk of renal ischaemia, but sometimes only effective drug
	Angioplasty
	Surgery
Phaeochromocytoma	Phenoxybenzamine
	Beta blocker
	Nifedipine
	Surgery (after adequate A and B blockade)
Endocrine (this category is low-renin hypertension)	Much depends on the specific disorder and treatment is complicated and generally may include:
	Spironolactone
	Triamterene/amiloride
	Dexamethasone
	Thiazide
Essential	Salt/weight/exercise
	Standard oral antihypertensives
Coarctation	Surgery
	Standard oral antihypertensives

Phaeochromocytoma

- Both alpha and beta blockade is required (Table 16.6).
- Surgical tumour removal should only be performed in experienced centres. The clinician should consult with the anaesthetist regarding discontinuation of drugs around the time of surgery. Drug would usually be given preoperatively and discontinued subsequent to the procedure.
- Maximizing alpha and beta blockade prior to surgery (to a stage where the patient may show postural hypotension) helps minimize intraoperative hypertension, when the tumour is manipulated and excessive catecholamine release can occur.

Additional medications

Drugs to be used when a combination due to any reason does not give full control of BP with acceptable side effects are shown in Table 16.7.

Table 16.6 Suggested treatment for hypertension in phaeochromocytoma

Drug	Route	Normal starting dose	Normal dose range (to maximum)	Divided doses/day	Preparations and comments
Phenoxy-benzamine	Oral	200 micrograms/kg/dose	1–4 mg/kg/day	2	Capsules 10 mg
Propranolol	Oral	1 mg/kg/dose	1–8 mg/kg/day	3	Tablets 10 mg, 40 mg, 80 mg

Table 16.7 Additional medications

Drug	Route	Normal starting dose	Normal dose range (to maximum)	Divided doses/day	Preparations and comments
Clonidine	Oral	2.5 micrograms/kg/dose to a maximum 25 micrograms	Maximum 200 micrograms/day	2	Tablets 25 micrograms, 100 micrograms Solution 5 micrograms/mL (made as extemporaneous preparation) May cause dry mouth and/or sedation Care in withdrawal due to rebound effect
Minoxidil	Oral	100 micrograms/kg/dose	200 micrograms/kg/day–1 mg/kg/day <12 years, maximum 50 mg/day; >12 years, maximum 100 mg/day	1–3	Tablets 2.5 mg, 5 mg, 10 mg Prolonged use can cause hypertrichosis
Prazosin	Oral	5 micrograms/kg/dose	50–400 micrograms/kg/day Maximum 500 micrograms/kg/day	2–4	Tablets 1 mg, 2 mg When GFR <50 start with a lower dose

Ambulatory blood pressure measurement in children

In recent years, ABPM has become an important additional tool in identifying hypertension and monitoring the effectiveness of antihypertensive medication. ABPM is well established in adult areas, but in children the results are variable, and validity and reliability are less consistent. Many of the established recommendations for ABPM apply to children, but substantial differences exist, especially in children <5 years of age.

Advantages

- Allows multiple measurements typically during a 24 h period.
- Provides a truer picture of BP trends.
- Provides better BP correlation with cardiac outcome.
- Identifies 'white coat hypertension'.
- Identifies nocturnal hypertension (non-dippers—absence of the normal physiological drop in BP when asleep).
- Provides arterial stiffness index.

Disadvantages

- Some of the most commonly used devices have failed the rigorous validation procedures to which they have been subjected, particularly in relation to children <5 years. ABPM is usually limited to children >5 years old. This is because it is necessary to keep the arm completely still during the measurement and young children do not usually manage this over a 24 h period, resulting in a 24 h record with very few successful readings during the awake periods. Monitors can be used in those <5 years for night monitoring if required.
- Lack of large series providing normative data, especially for infants and toddlers. Many of the trials relating to hypertension and outcome refer to casual BP readings, so interpretation of ambulatory readings may be problematic.
- Requires training and expertise in analysis and interpretation of data.
- Can cause discomfort with high inflation pressures if the child moves excessively during the measurement or has significant hypertension.

Measuring ambulatory blood pressure in children

- More difficult in children >6 months and <5 years. Great care must be taken when interpreting results due to the wide variations of activity and emotional states (situations that cause a sympathetic response, crying, falling over, and tantrums).
- The equipment selected must be validated for use in children and be lightweight with a selection of cuff sizes. The internal bladder size must cover 80–100% of the circumference of the arm.
- The software provided must allow for variations of frequency to be programmed into the monitor, and for the report to be customized to include actual sleep periods and paediatric reference data to calculated BP load automatically.
- The non-dominant arm is preferable, but the arm with the highest clinic reading should be used.

- Diaries should be given to the children to record activities, medication, and sleep periods; where possible, use the real sleep time to calculate nocturnal mean BP values. Recording activity and the emotional state is particularly relevant for children.
- Must avoid immersion in water while the monitor is attached.
- Normal daily activity would be encouraged during the monitoring period, but the arm must be still during the measurement.
- Avoid placing cuff too low on elbow as this is uncomfortable.
- Warn the child that they should call if the arm becomes painful (provide contact number, including out-of-hours contact details).
- Ensure that monitor is calibrated yearly, and should be within 5 mmHg of sphygmomanometry.

Interpretation of results

- The appropriate ABPM percentiles of mean day and night time systolic and diastolic BP, and sleeping and waking time should be programmed into the report settings. The overall summary, wake period, sleeping period, and night dip is provided.
- A diagnosis of hypertension can be based on a high daytime or night-time BP load and poor night dip. However, if only a few readings are obtained during the day, the 24 h report is of limited use. It is important to look at the number of readings while asleep and awake, and interpret only the successful ones. In children, intermittent extreme BP readings are unlikely to be valid and are most likely artefacts; an accurate diary can help to confirm this along with the activity setting which is available on some models

Definitions

- *BP load*: the percentage of valid ambulatory BP readings above the 95th percentile for age, sex, and height in a 24 h period. A load >25% is considered outside the normal range. If the mean BP in these children is only slightly elevated above the 95th percentile, these children should have their BP monitored periodically.
- *Mean BP*: the average of daytime, night-time, and 24 h BP measurement for systolic, diastolic, and mean arterial pressure (MAP; see Table 16.8).
- *Nocturnal dip*: the decline of BP during the sleeping period. A 'non-dipper' is a person whose night-time decline in mean systolic and diastolic ambulatory BP is <10%. A poor dip is typical for secondary hypertension unless due to sleep disorders
- *Number of readings*: half-hourly readings during the day and hourly readings during the night are usually acceptable. The final report should give a percentage of successful readings: >90% is considered to be a good result. The lower the success rate, the less valid the results.

All of these points need to be taken into consideration when reading an ABPM report. In children, the success of the test can be variable. In general, the accuracy of the test improves with age. Results for children <5 years should be interpreted with caution.

Table 16.8 90th and 95th percentiles of mean daytime and night-time ambulatory systolic and diastolic BP, stratified according to sex and height

Height (cm)	Systolic BP (mm Hg)				Diastolic BP (mm Hg)			
	Day		Night		Day		Night	
	90th pct	95th pct	90th pct	95th pct	90th pct	95th pct	90th pct	95th pct
Boys								
120	120.6	123.5	103.7	106.4	79.1	81.2	61.9	64.1
125	121.0	124.0	104.9	107.8	79.8	81.3	62.2	64.3
130	121.6	124.6	106.3	109.5	79.3	81.4	62.4	64.5
135	122.2	125.2	107.7	111.3	79.3	81.3	62.7	64.8
140	123.0	126.0	109.3	113.1	79.2	81.2	62.9	65.0
145	124.0	127.0	110.7	114.7	79.1	81.1	63.1	65.2
150	125.4	128.5	111.9	115.9	79.1	81.0	63.3	65.4
155	127.2	130.2	113.1	117.0	79.2	81.1	63.4	65.6
160	122.2	132.3	114.3	118.0	79.3	81.3	63.6	65.7
165	131.3	134.5	115.5	119.1	79.7	81.7	63.7	65.8
170	133.5	136.7	116.8	120.2	80.1	82.2	63.8	65.9
175	135.6	138.8	119.1	121.2	80.6	82.8	63.8	65.9
180	137.7	140.9	119.2	122.1	81.1	83.4	63.8	65.8
185	139.8	143.0	120.3	123.0	81.7	84.1	63.8	65.8
Girls								
120	118.5	121.1	105.7	109.0	79.7	81.8	64.0	66.4
125	119.5	122.1	106.4	109.8	79.7	81.8	63.8	66.2
130	120.4	123.1	107.2	110.6	79.7	81.8	63.3	66.0
135	121.4	124.1	107.9	111.3	79.7	81.8	63.4	65.8
140	122.3	125.1	108.4	111.9	79.8	81.8	63.2	65.7
145	123.4	126.3	109.1	112.5	79.8	81.9	63.0	65.6
150	124.6	127.5	109.9	113.1	79.9	81.9	63.0	65.5
155	125.7	128.5	110.6	113.8	79.9	81.9	62.9	65.5
160	126.6	129.3	111.1	114.0	79.9	81.9	92.8	65.4
165	127.2	129.8	111.2	114.0	79.9	81.9	62.7	65.2
170	127.5	130.0	111.2	114.0	79.9	81.8	62.5	65.0
175	127.6	129.9	111.2	114.0	79.8	81.7	62.3	64.7

pct, percentile.

Acute kidney injury

Background and pathophysiology

Background

Acute kidney injury (AKI) is a sudden, potentially reversible inability of the kidney to maintain normal body chemistry and fluid balance. It is usually accompanied by oliguria (urine output <0.5 mL/kg/h or <1 mL/kg/h in a neonate), but polyuric AKI can also occur.

The old term acute renal failure (ARF) has now been replaced by AKI.

Pathophysiology

* Renal insult causes vasoconstriction, desquamation of tubular cells (forming casts), intraluminal tubular obstruction, and back leakage of glomerular filtrate.
* Neutrophils adhere to ischaemic endothelium and release substances that promote inflammation.

The primary event is usually tubular damage, which leads to an adaptive fall in GFR due to renal vasoconstriction, to compensate for failure to reabsorb filtered solute. This vasoconstriction may then perpetuate renal damage. For this reason, research has focused on vasoactive compounds, such as angiotensin, prostaglandins, adenosine, endothelin, and nitric oxide. The role of inflammatory mediators has also been explored.

Early detection of AKI

Creatinine rises late in the evolution of AKI so there has been a search for biomarkers of injury.
* Cystatin C is a protease inhibitor produced at a constant rate from nucleated cells and is eliminated by glomerular filtration. It increases in parallel with creatinine but is independent of muscle mass.
* Plasma NGAL and KIM-1 increase prior to creatinine and, as well as other biomarkers of renal damage (IL-18, L-FABP) may be useful in the early detection of AKI but are not yet in routine clinical use.

Paediatric RIFLE (pRIFLE) and KDIGO criteria

Early detection of AKI would allow identification of a causative factor, avoidance of nephrotoxic drugs, and careful fluid management. AKI in children in intensive care, particularly if associated with fluid overload, is linked to increased mortality risk (Table 17.1). The pRIFLE system is used for detection and classification of AKI, risk stratification and for correlation with clinical outcomes:
* R = risk for renal dysfunction.
* I = injury to the kidney.
* F = failure of kidney function.
* L = loss of kidney function.
* E = end-stage kidney disease.

The KDIGO classification has three stages (Table 17.2).

Table 17.1 RIFLE criteria

	Estimated GFR	Urine output, mL/kg/h
R	Decreased by 25%	<0.5 for 8 h
I	Decreased by 50%	<0.5 for 16 h
F	Decreased by 75% or <35 mL/min/1.73 m^2	<0.3 for 24 h or anuric for 12 h
L	Renal failure >4 weeks	
E	Renal failure >3 months	

Table 17.2 KDIGO classification

Stage	Serum creatinine	Urine output, mL/kg/h
1	1.5–1.9 × baseline	<0.5 for 6–12 h
2	2–2.9 × baseline	<0.5 for ≥12 h
3	>3 × baseline	<0.3 for ≥24 h or anuric for 12 h

Causes

Causes are pre renal, renal (including acute-on-chronic kidney disease), and post renal. Pre-renal causes may lead to established renal AKI.

Pre-renal AKI

* Hypovolaemia: GI losses, burns, third-space losses (postoperative, sepsis, and nephrotic syndrome) and excess renal losses (renal tubular disorders).
* Peripheral vasodilatation: sepsis.
* Circulatory failure: congestive cardiac failure, pericarditis, cardiac tamponade.
* Bilateral renal arterial or venous thrombosis.
* Drugs (diuretics, ACE inhibitors, NSAIDs).
* Hepatorenal syndrome.

Renal AKI

* *Arterial*: embolic, arteritis, HUS.
* *Venous*: renal venous thrombosis.
* *Glomerular*: acute glomerulonephritis.
* *Tubular*: established acute tubular necrosis (ATN) due to prolonged pre-renal AKI, ischaemia, toxins or drugs; obstructive (crystals).
* *Interstitial*: TIN, pyelonephritis.
* *Acute-on-chronic*: decompensation of CKD due to intercurrent illness.

Post-renal AKI

* Obstruction in a solitary kidney.
* Bilateral ureteric obstruction.
* Urethral obstruction.
* Neuropathic bladder.

Obstruction may be congenital (e.g. at the PUJ, VUJ, ureterocoele, or PUVs), or acquired (e.g. calculi, external compression).

AKI due to dehydration is the commonest cause worldwide. In developed countries, admission to intensive care carries a high risk for AKI and is associated with an increased mortality risk. Sepsis and nephrotoxic mediations contribute.

AKI in neonates

➔ See Chapter 2.

Further reading

McCaffrey J, Dhakal AJ, Milford DV, et al. Recent developments in the detection and management of acute kidney injury. *Arch Dis Child* 2017;102:91–96.

Haemolytic uraemic syndrome: definitions

Definitions

- HUS is a triad of symptoms:
  - Haemolytic anaemia with fragmented erythrocytes.
  - Thrombocytopenia.
  - AKI.
- VTEC: verotoxin-producing *Escherichia coli*.
- STEC: Shiga toxin-producing *Escherichia coli* (the most commonly used abbreviation).
- MAHA: microangiopathic haemolytic anaemia.
- TMA: thrombotic microangiopathy. A microvascular occlusive disorder of capillaries, arterioles, and less frequently, arteries.
- TTP: thrombotic thrombocytopenic purpura. Microvascular aggregation of platelets causing ischaemic lesions mainly in the brain, and less frequently in the kidney and other organs.

The common event in HUS is endothelial injury resulting in MAHA, platelet aggregation, and local intravascular coagulation, particularly in the renal, mesenteric and brain vasculature.

Notes on terminology

- The D+ HUS/D− HUS terminology has been abandoned:
  - The terms Shiga toxin and verotoxin are equivalent.
  - Some patients with STEC infection do not have diarrhoea.
  - A diarrhoeal illness may trigger HUS in a patient with a genetic predisposition to HUS.
  - Thus, classifying patients only according the presence or absence of diarrhoea can lead to incorrect management.

Assessment and investigations: history, examination, and initial resuscitation

Important points in the history

The major differential diagnosis of AKI is the patient presenting for the first time with CKD, which may be either AKI on CKD or just advanced CKD, that was not previously recognized. The two may be difficult to distinguish from the biochemistry alone, so the history and US findings are particularly helpful. This is important because, as well as different investigations and fluid management, patients with CKD may need plans for long-term, more permanent dialysis access; and those with post-renal AKI need urgent urological review (Table 17.3).

Table 17.3 Points in the history and examination that assist in the differential diagnosis of AKI

Pre renal	Renal	Acute on chronic	Post renal
Diarrhoea and vomiting	Bloody diarrhoea (HUS)	Antenatally diagnosed anomaly	Antenatally diagnosed anomaly
Cardiac impairment	Drugs	Previous UTIs	Previous UTIs
Birth asphyxia	Birth asphyxia	Polydipsia and polyuria	Poor urinary stream
Drugs, e.g. ACE inhibitors or diuretics	Recent throat or skin infection	Poor urinary stream	Calculi
Acute weight loss	Prolonged convulsions	Family history	Palpable bladder or kidneys
Poor capillary refill	Systemically unwell	Long-standing malaise	Spinal abnormality
Low BP[a]	Associated symptoms/signs	Small/syndromic	
	Umbilical catheters	Renal osteodystrophy	

[a] It is possible for the BP to be paradoxically high if there is extreme vasoconstriction.

Initial assessment, examination, and resuscitation

- Attend to life-threatening features first, i.e. volume status (see Table 17.4), oxygenation (colour, respiratory rate, oxygen saturation), and electrolyte derangements (see later in topic).
- Oedema may not be helpful in deciding fluid replacement as it can be present with both intravascular overload and hypovolaemia due to third spacing.
- BP should not be viewed in isolation—hypertension with cool peripheries suggests intravascular depletion while hypertension with warm peripheries suggests fluid overload.

Investigations

Initial investigations

US scanning of the urinary tract is essential at the earliest opportunity (Fig. 17.1):

- To exclude obstruction: the absence of hydronephrosis does not rule out significant high-pressure obstruction, so any degree of dilatation should be considered significant, as dilatation will not occur if there is anuria and may be minimal with oliguria. Nephrostomy drainage may be necessary if there is no other clear diagnosis.
- To see if there are signs of CKD (small or cystic kidneys), although in some conditions, such as nephronophthisis, renal size may be preserved.
- In most cases of AKI the kidneys are enlarged and echo bright
- To look at vascular flow using Doppler studies if an abnormality of renal blood flow is suspected.
- Urine biochemistry is useful in distinguishing between pre-renal AKI and established ATN: urinary sodium <10 mmol/L (<20 in neonates), fractional excretion of sodium (➔ see 'Appendix') (FeNa) <1% (<2.5% in neonates), and urine osmolality >500 mOsm/kg (>400 in neonates) suggests pre-renal AKI.
- Urine for blood, protein, and casts.
- Urine MC&S.
- U&Es, creatinine, plasma bicarbonate, Ca, PO_4, Mg, ALP, albumin, LFTs, and glucose.
- FBC including blood film if low platelets (see later in topic).
- Coagulation screen.
- Blood culture and CRP.
- Chest X-ray if respiratory or cardiac signs.

Table 17.4 Assessment and management of intravascular volume status

Hydration status	Clinical features	Initial management
Dehydrated	Tachycardia, cool hands, feet, and nose (>2°C core–peripheral temperature gap), prolonged capillary refill time, low BP (late sign), dry mucous membranes, sunken eyes	Fluid resuscitation 10 mL/kg normal saline over 30 min, assess urine output and repeat if necessary
Euvolaemic		Fluid challenge 10–20 mL/kg 0.9% saline over 1 h, with furosemide 2–4 mg/kg IV, maximum 12 mg/kg/day
Intravascular fluid overload	Tachycardia, gallop rhythm, raised JVP and BP, palpable liver	Furosemide 2–4 mg/kg IV; maximum 12 mg/kg/day. Dialysis if no response

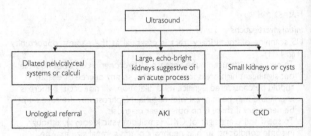

Fig. 17.1 US in the diagnosis of the cause of AKI.

Further additional investigations depend on clinical presentation

For *suspected HUS* (see p. 434):
* Blood film to look for fragmented cells, LDH.
* Group and save or crossmatch.
* Stool culture.
* STEC serology.
* HUS may be due to T-antigen exposure by: *Streptococcus pneumoniae*; influenza virus or HIV (see p. 438); SLE; abnormalities of complement regulation: factor H, autoantibodies to factor H, factors I and B, membrane cofactor protein and thrombomodulin (see p. 439); and von Willebrand factor protease deficiency (see p. 439).
* Haptoglobins

For *acute nephritis* (see Chapter 9):
* ESR.
* Throat or infected skin swab.
* Anti-Streptolysin O titre, anti-DNAse B.
* Complement (C3, C4, C3 nephritic factor if C3 low).
* Immunoglobulins including IgA.
* ANA, dsDNA, anti-GBM, ANCA, eNA, anti-cardiolipin antibodies.

Infections and AKI (see Chapter 12):
* Meningococcal septicaemia.
* Hepatitis B, hepatitis C, and HIV.
* Leptospirosis.
* Malaria.

For *suspected rhabdomyolysis* (e.g. prolonged convulsions) (see p. 444)
* Creatine kinase.
* Urine myoglobin.

For *tumour lysis* (see p. 446)
* Urate.

For *renal hypouricaemia* (a rare cause of AKI):
* History of loin pain and AKI post exercise.
* Low plasma urate and high urine urate.

For *acute-on-CKD*:
• PTH.
• Haemoglobin.

For *obstruction*
• Will depend on US findings and surgical intervention plan.

Renal biopsy

Is indicated as soon as possible when:
• renal function is deteriorating and the aetiology is not certain.
• nephritic/nephrotic presentation.

as these features are suggestive of rapidly progressive crescentic glomerulonephritis, which needs urgent treatment to prevent long-term renal
damage (➔ see Chapter 11).

Causes of microangiopathic haemolytic anaemia

In association with infections

- Enterohaemorrhagic *Escherichia coli* producing Shiga toxin.
- *Shigella dysenteriae* type 1 producing Shiga toxin.
- *Streptococcus pneumoniae* producing neuraminidase (Thomsen–Friedenreich antigen ('T antigen')).
- Influenza virus.
- HIV.

Thrombotic thrombocytopenic purpura

- Severe deficiency (<10%) of ADAMTS13 (von Willebrand factor-cleaving protease).

Cobalamin C deficiency (MMA)

- Defects of vitamin B12 intracellular metabolism.

Atypical HUS (defined as HUS without coexisting disease)

- Complement alternative pathway dysregulation, due to complement gene mutations and/or anti-complement factor H antibodies.
- Mutations in the gene encoding DGKe (diacylglycerol kinase e).

Drug-associated MAHA

- Ciclosporin, tacrolimus.
- Mitomycin, cytotoxic drugs, gemcitabine.
- Ticlopidine, clopidogrel.
- Oral contraceptives.
- Crack cocaine.
- Quinine.

MAHA secondary to other causes

- Malignant hypertension.
- Bone marrow transplant associated.
- Post renal transplantation.
- SLE and antiphospholipid syndrome.
- Collagen type III glomerulopathy.
- Cancer associated.
- Systemic sclerosis.
- Pregnancy associated.

Management

The kidneys usually provide volume and electrolyte homeostasis by adjusting urine output and composition in real time. In AKI, the medical team has to provide this critical homeostatic function to the patient mainly by adjusting fluid intake to output. Obviously, real-time adjustment is not possible, but frequent monitoring is necessary.

Monitoring

- Weigh twice daily.
- Hourly input–output recording.
- Hourly observations including BP and monitoring of toe–core temperature gradient.
- 6-hourly blood glucose levels if disease may affect blood sugar control (e.g. HUS).
- Neurological observations hourly.
- U&Es, creatinine and plasma bicarbonate, Ca, PO_4, FBC, frequency determined by clinical picture (may be appropriate to perform up to every 6 h).
- If not anuric: urine electrolytes. Urinary electrolytes will not be interpretable in children on furosemide.

Fluids

- Further boluses of crystalloid or colloid and/or furosemide as indicated by hydration and urine output.
- A furosemide infusion may be of benefit (maximum 12 mg/kg/24 h), if there is evidence for increased urine output in an oligoanuric patient. The maximum dose must not be exceeded due to the nephro- and ototoxicity of furosemide.
- If nephrotic, consider a bolus of albumin (➔ see Chapter 9).
- Give insensible losses (400 mL/m²/day or 30 mL/kg/day) plus urine output and other ongoing fluid losses. This can be given as feed if tolerated (see following section) or IV normal saline (half normal if hypernatraemia).
- Replace 100% of urine output if euvolaemic.
- Restrict to 50–75% urine output if intravascularly overloaded to allow a negative fluid balance.
- There is no evidence to support the use of renal dose dopamine.
- Be prepared to adjust fluid composition and rate in response to values provided from monitoring.

After 24 h, an assessment can be made as to whether to proceed to dialysis or to continue to manage conservatively, although this decision needs to be reviewed on a daily basis.

Monitoring

- Frequency of measurements of weight, fluid balance, and routine and neurological observations as for the first 24 h.
- U&Es, creatinine and plasma bicarbonate, Ca, PO_4, Mg, albumin, and FBC (usually daily but frequency is determined by the clinical picture).
- Urinalysis daily.

Conservative management

- With careful attention to diet and fluid restriction of the euvolaemic child to an intake of insensible fluid losses and urine output, even patients with oliguria can be managed without dialysis for a prolonged period of time. However it is difficult to maintain an adequate nutritional intake if the fluid allowance is very low, as catabolism (which also causes a high urea and hyperkalaemia) culminates in malnutrition.
- A suggested dietary approach is described in ⊃ 'Nutrition in acute kidney injury'.

Indications for dialysis

Indications are never absolute but vary according to residual urine output, i.e. oligoanuria/anuria/polyuria, and clinical judgement is required.

Oligoanuria with no response to furosemide

- Hyperkalaemia >6.5 mmol/L with T-wave changes on ECG.
- Severe fluid overload with pulmonary oedema.
- Urea >40 mmol/L (consider >30 mmol/L in a neonate).
- Severe hypo- or hypernatraemia or acidosis.
- Multisystem failure.
- Anticipation of prolonged oliguria, e.g. HUS, so that space can be made for blood transfusions if required and dietary intake.

Fluids for the patient on dialysis

- A fixed fluid intake can be prescribed when dialysis is established. A suggested starting volume would be half the normal maintenance fluid allowance (see Table 17.5), which can be increased depending on efficiency of dialysis or the development of urine output. The best form of fluid intake is oral feeds as guided by a dietician if possible.

Established AKI

- Monitoring of routine observations can be decreased to 4-hourly and weight and U&Es, creatinine and plasma bicarbonate, Ca, PO_4, and FBC to daily.
- A fixed fluid intake can be introduced for conservatively managed patients as urine output increases, using a regimen similar to patients on dialysis (see earlier in topic).

Table 17.5 Maintenance water and electrolyte allowance for healthy children

	Weight (kg)	Daily requirement
Water	<10	100 mL/kg
	11–20	1000 mL plus 50 mL/kg for each extra kg >10
	>20	1500 mL plus 20 mL/kg for each extra kg >20
Sodium, potassium, and chloride	<10	2.5 mmol/kg
	11–30	2.0 mmol/kg
	>30	1.5 mmol/kg

The recovery phase

- Polyuria may develop in the recovery phase, so during this time it may be necessary to return to twice-daily weights, hourly input–output recording, and hourly observations including BP and monitoring of the toe–core temperature gradient.
- Urine output and insensible losses should be replaced for 24 h with 0.9% saline, then a fixed fluid intake can be set. This can start at around two-thirds of the previous day's intake, if renal function continues to improve.
- Dialysis can be stopped when the urine output is sufficient to allow an adequate nutritional intake and the creatinine starts to decline.

Management of electrolyte abnormalities in AKI before dialysis

Hyperkalaemia

- K >6.5 mmol/L is an indication for emergency treatment until dialysis or urine output has been established.
- Monitor for signs of toxicity on ECG (peaked T waves, prolongation of PR interval, flattening of P waves, QRS widening) (➲ see Chapter 6).
- Toxicity of K is increased if there is hypocalcaemia.
- Only ion exchange resins remove potassium from the body, so it is important to check the serum K for rebound after 2–4 h.
- Of all the ways to reduce K, the simplest is to use a salbutamol nebulizer, which is familiar to all paediatric nurses, quick to prepare and administer, and rapidly effective (Table 17.6).

Hyponatraemia

- Mild hyponatraemia is often dilutional secondary to prior prescription of hypotonic fluids.
- A plasma Na concentration of >118 mmol/L will usually correct with fluid restriction ± dialysis and fluid replacement with normal saline.
- A plasma Na concentration of <118 mmol/L risks CNS damage so the Na should be raised to around 125 mmol/L with hypertonic saline (3%) according to the formula:

$$Na\ dose\ (mmol) = (125 - measured\ plasma\ Na \times weight\ in\ kg \times 0.6)$$

and given over 2–4 h (➲ see 'Disorders of sodium and water: hyponatraemia').

- Severe hyponatraemia with oliguria is an indication for dialysis.

Hypernatraemia

- Much less common than hyponatraemia.
- Most commonly due to severe dehydration, very occasionally due to diabetes insipidus. Salt poisoning (deliberate or iatrogenic) is another rare cause. Careful assessment of fluid status is therefore mandatory.
- Give furosemide 3–4 mg/kg IV (maximum 12 mg/kg/day) if salt retention is the cause and patient has urine output.
- Fluid replacement will depend on cause and hydration. Replace insensible losses as 0.45% saline.
- Severe hypernatraemia with oliguria is an indication for dialysis.

Table 17.6 Emergency management of hyperkalaemia

Effect on potassium	Treatment	Dose	Side effects
Reduces toxic effect of K by stabilizing the myocardium	10% calcium gluconate IV	0.5–1 mL/kg over 5–10 min	Bradycardia, hypercalcaemia
Shifts K into cells	Salbutamol nebulizer	2.5 mg if <25 kg 5.0 mg if >25 kg Maximum 2-hourly	Tachycardia, hypertension
	Salbutamol IV	4 micrograms/kg over 10 min	
	Sodium bicarbonate 8.4% IV	1–2 mmol (mL)/kg over 10–30 min	Hypernatraemia, reduces ionized calcium
	Glucose and insulin IV	0.5–1.0 g/kg/h glucose (2.5–5.0 mL/kg/h 10% glucose) and insulin 0.1–0.2 U/kg as a bolus or continuous infusion of 10% glucose at 5 mL/kg/h (0.5 g/kg/h) with insulin 0.1 unit/kg/h	Hypoglycaemia Monitor blood glucose every 15 min during bolus then at least hourly
Removal of K from the body	Calcium resonium orally or per rectum with oral lactulose	1 g/kg every 4 h 2.5 mL <1 year; 5 mL 1–5 years, 10 mL >5 years	Effect is slow. Large doses can become impacted in the gut if given orally
	Sodium resonium	As above	

Hyperphosphataemia

- Start treatment if plasma PO$_4$ >1.7 mmol/L (> 2.0 mmol/L in a neonate).
- Treatment is by dietary phosphorus restriction and phosphate binders which are given with oral intake.
- Calcium carbonate 250 mg tablets can be dissolved in feeds, starting dose:
  - Up to 2 years: 250 mg four times a day.
  - 2–5 years: 500 mg three times a day.
  - 5–10 years: 750 mg three times a day.
  - >10 years: 1000 mg three times a day.

These doses may need to be increased considerably, depending on plasma PO$_4$ levels.

Hypocalcaemia
- Hypocalcaemia, particularly in association with hyperkalaemia can lead to cardiac arrest, therefore cardiac monitoring is necessary if hypocalcaemia is severe.
- Corrected calcium can be estimated from total calcium and albumin as follows:

Corrected calcium = total plasma calcium + (36 – plasma albumin)/40.

- If the corrected calcium is <1.9 mmol/L or if bicarbonate therapy is required, treat with IV 10% calcium gluconate 0.1 mg/kg (0.5 mL/kg) over 30 min to 1 h.
- Hypocalcaemia will improve if hyperphosphataemia is treated.
- If AKI on preceding CKD, commence activated vitamin D (alfacalcidol or calcitriol) at a dose of 0.01 micrograms/kg/day.

Acidosis
- May be severe if the respiratory system is unable to compensate. Maximum respiratory compensation may take over 24 h. Correct with sodium bicarbonate if HCO_3^- <18 mmol/L. If the child is unwell, use IV bicarbonate.
- Calculate IV dose as:

mmol $NaHCO_3$ = (18 – measured HCO_3) × 0.6 × weight in kg.

- Give over 1 h.
- Oral dose is 1–2 mmol/kg/day for infants and 70 mmol/m^2/day for older children, to be divided into two to four doses.
- The ionized calcium must be checked and corrected before treatment since correction of acidosis further lowers ionized calcium.

If there is hypernatraemia or oliguria/fluid overload, dialysis may be the only treatment.

Hypertension

• Usually due to fluid overload, although it is important to be sure that it is not due to intense vasoconstriction because of hypovolaemia (very rare).
• First treatment is furosemide, and failure to respond is an indication for dialysis although it is usual to consider other first-line agents (e.g. calcium channel blockers, labetalol if severe hypertension with signs of encephalopathy) in addition, particularly since it usually takes several hours to establish emergency dialysis.
• If dialysis is adequate but hypertension persists, nifedipine is the first choice; the starting dose is 250 micrograms/kg, three times daily. Maximal daily dose is 3 mg/kg/day.

Nutrition in acute kidney injury

- Adequate nutrition will help:
  - prevent catabolism
  - control metabolic abnormalities (particularly potassium and phosphate)
  - recovery—it may delay or prevent the need for dialysis.
- The fluid restriction will limit the nutritional prescription. Dialysis allows a higher fluid intake and therefore better nutritional intake.
- Consider NG feeding if the child is unable to meet the nutritional goals orally, e.g. due to nausea or neurological impairment.
- Parenteral nutrition should only be considered if enteral nutrition is not tolerated.
- If on prolonged PD, a higher protein intake may be required (Table 17.7).

Table 17.7 Nutritional guidelines for the child with AKI

Boys and girls	Energy (EAR)	Protein (RNI)
0–6 months	95 –115 kcal/kg	1.5–2.1 g/kg
6–12 months	95 kcal/kg	1.5–1.6 g/kg
1–3 years	95 kcal/kg	1.1 g/kg
4–6 years	90 kcal/day	1.1 g/kg
7–10 years	1740 ♀, 1970 ♂ kcal/day	28 g/day
11–14 years	1845 ♀, 2220 ♂ kcal/day	42 g/day
15–18 years	2110 ♀, 2755 ♂ kcal/day	55 g/day ♂ 45 g/day ♀

EAR, estimated average requirement; RNI, reference nutrient intake i.e. amount of protein needed for maintenance and growth

Day 1

- High-energy, protein-free fluids using a glucose polymer, e.g. Maxijul® solution.
- Concentration depends on degree of nausea, vomiting, diarrhoea:
  - Infants: 15% Maxijul®.
  - 1–2 years: 20% Maxijul®.
  - >2 years: 25% Maxijul®.
- Full energy requirements will not be met if fluid restricted.
- Potassium and phosphate intakes may need adjusting.

Day 2

- Consider introduction of protein depending on degree of uraemia.
- If urea 30–40 mmol/L, start 0.5 g protein/kg dry weight/day:
  - Infants—diluted whey-based infant formula e.g. Cow & Gate 1® or SMA® 1 + Maxijul®.
  - Children—diluted paediatric enteral feed e.g. Nutrini® (paediatric sip feed e.g. Paediasure® if feeding orally) + Maxijul®.
- If urea >40 mmol/L continue protein-free high energy fluids for a further 24 h.

Day 3

Increase/introduce protein depending on degree of uraemia:

* If urea 20–30 mmol/L: increase protein to 1 g/kg dry weight/day.
* If urea 30–40 mmol/L: start 0.5 g protein/kg dry weight/day (see 'Day 2').
* Maximize energy intake using Maxijul® and fat emulsion, e.g. Calogen® as tolerated.

Day 4 onwards

* Normalize eating and drinking patterns as renal function improves.
* If urea 20–30 mmol/L: increase protein to 1 g/kg dry weight/day.
* Once urea <20 mmol/L: ensure intake provides at least the RNI protein for height age in infants/chronological age in children.

Drug therapy

(➔ See Chapter 22.)

- Correct drug doses according to GFR. The calculation for eGFR (➔ see 'Appendix') needs to be interpreted with caution as the formula assumes a stable situation.
- Change of GFR will necessitate regular revision of drug dosages.
- Many drugs require decreased doses or a prolonged dosage interval in renal failure.
- It is preferable to avoid known nephrotoxic drugs in AKI when an alternative is available.

Dialysis

(➔ see Chapter 19 and Chapter 20.)

Choice of dialysis

* Options are PD, HD, or haemofiltration.
* Most children requiring intensive care are managed with CRRT
(➔ see Chapter 20).
* HD is the preferred option if vascular access is needed for plasma
exchange as well. If the urea is very high, a short session (2 h) with
mannitol 1 g/kg IV to maintain plasma osmolality (➔ see Chapter 20)
will be necessary as intracerebral disequilibrium is most likely with
the first session. Thereafter, daily HD is likely to be needed until the
biochemistry improves, when it can be weaned accordingly.
* PD can be started immediately in the child with AKI:
  * Flush the catheter until the effluent is clear of blood and debris.
  * Use continuous, 24 h cycling, initially with 20 to 30 min cycles (10 min
    fill, 10 min dwell, 10 min drain) then varying according to response.
  * Start with 10 mL/kg fill volumes. This can be built up promptly if
    there is no leakage and the child tolerates it, to 40 mL/kg.
  * It is usual to start with 1.36% dialysate, but this can be increased if
    fluid removal is inadequate (Table 17.8).

Table 17.8 Advantages and disadvantages of the different types of renal replacement therapy

Dialysis modality	Benefits	Disadvantages
PD	Can be carried out by ward nurses	Risk of peritonitis/leakage/drainage problems
	Ease of access	
	May be continued indefinitely with Tenckhoff catheter	Rapid removal of a large volume of fluid is difficult so not recommended if pulmonary oedema present
		Potential risk of pulmonary compromise in patient with respiratory problems
HD	Gold standard solute clearance	Requires haemodynamically stable patient
	Bicarbonate is standard	
	Can be used to rapidly remove large volumes of fluid, e.g. with pulmonary oedema	Vascular access may be difficult
CRRT	Good ultrafiltration	Requires continuous anticoagulation
	Solute clearance may be improved with addition of dialysis (CVVHD)	Vascular access may be difficult
	Does not cause major fluid shifts and disturbances to BP and cardiac output	

Follow-up of acute kidney injury

Survival and renal recovery depends on the cause of the AKI. Long-term follow-up is necessary, with the exception of children with pre-renal AKI, in order to detect the development of proteinuria and hypertension which herald CKD, an increasingly reported issue after AKI.

* BP and Ua:UCr, (on the first urine of the morning taken on rising) should be monitored 12 months after AKI.
* Annual BP and Ua:UCr for life.
* Check creatinine if previous measurement elevated or if proteinuria or raised BP develops.
* For treatment of proteinuria, ⮕ see Chapter 18 and for hypertension, ⮕ see Chapter 16.

Reference

Kellumand JA, Lameire N, KDIGO AKI Guideline Work Group. Diagnosis, evaluation, and management of acute kidney injury: a KDIGO summary (Part 1). *Crit Care* 2013;17:204–219.

Shiga toxin-producing Escherichia coli haemolytic uraemic syndrome

Epidemiology and notes

- STEC-HUS represents 90% of HUS in children.
- It occurs mainly in children <3 years, almost never in neonates.
- The average annual incidence of STEC-HUS for the UK and Ireland is 0.71 per 100,000. In Western Europe or North America, its annual incidence rate is 2–3 per 100 000 children <5 years of age.
- Serotype *E. coli* 0157:H7 is the most frequent (70% of cases in the UK) but other serotypes (e.g. 0111, 0103) are also associated.
- Shiga toxin binds to the glycolipid receptor Gb3, highly expressed in the kidney and brain, explaining the specific organ involvement.
- Genetic differences in the Gb3 receptor likely explain the variable susceptibility to HUS.
- The risk of developing HUS in patients with intestinal *E. coli* 0157:H7 infection is 10%.
- Cows are the main vectors of *E. coli* 0157:H7 which can be present in their intestinal lumen and faeces. Cattle do not express the Gb3 receptor and thus do not develop disease.
- Humans are infected from contaminated undercooked ground beef, unpasteurized raw milk or milk products (cheese), contaminated water (well water, or lake water swallowed during bathing), fruits, fruit juice, or vegetables.
- Person-to-person transmission is possible.
- Transit-slowing agents and antibiotics (such as beta lactams or trimethoprim–sulfamethoxazole) increase the risk of HUS developing in infected individuals.
- STEC-HUS may occur simultaneously or a few days or weeks apart in several members of a family, mainly siblings, because of contamination from the same environment, or person-to-person transmission.
- Epidemics are well described.
- HUS caused by *Shigella dysenteriae* is important on a worldwide basis, but is an uncommon cause of STEC-HUS in the UK.

Clinical features of typical STEC-HUS

- Differentiation between post-infective and other causes of MAHA is, at presentation, on the basis of the history. Children with STEC-HUS are usually more systemically unwell.
- Diarrhoea (bloody) and vomiting (most, not all).
- Rectal prolapse, intussusception, toxic dilatation of colon, and bowel perforation.
- Hydration at the time of the diagnosis of HUS is variable—may be dehydrated or overhydrated (if anuric but able to drink, or perhaps most commonly from inappropriate IV fluids).
- Hypovolaemic shock in 2%.
- Oligoanuria appears between 1 and 14 days after the onset of diarrhoea.
- MAHA and thrombocytopenia precede the AKI.

- Jaundice in 35%.
- Hypertension in one-third.
- The most common extrarenal manifestation is CNS disturbance affecting up to 20%. Beware of early signs such as lip-smacking:
  - Seizures.
  - Cranial nerve palsy.
  - Cerebral oedema.
  - Encephalopathy.
  - Coma.
  - Decerebrate posturing.
  - Hindbrain herniation—causing respiratory arrest.
- Cardiomyopathy.
- Diabetes mellitus (due to necrotizing pancreatitis) affects up to 5%.
- Renal cortical necrosis:
  - Due to acute cortical ischaemia.
  - Mainly observed in the most severe forms of STEC-HUS.
  - Associated with prolonged anuria at the acute phase.
  - High risk of CKD.

Investigations

- FBC, platelets, blood film.
- Blood glucose monitoring
- Chemistry including renal and liver function, LDH, glucose, urate, lipase, and amylase.
- Clotting screen.
- Group and save blood.
- Urine dipstick for blood and protein.
- Ua:Ucr.
- STEC serology.
- Shiga toxin PCR.
- Stool microscopy and culture.

Selective investigations

- Direct Coombs test (positive in T-antigen HUS—➜ see 'Pneumococcal haemolytic uraemic syndrome').
- Erect chest X-ray, abdominal X-ray.
- Renal and abdominal (to include biliary tree and pancreas) US: to exclude preceding structural renal abnormalities and other organ involvement.
- CT abdomen (if pancreatitis or suspect collection).
- ECG: if severe electrolyte disturbance or cardiac failure.
- EEG: if seizures or altered conscious level.
- MRI brain (or CT): if seizures or altered conscious level.
- Renal biopsy very rarely required and risky in view of the low platelet count.

Treatment: general points

- Early diagnosis and supportive care are of major importance. There is no specific therapy for STEC-HUS (➜ see p. 434).
- Attention to the presence of hypovolaemia at presentation is important. There are studies suggesting that volume expansion may improve outcome.

Blood transfusion

- Packed red cell transfusion is indicated if Hb <60 g/L, or if <70 g/L but symptomatic (e.g. short of breath, shock). May worsen hyperkalaemia and volume overload.
- Platelet transfusion is rarely indicated unless invasive surgery is planned, or there is intracranial haemorrhage. If given, platelets are rapidly consumed in the haemolytic process and may worsen the damage.

Antibiotics

- It is generally accepted that antibiotics are not part of the routine management of STEC-HUS. Some suggest that antibiotics may make HUS worse, due to release of STEC from killed bacteria, although this remains controversial.

Plasma exchange

- Some advocate the use of plasma exchange if CNS signs develop in typical HUS. There are no controlled data to support this, and this recommendation remains anecdotal.

Eculizumab

- Is being used in some parts of the world in severely affected patients. There are clinical trials in progress but no results are available yet.

Prevention of HUS

- Ground beef must be cooked until the inside is no longer pink.
- Non-pasteurized products must not be given to young children.
- Children who touch cows or goats must wash their hands afterwards.
- Strict rules governing cattle slaughter to prevent contamination of meat by intestinal content.
- When E. coli 0157:H7 infection is suspected, information and surveillance of siblings and family is necessary. Handwashing with soap and water rather than alcohol-based gels is the most effective means of preventing person-to-person spread.
- Confirmed STEC-HUS is a notifiable disease.

Prognosis

- Acute mortality rate is currently 3–5%.
- 5–10% develop CKD stage 5.
- After 15 years or more of follow-up, 20–60% of patients have proteinuria and/or hypertension, with up to 20% having CKD. These problems may appear after several years of apparent recovery.

Poor renal prognostic factors

- Neutrophilia >20 × 10^9/L.
- Shock during the acute phase.
- Anuria >2 weeks.
- CNS involvement.
- Severe colitis and/or rectal prolapse.
- Cortical necrosis.
- >50% glomeruli with TMA lesions (best predictor, but biopsy is very rarely performed).

Outcome following renal transplantation for STEC-HUS

- In most retrospective series, no recurrence of HUS was observed.
- Occasional case reports of HUS recurrence in the graft are described, suggesting that some patients with aHUS have been misdiagnosed.
- Calcineurin inhibitors are not contraindicated in this setting.

Further reading

Spinale JM, Ruebner RL, Copelovitch L, et al. Long-term outcomes of Shiga toxin hemolytic uremic syndrome. *Pediatr Nephrol* 2013;28:2097–2105.

Pneumococcal haemolytic uraemic syndrome

The incidence of pneumococcal HUS is increasing so that in some countries it is overtaking STEC-HUS as the commonest cause.

* *Streptococcus pneumoniae* produces neuraminidase which cleaves N-acetylneuraminic acid from the glycoproteins on the cell membranes of red cells, platelets, and glomeruli. Current thinking is that this exposes the T antigen. The exposed antigen then reacts with anti-T antibody resulting in TMA.
* The antigen–antibody reaction is called T activation and occurs more commonly in infants and young children.
* Diagnosis is by testing for red-cell T activation; and the direct Coombs test will be positive.
* Although all *S. pneumoniae* produce neuraminidase, not all cause T-cell activation. Variation is likely to be due to different strains producing different quantities of neuraminidase with different enzymatic activity, and to individual patient variation in their amount of anti-T antibody.
* Anti-T antibody may be present in transfusions and plasma so red cells and platelets should be washed before transfusion (to remove anti-T antibody) and the use of plasma avoided as far as possible. Early diagnosis may prevent ongoing activation by the use of non-washed cells.
* HUS is typically associated with severe pneumococcal infections, such as empyema or meningitis, potentially because of higher neuraminidase production.
* Activation clears when the infection is controlled so antibiotic therapy is needed but the early commencement of antibiotics does not reduce risk or alter the severity of HUS.
* Initial reports suggested increased mortality and worse renal outcome than for STEC-HUS. However, much of the morbidity is due to the pneumococcal infection (e.g. meningitis) and more recently it appears that renal outcome is no worse.
* Influenza virus and HIV have also been associated with HUS.

Reference

Spinale JM, Ruebner RL, Kaplan BS, et al. Update on Streptococcus pneumoniae associated hemolytic uremic syndrome. *Curr Opin Pediatr* 2013;25:203–208.

Atypical haemolytic uraemic syndrome

Atypical haemolytic uraemic syndrome (aHUS) is HUS with no other coexisting disease. The diagnosis is based on the history and findings initially as genetic studies take time.

- STEC-HUS, pneumococcal and influenza-induced HUS, TTP, and cobalamin C defect HUS must be excluded.
- Represents <10% of HUS in children.
- Any age can be affected, including newborns.
- There is usually no prodromal diarrhoea, nor seasonal predominance, although infections (including viral or bacterial gastroenteritis) may trigger an episode of aHUS in a susceptible individual.
- Onset may be sudden, and is relapsing and remitting over weeks or months.
- Arterial hypertension is frequent.
- Deterioration in renal function of varying severity leads to CKD in most cases (and CKD stage 5 in some cases), after weeks, months, or years.
- Some children have relapses of HUS, often triggered by infectious diseases, which can occur even when there is CKD stage 5, i.e. extrarenal disease can continue, e.g. haemolytic episodes, pancreatitis, etc.
- Some have a presentation like TTP, with predominance of CNS symptoms which is the main clinical feature which differentiates TTP from HUS (although HUS can have CNS involvement, so this differentiation is not clear cut).
- aHUS is often familial, with AR or AD inheritance (➲ see 'Genetics of aHUS').
- Histological lesions are arteriolar TMA, with intimal cell proliferation, thickening of the vessel wall, and narrowed lumens of arterioles.
- Renal biopsy can be useful when diagnosis is uncertain.

Genetics of aHUS

Central to the pathogenesis of aHUS is overactivation of the alternative pathway (AP) of complement. Mutations that result in the loss of protection of endothelial cells and platelets from complement attack have been detected in 60–70% of cases in the following complement regulatory proteins:

- Complement factor H (CFH, the most important regulator of the AP), the commonest abnormality. Mutations may not result in a decrease in CFH levels.
- Complement factor I (CFI, up to 12% of cases). Again measured levels may be normal.
- Membrane cofactor protein (MCP, CD46), which protects cells from damage from complement and is present on podocytes.
- Thrombomodulin (THBD), an anticoagulant glycoprotein that plays a role in the inactivation of C3a and C5a.
- Autoantibodies to factor H (up to 10%).
- Deletions of CFHR1–5, CFH-related proteins, which are related to autoantibodies to CFH.
- Gain-of-function mutations of C3 and complement Factor B (CFB).

• There is incomplete penetrance such that first-degree relatives carrying the same mutation are often asymptomatic. Presumably, for HUS to develop there must be a combination of genetic and environmental factors. There are genetic causes of aHUS that are not related to the complement pathway (❯ see p.443).
  • Deficiency of ADAMTS13 (von Willebrand factor cleaving protease).
  • Cobalamin C defect (cblC)-associated HUS.
  • DGKe deficiency (diacylglycerol kinase-epsilon).

Genetic screening should be undertaken in:
• all patients with a diagnosis of aHUS
• where there is a family history of HUS
• if there is recurrence in a patient with presumed STEC-HUS
• if HUS occurs post transplant.

Specific tests to be considered for the investigation of aHUS

• Stool culture for verotoxin-producing E. coli (STEC).
• Serology for STEC both acute and convalescent.
• PCR for STEC.
• LFTs.
• Direct Coombs test (positive in 'T-antigen' associated cases).
• T antigen (if available).
• C3, C4, CH100, C3 nephritic factor, CFH, CFI, CFB plasma levels. C3 levels are low in 30–40% of cases (normal C4 and low C3 and CFB suggest activation of the AP).
• C5a and C5b-9 are raised in 50% of cases of acute aHUS.
• von Willebrand factor multimeric analysis.
• ADAMTS-13 enzyme activity.
• Urine for methylmalonic acidaemia and homocysteine.
• ANA, ds-DNA antibodies, ENA, anticardiolipin antibodies, lupus anticoagulant.
• HIV test.
• Renal biopsy if diagnosis unsure.
• Genetics (if pneumococcal HUS excluded): CFH, CFI, CD46, C3, CFB, DGKe, and THBD for mutations and genomic disorders. Serum for CFH autoantibodies (preferably before any plasma has been given to be sure the antibodies are primary and not secondary).

Treatment

Eculizumab

• A monoclonal anti-C5 antibody that prevents C5 cleavage and the formation of proinflammatory C5a and prothrombotic C5b-9.
• Complement blockade occurs within an hour of the first dose.
• For idiopathic (presumed genetic) aHUS, trials of eculizumab have shown it to result in prompt improvement in platelets, LDH, and haemoglobin, followed by improvement in renal function so that it is now the first-line treatment for aHUS in countries where it is available (Table 17.9).

Table 17.9 Eculizumab dosing

Eculizumab dosing weight (kg)	Induction	Maintenance
>40	900 mg weekly × 4 doses	1200 mg at week 5 then every 2 weeks
30–40	600 mg weekly × 2 doses	900 mg at week 3 then every 2 weeks
20–30	600 mg weekly × 2 doses	600 mg at week 3 then every 2 weeks
10–20	600 mg weekly × 1 dose	300 mg at week 2 then every 2 weeks
5–10	300 mg weekly × 1 dose	300 mg at week 2 then every 3 weeks

- NB: the drug is cleared by plasma exchange
- Immunity against *Neisseria meningitis* depends on C5b-9 so meningococcal vaccine must be administered and antibiotic prophylaxis given for at least 2 weeks after the vaccine and some think longer as the response to the vaccine may be impaired if there is an abnormality of the AP of complement.
- The duration of treatment with eculizumab needed to prevent relapse is unknown. Current recommendations are for lifelong treatment.
- The risk of relapse seems to be lower after withdrawal with CFI, MCP, or no identified mutations.
- There may be situations when a child does not respond to eculizumab and there is a need to establish whether the AP is suppressed:
  - Marker of complement blockade is CH50 <10%.
  - Soluble C5-b9 levels may be variable and are not helpful.
  - Eculizumab trough levels <50 micrograms/mL do not reduce CH50.
- It would not be expected that antibodies to CFH would respond to eculizumab and children with anti-CFH antibody-associated HUS may be better managed with a combination of plasmapheresis with cyclophosphamide, MMF, steroids, or rituximab if there is no response to eculizumab.
- Plasmapheresis and/or FFP may be used when eculizumab is not available. Plasmapheresis has been shown to be effective in some series, particularly if there is neurological involvement. Treatment is usually started daily and after 5–10 days the response assessed. Some children do not respond whereas others become dependent on plasma therapy and need regular ongoing treatments to prevent relapse.

Prognosis

Before eculizumab, the overall prognosis was poor, with a 25% mortality during the initial episode. 50% of survivors needed long-term dialysis. Outcome is affected by the genetic abnormalities, but even with known mutations outcome can be variable and affected by the presence of additional undefined modifiers.

Overall patient outcome before eculizumab:
- CFH mutations do the worst: 60–70% die or reach CKD stage 5 within 1 year.
- MCP mutations do better, with >80% remaining dialysis independent although recurrent episodes are common.
- CFI mutations are intermediate: 50% die or develop CKD stage 5 within 2 years.
- CFH antibodies: <50% develop CKD stage 5.

These figures have improved considerably with the use of eculizumab.

Post transcript

(➔ See 'Recurrent and de novo renal disease following renal transplantation'.)
- The risk of recurrent aHUS post transplant was 60% before eculizumab, with graft survival of 30% at 5 years.
- The risk of recurrence without eculizumab is:
  - highest with CFH, C3, or CFB mutations (80%) with graft loss of 80% by 2 years.
  - 50% with CFI.
  - 20% with no identified mutation.
  - MCP is corrected by an allograft bearing wild-type MCP so the recurrence rate is low (<10%).
  - increased with increasing anti-CFH antibody titres.
- Current recommendations are for prophylaxis with eculizumab at the time of transplant and its continuation post transplant until there is more information available about relapse after withdrawal in native kidneys.

Further reading

Loirat C, Fakhouri F, Ariceta G, et al. An international consensus approach to the management of atypical hemolytic uremic syndrome in children. Pediatr Nephrol 2016;31:15–39.

Genetic causes of haemolytic uraemic syndrome not related to the complement pathway

These disorders need to be diagnosed as soon as possible after presentation as the management is specific to each disorder and eculizumab is not a treatment.

Thrombotic thrombocytopenic purpura

- Due to deficiency of the enzyme ADAMTS13 (von Willebrand factor cleaving protease). This can be due to constitutional/familial deficiency or due to the presence of an inhibitor.
- The level is <10% normal and often much lower than this.
- This is predominantly a disease of adults but there are a few reports of ADAMTS deficiency in paediatric patients.
- Symptoms are mainly neurological but the kidneys can be involved.
- Treatment is with plasma exchange with FFP or its equivalent.

Cobalamin C defect (cblC)-associated HUS

- Methylmalonic aciduria with homocystinuria is the most common inborn error of vitamin B12 metabolism.
- HUS usually occurs during infancy but later onset has been reported.
- Treatment is supplementation with hydroxocobalamin and betaine.

DGKe deficiency (diacylglycerol kinase-epsilon)

- A lipid kinase expressed in endothelium, platelets, and podocytes.
- AR inheritance.
- Leads to an activated and prothrombotic phenotype.
- HUS usually presents before 1 year of age.
- Persistent proteinuria and hypertension and progression to CKD.
- DGKe mutations can also present with steroid-resistant nephrotic syndrome.

Rhabdomyolysis

Background

Rhabdomyolysis is the breakdown of striated muscle resulting in the release of myoglobin, which is nephrotoxic. Early recognition is important as aggressive hydration may prevent AKI.

Presentation

* Approximately half present with the triad of diffuse myalgia, weakness, and dark urine.
* Calf pain or muscle swelling.
* There may be a history of trauma, loss of consciousness, and prolonged immobilization or grand mal seizures.

There are acquired (more common) and hereditary causes:

Acquired causes

* Excess muscle activity in normal muscles: mechanical and thermal muscle injury and ATP depletion can occur with heat stroke, status epilepticus, status asthmaticus, myoclonus, and severe dystonia.
* Crush injury and other trauma: due to direct muscle injury and ischaemia reperfusion injury after prolonged ischaemia. Large numbers of cases have been reported following earthquakes.
* Drugs and toxins: many drugs have been reported to cause rhabdomyolysis, either via a direct toxic effect, or by inducing myositis or coma, or by excessive neuromuscular stimulation. Some toxins include snake venom and insect bites.

Hereditary causes

Disorders of muscle carbohydrate metabolism

McArdle disease is an AR disorder resulting in deficiency of myophosphorylase, and, as a result, defective generation of glucose from glycogen. Anaerobic type 2 muscle fibres are activated during vigorous exercise and are therefore particularly dependent on ATP. The rhabdomyolysis that results from ATP depletion causes muscle pain which is relieved by rest. Other inherited diseases affecting the glycolytic/glycogenolytic pathways include *phosphofructokinase deficiency (Tarui disease)*, and *phosphoglycerate mutase deficiency*.

Carnitine palmitoyltransferase deficiency

Carnitine palmitoyltransferase deficiency is an AR disorder resulting in abnormal production of energy from long-chain fatty acids. Aerobic type 1 muscle fibres are affected, so that muscle pain and rhabdomyolysis occur with prolonged exercise and inadequate energy intake. Frequent high-carbohydrate meals may help.

Malignant hyperthermia (hyperpyrexia)

Malignant hyperthermia is an AD disorder of the calcium release channel of the sarcoplasmic reticulum resulting in high resting sarcoplasmic calcium concentrations. Exposure to halothane, succinyl choline, and caffeine triggers further calcium release, resulting in muscle contraction, hyperthermia, and rhabdomyolysis.

Neuroleptic malignant syndrome

The neuroleptic malignant syndrome (NMS) is a central defect causing a gradual development of hyperthermia, muscle rigidity, fluctuating consciousness, autonomic instability, and rhabdomyolysis. Drugs which can cause NMS include phenothiazines, butyrophenones, and other antipsychotics.

General points

- Plasma myoglobin levels rapidly rise during injury, then fall within 6 h although plasma levels are not routinely measured.
- Plasma creatine phosphokinase levels rise 2–12 h after injury, and peak 24–72 h later.

Investigations

- Myoglobinuria:
  - Urinalysis—stick test strongly positive for blood but no or few red cells on urine microscopy.
  - Urine myoglobin positive.
- Elevated plasma creatine phosphokinase (MM band).
- Other plasma electrolyte disturbances:
  - Hyperkalaemia
  - Hyperphosphataemia
  - Hypocalcaemia.
  - Hyperuricaemia.

Management

Manage the patient on the basis of urine output and plasma electrolytes and not the plasma creatine phosphokinase.

- If urine output is reasonable (>0.5 mL/kg/h):
  - High fluid input = 3 L/m^2/day (0.45% saline/2.5% dextrose, may need adjustment: follow electrolytes regularly).
- If oligoanuric:
  - Consider first a fluid challenge (5–10 mL/kg).
  - Possibly with furosemide to establish urine output.
- If unsuccessful:
  - Dialyse for severe electrolyte disturbance.
  - CVVH clears myoglobin reasonably well.
  - Determine underlying condition. Muscle biopsy may be necessary for congenital enzyme defects.
  - Outcome depends on cause, but full recovery is usual

References

Elsayed EF, Reilly RF. Rhabdomyolysis: a review, with emphasis on the pediatric population. *Pediatr Nephrol* 2010;25:7–18.

Tumour lysis syndrome

Background

Tumour lysis syndrome (TLS) occurs in haematological malignancies and lymphoproliferative conditions. Rapid cell breakdown leads to hyperuricaemia (pre TLS). The development of urate nephropathy, with AKI, hyperphosphataemia, hyperkalaemia, and hypocalcaemia, indicates established TLS. Prevention is the aim of management, using high fluid intake and allopurinol or rasburicase. The advent of rasburicase (urate oxidase) has made TLS a rare occurrence. Rasburicase converts uric acid to allantoin, which is much more soluble. TLS can occur prior to chemotherapy because of autolysis of tumour cells but usually starts after induction of treatment. Duration depends on severity and supportive measures in place, but on average lasts for approximately 48 h.

The most important thing is to assess the risk of TLS.

Factors that predispose to TLS, i.e. high-risk patients:
- High cell count leukaemia (total white cell count usually in excess of $100 \times 10^9/L$).
- Burkitt's type lymphoma.
- Large tumour bulk.
- Bulky T-cell lymphoma.
- Bulky lymphoproliferative disease (LPD) or post-transplant lymphoproliferative disease (PTLD).
- Evidence of renal infiltration with tumour (e.g. on US).
- Evidence of renal impairment.

Management

- Increased hydration is important for all levels of risk:
  - Low-risk patients can be managed with monitoring of fluid status.
  - Medium-risk patients can be given allopurinol for 7 days.
  - High-risk patients should be given rasburicase.
- Patients already in established TLS at time of admission need insertion of a HD catheter at the time of anaesthetic for Hickman line or bone marrow followed by HD (➔ see 'Management after haemodialysis').
- Disturbances of calcium and magnesium homeostasis can occur (as a result of the hyperphosphataemia, renal impairment, changes in acid–base balance, or due to the diuresis) and can lead to tetany or seizures.
- It is important that potassium is not added to hydration fluids.

Prevention of tumour lysis syndrome

- Hydrate with 3 L/m²/day of 0.45% sodium chloride/2.5% glucose, or 0.9% sodium chloride, depending on plasma and urinary sodium. This can be increased to 4 L/m²/day if there is no evidence of fluid overload (tachycardia, tachypnoea, gallop rhythm, desaturation or oxygen requirement).
- Give allopurinol 100 mg/m², 8-hourly by mouth if no high-risk features (see earlier in topic); or rasburicase 200 micrograms/kg once per day if high risk or if poor response to allopurinol, starting 12 h prior to chemotherapy if possible.

- Review the patient clinically as appropriate (but at least every 4–6 h). Check for oliguria or fluid overload. Calculate the fluid balance and measure plasma biochemistry (Na, K, Ca, PO4, TCO_2, urate, urea, and creatinine) every 4–6 h. (If very high risk, monitor biochemistry 2- to 3-hourly). Give furosemide 1–2 mg/kg if there are signs of fluid overload. Use a cardiac monitor to look for evidence of peaked T waves and dysrhythmias secondary to hyperkalaemia.
- Alkalinization of the urine is not recommended. This is because although bicarbonate may render the urate more soluble, an alkaline urine is very difficult to achieve without a dangerously high blood pH. This, along with the arrival of rasburicase, has made bicarbonate therapy unnecessary.

Treatment of established TLS

- HD is the preferred treatment for established TLS; haemofiltration or haemodiafiltration are less efficient in the acute phase.

Indications for HD

- Rapid rise in plasma potassium, phosphate, or urate; or plasma potassium >5 mmol/L and/or plasma phosphate >4 mmol/L if there is ongoing TLS or anuria.
- Pulmonary oedema (give oxygen and consider ventilation as immediate measures).
- Oliguria unresponsive to furosemide (1–2 mg/kg but may need up to 5 mg/kg).

The rate of rise of these markers is very important—act before the patient reaches a critical state.

Management after haemodialysis

- Nearly all patients require two HD sessions; some need three or more.
- After HD there will be a rebound in biochemistry, therefore continue to review the patient every 2–4 h both clinically (for oliguria and fluid overload) and biochemically (Na, K, Ca, PO4, TCO_2, urate, urea, and creatinine).
- The indications for further HD are as previously listed.
- Some patients may benefit from going onto haemofiltration after the first HD session in an attempt to prevent the biochemical rebound. This therapy is unproven.

Prevention and treatment of TLS

Prevention and treatment of tumour lysis syndrome

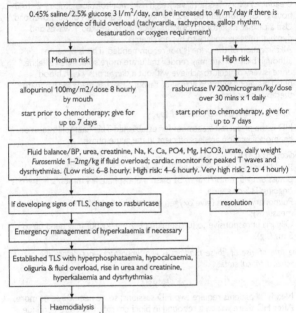

0.45% saline/2.5% glucose 3 l/m²/day, can be increased to 4l/m²/day if there is no evidence of fluid overload (tachycardia, tachypnoea, gallop rhythm, desaturation or oxygen requirement)

Medium risk

High risk

allopurinol 100mg/m2/dose 8 hourly by mouth

start prior to chemotherapy; give for up to 7 days

rasburicase IV 200microgram/kg/dose over 30 mins × 1 daily

start prior to chemotherapy, give for up to 7 days

Fluid balance/BP, urea, creatinine, Na, K, Ca, PO4, Mg, HCO3, urate, daily weight *Furosemide* 1–2mg/kg if fluid overload; cardiac monitor for peaked T waves and dysrhythmias. (Low risk: 6–8 hourly. High risk: 4–6 hourly. Very high risk: 2 to 4 hourly)

If developing signs of TLS, change to rasburicase

resolution

Emergency management of hyperkalaemia if necessary

Established TLS with hyperphosphataemia, hypocalcaemia, oliguria & fluid overload, rise in urea and creatinine, hyperkalaemia and dysrhythmias

Haemodialysis

Reference

Jones GL, Will A, Jackson GH, et al. Guidelines for the management of tumour lysis syndrome in adults and children with haematological malignancies on behalf of the British Committee for Standards in Haematology. *Br J Haematol* 2015;169:661–671.

Contrast-induced nephropathy

Radiocontrast agents are iodinated compounds that are removed from the body by renal excretion. They are potentially nephrotoxic, causing contrast-induced nephropathy (CIN):

Pathology of CIN

- Direct cytotoxic effect through the generation of reactive oxygen species.
- Renal vasoconstriction and medullary hypoxia
- Osmotic load and hyperviscosity.

CIN is characterized by

- a rise in serum creatinine within 24 h of the contrast exposure, peaking within 3–7 days and returning to baseline within 14 days
- oliguria is uncommon although there may be decreased urine output.

Risk factors

- Large volumes of contrast.
- Preceding CKD.
- Diabetes.
- Hypovolaemia.
- Anaemia.
- Concomitant nephrotoxic drugs.

Prevention

- Stop NSAIDs 3–4 days beforehand as they inhibit vasodilatory renal prostaglandins.
- Low-osmolality contrast media using the lowest dose possible.
- IV volume expansion with 0.9% saline 10 mL/kg when not on dialysis.
- Continue IV fluids for 6 h after the procedure if not a patient on a restricted fluid intake.
- acetylcysteine can be used in high-risk patients:
  - It is an antioxidant and vasodilates the renal medullary circulation.
  - 600 mg twice daily (scaled for patient size) for 24 h before and on the day of the procedure, oral or IV but oral route is preferable.
  - There is no proven benefit.
- Sodium bicarbonate, statins, and ascorbic acid have also been used but again with no proven benefit.
- Radiocontrast can be readily removed by dialysis so timing of the radiological procedure should be scheduled to precede a dialysis session. HD is better than PD at radiocontrast removal.

Gadolinium

- Gadolinium-based contrast agents are non-iodinated compounds given IV, primarily during vascular imaging with MRA.
- They are less nephrotoxic than iodinated agents.

- In patients with severe CKD, gadolinium can be deposited in dermal vessels. Skin findings vary and can look like either systemic sclerosis or a localized scleroderma (morphea). This occurs 2 days to 18 months after exposure, particularly if there is acidosis.
- They should not be used if the GFR is <15 mL/min/1.73 m^2 and only if there are no suitable alternatives in less severe CKD.

Further reading

Cronin RE. Contrast-induced nephropathy: pathogenesis and prevention. *Pediatr Nephrol* 2010;25:191–204.

Chronic kidney disease

Background

- CKD occurs when there are irrecoverable, bilateral abnormalities of the renal parenchyma.
- KDIGO defines CKD as either GFR <60 mL/min/1.73 m² or GFR >60 mL/min/1.73 m² with evidence of renal structural damage.
- Progressive decline in GFR does not happen if only one kidney is abnormal.
- Progressive decline in renal function to the need for renal replacement therapy (RRT, i.e. dialysis and/or transplantation) occurs in moderate to severe cases (Table 18.1), but it is not known if all milder cases progress.
- Many children, particularly those with renal dysplasia, can have stable renal function even in the worst stages of CKD for many years. Over the first 4 years of life, an improvement in GFR often occurs.
- Children with glomerular disease, proteinuria, and/or hypertension are more likely to have a progressive fall in renal function regardless of age.
- Puberty is associated with a decline in renal function.
- More rapid decline in GFR is often heralded by the onset or worsening of proteinuria.

Table 18.1 The probability of needing renal replacement therapy at age 20 years according to GFR in early childhood

GFR in early childhood (mL/min/1.73 m²)	Probability of needing RRT at age 20 years (%)
51–75	37
25–50	70
<20	97

Epidemiology

The true incidence of CKD in childhood is not known. Figures quoted range from 2 to 16 per million child population (pmcp) per year depending on area, reflecting local resources. These figures are likely to be underestimates throughout the world, because many children go undiagnosed and may not present even until adulthood. The incidence of children needing RRT is collected by national registries, and in the developed world is similar at 9–10 pmcp per year in the UK, Australia, and New Zealand, and slightly higher at 15 pmcp per year in the USA.

The incidence of CKD is higher in boys (who have a higher incidence of CAKUT) and in ethnic minorities. In the African American population this may be partly explained by the high-risk genotype for apolipoprotein L1 (*APOL1*), which is associated with an increased occurrence of FSGS. CAKUT is the commonest cause in younger children, although glomerular diseases become the commoner cause with increasing age.

Mortality

- CKD is associated with a decrease in life expectancy, and even early CKD is associated with an increased risk of premature death from CVD.
- Mortality risk increases with the severity of CKD, and has been estimated to be 1.4% higher than the age-matched population for children before RRT is needed, but much higher for children on chronic dialysis, when lifespan is reduced by 40–60 years, and by 20–30 years for patients with renal transplants.
- Mortality risk is highest during the first year of dialysis; if referral to paediatric nephrology care is late during the course of the disease; and in the presence of co-morbidities, lower socioeconomic status, and poor macroeconomic factors.
- Mortality rates in the first year post transplant are 15 times higher than the normal population in those 16–21 years old at transplant, and 130 times higher in those 0–4 years old at transplant.
- Mortality on RRT is also higher in young children in whom associated co-morbidities contribute. The 20-year overall survival is around 83%, being 76% in those <1 year, 81% in 2–5-year-olds, and 85% in 6–18-year-olds.
- Survival is improving with time, both for dialysis and post transplant.
- Causes of death on RRT are principally CVD (30%) and infection (20%).
- Malignancy represents 14% of deaths post transplant, mostly after 10 years.

Further reading

Chesnaye NC, van Stralen KJ, Bonthuis M, et al. Survival in children requiring chronic renal replacement therapy. *Pediatric Nephrol* 2018;33:585–594.

Assessment of renal function

Plasma creatinine

- The easiest way to assess renal function on a day-to-day basis is by measuring the plasma creatinine level. This is produced at a constant rate from the breakdown of creatine phosphate in muscle at a rate of ~10–25 mg/kg/day (90–210 µmol/kg/day).
- Normal plasma creatinine levels, therefore, increase progressively with growth and, in particular, muscle mass.
- Creatinine is excreted by filtration without reabsorption, except in the premature infant, when 'back-diffusion' can occur.
- Tubular secretion of creatinine increases early in CKD so that the plasma level may not rise until saturation of tubular secretion occurs, usually when renal function falls to about half of normal. Thus, plasma creatinine may overestimate GFR.
- As renal function declines, decreasing muscle mass due to malnutrition may lead to a fall in the plasma creatinine level, which may underestimate the severity of CKD.
- Conversely, the child starting recombinant growth hormone therapy (rhGH) may show a rise in plasma creatinine due to the effects of rhGH on muscle bulk.
- Plasma creatinine levels may also be affected by dietary meat intake and drugs that interfere with its tubular secretion, e.g. trimethoprim.
- Plotting of the reciprocal of creatinine against time may be useful to illustrate the rate of decline in renal function. However, the constraints already mentioned apply to this method too.

Clearance

- Clearance is the volume of blood cleared of a substance in unit time (mL/min). It is corrected for size by conversion to a surface area of 1.73 m^2.
- An estimate of GFR (mL/min) can be obtained by measuring the clearance of a solute, e.g. creatinine, which is:

$$UV / P$$

where U is the urine creatinine, V is the urine flow rate (mL/min), and P is the plasma creatinine.
- Given the difficulties of a timed urine collection in children, this is not often undertaken. Also, since creatinine is excreted by tubular secretion as well as glomerular filtration, GFR may be overestimated. Cimetidine inhibits tubular secretion of creatinine and estimates of GFR obtained from cimetidine-primed creatinine clearance have been shown to equate better with inulin clearance.

Inulin method to measure clearance

- Currently the gold standard but very difficult in children.
- An IV bolus of inulin is followed by a continuous infusion to maintain the plasma inulin concentration at a constant level. After a period of equilibration, a diuresis is induced by oral or IV fluid administration, and serial timed urine collections are commenced. Inulin concentration is measured in plasma samples obtained at approximately the midpoint of

each urine collection period. The inulin excretion rate ($U_{inulin} \times V$) and plasma inulin concentration for each time period are used to calculate GFR. A mean value is calculated from the serial GFR results.

Plasma disappearance method

* For a marker substance that is filtered at the glomerulus, but not reabsorbed by the tubules, the rate of decline of plasma concentration after an IV bolus will reflect the rate at which the substance is cleared from the plasma by glomerular filtration. This technique avoids the need for timed urine collections. [^{51}Cr]EDTA and iohexol are the commonest substances to be used for this technique. The more samples that are taken, the more accurate the disappearance slope, and therefore the more accurate the GFR calculation.
* Mathematical modelling allows estimation of the GFR. The accuracy of this technique is dependent upon knowledge of the exact dose administered and errors of volume of distribution which occur with oedema or dehydration. Time between plasma samples may need to be extended at low GFR in order to have a significant decline in the plasma concentration. This method tends to overestimate the GFR at high–normal levels of renal function.

Formulae for calculation of estimated GFR (eGFR)

* GFR (mL/min/1.73 m^2) in childhood can be estimated (eGFR) using the modified Schwartz formula, which has used results from children with CKD and the enzymatic method for measuring creatinine to develop the equation:

$$0.143 \times \text{height (cm)} / \text{plasma creatinine (mg/dL)}$$

* If the creatinine is µmol/L it needs to be converted to mg/d: so the formula would be:

$$0.143 \times \text{height (cm)} / \text{plasma creatinine (mmol/L/88.4)}$$

$$\text{or } 0.365 \times \text{height (cm)} / \text{creatinine (mmol/L)}$$

* However, this formula has not been validated outside the range of GFR between 15 and 75 mL/min/1.73 m^2.

Cystatin C

* Milder cases of CKD may go undiagnosed in childhood because:
  * creatinine increases progressively with increasing height and muscle bulk so may not be raised in a child who is small and thin due to CKD.
  * plasma creatinine does not rise until renal function has fallen to less than half of normal.
* For these reasons, cystatin C can be used to assess renal function. Cystatin C is a small protein that is freely filtered at the glomerulus and produced by all nucleated cells. It is not affected by muscle mass (although large doses of steroids increase production).
* It is, therefore, of particular use in children with very low muscle bulk in whom creatinine measurements are unreliable (e.g. neurological diseases, anorexia nervosa).

- It can be used for eGFR but there are no studies showing a benefit over creatinine eGFR in circumstances other than low muscle bulk.
- Currently the cost of the cystatin C assay is about ninefold greater than creatinine.
- There are different assays making standardization difficult and creating the need for different formulae for eGFR.
- The simplest validated formula for eGFR in children is the Berg formula:

$$Berg_{Cyst}\,eGFR = 91 \times cystatin\ C^{-1.213}$$

- Newer formulae using both creatinine and cystatin C are being developed and there is much debate about the optimum formula.

CKD should be suspected in any child with

- plasma creatinine above the normal range for age.
- bilateral renal defects on antenatal scans.
- bilateral renal defects on scans, e.g. for UTIs.
- a family history of CKD.
- persistent proteinuria.
- previous AKI.
- hypertension.

Presentation of chronic kidney disease

- Most present in the newborn period, usually following antenatal diagnosis (~50% of cases), although some abnormalities may be missed without a third-trimester scan.
- UTI.
- Decompensation of CKD causing AKI (precipitated by infection or dehydration).
- Polydipsia and polyuria.
- Family history.
- Poor nutritional intake and short stature.
- Pallor (anaemia), lethargy, and nausea.
- Bony abnormalities from renal osteodystrophy.
- Incidental finding of proteinuria.
- Hypertension.
- Mild cases are frequently asymptomatic.

The current classification is shown in Tables 18.2 and 18.3.

Children <2 years of age

This staging system does not apply in the first 2 years of life, when GFR is increasing from intrauterine levels. The plasma creatinine must be compared to age matched levels.

Causes of chronic kidney disease in children

In order of frequency:
- CAKUT.
- Renal cystic diseases.
- Nephrotic syndromes.
- Nephronophthisis (isolated or in association with syndromes).
- Glomerulonephritides.

Table 18.2 The current classification

Stage	GFR (mL/min/1.73 m²)	Features
1	>90	Renal parenchymal disease present
2	60–89	Usually no symptoms, but may develop biochemical abnormalities at the lower end of the GFR range
3A	45–59	Biochemical abnormalities and anaemia, and
3B	30–44	in addition may develop poor growth and appetite
4	15–29	Symptoms more severe
5	<15 or dialysis	Renal replacement therapy will be required

Table 18.3 Table showing addition of albuminuria staging to CKD stage

Albuminuria	mg albumin/g creatinine
A1	<30
A2	30–300
A3	>300

Addition of the letter 'A' to any stage implies proteinuria and therefore greater likelihood of progression of CKD.

- Vascular events.
- Atypical haemolytic uraemic syndrome (aHUS).
- Renal stone diseases.
- Familial nephropathies.
- Systemic diseases (SLE, vasculitis).
- Following AKI.

Pathogenesis

Despite these different causes of CKD, progressive destruction of renal tissue works through a common pathway. Abnormal intrarenal haemodynamics, chronic hypoxia, inflammation, cellular dysfunction, and activation of fibrogenic biochemical pathways lead to replacement of normal structures with extracellular matrix, culminating in fibrosis. For this reason, biopsy of a kidney at CKD stage 4/5 may not help in making a diagnosis as this common final pathway has a uniform histological appearance.

Further reading

KDIGO. 2012 Clinical practice guideline for the evaluation and management of chronic kidney disease. *Kidney Int Suppl* 2013;3:1–150.

Pottel H. Measuring and estimating glomerular filtration rate in children. *Pediatr Nephrol* 2017;32:249–263.

Investigation of the cause of chronic kidney disease

After the history and examination, US and stick testing of the urine for protein may be enough to provide a diagnosis, and will guide further investigations as necessary (Table 18.4). The kidneys are usually echo bright with poor corticomedullary differentiation in all causes of CKD (and AKI). Further imaging may be necessary if structural or cystic lesions or calculi are the cause and will depend on US appearances.

* Urine stick testing:
  * Heavy proteinuria without significant haematuria suggests a nephrotic syndrome.
  * Less protein is filtered as the GFR declines so that proteinuria may seem to improve as renal function worsens.
  * Proteinuria and haematuria suggest a glomerulonephritis or familial nephropathy.
  * Proteinuria may be tubular (tubulopathy), such as in Dent disease—if suspected, send urine for low-molecular-weight proteins, such as Urbp:Ucr or beta-2-microglobulin.
  * Proteinuria may result from any cause of CKD because of hyperfiltration due to raised intraglomerular pressure as a result of glomerular hypertrophy, which occurs in response to decreased glomerular numbers.
  * No proteinuria may be present with cystic diseases and dysplasias.
* Complement levels, ANA, anti-double stranded DNA (anti-ds-DNA), antineutrophil cytoplasmic and anti-GBM antibodies, IgA levels, ASOT/anti-DNAase if glomerulonephritis suspected.
* Plasma and urine Ca, oxalate, and purines if calculi.
* Urine pH and white cell cystine if tubulopathy suspected.
* Renal biopsy may be necessary if the cause of CKD is not clear, but should be avoided in advanced CKD when the kidneys are small (<5 cm bipolar length) as there is a significantly increased risk of bleeding, and histology may show ESKD without being able to identify the cause.
* More and more causes of CKD can be diagnosed by looking for genetic mutations (➔ see 'Genetic testing and antenatal diagnosis', p. 39).

Table 18.4 Appearance of kidneys on renal US and guide to differential diagnosis

Cystic	Small	Normal sized	Obstruction	Calculi
Dysplasia	Dysplasia ± VUR	Glomerulo-nephritides	Dysplasia with posterior urethral valves	Recurrent UTIs ± obstruction/reflux
Autosomal recessive polycystic kidney disease	Vascular insults (venous or arterial)	Familial nephropathies	Dysplasia with vesicoureteric junction obstruction	Calcium disorders
				Dent disease
Autosomal dominant polycystic kidney disease	All causes may result in small kidneys by stage 5 CKD	Nephrotic syndromes	Dysplasia with PUJ obstruction	Hyperoxaluria
Tuberous sclerosis		Nephronophthisis (may be cystic)	Neuropathic bladder	Purine disorders
Glomerulocystic diseases		Tubulopathies		Cystine

Management: overall aims

Aims of management of CKD

- Slow progression.
- Prevent biochemical and haematological derangements.
- Maintain normal growth and development.
- Preserve the limb vasculature—when possible avoid use of:
  - antecubital veins as they will be needed for fistula formation
  - subclavian veins, stenosis of which would preclude creation of a fistula in that arm.

Outpatient checks in the child with CKD

- Height, weight and head circumference.
- Pubertal stage.
- BP.

Investigations at each clinic visit

- FBC and estimation of iron (Fe) stores (transferrin saturation or reticulocyte haemoglobin) if needing an erythropoiesis-stimulating agent (ESA)).
- U&Es, bicarbonate, and creatinine.
- Ca, ionized Ca, phosphate, albumin, ALP, and intact PTH.
- Up:Ucr or Ua:Ucr measured in the first urine of the morning (to standardize measurements and reduce the orthostatic element).
- Fasting high- (HDL) and low-density lipoprotein (LDL), total cholesterol, and triglycerides 6-monthly.

Management

- Nutrition.
- Fluid and electrolyte balance.
- Growth.
- Anaemia.
- Hypertension (HTN).
- CKD–mineral and bone disorder (CKD-MBD).
- Immunizations.
- Preparation for RRT.

See individual sections for further details.

Slowing the progression of chronic kidney disease

Proteinuria
The rate of decline of kidney function is associated with the quantity of proteinuria, which in turn is related to the degree of hyperfiltration and glomerular hypertension. Proteinuria may itself be toxic to the tubulointerstitium. The level at which to start treatment is unknown; some would suggest that any proteinuria should be treated.

- The aim is to reduce proteinuria by progressively increasing the dose of an ACE inhibitor (which dilates the glomerular afferent arteriole, reducing intraglomerular pressure), stopping if there are side effects or abnormal biochemistry. Usually, it is possible to reduce proteinuria by half.

- An AT1 receptor blocker can be used as an alternative to an ACE inhibitor (see Table 18.5) or if there are side effects with the ACE inhibitor.
- Most centres use enalapril or captopril as their ACE inhibitor of choice. Plasma creatinine and K and BP should be measured at each clinic visit and 4–7 days after each increase in dose.

Table 18.5 Commonly used renin–angiotensin system blockers

Drug	Route	Normal starting dose	Normal dose range (to maximum)	Divided into doses/day	Preparations and comments
Captopril	Oral	50 micrograms/kg/dose	0.5–3 mg/kg/day (maximum 6 mg/kg/day)	3	Tablets 2 mg, 6.25 mg. Very soluble in water. Caution in renal artery stenosis, hyperkalaemia, and when GFR <30
Enalapril	Oral	100 micrograms/kg/dose	200–500 micrograms/kg/day (maximum 600 micrograms/kg/day up to 40 mg/day)	1	Tablets 2.5 mg, 5 mg, and 10 mg. Contraindicated commencing treatment in pregnancy and hyperkalaemia. Caution in renal artery stenosis and when GFR <30
Irbesartan	Oral	2 mg/kg/dose	6–12 years: 75–150 mg/day; >13 years: 150–300 mg/day	1	Tablets 75 mg, 150 mg
Losartan	Oral	Initially 700 micrograms/kg once daily (maximum per dose 25 mg). Initially 50 mg once daily, adjusted according to response to 1.4 mg/kg once daily; maximum 100 mg per day.	6–17 years Body-weight 20–49 kg >50 kg		Maximum 50 mg per day. Maximum 100 mg per day.

- Check Up:Ucr or Ua:Ucr for evidence of benefit; aim for maximum reduction of proteinuria without hypotension or hyperkalaemia.
- There may be a rise in plasma creatinine as the total renal blood flow is decreased. A rise of up to 25%, if not increasing, may be acceptable.
- ACE inhibitors carry a risk of severe hypotension, especially when other risk factors, such as nephrotic syndrome or when salt depleted (e.g. with gastroenteritis) are present. Consider stopping the ACE inhibitor during these episodes.
- ACE inhibitors may depress erythropoiesis so watch FBC.
- Cough is a side effect of ACE inhibitors.
- There is a risk of fetal malformations, particularly if used during the second and third trimesters. All teenage girls need to be informed of this risk.

Hypertension

Hypertension is another important contributor to the progression of CKD. The BP should be maintained within the normal range for age and height. European guidelines recommend <75th centile if there is CKD and no proteinuria and <50th centile in CKD with proteinuria.

Dyslipidaemia

- Dyslipidaemia may contribute to the progression of CKD. Increased LDL cholesterol is a particular problem for children with nephrotic syndrome. Hypertriglyceridaemia and abnormal apolipoprotein metabolism is a feature of CKD.
- Dietary intervention may be necessary, and some children (particularly those with nephrotic syndrome) may need lipid-lowering agents. The recent SHARP study has reported a reduction in cardiovascular events in adult CKD patients treated with statins. No comparable data exist in children and concerns remain about the toxicity of statins in young children, particularly those <8 years of age.

Low-protein diet

There is no evidence that a low-protein diet is beneficial in children and this is not recommended.

Treatment of anaemia

Anaemia and subsequent tissue hypoxia may contribute to the progression of CKD. Increasing oxygen delivery to tubular cells may decrease tubular damage and protect against nephron loss induced by tubular injury (➔ see 'Management: anaemia').

Further reading

Lurbe E, Agabiti-Rosei E, Cruickshank JK, et al. Consensus statement 2016 European Society of Hypertension guidelines for the management of high blood pressure in children and adolescents. J Hypertens 2016;34:1887–1920.

Management: fluid and electrolytes

Background

- Many children with CAKUT are Na, bicarbonate, and water losers, and need salt and bicarbonate supplementation, and free access to water.
- A low-K diet may be necessary when the GFR falls to <10% of normal.
- Ca absorption is poor and vitamin D may be needed to improve this.
- Phosphate retention needs early dietary intervention.

Table 18.5 gives the recommended nutrient guidelines for populations of healthy children. They are not, however, always appropriate for the individual child with CKD, and should not be considered as nutritional targets.

Sodium, bicarbonate, and water

Requirements for salt, water, and bicarbonate vary with the type of renal disease. Children with dysplasia and CAKUT are usually Na, bicarbonate, and water losers. This is because the predominant effect is on the renal tubule, so that reabsorption of Na, bicarbonate, and water from the glomerular filtrate is inadequate. Therefore, these children are often polyuric and polydipsic, and are prone to episodes of decompensation with hypovolaemia and AKI, unless they have salt and bicarbonate supplementation and free access to water (Table 18.6).

Sodium

- Requirements can be very high in early CKD, but fall as the glomerular disease progresses such that by stage 4–5 CKD, salt restriction may become necessary.
- The heaviest electrolyte losers are those with tubulopathies, in particular cystinosis; replacement of adequate Na and bicarbonate may be difficult.
- Salt depletion leads to chronic volume depletion and contributes to poor growth; NB: hyponatraemia is not a feature of salt depletion.

Table 18.6 Recommended nutrient intake (RNI) for calcium, sodium, potassium, and phosphorus

Age	RNI for Ca (mmol/day)	RNI for Na (mmol/day)	RNI for K (mmol/day)	RNI for P (mmol/day)
0–3 months	13.1	9	20	13.1
4–6 months	13.1	12	22	13.1
7–9 months	13.1	14	18	13.1
10–12 months	13.1	15	18	13.1
1–3 years	8.8	22	20	8.8
4–6 years	11.3	30	28	11.3
7–10 years	13.8	50	50	13.8
11–18 years	25 ♂ 20 ♀	70	80 (11–14 years) ♂ 90 (15–18 years) ♀	25 ♂, 20 ♀

* Children with CKD due to predominantly glomerular disease may retain salt and water and develop hypertension. Such children should be managed with a 'no added salt' diet (avoidance of foods particularly high in salt and no salt added to food in cooking or at the table).
* Many infants on peritoneal dialysis (PD) lose excessive amounts of Na in urine and dialysate and need supplementation.

Bicarbonate

As well as urinary bicarbonate losses there may be an inability to acidify, and bicarbonate replacement, starting dose 1 mmol/kg/day in two to four divided doses, may be needed.

Water

Children who are unable to concentrate their urine require free access to water.

Potassium

* CKD can be associated with K retention, but hyperkalaemia does not usually occur until the GFR is <10% of normal.
* Possible causes of hyperkalaemia include:
  * inadequate energy intake.
  * antihypertensive and K-sparing drugs, e.g. captopril and spironolactone.
  * high dietary intake of K.
  * acidosis.
* Adequate control of plasma K can usually be achieved by improving energy intake, avoiding foods that are very high in K, while allowing foods containing moderate amounts of K.
* Furosemide may be of benefit, but must be used with care as the change in circulating blood volume can destabilize renal function in severe CKD.
* Oral K chelators are available.

Calcium and phosphate

➔ See 'Management: mineral and bone disorder', p. 479.

Further reading

Department of Health Report on Health and Social Subjects. *Dietary Reference Values for Food, Energy and Nutrients for the United Kingdom*, No. 41. London: Stationery Office, 1991.

Royle J. The kidney. In: Shaw V, Lawson M, Eds, *Clinical Paediatric Dietetics*, 3rd edn. Oxford: Blackwell Sciences Ltd, 2007:211–226.

Management: growth

Background

- Growth retardation occurs in up to 50% of children with CKD stage 3B and below.
- Children with congenital nephropathies are particularly severely affected, because growth in the first 2 years of life is faster than at any other time, and is principally dependent on nutrition, which is very difficult to maintain because the infant with CKD is anorexic and frequently vomits.
- After this age, when the role of growth hormone (GH) becomes more important, the rate of growth can be normal.
- Growth may also be adversely affected at the time of puberty, which may be delayed, with an abnormal pubertal growth spurt.
- Growth retardation increases with CKD stage, but it has to be remembered that many children have associated syndromes that in themselves affect growth.
- Successful renal transplantation can normalize growth in some children, particularly the younger ones, but may be counteracted by corticosteroid therapy used as immunosuppression.

Important points

- Length and weight must be measured at each clinic visit, and head circumference and pubertal stage when appropriate. Results should be plotted on growth charts. This enables calculation of the rate of growth, a decline requires urgent action.
- The best described cause of poor growth is inadequate intake of calories and protein leading to malnutrition. Water, electrolyte, and acid–base imbalances, bone disease, and GH resistance are also important.
- Many children need dietary supplements orally or enterally.
- Gastrostomy feeding delivered overnight by an enteral feeding pump is associated with reduced vomiting.
- Vomiting needs evaluation for gastro-oesophageal reflux; antireflux medications may help. If not, Nissen fundoplication may be necessary.
- Correction of biochemical abnormalities is necessary for normal growth.
- Many children are salt losers and need salt supplementation.
- Children who fail to respond to all these measures may benefit from rhGH.
- Steroid therapy, particularly if daily, is an important cause of poor growth post transplantation.

Investigations

- Dietary assessment of calorie and protein intake.
- Assessment of salt and water intake.
- In infants with a history of vomiting, barium swallow for reflux and malrotation, and gastro-oesophageal pH studies.
- Bicarbonate, PTH, and thyroid function tests.

Management

- Act on any decline in rate of growth by addition of dietary supplements, either orally or enterally, via nasogastric (NG) tube or gastrostomy, if anorexic.
- Gastrostomy may be placed by percutaneous endoscopy (PEG) or open placement surgically, when the stomach is sewn to the abdominal wall.

Open gastrostomy is necessary in:

- The child on PD, to reduce the risk of peritonitis (➲ see 'Management: nutrition', p. 467 and 'Management: enteral feeding', p. 475). Careful consideration must be given to a PEG if there may be an abnormal position of intraabdominal organs; e.g. post intraabdominal surgery or severe kyphoscoliosis; and if the child has varices or other intragastric pathology, e.g. ulcer.
- The child in whom intraabdominal organs may be in an abnormal position, e.g. post surgery or severe kyphoscoliosis.
- With gastric pathology, e.g. varices (such as in ARPDK) or ulcer.
- Salt supplementation may be necessary in children with renal dysplasia, which is predominantly a tubular lesion.
- Correct acidosis, hyperparathyroidism (➲ see 'Management: mineral and bone disorder', p. 479), and abnormal thyroid function.
- Vomiting can be a very big problem for infants. It may be so severe that nutritional intake is compromised. There may be benefit from prokinetic agents such as alimemazine and erythromycin. Reduction of gastric acid secretion with H2-receptor antagonists (e.g. ranitidine) and proton pump inhibitors (e.g. lansoprazole) may also be of benefit in symptom reduction. 5HT3 receptor antagonists (e.g. ondansetron) may help with anorexia and vomiting.
- Vomiting is usually less with a gastrostomy than a NG tube.
- If vomiting persists despite oral medication and there is gastro-oesophageal reflux, Nissen fundoplication is indicated.
- rhGH can be offered to the child whose growth has failed to respond to all these measures (➲ see 'Management: growth', p. 465).

Further reading

KDOQI Work Group. KDOQI Clinical practice guideline for nutrition in children with chronic kidney disease: 2008 update. *Am J Kidney Dis* 2009:53:S11–104. ℘ http://www.kidney.org/professionals/KDOQI/

Rees L, Shaw V. Nutrition in children with CRF and on dialysis. *Pediatr Nephrol* 2007;22:1689–1702.

Management: nutrition

Background

Ensuring appropriate nutrition is one of the most important aspects of care of the child with CKD. Involvement of the paediatric renal dietitian is crucial to:
- control symptoms and prevent complications, particularly uraemia and renal bone disease (thereby delaying the need for dialysis).
- promote optimum growth.
- preserve residual renal function.

Causes of poor nutritional intake

Anorexia and vomiting are characteristic of CKD:
- Poor appetite may be due to abnormal taste sensation, the requirement for multiple medications, the preference for water in the polyuric child, and elevated circulating cytokines such as leptin, tumour necrosis factor (TNF)-alpha, and IL-1 and -6, which act through the hypothalamus to affect appetite and satiety.
- Vomiting may result from gastro-oesophageal reflux and delayed gastric emptying in association with decreased clearance of polypeptide hormones.
- Insufficient intake may be due to episodes of fasting surrounding surgical procedures and episodes of sepsis.
- Many children with CKD have associated co-morbidities that influence feeding (and growth) in their own right.

Important general points

Energy
- Inadequate energy from non-protein sources will result in the use of dietary protein for energy, rather than growth, and also result in increased plasma urea and K levels.
- Oral supplements and/or enteral feeding may be necessary to achieve optimum energy intake.
- Enteral feeding is indicated in both infants and children when oral intake is inadequate to maintain growth and should be considered as soon as the growth rate falls below normal.
- Children on PD having glucose-containing dialysate will absorb glucose during the dwell time (average 10 kcal/kg body weight/day).

Protein
- Protein intake above the reference nutrient intake (RNI) is recommended to ensure adequate intake for growth.
- Protein intake often needs adjustment to nearer the RNI when GFR is <25 mL/min/1.73 m² (see Table 18.7). Kidney Disease Outcomes Quality Initiative (KDOQI) recommends 100–140% dietary reference intake (DRI; CKD stage 3); 100–120% DRI (CKD stage 4–5).
- Aim for plasma urea levels <20 mmol/L in infants and children under 10 years and <30 mmol/L in older children (>10 years) with a normal serum albumin.

Table 18.7 Guidelines for energy intake and protein requirements in children with conservatively managed CKD

Age	Energy[a]	Protein[b] (use height age for infants and children <2nd centile for height)
Preterm	120–180 kcal/kg	2.5–3.0 g/kg
0–3 months	115–150 kcal/kg	2.1 g/kg
4–6 months	95–150 kcal/kg	1.6 g/kg
7–12 months	95–150 kcal/kg	1.5 g/kg
1–3 years	95–125 kcal/kg	1.1 g/kg
4–6 years	90–110 kcal/kg	1.1 g/kg
7–10 years	1740 ♀, 1970 ♂ kcal/day	28 g/day
11–14 years	1845 ♀, 2220 ♂ kcal/day	42 g/day

[a] Depending on losses through vomiting and underlying diagnosis; [b] reference nutrient intake (except for preterm).

Table 18.8 Guidelines on protein intake for children on peritoneal dialysis and haemodialysis

Age	Peritoneal dialysis[a]	Haemodialysis[b]
Boys and girls	Protein (g/kg/day; use height age for infants and children <2nd centile for height)	Protein (g/kg/day; use height age for infants and children <2nd centile for height)
Preterm	3.0–4.0	3.0
0–3 months	≥2.4	≥2.2
4–6 months	≥1.9	≥1.7
7–12 months	≥1.8	≥1.6
1–6 years	≥1.4	≥1.2
7–14 years	≥1.3	≥1.1
15–18 years	≥1.2	≥1.0

[a] RNI + 0.3 g/kg/day to compensate for peritoneal losses; [b] RNI + 0.1 g/kg/day to compensate for dialytic losses.

* The blood urea level is a reflection of protein intake, unless there is a catabolic state, when it reflects tissue breakdown.
* Symptoms of nausea and anorexia increase when the urea starts to climb >20 mmol/L.
* A very low urea suggests protein malnutrition.
* Dietary protein intake is rarely inadequate in CKD stages 1–4 as it is easily achieved from the diet.
* Protein intakes on dialysis are 100% RNI with an allowance to replace dialysate losses (see Table 18.8)—these are greatest in infants and after peritonitis.

Vitamins and minerals

See Table 18.9.

Few data are available on the micronutrient requirements of children with CKD.

- Vitamin supplements should not be routinely prescribed, as most contain vitamin A (e.g. Abidec®, Dalivit®). Renal excretion of vitamin A metabolites is impaired in CKD and high plasma levels can be associated with hypercalcaemia, anaemia, and hyperlipidaemia.
- Intake from diet, infant formula, enteral feeds, or nutritional supplements and any 'self-prescribed' micronutrient supplement must be considered before any supplement is prescribed.
- In patients with CKD not requiring RRT and those on HD, the aim is to achieve RNI for all micronutrients except vitamin A.
- Children on PD require supplements of vitamin C, pyridoxine, and folic acid to offset dialysate losses, e.g. Dialyvit® Paediatric (½ capsule <5 years of age; 1 capsule >5 years of age) or three Ketovite® tablets daily, adjusted after assessment of the individual's intake of micronutrients. Ketovite® liquid is not appropriate as this provides high doses of vitamin A.
- If a Fe preparation is prescribed, this should ideally be given in two or three divided doses and taken in the absence of food, antacids, and phosphate binders. Fe preparations available include:
  - sodium feredetate (Sytron®) (55 mg Fe in 10 mL).
  - ferrous sulfate 200 mg (65 mg Fe).
  - ferrous fumarate 210 mg (68 mg Fe).
- *Nutritional vitamin D (25(OH)D)*: a very large proportion of patients with CKD are deficient. The daily requirement in children with CKD is unknown.

Table 18.9 Selected micronutrient content of vitamin and mineral preparations

Vitamin and minerals	Paediatric Dialyvit®	Ketovite® tablets (3)	Ketovite® liquid (5 mL)	Abidec® (0.6 mL)	Dalivit® (0.6 mL)
Vitamin A (micrograms)			750	400	1500
Pyridoxine (mg)	2	1		0.8	1
Folic acid (micrograms)	1000	750			
Vitamin C (mg)	40	50		40	50
Vitamin D (micrograms)			10	10	10
Iron (mg)					
Zinc (mg)	8				
Suitable in CKD?	✓ All children on PD	✓ All children on PD	✗ Caution vitamin A	✗ Caution vitamin A	✗ Caution vitamin A

UK Department of Health guidelines recommend the following vitamin D supplementation for all children and it is logical to follow this advice for children with CKD:

- Aged 1–4 years: 10 micrograms (400 IU) daily.
- Aged <1 year: 8.5–10 micrograms daily.
- Children who have >500 mL of infant formula a day do not need any additional vitamin D as formula is already fortified.
- Older children who are rarely exposed to sunlight may need to continue with a 10-microgram supplement.

Practical management of feeding

There are various types of supplements, with different ratios of calories and protein. In the young child with vomiting, it is possible to increase the feed concentration and therefore decrease the feed volume. However, the vomiting may worsen and diarrhoea can occur with increasing feed density so changes should be introduced gradually.

Diet in infancy

- Breast milk or whey-based infant milk (e.g. SMA® 1 or Cow & Gate® 1) are best as they have a low renal solute load.
- Infants with uncontrolled plasma urea levels may need a higher-energy feed. Infant formula can be supplemented with glucose polymer (e.g. Vitaijul®) and/or fat emulsion (e.g. Calogen®).
- If the urea level remains raised despite optimizing energy intake then protein intake should be reduced in 0.2 g/kg increments towards the RNI.
- Raised plasma K levels (>6.0 mmol/L) are most often due to inadequate energy; energy intake should therefore be optimized.
- If hyperkalaemia is more severe (>6.5 mmol/L) or persistent, Renastart® or Kindergen® (low-K, low-phosphate formula) can be used to replace part of the standard infant formula base of the feed.
- If hypercalcaemia is persistent, Locasol® (low Ca formula) can be useful, although consideration of reduced doses of activated vitamin D and/or Ca containing phosphate binders must be adjusted first.

Weaning solids

- These should be low in protein and phosphate to start, i.e. baby rice, pureed fruits, and vegetables.
- As the infant takes more protein from solids, protein intake from the milk should be adjusted as needed.
- Cows' milk and cows' milk products may need to be restricted to prevent plasma phosphate levels increasing.

Diet in children

- The diet will normally be high in energy and restricted in phosphate.
- Protein and K may need to be restricted, particularly in CKD stage 4 and 5.

Protein

- Requirements are based on chronological age. If <2nd centile for height, requirements are based on height age (i.e. the age at which the child's height would be on the 50th centile) to ensure adequate protein intake.
- About 70% of protein intake should be from high biological value sources, e.g. meat, fish, cheese, eggs, or milk (NB: phosphate content may limit use of these foods).
- The remaining protein is given as lower biological value sources, e.g. bread, rice, potatoes, pasta, and biscuits. These foods are usually allowed freely.
- Strict protein restriction is not necessary, and simple dietary advice about reducing the size of protein portions in meals and limiting protein to two meals/day is usually adequate to keep the urea at an acceptable level. A small number of patients will require specific protein portion advice if urea levels cannot be controlled.
- On the other hand, sufficient protein intake may be difficult to achieve in the child on dialysis. Protein supplements over and above the normal RNI for protein for age are usually needed, as protein in PD and amino acids in HD are lost in the dialysate effluent.

Energy

- High-energy foods/diet are recommended.
- High-energy drinks are encouraged (e.g. flavoured Vitajoule® or Maxijul® water, sugar-containing squashes, and fizzy drinks such as Lucozade® High Energy).
- Children with poor appetites can benefit from nutritional supplements (a paediatric sip feed, e.g. Paediasure®, Fortini®, Paediasure Plus Juce®; older children may have an adult sip feed, e.g. Fresubin®, Fortisip®, Ensure Plus Juce®, ProvideXtra®).
- For children on enteral feeds, infant formula is changed to a paediatric enteral feed, e.g. Nutrini® or Paediasure® between 1 and 2 years of age (greater energy and protein density).
- For children on a fluid restriction, HD, PD, or for those who need a more energy- and protein-dense feed, Nepro® or Suplena® are available (also low in K and phosphate). Renilon® 7.5 is an alternative oral high-energy and protein supplement (although not nutritionally complete).

More recently, evidence is emerging that, as in much of the rest of the world, there are increasing numbers of children with CKD who are developing obesity, and that obesity may become a health issue for children with CKD as well.

Further reading

KDOQI Work Group. KDOQI clinical practice guideline for nutrition in children with chronic kidney disease: 2008 update. *Am J Kidney Dis* 2009;53(Suppl. 2): S11–124. ℬ http://www.kidney.org/professionals/KDOQI

Management: use of recombinant human growth hormone

Background

The use of rhGH has been shown to be safe and effective over 2 years of treatment, and uncontrolled studies suggest that its benefits may continue over subsequent years. rhGH should be considered when growth has failed to respond to correction of inadequate diet and biochemical abnormalities, and optimization of dialysis. For children on steroid therapy, the dose of steroids should be reduced to the lowest possible.

Important points

* There is GH resistance in CKD as circulating GH are levels are high and bioavailability of insulin-like growth factor 1 (IGF-1) is low.
* rhGH is licensed in prepubertal children whose GFR is reduced by 50% and in children after 1 year post transplant.
* rhGH has the most beneficial effect in the youngest, most growth-retarded patients. Children with less severe CKD do better than those on dialysis. After transplantation, those with the best renal function, on low doses of steroids have the greatest response to rhGH.
* Some children are small and have CKD as part of a syndromic diagnosis. These children respond poorly to rhGH.

Indications for the use of recombinant human growth hormone

Children with CKD (including post transplant) of all ages who have a height (Ht) standard deviation score (SDS) <–2 SD and a Ht velocity SDS <–1 SD below the mean, after adequate nutrition has been established, metabolic abnormalities have been corrected, dialysis adequacy ensured, and steroid therapy reduced to a minimum.

Examination

* Assessment of Ht SDS, Ht velocity, and Ht velocity SDS over the previous year.
* Assessment of pubertal staging.
* Dietary review to ensure adequate calorie and protein intake.
* Parental heights should be measured and the target height calculated (95% of children will have a final height within 8.5 cm on either side of the mid-parental height).
* Fundoscopy, as benign intracranial hypertension is a recognized side effect.

Investigations at start of therapy

* Fasting plasma glucose and insulin levels.
* Fasting triglycerides and cholesterol.
* Thyroid function tests.
* IGF-1.
* Bone age.

Follow-up and further investigations
- Fundoscopy 3-monthly.
- Calculation of Ht SDS and Ht velocity 6-monthly, and Ht velocity SDS after 1 year.
- Pubertal staging 6-monthly.
- Fasting plasma glucose and insulin, triglycerides, and cholesterol 6-monthly.
- IGF-1 and bone age annually.

Management

The recommended dose of rhGH is 45–50 micrograms/kg or 1.4 mg/m^2 daily by SC injection. Higher doses may be needed and can be adjusted if necessary after 6 months.

Do not commence treatment if
- within 1 year post transplant (as spontaneous catch-up may occur).
- inadequate dietary intake.
- the PTH is more than twice the upper limit of normal, as the extra demands for Ca may worsen osteodystrophy. There is an increased incidence of avascular necrosis of the hip, which may be related to high PTH levels.
- post transplant the prednisolone has not been reduced to the minimum possible dose.
- post transplant there have been rejection episodes within the preceding year, as there is an association with continuing rejection in patients treated with rhGH.
- dialysis adequacy is not optimized.
- there is X-ray evidence of epiphyseal fusion (i.e. growth is complete).

rhGH should be stopped when
- the child receives a renal transplant (to assess growth in the first year post transplant) unless the child has GH deficiency.
- there are side effects.
- there is no increase in Ht SDS or Ht velocity after 1 year.

Consideration should be given to stopping rhGH when
- there is non-compliance.
- the increase in Ht velocity is <50% from baseline in the first year of treatment.
- after the first year if the Ht velocity falls to the pre-rhGH value. However, Ht velocity SDS may be more useful than Ht velocity during puberty, when a spontaneous increase in Ht velocity would be expected.
- when the target height is approached and Ht velocity is <2 cm/year.

Factors that increase the chances of a response to rhGH
- Young age.
- More growth retarded.
- Less severe CKD, including post transplant.
- Post transplant, on low doses of steroids.

Side effects

There should be regular surveillance for efficacy and side effects

* Avascular necrosis of the femoral head and slipped femoral epiphysis, particularly if there is CKD-MBD.
* Intracranial hypertension post-transplant and in children on dialysis.
* There is a possible slight increase in the risk of transplant rejection in patients who have had previous rejection episodes.
* There have previously been concerns about using rhGH post transplant for fear of inducing malignancy. However, the consensus view is that the risk of this is negligible.
* Any potential side effects must be reported.

Further reading

Rees L. Growth hormone therapy in children with CKD after more than two decades of practice. *Pediatr Nephrolo* 2016;31:1421–1435.

Management: enteral feeding

Background

- Enteral feeding is indicated when calorie or protein intake is inadequate, or when struggling with oral intake in an anorexic child causes intolerable strains within the family.
- Although a NG tube is acceptable for a short time, most families prefer the placement of a gastrostomy, which cannot be seen beneath clothing.
- Vomiting may improve following insertion of a gastrostomy, but in children with persistent vomiting a Nissen fundoplication may be indicated.
- Although it is customary to undertake a barium swallow before a Nissen, it is not uncommon for this to be negative, and most would proceed with a Nissen despite this if vomiting is profuse.
- A barium swallow has the additional advantage of excluding gut malrotation.

Nasogastric tubes

Advantages

- The method of choice in the infant weighing <4 kg.
- Placement is simple and easily taught to families.
- There is no risk of peritonitis in children on PD.

Disadvantages

- The trauma of frequent replacement is considerable, for the child and family.
- They may inhibit the development of oromotor skills causing subsequent problems with speech and swallowing.
- Appearance is altered, giving the obvious demonstration of a 'sick child'.
- Rarely, may result in oesophageal or gastric perforation.
- Increased risk of gastro-oesophageal reflux, vomiting, and aspiration because the tube stents open the lower oesophageal sphincter.

Transpyloric tubes

It is possible to advance the feeding tube beyond the stomach, either into the duodenum or jejunum, to try to reduce vomiting. However:

- they are easily displaced and require interventional radiology for insertion and replacement, with frequent radiation exposure.
- they cannot be used for bolus feeds, only continuous feeds.

Gastrostomies

Insertion of a gastrostomy may be percutaneous endoscopic (PEG), percutaneous radiological, or percutaneous laparoscopic. It may also be 'open', of which the commonest type is the Stamm. Whatever the type of placement, the gastrostomy tube exit site is limited to the left upper quadrant of the abdomen or the midline because of the anatomy of the stomach. As a result, PD catheters should not be placed in the left upper quadrant in children who may subsequently need gastrostomy placement.

Perioperative management

- All types require perioperative antibiotic cover.
- Stop medications that reduce gastric acid production as patients on these drugs may have bacteria in their stomachs.

- Leave unused, with the tube left to gravity drainage, for 24–48 h before starting feeds.
- Start with clear fluids administered continuously over 24 h by pump, changing to the appropriate feed when this is tolerated.

Techniques of insertion

Percutaneous endoscopic gastrostomy

The 'pull technique'

- An endoscope is introduced into the stomach and the stomach is insufflated.
- An IV catheter is inserted percutaneously and a wire is passed into the stomach.
- The wire is grabbed and pulled out through the mouth, and the wire is used to pull the gastrostomy tube from the mouth into the stomach and through the abdominal wall.
- The PEG is secured by rigid phalanges inside and outside the abdominal wall.

The 'push technique'

- The wire is passed into the stomach, and used to pass dilators and then the gastrostomy tube.
- Interventional radiological placement uses the push technique:
  - Barium sulphate suspension is given the night before the procedure for colonic opacification.
  - The NG tube is used to insufflate the stomach and screening is used to check that the bowel is satisfactorily displaced.
  - The stomach bubble is identified on fluoroscopy or US, and a needle is introduced and used to pass dilators for the gastrostomy tube.
- Percutaneous laparoscopic procedures use the push technique, but are done under direct vision using a laparoscope. It is difficult to combine with an endoscopic approach due to insufflation inside and outside the stomach.

Open gastrostomy

- A small incision is made and the greater curvature of the stomach is pulled out of the peritoneal cavity.
- A purse-string suture (or two) is placed in the stomach.
- A hole is made in the middle of the purse-string suture and a tube (latex tube such as a Malecot) or a button is placed through purse string, which is then tied.
- The stomach is sewn onto abdominal wall, usually with at least four separate sutures.
- If a latex tube is used, it can be replaced by a button after 3–4 weeks.
- There are different types of button, e.g. MIC-KEY®, Bard Button®, or Mini Button®. The principle is the same—they all have a 'stalk' to insert through the abdominal wall and something to hold the distal (intragastric) portion in the stomach. The internal fixing device can vary, although usually it is a water-filled balloon.
- All buttons have a valve in the lumen to prevent leaking of stomach contents from the lumen of the tube.

Complications

Are reported to be minor in 10–15%, major in 3–5%, and the mortality is up to 1%.

Specific to percutaneous endoscopic gastrostomy

- Intra-abdominal leakage because the tube is held against the abdominal wall with no suturing. Peritonitis can develop in the child on PD.
- Tube blockage.
- Gastrocolic fistula, due to accidental snaring of the colon between the stomach and abdominal wall—the child may present with stools that look like the feed, and weight loss.
- Routine replacement is needed every 2 years under general anaesthetic due to the rigid intragastric portion of the tube. Alternatively, some physicians cut this off and allow it to pass through the GI tract.

Specific to open gastrostomies

- *Balloon rupture*: if the balloon has burst or is leaking, the button needs to be replaced. Parents can be taught to replace the button at home. A smaller lumen tube should be provided in case the button cannot be reinserted by the family.
- *Tube displacement*: if displacement occurs within 2 weeks of surgery, the tract will not be well formed, and forcing a tube may disrupt the stomach from the abdominal wall. The tube should, therefore, be replaced under radiological cover.
- *Closure of the tract*: this can happen very quickly or can take time. In general, the longer the feeding gastrostomy has been in place, the longer the time for the tract to spontaneously close. It is important, therefore, that parents are taught to come to the hospital straight away should there be problems.
- *Tract too large*: the button can be taken out for progressively more hours to allow the tract to shrink.

Of both percutaneous endoscopic and open gastrostomies

- *Leakage around the gastrostomy exit site*: do not put in a bigger tube, pull the balloon tight to the abdominal wall or blow up the balloon more. Wait for the tract to epithelialize, keep the skin in good condition, and cauterize any granulomas.
- *Skin irritation and itching, particularly if there is leakage*: the skin should be kept clean and dry, a barrier cream used, and *Candida* treated if necessary. Skin irritation may progress to 'gastrostomy dermatitis'. The skin should be cleansed each day with soap and water only, avoiding hydrogen peroxide, alcohol, povidone-iodine, and other lotions. Occlusive dressings should not be used.
- *Exit site infection*: swab and use topical antibiotic cream and oral antibiotics if severe. Granulomas can be treated with application of silver nitrate twice a week.
- Failure of the tract to close after tube removal, resulting in a permanent gastrocutaneous fistula, which needs to be surgically closed.
- *Haemorrhage*: most commonly, this is due to bleeding from a granuloma, but can also be due to trauma, or rarely, GI bleeding. It is, therefore, important to differentiate bleeding through the lumen of the tube (GI bleeding) from bleeding around the tube (skin irritation or granulation tissue).

- *Exacerbation of reflux due to distortion of gastric anatomy (rare)*: this may be counteracted by the use of a gastrojejunal tube, entering via the gastrostomy site. Many of these patients may need a subsequent fundoplication.

Open gastrostomy

Indicated in:
- children who have had previous abdominal surgery
- children on PD as there is a risk of PEG formation causing peritonitis. PD should be withheld for a few days after the procedure
- children undergoing Nissen fundoplication
- in the presence on varices (e.g. ARPKD).

Management of a gastrostomy button
- The button is held in place by a water-filled balloon. Parents are taught to test whether the balloon is intact by withdrawing the water from it each week. If the balloon has burst, the button needs to be replaced.
- Parents can be taught to replace the button at home. If they prefer not to, they should be provided with a NG tube in case the button falls out. This should be inserted 2.5 cm (1 inch) into the gastrostomy and strapped in place to keep the tract open until they get to the hospital. Closure of the tract can happen very quickly or may take time. It is important, therefore that parents are taught to contact the hospital straight away should there be problems.
- If there are no complications, the life of the button depends on the make, but some can last for up to 3 years.

Timing of gastrostomy insertion in the child who is about to start or on peritoneal dialysis
- It is better to insert a gastrostomy prior to commencement of PD in order to decrease the risks of peritonitis, because placement of a PEG leads to a small leak of stomach contents into the peritoneal cavity. Dialysate, due to its high dextrose content, will encourage any organisms to rapidly multiply and result in peritonitis.
- The open procedure limits contamination of the peritoneal cavity by entering the gastric lumen outside of the abdomen and by securing the stomach to the abdominal wall with sutures.
- There is no evidence that there is an increased risk of peritonitis in children on PD with an established gastrostomy.

Post-transplant management

In the majority of children, appetite improves post transplant so that the gastrostomy can be removed, although some continue to need it for the administration of fluids and medications. Its continued use will also be affected by the success of the transplant.
- Assess dietary intake 4–6 weeks post-transplant.
- Proportionately decrease feed as oral intake increases.
- Remove gastrostomy when diet, growth, fluids, and medication intake satisfactory, if the transplant is functioning well.

Further reading

Rees L, Brandt ML. Tube feeding in children with CKD: technical and practical issues. *Pediatr Nephrol* 2010;25:699–704.

MANAGEMENT: MINERAL AND BONE DISORDER 479

Management: mineral and bone disorder

CKD leads to abnormal vitamin D, Ca, phosphate, fibroblast growth factor 23 (FGF23), and PTH metabolism as follows:

- Decreased plasma 25(OH)D: due to dietary restrictions, decreased manufacture in skin because of reduced activity and sun exposure in children with CKD, and urinary losses of vitamin D-binding protein if proteinuria.
- Decreased Ca intake due to dietary restrictions.
- Increased FGF23 and decrease of its co-receptor Klotho in response to an increased phosphate load, resulting in phosphaturia, and maintaining a normal plasma phosphate in early CKD.
- Increased Plasma phosphate (when increased FGF23 can no longer compensate) due to decreased clearance and increased GI absorption if the active form of vitamin D, 1,25-dihydroxyvitamin D (1,25(OH)$_2$D) is prescribed.
- Decreased 1α hydroxylation of 25(OH)D to the active form, 1,25(OH)$_2$D.
- Decreased Ca absorption due to decreased 1,25(OH)$_2$D.
- Increased PTH due to low plasma Ca, high phosphate, and low 1,25(OH)$_2$D.

Untreated, CKD-MBD results, which is a constellation of:

- disordered bone turnover, mineralization, volume, and strength.
- bone pain and fractures.
- abnormal growth.
- vascular and soft tissue calcification.
- increased mortality from cardiovascular disease.

The term CKD-MBD is used to encompass all these abnormalities; renal osteodystrophy should be reserved for the bony abnormalities that are seen on histology.

Sequence of the events that cause chronic kidney disease–mineral bone disorders

Early CKD

See Fig. 18.1.

- Increased plasma 25(OH)D results in decreased 1,25(OH)$_2$D.
- Decreased 1,25(OH)$_2$D leads to low Ca absorption and (beneficially) low phosphate absorption.
- Low dietary Ca intake along with low absorption lead to low plasma Ca.
- The decrease in GFR and renal tubular phosphate excretion would be expected to cause hyperphosphataemia early in CKD. However, this is prevented by the FGF23–Klotho axis.

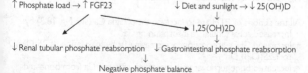

Fig. 18.1 Phosphate balance in early CKD.

FGF23

- Acts with its co-receptor Klotho, expression of which is decreased in early CKD.
- Requires Klotho to activate FGF signalling.
- Increased in early CKD in response to a high phosphate load.
- Produced by osteocytes and acts on the renal tubules to decrease phosphate reabsorption.
- Able to maintain plasma phosphate in the normal range in early CKD.
- Suppresses the renal 1α hydroxylase receptor, thereby reducing the synthesis of 1,25(OH)$_2$D and therefore GI phosphate absorption (and, adversely, Ca).
- Significantly linked with cardiovascular mortality.

CKD progression

- FGF23 is no longer able to compensate for the decreased glomerular filtration of phosphate and the plasma phosphate rises.
- The high plasma phosphate stimulates the secretion of PTH, which is also a phosphaturic hormone.
- Decreased renal 1α hydroxylase activity results in decreased conversion of 25(OH)D to 1,25(OH)$_2$D.
- Decreased 1,25(OH)$_2$D levels stimulate PTH secretion via the vitamin D receptors (VDR) in the PTH gland.
- Decreased plasma Ca stimulates PTH via the Ca sensing receptors (CaSRs).

See Fig. 18.2.

CaSR

- Vital to the minute-to-minute control that maintains the plasma ionized Ca within a narrow physiological range.
- If there is a small fall in ionized Ca, the PTH increases steeply, resulting in normalization of the serum Ca.
- In contrast, a rise in ionized Ca acts via the CaSR to shut off PTH secretion.
- Present in high concentrations on parathyroid cells and is also on bone cells and along the nephron.
- Stimulated by magnesium (to suppress PTH).

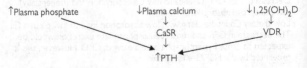

Fig. 18.2 Factors that stimulate PTH production.

All the actions of PTH are to increase the plasma Ca (see Fig. 18.3) by:
- Increased renal tubular reabsorption of Ca.
- Increased GI Ca absorption by increasing 1α hydroxylation of 25(OH)D to 1,25(OH)$_2$D.
- Increased bone turnover and, therefore, efflux of Ca from bone and decreased renal tubular reabsorption of phosphate.

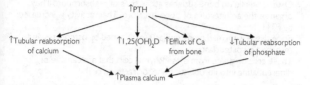

Fig. 18.3 Effects of PTH.

However, this creates a vicious circle of ongoing PTH stimulation, because:
- the increase in 1,25(OH)$_2$D augments phosphate absorption (alongside Ca), which in turn, stimulates PTH secretion further.
- CKD decreases the expression of the CaSR in the parathyroid glands so that Ca sensing is altered so that there is an increase in the set point for Ca (the Ca level at which there is a 50% reduction in PTH) and a change in the degree of suppression by Ca throughout the Ca-sensitive range.
- high plasma phosphate levels also increase the set point for Ca.

Persistent stimulation of the parathyroid glands leads to PTH resistance (Fig. 18.4). The logic, therefore, has to be that prevention of the process starting by early dietary intervention with phosphate restriction, and the use of phosphate binders and vitamin D as soon as metabolic derangements are detected, must be beneficial.

Persistent parathyroid stimulation

↓   Half-life of parathyroid cells is 30 years

Parathyroid hyperplasia

↓

Reduced VDR and CaSR expression

↓

Less suppression of PTH by 1,25(OH)$_2$D and calcium

↓

Nodular hyperplasia

↓

Need for parathyroidectomy

Fig. 18.4 The evolution of resistance to PTH.

Renal osteodystrophy

Normal bone turnover

During normal bone turnover:
- Osteoblasts form a layer at the site of new bone formation. Some become trapped in new bone and become osteocytes.
- Osteocytes enable metabolic exchange between the tissue fluids and bone, and withdraw or deposit minerals.

- Osteoclasts lie on bone surfaces at the sites of reabsorption. They organize the architecture of bone structure. Their activity is increased by PTH.
- Bone tissue is formed by osteoblasts, maintained by osteocytes and resorbed by osteoclasts.
- These cells originate from mesenchymal cells that are capable of differentiating into fibroblasts, bone, or cartilage cells.

The effect of PTH on the skeleton is to increase the activity of osteoclasts and osteoblasts:
- High PTH levels cause high bone turnover (osteitis fibrosa) with:
  - increased osteoclasts and bone resorption.
  - increased osteoblasts and bone formation, with increased osteoid and non-lamellar bone.
  - marrow fibrosis.
- Low PTH levels cause low-turnover (adynamic) bone disease:
  - normal or reduced osteoid.
  - low or diminished numbers of osteoclasts and osteoblasts.

Both low and high bone turnover lead to bone pain, fractures, deformities, and growth problems, and contribute to CVD.

Radiological changes

Radiological changes of CKD-MBD include rickets, hyperparathyroidism, and osteosclerosis, with:
- periosteal erosions.
- elevation and widening of the zone of provisional calcification with a coarse trabecular pattern.
- vertebral collapse, alternating with areas of osteosclerosis, giving the appearance called rugger jersey spine.

Radiological changes occur late and bone X-rays may be normal even with moderate hyperparathyroidism.

Vascular calcification

Cardiovascular disease (CVD) is the major cause of mortality in patients with CKD. Risk is increased 30-fold in comparison with the age-matched population, and much more in patients on dialysis. Calcification of the vascular media is characteristic of CKD.
- The most important factor contributing to this is the plasma phosphate.
- Plasma phosphate is an independent predictor of mortality in adults with CKD.
- Hyperphosphataemia causes osteoblastic differentiation of vascular smooth muscle cells that leads to vascular calcification.
- Resultant stiffening of the blood vessels causes diastolic dysfunction, hypertension, and increased cardiac work.
- Plasma calcium, PTH, and FGF23 also contribute to CVD in CKD-MBD.
- Vitamin D levels both above and below the normal range are associated with vascular calcification.

Aims of management of chronic kidney disease-mineral bone disorders

- To maintain normal bone turnover and therefore prevent symptoms of bone pain and fractures.
- To allow normal growth.
- To prevent CVD and soft tissue calcification.

It is important to intervene early in the course of CKD to prevent escape of the parathyroid glands from normal control mechanisms.

Phosphate control

Phosphate has probably the best described spectrum of toxicity of all molecules that circulate in excess in CKD:

- Decreased renal phosphate excretion plays a major role in the onset of hyperparathyroidism.
- Plasma phosphate levels are positively and independently correlated with an increasing risk of death from CVD: as phosphate levels increase above 5.6 mg/dL (= 1.8 mmol/L), the hazard ratio for mortality increases by 6% for every 1 mg/dL (= 0.3 mmol/L) increase in serum phosphate.
- Phosphate causes vascular calcification, which leads to diastolic dysfunction, hypertension, and increased cardiac work.

What phosphate level should we aim for?

- There is an association between phosphate levels and coronary artery calcification even in young adults without kidney disease.
- In patients with CKD, rising phosphate levels within the normal range are associated with a greater prevalence of vascular and valvular calcification.
- There are no clinical trials addressing the issue of plasma phosphate levels and mortality, although one study has demonstrated that the use of any type of phosphate binder, even with phosphate levels in the normal range, is associated with decreased mortality in patients on HD.
- Plasma phosphate varies throughout childhood, falling steeply from birth until the age of 1–2 years, then continuing to fall more slowly until the age of 7 years (Fig. 18.5).
- The optimum target is not clear, but a plasma phosphate level that is persistently at the upper limit of normal (ULN) implies that there are times when it is above normal. It makes sense, therefore, to try to keep the plasma phosphate around the 50th centile.

Dietary phosphate is principally in protein-containing foods, and dairy products in particular. Processed foods contain phosphate in significant quantities as it is a component of moisture and flavour enhancers.

- A normal adult diet contains ~800–1500 mg of phosphate, of which 50–70% is absorbed, depending on serum phosphate and vitamin D levels.
- $1,25(OH)_2D$ increases phosphate absorption to as much as 80–90%.
- In early CKD, dietary restriction may be sufficient to control plasma phosphate levels.
- Table 18.10 shows a suggested weight-related daily dietary phosphate intake for children with CKD.

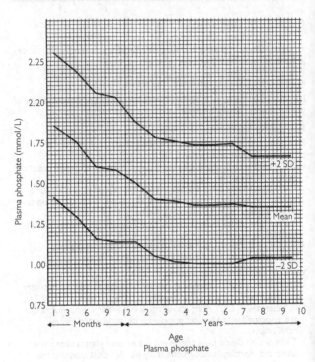

Fig. 18.5 Phosphate centiles according to age. Dietary control of phosphate.
Reproduced with permission from Clayton BE, Jenkins P, Round JM, (eds). (1980). *Paediatric Chemical Pathology: Clinical tests and reference ranges.* Oxford, UK: Wiley-Blackwell. Copyright © 1980 Wiley-Blackwell.

Table 18.10 Weight-related suggested daily dietary phosphate intake for children with CKD

Body weight (kg)	Phosphate allowance (mg)
<10	<400
10–20	<600
20–40	<800
>40	<1000

- Because restriction of dietary phosphate has its principal effects after meals, there may be no change in the morning plasma phosphate levels, so plasma values obtained in the afternoon are more useful in monitoring the effect of phosphate restriction or phosphate binders.
- The problem with dietary intervention is that foods high in phosphate are also usually high in Ca and vitamin D, so that nutritional 25(OH)D and Ca deficiency is common.

Phosphate binders

As CKD progresses, the majority of patients need a phosphate binder to reduce phosphate absorption. Phosphate binders are divided into Ca containing and non-Ca containing:

- Ca-containing preparations have been used the longest and are by far the most widely used phosphate binder, but have fallen out of favour because of their theoretical link with soft tissue calcification; the fear of ectopic calcification with excess Ca intake has led to a switch to newer non-Ca-containing drugs.
- Phosphate binders must be given with food and must not be given at the same time as Fe preparations as they form insoluble compounds in the gut. All the phosphate binders may have GI side effects. Preparations and cost of commonly used phosphate binders are shown in Table 18.11.

Calcium-containing phosphate binders

- Dissociation of $CaCO_3$ is maximal below a pH of 5, whereas maximal binding of Ca to phosphate is at a higher pH. It is not, therefore, as effective when given with H2 blockers or proton pump inhibitors.
- Ca acetate has better solubility over a wider range of pH. This means that Ca acetate has a greater binding capacity for the same elemental Ca content so that less Ca is absorbed (Table 18.12).
- Ca absorption is greater if the binder is taken between meals, when it acts as a Ca supplement.
- Absorption varies with plasma $1,25(OH)_2D$ levels, being as low as 3% in deficiency to presumably higher than the expected normal range in patients who are prescribed activated vitamin D, when hypercalcaemia may occur.
- The main issue with Ca-containing binders is the risk of absorption of Ca that cannot be excreted if urine production is reduced, resulting in hypercalcaemia and a risk of ectopic calcification.

Non-calcium-containing phosphate binders

Magnesium carbonate

- $MgCO_3$ is not commonly used, due to its propensity to cause diarrhoea.
- It is less effective than Ca salts.
- It may be a problem for children on dialysis, who are often already hypermagnesaemic.

Sevelamer hydrochloride

- Sevelamer is a non-absorbable polymer of allylamine hydrochloride.
- It functions best at pH 6–7 in the small intestine.
- It acts like an exchange resin; organic anions, and in particular phosphate, bind to cationic amine groups, displacing the chloride

Table 18.11 Preparations and cost of commonly used phosphate binders. Only calcium carbonate and acetate are licensed in all ages, and sevelamer hydrochloride for those >12 years of age

Preparation	Relative cost per capsule/tablet
Calcium containing	
Calcium acetate	n
Calcium carbonate	n × 1 to 2
Non-calcium containing	
Sevelamer hydrochloride	n × 6
Sevelamer bicarbonate	n × 6
Sevelamer bicarbonate sachets	n × 20

Table 18.12 Calcium-containing phosphate binders

	Elemental Ca content %	% Ca absorbed	Phosphate (mg) bound per mg Ca absorbed	Phosphate (mg) bound by 1 g
Calcium carbonate	40	20–30	1 mg P per 8 mg Ca	39
Calcium acetate	25	20 with meals, 40 between meals	1 mg P per 1–3 mg Ca	45

moiety. For this reason, an associated metabolic acidosis is common. Sevelamer is now available as the carbonate, which may remove this side effect.

- As well as phosphate, sevelamer binds bile salts, thereby exerting a beneficial effect on plasma total and low density cholesterol, but on the other hand, sevelamer also binds fat-soluble vitamins.
- The tablets need to be swallowed, and are difficult to use in children who are dependent on tube feeds because they form a gel that swells inside the tube causing a blockage.
- Hypercalcaemia is less common, but many children need Ca supplements.
- Sevelamer may attenuate the progress of coronary and aortic calcification when it is already established, probably through its effects on blood lipids, but there is no proven benefit over other binders in its prevention in patients in whom calcification has not started.
- Sevelamer is of benefit in patients who have a high dietary Ca intake. However, children on a low-phosphate diet who are not receiving a Ca-containing phosphate binder probably do not have a positive Ca balance when they are on maintenance dialysis.
- KDOQI recommends that in children exclusively on sevelamer, a higher dialysate Ca concentration and/or Ca supplementation with a Ca-containing phosphate binder is used.

Lanthanum carbonate
- Lanthanum is a trivalent cation that binds phosphate ionically and is active over a wide pH.
- Concerns centre on its safety because of the potential for its accumulation in the body, particularly in bone and liver, but absorption is low; <0.0013% is absorbed and is then excreted in bile.
- Studies in adults show that binding is similar to other Ca binders, and there is less hypercalcaemia and a similar incidence of hypocalcaemia to sevelamer.
- Lanthanum has now been used for 6 years with no evidence of significant side effects. There are no studies in children.

Case for and against calcium-containing phosphate binders
Recently, there has been a swing away from Ca-containing phosphate binders towards the routine use of sevelamer. The concern is that with the large doses of Ca from Ca-containing phosphate binders, coupled with decreased urinary excretion of Ca, particularly in the face of low bone turn-over, hypercalcaemia will occur and cause soft tissue calcification. Although this is a theoretical possibility, evidence of an improvement in survival in patients taking sevelamer is lacking.

Evidence for the use of calcium-containing phosphate binders in children
- Vascular calcification in paediatric patients is not a new phenomenon, and was seen at a time when aluminium hydroxide was the only commonly used phosphate binder.
- Coronary artery abnormalities were identified at postmortem in 12 children who had been on HD in the 1970s, and soft tissue calcification was present in 60% of autopsies undertaken in 120 children with uraemia, dialysis, or renal transplants who died between 1960 and 1983.
- Most studies are in adults, but there are dangers in extrapolating adult data to children, in whom there is the added dimension of a need for a positive Ca balance in the growing skeleton.
- It has to be remembered that not all hypercalcaemia is due to intestinal Ca absorption, and that high bone turnover itself can do this by increasing the efflux of Ca from bone. Indeed, hypercalcaemia is described with both sevelamer and lanthanum and vascular calcification is seen in adult pre-dialysis CKD patients who are not prescribed any phosphate binder.

Evidence against calcium-containing phosphate binders in children
- Some, but not all paediatric studies have identified a relationship between Ca-containing phosphate binder intake and cardiac calcification, left ventricular mass and/or carotid intima–media thickness.
- The serum Ca level does not reflect the total body Ca load.
- It is likely that episodes of hypercalcaemia in patients on dialysis, in whom calcification inhibitors are compromised, will worsen vascular calcification, particularly in association with high plasma phosphate.

Calcium

Of the total body Ca, 99% is in the skeleton, 0.6% in soft tissues, and 0.1% in ECF. Total skeletal Ca increases from ~25 g at birth to 900 and 1200 g in adult females and males, respectively.

* At low dietary Ca intakes, a greater proportion is absorbed (~34%), and is proportional to circulating 25(OH)D levels.
* At higher dietary intakes, there is less influence of vitamin D on Ca absorption, and less Ca is absorbed (~29%), i.e. there is adaptation to low 25(OH)D levels and dietary Ca intake.
* The amount of Ca incorporated into the skeleton increases up to a threshold dietary intake, above which no further bone accumulation occurs. This threshold is influenced by age such that during periods of rapid growth, i.e. infancy and adolescence, Ca balance is at its highest. These high Ca requirements are in comparison with the much lower values in adults (Table 18.13).
* The normal range for Ca parallels that of phosphate throughout childhood (Fig. 18.6).
* A low-phosphate diet is by definition also low in Ca (and 25(OH)D), and many children may be relying on their phosphate binder to provide adequate Ca intake.
* KDOQI recommends intake of 100% of the DRI for Ca, and limitation of the Ca intake from binders and dialysate solutions to <2 × DRI or <2500 mg elemental Ca.
* Ca balance is difficult in oliguric patients on dialysis. A dialysate Ca concentration of 1.75 mmol/L provides an influx of around 800 mg; 1.25 mmol/L will maintain neutral Ca balance.

Vitamin D

Evidence is emerging that the benefits of vitamin D extend beyond its effect on bone:

* It has anti-inflammatory properties and beneficial effects on the cardiovascular system.
* This has to be balanced against the risks of increased Ca and phosphate absorption, and hypercalcaemia and hyperphosphataemia.
* If it is possible to measure 25(OH)D, and this proves to be low, replacement doses of ergo or colecalciferol should be prescribed. Maintenance doses can be safely prescribed without routine measurement of levels.

Table 18.13 The calcium intake above which no further incorporation of calcium into bone occurs and the calcium balance per day at different ages

Age (years)	Ca threshold (mg/day)	Balance per day (mg/day)
0–1	1090	503 ± 91
2–8	1390	246 ± 126
9–17	1480	396 ± 164
18–30	957	114 ± 133

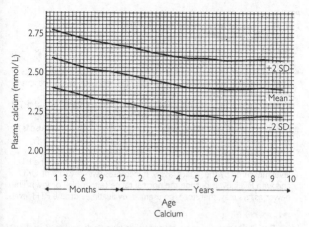

Fig. 18.6 Calcium centiles according to age.

Reproduced with permission from Clayton BE, Jenkins P, Round JM, (eds). (1980). *Paediatric Chemical Pathology: Clinical tests and reference ranges.* Oxford, UK: Wiley-Blackwell. Copyright © 1980 Wiley-Blackwell.

- If the PTH is high despite 25(OH)D supplementation and phosphate control, the smallest possible dose of 1,25(OH)$_2$D to suppress the PTH (0.01 micrograms/kg/day) can be introduced and then the dose titrated against the PTH level. The lowest possible dose is used to prevent its depressant effect on osteoblasts and hypercalcaemia.
- If hypercalcaemia develops, the 1,25(OH)$_2$D should be stopped.
- New vitamin D analogues may suppress hyperparathyroidism without inducing hypercalcaemia.

Parathyroid hormone

Guidelines for the management of CKD-MBD hinge on the need to keep the PTH level within a fixed range, which is one that maintains normal bone turnover. Current guidelines were written as our understanding of the interplay with CVD was emerging, are largely opinion based as they are extrapolated from adult studies and a small number of paediatric studies, and are largely out of date. The area is controversial, but there is a swing away from currently recommended very high levels in dialysis patients towards levels that are up to twice the upper limit of normal.

- European guidelines recommend maintaining the PTH in the normal range until dialysis, when up to 3 × ULN is acceptable.
- KDOQI recommends the normal range until CKD 4, when 1 to 2 × ULN is recommended and then 3–5 × ULN for patients on dialysis.
- When hyperparathyroidism becomes tertiary, with persistent hypercalcaemia, radiological changes, and no response to treatment, parathyroidectomies may become necessary.
- CaSR blockers (e.g. cinacalcet) are effective in reducing plasma Ca, phosphate, and PTH, and may be useful to try in the treatment of tertiary hyperparathyroidism before considering parathyroidectomy.

PTH assays

- PTH consists of 84 amino acids, 1–84PTH.
- Fragments of 1–84PTH circulate in CKD.
- Actions of the fragments depend on the presence of the amino or C terminal.
- 7–84PTH is the most important quantitatively in CKD. It antagonizes 1–84 PTH, acts at a specific C-terminal PTH receptor, and is present in the parathyroid gland.
- Current 'intact' immunoradiometric assays (IRMAs) measure 1–84PTH and also its fragments. The term 'intact' is therefore a misnomer.
- Newer assays (CAP-IRMA) measure only 1–84 PTH, but their use is not yet fully validated.
- The proportion of circulating PTH fragments can be calculated by subtracting the PTH level as measured by the new assay from the PTH level measured by the 'intact' assay. It increases with severity of CKD and with PTH levels outside the normal range (either high or low). The newer assays may, therefore, be useful in evaluating extreme PTH levels.

Further reading

Rees L, Shroff R. The demise of calcium-based phosphate binders-is this appropriate for children? *Pediatr Nephrol* 2015;30:2061–2071.

Management: anaemia

Background

The anaemia of CKD begins when the GFR falls below 35 mL/min/1.73 m^2. It is a normochromic, normocytic anaemia, with a low reticulocyte count. Causes are:

- decreased production of erythropoietin.
- decreased red cell survival.
- bone marrow inhibition due to uraemia or chronic inflammation.
- iron, vitamin B12, or folate deficiency.
- osteitis fibrosa.
- ACE inhibitors.
- blood loss during HD, from the GI tract or from repeated blood sampling.
- aluminium toxicity.

Important general points

- ESAs are effective in improving the anaemia of CKD and the failing renal transplant.
- The requirement relative to body weight decreases with age, being highest in infants.
- Dosage intervals can be determined by response and vary with the product.
- Erythropoietin is conventionally given weekly SC and more frequently in HD patients when it is given IV up to 3 times per week.
- Darbepoetin alfa has a longer half-life than erythropoietin, and is usually given every 2–4 weeks SC in pre-dialysis patients, every 1–2 weeks SC in PD patients, and weekly IV in HD patients. Pain at the injection site has been reported.
- Newer products being tested in children may enable administration as infrequently as monthly.
- Fe supplementation (oral or IV) is required.
- Oral Fe must be separated from phosphate binders and food by 2 h before or 1 h after. Proton pump inhibitors decrease absorption.
- All children should achieve a haemoglobin level above the lower limit of the normal range for age, but the upper limit is not known. An increase in cardiovascular events in adults with higher haemoglobin levels has led to a non-evidence-based recommendation of 10–12 g/dL for children. Recent evidence suggests better outcomes for children with levels at the higher end of the normal range.
- The normal range for haemoglobin for age and the level at which to begin evaluation for anaemia (when the haemoglobin is approaching the lower end of the normal range) by the measurement of Fe and folic acid levels and commencement of Fe therapy are shown in Table 18.14.

Assessment of iron stores

As well as absolute Fe deficiency, functional deficiency occurs when there is a need for a greater amount of Fe to support haemoglobin synthesis than can be released from Fe stores:

- High Fe availability is required to maximize the response to ESAs.

- Serum ferritin reflects body Fe stores and needs to be kept between 100 and 500 micrograms/L. However, it is an acute phase reactant so results may be difficult to interpret in the infected child, and CRP should be measured at the same time.
- Transferrin saturation is a marker of the amount of Fe available for incorporation into haemoglobin and should be >20%.
- Reticulocyte haemoglobin content is an indirect measure of the functional Fe available.

Management

See Fig. 18.7 and Table 18.15.

Darbepoetin alfa

- Darbepoetin alfa is a hyperglycosylated derivative of erythropoietin with a longer half-life.
- Darbepoetin alfa is available in the following strengths—20, 40, 60, 80, 100, 150, 300, and 500 micrograms as prefilled syringes or a prefilled disposable injection pen device (pen not advised if <25 kg as easy bruising).
- The complete vial always needs to be used; due to the unpredictability of mixing of the active drug in its suspension, incomplete use of the total dose will lead to administration of an unknown quantity of darbepoetin. Therefore, an increase in dose can only be according to the strengths available.
- The withdrawal of some preparations of erythropoietin beta (cartridges for use with the RecoPen® and prefilled syringes 1000 U) necessitates a change to darbepoetin for most children excluding infants.
- Darbepoetin alfa is approved for correction of anaemia and maintenance of a normal haemoglobin level in children age >11 years and haemoglobin maintenance if age >1 year and converting from stable doses of erythropoietin. It can be used off licence for anaemia correction at age 3–11 years. There is minimal information on the use of darbepoetin alfa in infants aged <1 year who should be treated with erythropoietin beta and then remain on erythropoietin beta or converted to darbepoetin alfa at age >1 year.

Table 18.14 Normal range for haemoglobin throughout childhood

Age range (years)	Mean haemoglobin level (g/dL)		Range or SD	5th percentile	
	Boys	Girls		Boys	Girls
0–0.5	11.5		9.5–13.5	9.5	
0.5–1	12.0		10.5–13.5	10.5	
1–2	12.0	12.0	±0.8	10.7	10.8
3–5	12.4	12.4	±0.8	11.2	11.1
6–8	12.9	12.8	±0.8	11.2	11.5
9–11	13.3	13.1	±0.8	12.0	11.9
12–14	14.1	13.3	±1.1	12.4	11.7
15–19	15.1	13.2	±1.0	13.5	11.5

Haemoglobin lower end of normal range
↓
Start oral Fe if ferritin <100 micrograms/L at dose of up to 6 mg/kg elemental Fe per day
or 1–2 mg/kg of elemental Fe per week IV
to maintain ferritin at 100–500 micrograms/L and TSAT 20–50%
check B12 and folate

↓   ↓

Erythropoietin beta 100 U/kg/week   **or**   Darbepoetin alfa 0.75 micrograms/kg every
subcutaneously or 50 U/kg three   2 weeks predialysis or 0.45 micrograms/kg
a week if IV   /week if on dialysis

↓

Measure haemoglobin, retics and ferritin monthly
Transferrin saturation if poor response
↓
If haemoglobin response <1gdL/month, consider:

↓   ↓

Functional iron deficiency;   Occult infection,
if transferrin saturation <20%   blood loss, or low vitamin B12
give IV iron   or folate

↓

If no cause found: erythropoietin↑ dose by 25%
Darbepoetin ↑ to the next syringe dose strength
↓
When stable haemoglobin, check every 2–3 months with ferritin TSAT and retics,
but if on IV Fe, check monthly

Fig. 18.7 Commencement of an ESA.

- Starting dose for children not previously receiving an ESA:
  - *Pre-dialysis*: 0.75 micrograms/kg SC every 2 weeks.
  - *PD*: 0.45 micrograms/kg SC weekly.
  - *HD*: 0.45 micrograms/kg IV weekly.
- Check the haemoglobin 2 weeks after starting darbepoetin alfa. If the haemoglobin has risen >1 g/dL, withhold the dose for a week and then give the next smallest dose strength, e.g. if receiving 30 micrograms go to 20 micrograms.
- If the haemoglobin increase is <1 g/dL after 2 weeks, do not change dose. However, if after 4 weeks the increase is still <1 g/dL, increase the dose to the next syringe strength. Do not increase dose more frequently than every 4 weeks.
- Continue until the target haemoglobin is reached.
- *Maintenance dose when target Hb achieved*: decrease the frequency of injections for predialysis or PD and increase proportionately the total dose at each injection: e.g. predialysis patient (25 kg) requiring 20 micrograms darbepoetin alfa every 2 weeks will need 40 micrograms every 4 weeks:
  - *Pre-dialysis*: SC every 3–4 weeks.
  - *PD*: SC every 2–3 weeks.
  - *HD*: IV every 1–2 weeks.
- *Conversion from erythropoietin beta*:

Weekly EPO dose (U) ÷ 240 = weekly darbepoetin alfa dose (microgram)

- I.e. PD patient maintained on 5000 U erythropoietin beta weekly will need 20 micrograms darbepoetin alfa weekly or 40 micrograms every 2 weeks (note adjustments of dose to correlate with prefilled syringe doses available).
- Children must be on a minimum weekly erythropoietin beta dose of 1200 U (~) to convert to an equivalent minimum available dose of darbepoetin alfa, i.e. 10 micrograms every 2 weeks (Table 18.15).

Table 18.15 Dose of IV iron according to ferritin and TSAT levels

	Ferritin (micrograms/L)	TSAT	Dose	Maximum single dose
Maintenance dose	>100 and <500	>20%	2 mg/kg/dose given every 2 weeks	100 mg
Accelerated dose	<100	<20%	7 mg/kg/dose × 1 dose for first week then 2 mg/kg/dose given once every 2 weeks	200 mg 100 mg
No treatment	>500	>50%		

Maintenance intravenous iron therapy for children on haemodialysis

All IV Fe formulations may be associated with immune-mediated reactions that may lead to anaphylaxis (more common with Fe dextran formulations) and the release of bioactive and partially unbound Fe into the circulation by the Fe agent, causing oxidative stress and hypotension (non-dextran forms). Most centres now use Fe sucrose, which carries less risk:

- Fe substitution is critical for optimal response to ESAs. Oral Fe may be poorly absorbed and may not be able to keep pace with the requirements of the marrow.
- IV Fe can be easily given to children on HD.
- Children on maintenance IV Fe therapy do not need oral supplements.
- The serum ferritin (micrograms/L) should be measured monthly. Fe (μmol/L) and transferrin (μmol/L) should be measured if response to the ESA is poor.
- Transferrin saturation (TSAT) can be calculated as follows:

$$TSAT = Fe \ (\mu mol/L)/2 \times transferrin \ (\mu mol/L) \ (\%)$$

- Treatment depends on the results of the serum ferritin and TSAT (Table 18.15).

Administration of IV iron

Fe (III)-hydroxide sucrose complex (Venofer®)—'off-label' use in children:

- Venofer® must only be administered by the IV route, either by slow IV injection at a rate of 1 mL undiluted solution/min (i.e. 5 min/100 mg ampoule), or by IV infusion.
- Extravasation of IV Fe causes a painful tissue reaction; secure IV access must be obtained prior to administration.
- Before administering the first dose to a new patient, a test dose of Venofer® must be given as follows:
  - *IV injection*: 0.5–1 mL (10–20 mg,) should be injected slowly over a period of 1–2 min. If no adverse events occur within 15 min of completing the test dose, then the remaining portion of the injection may be given.
  - *IV infusion*: preferred route for patients not on HD. Dilute 5 mL Venofer® (100 mg Fe) in 100 mL 0.9% NaCl. No other solution should be used. Infuse the first 25 mg Fe (i.e. 25 mL solution) as a test dose IV over a period of 15 min; if no adverse reactions occur during this time then the remaining portion of the infusion may be given at a rate of not more than 50 mL in 15 min. (Suggested infusion rate = 2 mg Fe (2 mL solution) per min.)
- Facilities for cardiopulmonary resuscitation must be available because allergic or anaphylactoid reactions, and hypotensive episodes may occur.
- Venofer® may be administered during the middle of the HD session directly into the venous limb of the dialyser under the same procedure as for IV administration.

Contraindications to IV iron

- Fe overload or disturbances in utilization of Fe.
- History of hypersensitivity to parenteral Fe preparations.
- History of asthma, eczema, or other allergic disorders or anaphylactic reactions.
- Clinical or biochemical evidence of liver damage.
- Acute or chronic infection.

Side effects of IV iron

- Very rarely, anaphylaxis or other allergic reactions can occur—if so, discontinue promptly. Allergic reactions have been more commonly observed when the recommended dosage is exceeded.
- Occasionally, metallic taste, headache, nausea, and vomiting.
- Hypotension may occur if the injection is administered too rapidly.
- Less frequently, abdominal disorders, paraesthesia, muscular pain, fever, urticaria, flushing, oedema of the extremities, phlebitis, and venous spasm at site of injection.

Pure red cell aplasia with anti-erythropoietin antibodies

- Consider diagnosis if escalating dose of ESA or epoetin dose >350 U/kg/ darbepoetin alfa >1.5 micrograms/kg/week.
- Occurred particularly in association with epoetin alfa (Eprex®), mostly if given SC. The incidence has decreased since the method by which Eprex® is stored and reconstituted was changed.
- Has also been reported rarely with epoetin beta and darbepoetin.
- Usually recovers, but may need immunosuppression.

Benefits of treatment of anaemia

- Anaemia may contribute to the progression of CKD.
- Amelioration of left ventricular hypertrophy.
- Improved quality of life and decreased hospitalization.
- Reduced need for transfusion, with its risks of infection and human leucocyte antigen (HLA) sensitization.

Further reading

Warady BA, Silverstein DM. Management of anemia with erythropoietic-stimulating agents in children with chronic kidney disease. *Pediatr Nephrol* 2014;29:1493–1505

Preparation for renal replacement therapy

Background

The general principle is that transplantation should be the ultimate aim for the overwhelming majority of children with CKD stage 5 in whom active treatment is felt appropriate. Preferably transplantation should be performed within the 6-month period prior to the need for dialysis (pre-emptive transplantation). Children should be prepared for a living or deceased donor transplant once the GFR is <15 mL/min/1.73 m² and it is clear that they are likely to require dialysis in the near future and/or are experiencing significant complications of their CKD, including growth failure. In this way dialysis may be avoided.

It is preferable to avoid dialysis because:
- dialysis is disruptive to family lifestyle, schooling, and social interactions, and places huge demands on the family.
- dietary and fluid restrictions are necessary on dialysis.
- mortality is higher on dialysis than post transplant.
- avoidance of dialysis preserves vascular and peritoneal access sites for future use.
- dialysis is associated with vascular calcification and risk of cardiovascular events.
- well-being, growth, and development are improved post transplant.

Discussions on choice of modality of RRT should begin at least 1 year before the anticipated date of starting. This enables:
- preparation of child and family for RRT.
- preparation of a living donor.
- pre-emptive transplantation.

Preparation for transplantation

Investigations and procedures that need to be completed before transplantation (Table 18.16) are as follows:
- Blood group and tissue typing.
- Is this to be a deceased donor or living related donor (LRD) transplant?
- If LRD, blood group potential donors and tissue type those with compatible blood group (group O is the universal donor, group AB the universal recipient).
- ABO incompatible transplant can be considered; check ABO antibody titres.
- Check immunity to hepatitis B and C, measles, mumps, varicella, HIV, CMV, and EBV.
- Ensure immunizations are complete (➔ see 'Immunization schedule for children with chronic kidney disease', p. 509).
- Ensure bladder is safe for transplantation:
  - If there is complete bladder emptying on US it is likely to be satisfactory.
  - Urodynamics will be necessary in children with structural renal anomalies that involve the bladder (e.g. severe VUR, posterior urethral valves, neuropathic bladder).
  - Decide where the transplant ureter will be anastomosed.

Table 18.16 A suggested pre-transplant assessment check list

	Date	Comment/result
Previous transplants		
LRD/deceased donor		
Blood group		
Tissue typing		
Cross-match (LRD)		
Immunization history		Separate sheet
Antibody results	Varicella	
	Measles	
	CMV repeat every 3 months if negative	
	EBV repeat every 3 months if negative	
	Hepatitis B	
	Hepatitis C	
	HIV	
US of aorta, IVC, and iliac vessels		
MRV/MRA (if previous femoral lines, transplant or child with VATER)		
Coagulation and procoagulation screen		
Bladder US		
Urodynamics		
Transplant ureter to be transplanted into		
Dental review		
Dialysis access		
Details of previous abdominal surgery		
Detailed interview with nephrology consultant		
Detailed interview with transplant surgeon		
Detailed interview with transplant sister		
Psychosocial assessment		

LRD, living related donor.

- If there have been previous lines into iliac vessels, or a previous transplant, US and MRA and MRV to ensure vessel patency.
- Children with VATER (vertebral defects, anal atresia, trachea-oesophageal fistula with (o)eosophageal atresia, renal defects, and radial dysplasia) may have a high dividing aorta and need MRA and MRV.
- HLA antibody measurement.
- Dental review, particularly looking for infection.
- Ensure that parents and child are fully informed.
- Ensure that the family and child have been offered a psychosocial assessment.

Coagulation and thrombosis screening prior to renal transplantation

Most important is the patient and family history.

Abnormalities of coagulation

- Is there a history of bleeding (e.g. delayed separation of the umbilical stump, bleeding post Guthrie test, severe/recurrent nosebleeds, surgical bleeding, easy bruising, menorrhagia)?
- Is there a history of bleeding in family members?
- Has the child had previous invasive procedures without bleeding complications?

Management

- All patients should have a coagulation screen.
- In the absence of a personal or family history of bleeding, a child with a normal coagulation screen does not require further coagulation testing prior to surgery (including renal biopsy)—a normal activated prothrombin time (APPT) will exclude any factor deficiency (and abnormal lupus anticoagulant or anticardiolipin antibodies).
- If the APPT has been normal on a previous screen, then it is not possible for the patient to have a factor deficiency. If the APPT is acquired, it is usually due to vitamin K deficiency or heparin contamination.
- In the event of an abnormal coagulation screen, follow Fig. 18.8.

Thrombotic abnormalities

- Does the patient have nephrotic syndrome?
- Is there a history of clotting?
- Is there a history of multiple miscarriages in the mother?
- Is there a history of clotting in family members?
- Is there a history of deep vein thrombosis in any relative aged <40 years?
- Is there a personal or family history of autoimmune disease?

Management

If any of the thrombotic abnormalities responses are positive, check a thrombophilia screen:

- This screens for thrombotic tendency and for lupus anticoagulant, which is an acquired abnormality.
- A positive lupus anticoagulant is a common finding in children with renal disease and is not always clinically significant. If it is positive, follow Fig. 18.9.

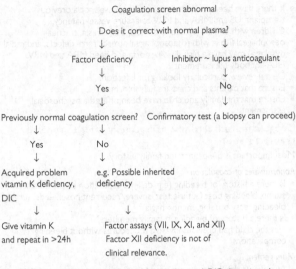

Fig. 18.8 Procedure if the coagulation screen is abnormal. DIC, disseminated intravascular coagulation

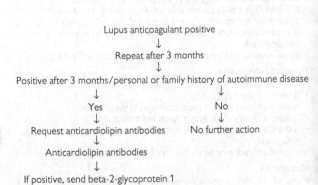

Fig. 18.9 Procedure if lupus anticoagulant positive.

- Inherited thrombophilias are rare:
  - Deficiencies of protein C, protein S, and antithrombin III, and the prothrombotic polymorphisms factor V G1691A and factor II G20210A predispose to venous thromboembolism.
  - Factor V Leiden and the G20210A mutation, along with antiphospholipid antibodies, lupus anticoagulant, and anticardiolipin antibody increase the risk of renal allograft thrombosis. It is not known whether other hypercoagulable states, such as hyperhomocysteinaemia or the C677T polymorphism of the methylenetetrahydrofolate reductase gene affect risk.
  - Anticoagulation has to be balanced against risk of bleeding; in patients with an identified thrombophilic risk factor, previous thrombosis or SLE, a plan for perioperative heparin until the graft is well functioning and the child is mobile should be considered.
- Aspirin 1 mg/kg body weight/24 h as a single daily dose (maximum 75 mg) is recommended for all children at the time of transplant and continued for 4 weeks post transplant.
- Families should be fully informed about the risks of transplantation. A suggested checklist is given in Box 18.1.

Preparation for dialysis

Background and principles

If a pre-emptive transplant is not possible, the type of dialysis to be used must be discussed with the family. At any time, ~20% of children on RRT are dialysed. Choice of dialysis modality varies around the world; PD is usually the first choice in Europe, whereas in the USA HD is more common. There are some universal rules:

- Avoidance of HD in the infant due to difficulties with vascular access.
- Intra-abdominal pathology, social difficulties, or technique failure may preclude PD.

When should dialysis be started?

There is no absolute GFR when dialysis should be started. The need should be considered when the GFR falls to <15 mL/min/1.73 m^2. However, some children with maintained urine output can do well with very low GFRs if there is good nutritional management. Indications for dialysis are:

- fluid overload.
- uraemic symptoms (nausea, anorexia, lethargy, itching).
- biochemistry cannot be controlled.
- growth rate is decelerating.

Points to discuss when considering dialysis

- Will the dialysis be at home? If yes, a home visit is necessary to see if the housing is suitable.
- If HD, is the child of a size for a fistula? Will this be home HD or, if in a centre, standard or haemodiafiltration (HDF).
- For preparation for dialysis access, ➔ see Chapter 19 and 'Dialysis', p. 432.

Box 18.1 Information for parents of children going forward for renal transplantation

Patient survival

* Transplant survival for:
  * living donor.
  * deceased donor.
  * effect of HLA matching.
  * effect of donor age.
* Risks post surgery:
  * Fluid overload and the risk of need for ventilation.
  * Hypertension, insulin-requiring (diabetes mellitus), and fits (convulsions/seizures).
  * The routine use of aspirin and renal venous thrombosis.
  * Postoperative bleeding (from transplant surgery or gut) and lymphocoele.
  * Primary non-function, delayed graft function, and the need for dialysis.
  * Management of disease recurrence and bacterial infection.
  * The need for scans/biopsies and the occasional need for return to theatre.
  * Other complications (including increased co-morbidity).

Complications that may occur, usually not postoperative

* Acute rejection, drugs used to treat it, and the use of transplant biopsy.
* Chronic transplant loss (UTIs, chronic rejection, recurrent disease).
* Bacterial infection (line, UTI).
* Viral infection (chickenpox, CMV, EBV, and PTLD).
* Transplant artery stenosis.
* Urological complications needing surgery or intervention by a radiologist.
* Malignancy (including care with sun exposure).

Immunosuppressive drugs used and their side effects

  (➔ See Chapter 21.)
* Steroids.
* Azathioprine.
* Tacrolimus.
* MMF.
* Basiliximab.
* Antithymocyte globulin (ATG).
* Sirolimus.
* Ciclosporin.

Effectiveness of types of dialysis

Only a well-functioning renal transplant can restore renal function, although most transplants do not maintain a normal GFR.

- Home nocturnal HD can deliver the equivalent to 50% normal renal function.
- HDF is the next most effective type of dialysis.
- Short daily HD delivers the equivalent of 25% of normal renal function.
- Conventional HD (4 h × 3 per week) and PD deliver ~15% of normal renal function.

Gout and hyperuricaemia

Presentation

Children with CKD can develop hyperuricaemia and this can lead to gout. The risk worsens as CKD progresses and with diuretic use. Moreover, some underlying diseases, such as HNF1B nephropathy can predispose to gout. Urate crystals are deposited in joints and other tissues. The development of an acutely painful, red, hot joint or surrounding tissues in a child with CKD suggests gout.

Differential diagnosis

* Septic arthritis (NB: the most important differential diagnosis is septic arthritis. Time to diagnosis is the major prognostic factor in infectious arthritis which can result in significant joint damage if not promptly treated).
* Cellulitis.
* Arthritis due to underlying cause of CKD, e.g. SLE.
* Trauma.
* Other crystal arthropathies i.e. calcium pyrophosphate dihydrate, calcium oxalate crystals (rare).
* Severe renal osteodystrophy.

These can usually be differentiated clinically. The child with gout is usually well otherwise.

Initial investigations

* Serum urate level:
  * Serum urate levels can fall into the normal range during an acute flare.
  * The urate level may not be higher than is usually found in CKD stage 4/5.
* Blood culture and CRP.
* Synovial fluid aspiration of affected joint for analysis by polarized light microscopy and culture:
  * The gold standard for gout diagnosis is demonstration of monosodium urate crystals by polarizing light microscopy in synovial fluid (specificity >85%, sensitivity 100%).
  * Gout and septic arthritis can coexist so Gram stain and culture of synovial fluid should still be done if infection is suspected even if crystals are identified.
* X-ray of affected area (this is not useful for diagnosis of acute gout but may help exclude trauma).

Additional investigations

* Laboratory findings during a gout attack are often non-specific and may include increased neutrophil count, increased ESR, and increased CRP.
* US of the affected joint can show hyperechoic cloudy areas or a linear density overlying the cartilage (specificity 95%, sensitivity 79%).
* Dual-energy CT can identify urate crystals and differentiate them from Ca depositions.

Background

Urate

- Urate is the final end product of purine metabolism.
- Urate is reabsorbed in the proximal tubules by URAT1.
- Children have a higher fractional excretion of urate (15–30%) compared to adults (10%), and are thus less prone to develop gout.
- CKD decreases the renal clearance of urate, therefore increasing the risk of gout.
- Urate clearance is further hampered in cystic kidney disease, hyperparathyroidism, the use of loop or thiazide diuretics, and the use of calcineurin inhibitors.
- A high dairy intake is associated with low serum urate levels. However, in children with severe CKD dairy is often avoided, thus again making these children more prone to develop gout.

High serum urate levels are thought to increase the progression of CKD in adults.

Hyperuricaemia

- Gout is associated with hyperuricaemia, although at the moment of a gout attack the serum urate can be normal.
- The most accurate time to measure baseline serum urate is at least 2 weeks after a gout attack, when symptoms have completely subsided.
- The initiation of urate-lowering therapy can precipitate a gout attack.
- Adequate long-term treatment with urate-lowering medication prevents progression of acute gouty arthritis into interval gout or chronic recurrent tophic gout.
- Hyperuricaemia subsequently causing hyperuricosuria can result in nephrolithiasis due to uric acid stone formation (especially in low urinary pH) or urate nephropathy due to urate crystal depositions in the renal medullary interstitium.

Not everyone with hyperuricaemia develops gout; individual differences in the formation of urate crystals and/or the inflammatory response to crystals may play a role.

Gouty arthritis

- This is an inflammatory arthritis caused by urate crystal formation in the synovial fluid of the affected joint.
- There are three stages: acute gouty arthritis, interval gout, and chronic recurrent tophic gout (the latter is rarely seen in children).
- A typical attack includes severe pain, redness, swelling, and disability, with a maximal severity of the attack after 12–24 h.
- Inflammation can extend beyond the affected joint (tenosynovitis, dactylitis, and cellulitis).
- Any joint can be involved (including the spine), but the lower limbs are most often affected.

Treatment

Management of gout includes both rapid treatment of acute flares and an effective long-term strategy to reduce serum urate to a concentration that achieves dissolution of monosodium urate crystals.

Acute treatment

Colchicine or a corticosteroid can be used to relieve acute attacks of gout. Treatment should be as early as possible and patients should be provided with an action plan and adequate drug supplies to facilitate early therapy.

Colchicine

Colchicine is anti-inflammatory and should be started at the first sign of acute gout. Treatment should be commenced if there is a high index of clinical suspicion. Treatment with colchicine should be stopped if nausea, vomiting, or diarrhoea occurs.

* <20 kg: 0.25 mg oral once or twice daily.
* 20–45 kg: 0.25 mg oral twice or three times daily.
  * Dose per course of acute treatment in paediatric patients <45 kg should be no more than 3 mg.
* >45 kg: 0.5 mg oral twice daily up to four times daily.
  * Dose per course of acute treatment in paediatric patients >45 kg should be no more than 6 mg.

Additional courses of colchicine therapy for treatment of an acute gout flare should not be repeated within 3 days.

Dose modification according to GFR (GFR in mL/min/1.73 m²)

There is increased risk of toxicity in patients on dialysis (PD or HD) as colchicine can accumulate. The signs of overdose may be delayed and therefore close monitoring is vital.

For GFR <50 mL/min/1.73 m², treatment course should not be repeated more than once every 2 weeks:

* <15 years or <45 kg:
  * GFR >50: no dose adjustment.
  * GFR 10–50: halve dose or increase interval.
  * GFR <10 or on dialysis (continuous ambulatory peritoneal dialysis (CAPD), HD): total dose per course of treatment should be no more than 1.5 mg.
* ≥15 years or ≥45 kg:
  * GFR >50: no dose adjustment.
  * GFR 10–50: halve dose or increase interval, e.g. 0.5 mg once daily.
  * GFR <10 or on dialysis (CAPD, HD): total dose per course of treatment should be no more than 3 mg

Adverse reactions

Diarrhoea and pharyngolaryngeal pain are common but mild and resolve with dose reduction. Less commonly, bone marrow suppression with agranulocytosis, myopathy, or rhabdomyolysis has been reported.

Interactions

Colchicine is metabolized by cytochrome P450 (CYP) 3A4 enzyme and is a substrate for the P-glycoprotein 1 (P-gp) efflux transporter. Therefore, drugs such as ciclosporin, tacrolimus, ketoconazole, protease inhibitors, imidazole, clarithromycin, simvastatin, Ca channel blockers (verapamil and diltiazem), and digoxin, may increase colchicine accumulation, requiring dose adjustment.

Prednisolone

Systemic corticosteroids have been used as a second-line alternative to NSAIDs or colchicine in the treatment of acute gout. For one or two large joints, intra-articular corticosteroids can be used.

- Dose (prednisolone):
  - Acute phase: 0.5–1.0 mg/kg/day orally in one or two doses (maximum 50 mg/day) at full dose for 2–5 days, taper over 7–10 days, and then stop or give at full dose for 5–10 days then stop.
  - Prophylaxis (during urate-lowering therapy): 5–10 mg once daily for 4 to 12 weeks (depending on clinical need and response).

Long-term management

The goal of long term therapy is to achieve a target serum urate level that prevents chronic monosodium urate crystal formation and deposition. Education of patients about the rationale for long-term urate-lowering therapy is crucial to successful gout management.

Preventative treatment: allopurinol

Allopurinol is a xanthine oxidase inhibitor. Xanthine oxidase catalyses oxidation of hypoxanthine to xanthine and subsequently uric acid. By inhibiting this enzyme, allopurinol and its main metabolite oxypurinol lower the level of uric acid in plasma. Chronic preventative treatment is recommended if there have been two or more acute episodes within one year or after the first attack if there are additional risk factors such as significantly raised urate levels or those on loop or thiazide diuretics or calcineurin inhibitors.

For patients already established on allopurinol, it should not be stopped during an acute attack. The acute episode should be treated appropriately.

Allopurinol dosing

- 1 month–15 years: 10–20 mg/kg daily (maximum 400 mg daily).
- 15–18 years: initially 100 mg daily, increased according to response (maximum 900 mg daily) (highest dose approved by US FDA is 800 mg).

Doses are preferably given after food. Doses >300 mg daily should be given in divided doses.

Monitor urate levels at routine blood checks (not less than every 3 months in the first year and ideally every month until target serum urate level achieved). The goal in children with normal renal function is a serum urate level of <350 µmol/L but this needs to be interpreted alongside the stage of CKD when urate levels are higher.

Dose modification according to GFR (GFR in mL/min/1.73 m²)

- <15 years:
  - GFR >60: no dose adjustment.
  - GFR 30–60: 5–10 mg/kg daily (maximum 50 mg/daily).
  - GFR 15–30: 5–10 mg/kg on alternate days (maximum 50 mg on alternate days).
  - Dialysis: 2.5–5 mg/kg weekly (maximum 50 mg weekly) and check levels.

- ≥15 years:
  - GFR >60: no dose adjustment.
  - GFR 30–60: 50–100 mg/day maximum 100 mg daily.
  - GFR 15–30: 50–100 mg on alternate days maximum 100 mg on alternate days.
  - Dialysis: 100 mg weekly and check levels. Give dose after dialysis.

If there are facilities for measurement of the concentration of the main metabolite of allopurinol, oxypurinol, the allopurinol dose can be adjusted to maintain the plasma oxypurinol levels at <100 µmol/L (15.2 mg/L).

Adverse reactions

Skin reactions are the most common reaction and may occur at any time during treatment.

Interactions

Allopurinol enhances effects and increases toxicity of azathioprine and mercaptopurine (reduce dose of affected drug by 50%). There is an increased risk of rash when given with penicillin antibiotics. There is a possible increase in the plasma concentration of ciclosporin and the anticoagulant effect of coumarins may be enhanced.

Contraindications

Traditionally, allopurinol has not been started during an acute attack. However, recent studies indicate that starting urate-lowering therapy during an acute flare does not prolong the flare provided the acute episode has been adequately treated. Coverage with anti-inflammatory prophylaxis as described previously should be used in these situations.

Other treatment options

Losartan

Losartan increases uric acid excretion by reduction of reabsorption of uric acid in the proximal tubule. This effect is specific to losartan and is not an ARB class effect.

- Initial dose: 0.5–0.7 mg/kg orally once daily. Adjust according to response.
- 20–50 kg: maximum 50 mg once daily.
- >50 kg: maximum 100 mg once daily.
- A lower starting dose should be considered in patients with:
  - intravascular volume depletion
  - creatinine clearance <20 mL/min/1.73 m^2.
- Monitor serum creatinine and potassium.

Further reading

Dalbeth N, Merriman TR, Stamp LK. Gout. *Lancet* 2016;388:2039–2052.

Immunization schedule for children with chronic kidney disease

Background

All children must complete all routine childhood vaccines. For those approaching dialysis and transplantation, also consider the following vaccines:
- BCG (if available).
- Hepatitis B.
- Annual influenza.
- Pneumococcal polysaccharide (PPV).
- Varicella.

Immunizations must begin as soon as possible in the child born with severe CKD (including infants with CNS) as the schedule can rarely be completed before 16 months of age. Only in exceptional circumstances can transplantation occur without completing the full vaccination schedule.

Important general points

Vaccination information changes frequently. Check the following online information sources for the most up-to-date information:
- Routine immunization information: ℘ https://www.gov.uk/government/publications/routine-childhood-immunisation-schedule
- *British National Formulary for Children*: ℘ https://www.medicinescomplete.com/mc/bnfc/current/
- Public Health England 'The Green Book'—*Immunization Against Infectious Disease*: ℘ https://www.gov.uk/government/collections/immunisation-against-infectious-disease-the-green-book
- Individuals with uncertain or incomplete immunization status: ℘ https://www.gov.uk/government/uploads/system/uploads/attachment_data/file/463433/HPA-algorithm-September-2015-04b.pdf
- US guidelines: ℘ https://cdc.gov search for immunization schedules

Live vaccines
- The following vaccines are live:
  - BCG.
  - MMR.
  - Rotavirus.
  - Varicella.
  - Influenza (intranasal preparation only).
- If MMR and varicella vaccines are not given at the same time, leave a 4-week interval between each vaccine (there is no minimum suggested time interval for any other combination of the live vaccines listed here).
- Delay transplantation for 1 month after a live vaccine (3 months for BCG).
- Live vaccines should not be given to the following patients:
  - Patients receiving systemic high-dose steroids, until at least 3 months after treatment has stopped. This includes children who receive prednisolone, orally or rectally, at a daily dose (or its equivalent) of 2 mg/kg/day for at least 1 week, or 1 mg/kg/day for 1 month. Occasionally, individuals on lower doses of steroids may be immunosuppressed and at increased risk from infections.

In those cases, live vaccines should be considered with caution. Non-systemic corticosteroids, such as aerosols or topical or intra-articular preparations, do not cause systemic immunosuppression. Therefore, administration of live vaccines is not contraindicated.

* Patients who have received immunoglobulin, until at least 3 months after the last injection or who are due to receive an injection of immunoglobulin in 3 weeks after the live vaccine. Immunoglobulin may interfere with the immune response to live vaccine viruses because it may contain antibodies to measles, varicella, and other viruses.
* Patients receiving other types of immunosuppressive drugs (e.g. azathioprine, ciclosporin, methotrexate, cyclophosphamide, leflunomide, and the newer cytokine inhibitors) alone or in combination with lower doses of steroids, until at least 6 months after terminating such treatment. The advice of the physician in charge or immunologist should be sought.
* Patients with immunosuppression due to HIV infection: take specialist advice.

Many patients with relatively minor immunodeficiencies can, and should, receive all recommended vaccinations, including live vaccines. Where there is doubt or a relatively severe immunodeficiency is present, it is important to obtain individual specialist advice.

Replacement schedules of corticosteroids for people with adrenal insufficiency do not cause immunosuppression and are not, therefore, contraindications for administration of live vaccines.

Live vaccines are likely to be safe in those receiving other immunomodulating drugs, e.g. interferon. However, advice should be sought from the specialist in charge of the therapy to ensure that the patient has not been immunosuppressed by the treatment.

Inactivated vaccines

May be administered to immunosuppressed individuals, although they may elicit a lower response than in immunocompetent individuals.

Vaccines required in addition to routine childhood immunizations

BCG SSI (Statens Serum Institut) (live vaccine)

BCG vaccine is not given routinely throughout the world but may be given to newborns in endemic areas. Availability of the vaccine is decreasing. BCG attenuates TB but does not prevent it. BCG is most effective in infants and after that effectiveness deceases with age. BCG can be given to children up to the age of 6 years without a prior skin test for hypersensitivity to tuberculin, unless they were born in or visited (>3 months) a high-incidence country. The diagnostic test to screen for latent TB in renal patients is QuanitFERON® (an interferon gamma release assay test).

The vaccine is usually recommended for children over the age of 6 years with a negative skin test. (NB: tuberculin testing should not be carried out within 4 weeks of receiving an MMR vaccine as the response may be falsely negative). However, difficulties with supply and decreased effectiveness with age means that some centres do not use it routinely.

BCG SSI dosing information

This is a *live* vaccine

- *<12 months*: 0.05 mL.
- *12 months and older*: 0.1 mL.
- *Route of administration*: intradermal injection, at the insertion of deltoid muscle (preferably left) onto humerus. The same arm should not be used for further immunization for at least 3 months due to the risk of regional lymphadenitis.
- BCG may be given simultaneously with another live vaccine but, if not given at the same time, allow an interval of 4 weeks.
- Transplantation: delay for 3 months.

Hepatitis B

Hepatitis B vaccine is given routinely in some parts of the world (including the USA) and will be introduced soon for babies in the UK. All patients who will need ESKD management should be immunized against hepatitis B, at any age, preferably pre-emptively while the GFR remains relatively high. An *accelerated course* can be used so that the third dose is given 2 months after the first dose (i.e. doses at 0, 1, and 2 months and a booster dose at 12 months). The accelerated schedule is recommended in high-risk groups where rapid protection is required. The immunization schedule and booster doses may need to be adjusted in those with low antibody concentration.

Hepatitis B dosing information: Engerix B® (GlaxoSmithKline)

Accelerated schedule for renal insufficiency and HD patients:

- *Neonate*: 10 micrograms every 1 month for 3 months, followed by 10 micrograms after 10 months for one dose (i.e. 0, 1, 2, and 12 months).
  - *Route of administration*: intramuscular (anterolateral thigh preferred (*not* buttock)).
- *Child 1 month–15 years*: 10 micrograms every 1 month for 3 months, followed by 10 micrograms after 10 months for one dose (i.e. 0, 1, 2, and 12 months).
  - *Route of administration*: intramuscular (anterolateral thigh (infants and young children) or deltoid muscle (older children) preferred (*not* buttock)).
- *Child 16–17 years* (not listed as accelerated schedule): 40 micrograms every 1 month for 3 months, followed by 40 micrograms after 4 months for one dose (i.e. 0, 1, 2, and 6 months).
  - *Route of administration*: intramuscular (deltoid muscle preferred, *not* buttock).
- *Check*: anti HBsAg antibodies 2–3 months after the final dose. Dialysis patients should be monitored annually and revaccinated if necessary (see Table 18.17).

Hepatitis B dosing information: HBvaxPRO® (Sanofi Pasteur MSD Limited)

Immunization against hepatitis B infection (accelerated schedule):

- *Neonate*: 5 microgram every 1 month for 3 months, followed by 5 microgram after 10 months for 1 dose (i.e. 0, 1, 2, and 12 months).
  - *Route of administration*: intramuscular (anterolateral thigh preferred (*not* buttock)).

Table 18.17 Revaccination for hepatitis B

100 IU/L	Protective	Give booster at 5 years
10–100 IU/L	Poor responder	Give booster at 1 and 5 years
<10 IU/L	Non-responder	Repeat course of vaccine

- *Child 1 month–15 years*: 5 micrograms every 1 month for 3 months, followed by 5 micrograms after 10 months for 1 dose (i.e. 0, 1, 2, and 12 months).
  - *Route of administration*: intramuscular (anterolateral thigh (infants and young children) or deltoid muscle (older children) preferred (*not* buttock)).
- *Child 16–17 years*: 10 microgram every 1 month for 3 months, followed by 10 micrograms after 10 months for 1 dose (i.e. 0, 1, 2 and 12 months).
  - *Route of administration*: intramuscular (deltoid muscle preferred, *not* buttock)

Chronic haemodialysis patients
- *Child 16–17 years*: 40 micrograms every 1 month for 2 months, followed by 40 micrograms after 5 months (i.e. 0, 1, and 6 months).
  - *Route of administration*: intramuscular (deltoid muscle preferred, *not* buttock).
- *Check*: anti HBsAg antibodies 2–3 months after the final dose. Dialysis patients should be monitored annually and revaccinated if necessary (see Table 18.17).

If Engerix B® is not available, use HBvaxPRO® brand.

Varicella vaccine (live vaccine)
- Can be given with, or 4 weeks after, MMR vaccine if non-immune (check titres).
- Ensure lymphocyte count >1.2×10^9/L.
- Delay for 3 months if patient has received immunoglobulin or a blood transfusion because of likelihood of vaccine failure due to passively acquired varicella antibodies.
- Salicylates should be avoided for 6 weeks after varicella vaccination as Reye syndrome has been reported following the use of salicylates during natural varicella infection. Vaccination with varicella vaccine is not contraindicated in individuals aged 16 years or over who need to take aspirin.
- If a measles-containing vaccine is not given at the same time as the varicella vaccine, an interval of at least 1 month must lapse between vaccines. Measles vaccination may lead to short-lived suppression of the cell-mediated response.

Varicella dosing information: Varilrix® or Varivax®
This is a *live* vaccine:
- *From the age of 12 months*: two doses (0.5 mL) with an interval between doses of 4–8 weeks but many need three doses.
- *Route of administration*: SC or intramuscular injection into the high anterolateral thigh (younger children) or deltoid region (older children).
- *Check*: titres (ELISA) 2–3 months after completing course.
- *Transplantation*: delay for 1 month after vaccination course if seroconversion demonstrated.

Pneumococcal vaccine

Pneumococcal polysaccharide vaccine-23 valent: Pneumovax II®
- Not to be used for primary vaccination in children <2 years old.
- Children over 2 years old who have received the conjugate (PCV—Prevenar 13®) vaccine need a dose of 23-valent vaccine (PPV—Pneumovax II®) to provide protection against the serotypes of *Streptococcus pneumoniae* not covered in the conjugate vaccine.

Pneumococcal polysaccharide dosing information: Pneumovax II®
- *>2 years and received primary immunization with the conjugate vaccine (PCV)*: 0.5 mL (one dose)—at least 2 months from last PCV dose.
- *At-risk children who are eligible for 1 or 2 doses of PCV but have already received a dose of PPV*: leave an interval of at least 6 months between PPV and PCV vaccines.
- *>5 years and high risk (e.g. nephrotic syndrome)*: 0.5 mL every 5 years (no antibody levels required).
- *Route of administration*: intramuscular injection.

See Table 18.18 for an immunization schedule for paediatric patients with chronic kidney disease.

Table 18.18 Immunization schedule for paediatric patients with chronic kidney disease

When to immunize (age)	RCI[a]	What vaccine to give	Vaccine given	Date given
From birth onwards	X	Bacillus Calmette–Guérin (BCG) (live vaccine) (if available)		
	X	Hepatitis B (use Engerix B® accelerated schedule for patients with renal insufficiency) 4 doses at: 0 month 1 month from 1st dose 2 months from 1st dose 12 months from 1st dose (0–15 years old)	1st dose 2nd dose 3rd dose 4th dose	
2 months	✓	5-in-1 (DTaP/IPV/Hib) vaccine: diphtheria, tetanus, whooping cough (pertussis), polio, and Haemophilus influenzae type b (known as Hib) (Pediacel® or Infanrix®-IPV Hib)		
	✓	Pneumococcal (PCV) vaccine (Prevenar 13®)		
	✓	Rotavirus vaccine (live vaccine) (Rotarix®)		
	✓	Meningococcal group B vaccine (MenB) (Bexsero®)		

3 months	✓	5-in-1 (DTaP/IPV/Hib) vaccine (second dose) (Pediacel®, Infanrix®-IPV Hib)
	✓	Meningococcal group C (Neisvac-C® or Menjugate®) Note: not required from 1 July 2016
	✓	Rotavirus vaccine (*live vaccine*) (second dose) (Rotarix®)
4 months	✓	5-in-1 (DTaP/IPV/Hib) vaccine (third dose) (Pediacel®, Infanrix®-IPV Hib)
	✓	Pneumococcal (PCV) vaccine (second dose) (Prevenar 13®)
	✓	Meningococcal group B (MenB) vaccine (second dose) (Bexsero®)
6 months (and then annually)	✗	Inactivated (injectable) influenza (flu) vaccine NB: nasal flu vaccine is a *live vaccine* (offered as part of routine immunization schedule at 2, 3, and 4 years)
12–13 months	✓	Hib/Men C booster: meningitis C (second dose) and Hib (fourth dose) (Menitorix®).
	✓	Measles, mumps and rubella (MMR) vaccine (*live vaccine*) (MMR VaxPRO® or Priorix®)

(Continued)

Table 18.18 (Contd.)

When to immunize (age)	RCI[a]	What vaccine to give	Vaccine given	Date given
	✓	Pneumococcal (PCV) vaccine (third dose) (Prevenar 13®)		
	✓	Meningococcal group B vaccine (third dose) (Bexsero®)		
	✗	Varicella-zoster vaccine (live vaccine) Varilrix® or Varivax® (2 doses: 4–8 weeks apart)	Check status before giving	
From 2 years	✗	Pneumococcal polysaccharide vaccine (PPV) (Pneumovax II®) (Single dose—at least 2 months after the final dose of PCV.) Revaccination after 5 years may be necessary in patients with nephrotic syndrome		
3 years and 4 months (up to starting school)	✓	Measles, mumps, and rubella (MMR) vaccine (live vaccine) (second dose) (MMR VaxPRO® or Priorix®)		
	✓	4-in-1 (DTaP/IPV); preschool booster of diphtheria, tetanus, whooping cough (pertussis), and polio (Infanrix®-IPV or Repevax®)		
12–13 years (girls only)	✓	Human papillomavirus (HPV) vaccine: two injections given 6–12 months apart (Gardasil®) for patients aged 11–14 and 3 doses for ages 15–26 years.		

		Vaccine given	Date given	Notes
From 14 years ✓	3-in-1 (Td/IPV) teenage booster, given as a single jab and contains vaccines against diphtheria, tetanus, and polio (Revaxis®)			
✓	Meningococcal groups A, C, W, and Y disease, Men ACWY vaccine (Nimenrix® or Menveo®)			
✓	Check MMR status			

Miscellaneous

Other vaccines that may be needed based on need include varicella (against chicken-pox).

For patients with atypical haemolytic uraemic syndrome (aHUS) where eculizumab is to be initiated, discuss vaccine requirements with pharmacy.

Where routine immunization has not been completed, outstanding doses should be given according to the recommended schedule.

Others	RCI[a]	Vaccine required	Vaccine given	Date given	Notes
Complement disorders, e.g. aHUS (including those receiving complement inhibitor therapy)	X	Hib/MenC MenACWY MenB PCV13 (to any age) PPV (from 2 years of age) Annual flu vaccine	Check status before giving		
Chronic liver condition (from 12 months)	X	Hepatitis A (Havrix®, Epaxal®, Vaqta paediatric®: refer to relevant prescribing schedule)			

This table includes vaccines that are not part of the routine immunization schedule i.e. includes those for 'at-risk' groups.

[a] RCI = UK Routine childhood immunization; ✓ = included in RCI, X = not part of RCI = *live vaccine*.

References

Joint Formulary Committee. *British National Formulary for Children*. London: BMJ Group and Pharmaceutical Press. ℘ https://www.medicinescomplete.com/mc/bnfc/current/

Public Health England. Immunisation Against Infectious Diseases: 'The Green book' and updates from the Department of Health ℘ https://www.gov.uk/government/collections/immunisation-against-infectious-disease-the-green-book

Public Health England. Revised recommendations for the administration of more than one live vaccine. April 2015. ℘ https://www.gov.uk/government/uploads/system/uploads/attachment_data/file/422798/PHE_recommendations_for_administering_more_than_one_live_vaccine_April_2015FINAL_.pdf

Joint Formulary Committee. *British National Formulary for Children*. London: BMJ Group and Pharmaceutical Press. ℘ https://www.medicinescomplete.com/mc/bnfc/current/

Public Health England. Routine childhood immunisations from summer 2016 (born on or before 31 July 2017. 2014. ℘ https://assets.publishing.service.gov.uk/government/uploads/system/uploads/attachment_data/file/533863/PHE_2016_Routine_Childhood_Immunisation_Schedule_SUMMER2016.pdf

Peritoneal dialysis in end-stage kidney disease

Principles of peritoneal dialysis

* Solute moves down the concentration gradient across the peritoneal membrane by diffusion and water by osmosis (ultrafiltration (UF)).
* UF causes movement of solutes by convection, so that solutes may be carried across the membrane (solvent drag) even in the absence of a concentration gradient.
* Both solute and water transport are bidirectional as pressure and osmotic gradients equilibrate.

Transport of solute

Diffusion depends on:

* the solute concentration between blood and dialysate.
* the molecular weight of the solute as diffusion is dependent on size.

Diffusion is increased by increasing the fill volume which:

* increases the volume available for diffusion.
* increases recruitment of peritoneal surface area.
* prolongs the osmotic gradient.

Transport of water

* Water moves from capillaries to peritoneal cavity down a pressure gradient.
* The force is osmotic pressure.

UF is increased by:

* increasing the osmotic concentration of the dialysate (usually by glucose).
* smaller fill volumes (lowers intraperitoneal pressure (IPP)).
* shorter dwell times (each fill freshly establishes osmotic gradient).

Convective mass transfer

* Depends on amount of fluid removed by UF and on membrane permeability.
* Contributes more to movement of larger solutes.

Convective mass transfer is increased by:

* longer dwells.
* less reabsorbable osmotic agents, e.g. icodextrin.

The physiology of water and solute transport: the three-pore model

The frequency of peritoneal pores is inversely related to their size.

The ultra-small pores

* Are the most abundant.
* Are endothelial water channels (AQP1), so allow sodium-free water transport.

The small pores

* Allow diffusion of solutes and water.

The large pores
- Low numbers (<1% of AQP1 channel numbers).
- Facilitate convective mass transport and macromolecular leakage into the peritoneal cavity.

Reabsorption of sodium and water and macromolecules

Is driven by:
- loss of osmotic gradient.
- increasing IPP.

It occurs via:
- small pores.
- lymphatics under the diaphragm.
- lymphatics and blood vessels in the peritoneal cavity.

During a PD cycle
- Sodium-free water transport occurs first through AQP1 channels, generated by the osmotic gradient.
- This causes an initial dilution of the dialysate sodium (called sodium sieving).
- Sodium and water flow from blood to dialysate through the small pores, generated by the concentration and pressure gradient.
- Glucose diffuses back into plasma via small pores so free water clearance decreases.
- Sodium and water diffuse back through the small pores as the concentration gradient decreases and IPP increases.

Efficiency of peritoneal dialysis

The efficiency of PD is affected by:

The peritoneal membrane
- The capillary wall.
- The interstitium.
- Mesothelial cells.
- Density of pores.

The peritoneal microcirculation
- Capillary blood flow.
- Lymphatics.

The dialysis compartment
- The type of osmotic agent.
- The concentration of the osmotic agent.

Reference

Fischbach M, Zaloszyc A, Sbhaefer B, et al. Optimising peritoneal dialysis prescription for volume control: the importance of varying dwell time and dwell volume. *Paediatr Nephrol* 2014;29:1321–1327.

Insertion of the peritoneal dialysis catheter: the surgical technique

Preoperative management

- Screen for nasal carriage of *Staphylococcus aureus* with a nasal swab. If positive, check carers and treat if necessary. Use mupirocin 2% ointment to each nostril for 5 days and then for 5 days per month each month. Follow-up swabs should be at least 2 weeks post treatment.
- Ensure that the child is not constipated, which may cause the catheter to be pushed up out of the pelvis and/or affect dialysate circulation.
- IV antibiotic cover preoperatively. One choice would be amikacin 10 mg/kg (maximum 500 mg) and teicoplanin 10 mg/kg (maximum 400 mg) one dose of each IV.

Catheter types

- Catheters with two cuffs (to prevent tracking of organisms from the exit site down the tunnel) and a downward pointing exit site (to prevent collection of debris) are preferable.
- A catheter that spirals at the intraperitoneal end reduces the risk of blockage of the catheter by bowel or omentum.
- A swan-neck catheter/tunnel reduces the risk of catheter displacement.

The surgery

- Consider gastrostomy placement and healing before PD catheter insertion.
- Insertion of a PD catheter needs a skilled and experienced surgeon.
- Omentectomy will reduce the chances of catheter blockage.
- The tip of the catheter should be in the lowest part of the pelvis without bending.
- The distal cuff should be 2 cm from the exit site and the proximal cuff embedded in fascia.
- Any hernia should be repaired at the time of catheter placement.
- The exit site should be as small as possible, above the nappy in young children, and away from other stoma, e.g. gastrostomy, ureterostomy, etc.
- The catheter drainage should be checked before leaving theatre.

Postoperative management

- The catheter should be flushed continuously with 10 mL/kg dialysate until the dialysate is clear, then capped off with heparinized saline (instil 20 mL heparinized saline (1000 IU heparin + 19 mL 0.9% NaCl).
- Thereafter the catheter can be flushed weekly until use.
- The catheter must be securely fixed with dressings to prevent movement at the exit site and these dressings should not be removed for the first week as movement of the catheter within the tunnel prevents healing and results in leaks, exit site infection, and granulomas.
- Thereafter the exit site should be cleaned once a week for the first 3 weeks.
- It is preferable to leave the catheter for 3 weeks to allow healing of the tunnel before use.

Complications of peritoneal dialysis catheters

- Exit site and tunnel infections will result from inadequate catheter immobilization post insertion (➔ see 'Care of the exit site and exit site infection'). They can lead to peritonitis by tracking of infection down the tunnel. A new catheter cannot be inserted until the abdominal wall is free from infection.
- If exit site or tunnel infection is suspected, a US of the tunnel might show hyperaemia or collections, and be able to identify the position of any collection relative to the cuffs.
- Postsurgical leakage of fluid may be due to:
  - an SC tunnel that is too large.
  - a perpendicular tunnel.
  - fluid retention and abdominal wall oedema.
  - catheter blockage (PD fluid will flow along the path of least resistance).
  - early commencement of dialysis before healing.
- Leakage can be treated by suspending dialysis and immobilizing the catheter. When dialysis is started, low volumes (10 mL/kg) should be used. If leakage persists, the catheter should be replaced.
- It has been established that leakage after dialysis is often due to catheter blockage.
- Catheter migration from out of the pelvis (seen on abdominal X-ray) can be due to:
  - torque placed on the catheter at the time of insertion which causes it to try to undo the bend inflicted on it.
  - too acute an angle of entry of the catheter to the peritoneal cavity.
  - the shallow pelvis of infants.
  - constipation.
  - adhesions or sclerosing peritonitis.
- The catheter can be repositioned laparoscopically and it can be sutured in position in the pelvis if there is not too much torque. If there is, however, the catheter needs to be replaced.
- Cuff extrusion may be caused by:
  - torque.
  - placement of the catheter cuff too near the exit site.
  - exit site or tunnel infection.
  - weakness of the abdominal wall.
- The cuff may be shaved if there is no infection but the catheter must be replaced if there is infection.
- Poor catheter drainage may be due to blockage by omentum. Many surgeons undertake routine omentectomy at the time of catheter insertion although it is not always possible to identify it all. If blocked, a laparoscopic approach can be taken to unblock it.

Care of the exit site and exit site infection

Catheter-related infections (exit site or tunnel) with subsequent peritonitis account for up to 20% of transfers to HD. These infections are strongly linked to the nasal carriage of *Staphylococcus aureus*.

- The most important way to prevent infection and granuloma formation is immobilization of the catheter.
- In the first 3 weeks post catheter insertion:
  - Post insertion the PD catheter should be securely dressed to immobilize it and the dressings should not be removed for the first week.
  - The exit site should be cleaned once a week.
  - The exit site is likely to look red during this time. However, a swab must be taken if infection is considered.
- After 3 weeks post catheter insertion:
  - The exit site should be cleaned every other day, or daily if there is colonization or infection. A strict aseptic technique should be used. Aqueous chlorhexidine 0.05% can be used until the exit site is clean and the chlorhexidine is then removed with sterile water.
  - Immobilization of the catheter remains paramount.
  - Screen 3-monthly for nasal carriage of *Staphylococcus aureus* and treat with mupirocin 2% ointment (and swab carer) if positive.
  - The exit site should be swabbed monthly on a routine basis or if there are signs of infection.
  - If the exit site is positive for *S. aureus*, but no clinical signs of infection (i.e. colonized), apply mupirocin 2% ointment once daily to the exit site for 4 weeks and eradicate nasal carriage in child and carer if present.
  - If the exit site looks infected (red, tender, swollen, discharge, or granuloma), an US can determine whether there is extension of infection down the tunnel. Topical mupirocin, oral antibiotics (usually flucloxacillin or ciprofloxacin if a history of *Pseudomonas*) and an antifungal (usually nystatin 100,000 U four times daily orally) should be prescribed. Granuloma can be treated with silver nitrate sticks once daily for 5 days.
- Flucloxacillin dose for PD patients:
  - 62.5 mg three times a day age <1 year.
  - 125 mg three times a day age 1–5 years.
  - 250 mg three times a day age 5–10 years.
  - 250 mg three times a day to 500 mg age >10 years.
- Ciprofloxacin dose for PD patients:
  - 20 mg/kg once a day age 4 weeks onwards (maximum dose 750 mg/day) for 2 weeks.
  - 10 mg/kg once a day thereafter.
- If there is tunnel infection beyond the external cuff, consider removal of catheter.
- If there is no response at 4 weeks, repeat tunnel US. If no tunnel infection, treat for a further 2 weeks and then consider removal if treatment failure.
- If there is no response at 4 weeks and tunnel infection, consider removal of catheter.

Prevention and treatment of Exit Site Infection in peritoneal dialysis

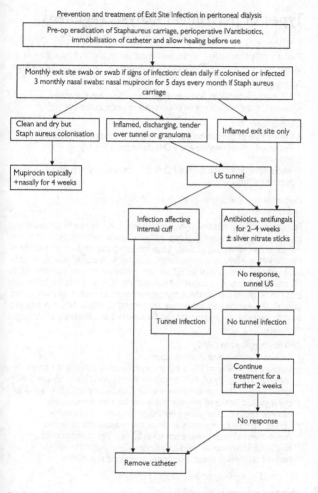

Reference

Warady BA, Bakkaloglu S, Newland J, et al. Consensus guidelines for the prevention and treatment of catheter-related infections and peritoneal dialysis: 2012 update. *Perit Dial Int* 2012;32(Suppl 2):S32–86.

Types of peritoneal dialysis regimens

Continuous ambulatory peritoneal dialysis (CAPD)

Fluid is instilled manually into the peritoneal cavity, and drained and replaced usually four times a day. The types of dialysate can be individually adjusted.

Advantages
* No machine required and less dialysate used so less expensive.
* Good for the adolescent who wants to socialize in the evening.

Disadvantages
* Higher rate of peritonitis due to more frequent catheter access.
* Increased risk of herniae and PD leaks as the IPP is higher when ambulant.
* Abdominal distension due to PD fluid in the daytime may affect nutritional intake.

Automated peritoneal dialysis (APD) using cycling machines

Peritoneal dialysis machines (cyclers) for use at home can be programmed to deliver a personalized regimen using computer technology. Information can be obtained retrospectively from the computer chip on all aspects of the dialysis at home (e.g. compliance, lost dwell times, catheter flow rates, etc.). Fill volumes as low as 60 mL can be delivered and can change by 10 mL increments if necessary. Machines are now available for home use that can be connected to the managing centre via a modem, allowing collection of information about the treatment regimen, drains, BPs, weights, etc. so that the program and results can be accessed and the program changed remotely.

Benefits compared to CAPD
* Less connections and disconnections.
* Increased flexibility of PD program enables more solute and water removal. The ability of APD to deliver short cycles, high dialysate flow rates, and variable intraperitoneal volumes make it particularly good for the high fluid intake of the infant diet and for high transporters.
* No interruption to schooling by dialysis procedures in the day.
* Lower daytime fill improves appetite and reduces risk of hernia.
* Assessment of membrane transport (➔ see 'Peritoneal equilibrium test') characteristics enables calculation of the optimum dialysis regimen, for which there are computer programs available.

Types of automated peritoneal dialysis

Nocturnal intermittent PD (NIPD)

The child is on PD overnight and the abdomen is left empty during the daytime.

Advantages in the day
* No glucose absorption.
* No loss of proteins.
* No interference with nutrition.

- Preservation of the peritoneal membrane due to decreased peritoneal exposure to dialysate. The peritoneal cells and immunoglobulins may be reconstituted during the dry phase.
- Body image may be better as there is no abdominal distension in the day.

Disadvantages

- Significantly reduced clearance of solute and water due to decreased dialysis time. The clearance of both large and small molecules may be reduced by as much as one-third.
- Reduced clearance of larger molecules (phosphate) as no long daytime dwell.
- No flush of the PD catheter at the start of the session.
- No intraperitoneal fluid that can be collected if peritonitis is considered.

Continuous cycling PD (CCPD)

This provides 24 h of dialysis/day using a nocturnal program along with a daytime dwell of ~60% of the nocturnal fill volume. The daytime dwell is drained at bedtime when the cycler is reconnected

Advantages

- The daytime dwell (called the last bag fill) increases overall clearance of larger molecules.
- A daytime dwell of glucose polymers (icodextrin) offers sustained UF.
- An extra cycle can be programmed to give an additional day time exchange prior to the overnight dialysis, and usually on return from school.

Disadvantages

- Equilibration may occur during the day resulting in reabsorption of sodium and water.
- PD fluid in the abdomen all day may adversely affect the peritoneum, nutrition and body image.

Tidal peritoneal dialysis

Tidal PD, when only a proportion of the fill volume is drained at each cycle, is useful when there is abdominal pain on draining; when there are lost dwell times due to repeated alarms because of poor returns (due either to catheter problems or in the polyuric child who absorbs dialysate); and for clearance of larger molecules such as phosphorus.

- A fixed proportion, usually 50–80% of the fill volume, is drained at each cycle, The optimum percentage drain can be calculated by observing the drainage flow rate and using the point at which this declines.
- A complete drain is usually programmed for the middle of the night.
- Continuous contact between dialysate and peritoneal membrane aids clearance.
- As the abdomen always contains dialysate, time without any dialysis is reduced.
- It avoids alarms due to low flow if there is catheter malfunction.
- It is best for high transporters.

Adapted automated peritoneal dialysis

Some cyclers are able to individualize each exchange. This can therefore be used to improve UF and solute removal.

* The cycles start with short dwells with small fill volume to favour sodium free UF.
* This results in haemoconcentration and an increase in diffusion capacity in subsequent long exchanges.
* Sodium free water transport dilutes the sodium concentration of the residual dialysate prior to switching to long high volume dwells.
* This further increases the plasma/dialysate sodium gradient promoting diffusive sodium removal.

The peritoneal dialysis prescription requirements

The optimum prescription provides ideal solute clearance and fluid removal.
Requirements for a CAPD prescription:
- Fill volume.
- Number, dwell time, and time of each exchange.
- Dialysate:
  - Glucose based, or a combination of glucose based, amino acid based, or icodextrin.
  - Glucose concentration.
  - Calcium concentration (for glucose based dialysate).

Requirements for an APD prescription—overnight:
- Fill volume.
- Number of hours, cycles, and dwell time.
- Dialysate:
  - Glucose based, or a combination of glucose based, amino acid based, or icodextrin.
  - Glucose concentration.
  - Calcium concentration (for glucose-based dialysate).

Daytime dwell (last bag fill):
- Fill volume.
- Dialysate.
  - Glucose based, amino acid based, or icodextrin.
  - Calcium concentration (for glucose based dialysate).

Fill volume

A fill that is too low in volume will cause:
- rapid solute transfer and loss of UF capacity, i.e. the larger the dialysate volume, the longer the osmotic difference will continue
- inadequate drainage from the previous fill, which will affect the concentration gradient.

A fill that is too large in volume results in raised IPP causing:
- pain.
- diaphragmatic splinting.
- hydrothorax.
- herniae.
- gastro-oesophageal reflux, vomiting, and anorexia.
- enhanced lymphatic drainage and loss of UF.

Optimum fill volume
- Peritoneal membrane recruitment (utilization) increases until 1100–1400 mL/m^2 body surface area (BSA) in >2-year-olds. Do not exceed 50 mL/kg.
- This corresponds to an IPP of 18 cmH$_2$O.
- There is better peritoneal recruitment when lying down.
- Use 800 mL/m^2 BSA for <2-year-olds.

Optimum intraperitoneal pressure
- 7–14 cmH$_2$O.

Day-time fill
- 600–800 mL/m^2 enhances clearance.
- If there is poor return on the initial drain from the daytime dwell when starting back on overnight PD (< two thirds of the last bag fill), Icodextrin can be used to optimize solute and water clearance.

The characteristics of the peritoneal membrane influence the peritoneal dialysis prescription

(➔ See 'Peritoneal equilibrium test'.) The program can be adjusted according to results of the peritoneal equilibrium test (PET), in conjunction with weight, BP, and UF.

High transporters
Reach small solute equilibration more quickly:
- Solutes and UF are reabsorbed.

Treat with:
- short dwell times: APD.
- icodextrin in day.

Low transporters
- Solute dialysate/plasma (D/P) ratio increases linearly.
- UF continues during the dwell.

Treat with:
- long dwell times: CAPD or APD.

As a rule
- Infant and young children are high transporters.
- Older children and young adults are low transporters.

Number of hours, cycles, and dwell time

Influenced by:
- size.
- residual renal function.
- biochemistry.
- transporter type.

Hours
- Usually 9–14, but the school and family routine need to be taken into consideration.
- An additional daytime exchange can be programmed, usually on returning from school prior to the overnight dialysis, to increase fluid removal.
- A suggested schema to start PD would be as illustrated in Table 19.1.

Table 19.1 Suggested schema to start PD

	Hours	Ratio of cycles to hours
Infant	12–14	1:1 or more
Polyuric child	Up to 12	2:3
Oliguric/anuric child	Up to 12	1:1

- The risk of recirculation is more significant in infants on PD, due to their low fill volumes. Low-volume lines should be used where available, to reduce the volume of 'used' effluent returned back to the infant, by up to one-half.

Influences on drain time

- Catheter drainage is not linear.
- A high flow rate is maintained until a critical intraperitoneal volume is reached.
- After this critical point the flow rate drops.
- The final part of the drain takes much longer.
- The critical intraperitoneal volume is individual and can be obtained from the computer chip record from the cycler. This can be used to optimize drain time, e.g. if the drainage is very fast, the minimum drain time can be set correspondingly low with some makes of machine.

Tidal peritoneal dialysis

Indications

- Patients with adhesions and poor drainage.
- Patients who experience significant drain pain on all cycles.
- Patients approaching peritoneal membrane failure.

How it works

- The peritoneum is filled with the child's usual fill volume.
- At the first drain, a programmed percentage of the fill volume is removed, leaving some dialysate in the peritoneum all the time.
- If trying tidal for the first time, consider starting on 85% tidal volume.
- If tidal is being used for drain pain, and the pain persists, the tidal volume can be reduced in 5% steps.
- The number of times the abdomen is fully drained needs to be programmed—if the patient is not polyuric, this should be at least three times—on the initial drain, at the mid-point of the program duration, and again at the end of the program, prior to their last bag fill.
- The tidal program and strength of glucose bags used need to be closely monitored and adjusted more often, to ensure the patient continues to ultrafiltrate sufficient amounts.
- The amount of time spent filling and draining is reduced, so improving clearance time.
- Tidal PD reduces catheter contact with peritoneum so improves pain on filling/draining.

Additional program settings on the dialysis machine

- Each dialysis machine will have default safety alarms set within it. These can be individualized for specific patients, if deemed appropriate. Reasons to consider adjusting these alarm settings may include:
  - to optimize a patient's drain volume.
  - to optimize drainage in patients who may pocket fluid, e.g. with prune belly, adhesions, suboptimal PD catheter position, bad sleep positions.
  - to reduce risk of fluid retention in anuric patients.
  - to reduce drain alarms in polyuric patients.
  - to notify carer if a polyuric patient ultrafiltrates too much.

Peritoneal dialysis solutions

Dialysate solutions contain an osmotic agent, which is usually glucose. Osmotic UF can be increased by increasing the concentration of glucose. The rate of absorption of glucose from the peritoneum into the peritoneal capillaries varies; this affects the length of time for which the gradient remains effective. Other osmotic agents can be used, including amino acids and glucose polymers.

Glucose

* Standard solutions are available at glucose concentrations of 1.36%, 2.27%, and 3.86%. This means 1360–3860 mg/dL, i.e. supraphysiological levels.
* Exposure of the peritoneum to glucose-containing dialysate damages the peritoneum in the long term by inducing mesothelial denudation, submesothelial fibrosis, hyaline vasculopathy, and neoangiogenesis. The latter leads to an initial increase in the vascular surface area, which causes an increase in the peritoneal transport rates of small solutes and UF failure. This can be treated with short dwells and icodextrin (➔ see 'Icodextrin'). However, subsequent membrane thickening and scarring of blood vessels causes irreversible membrane failure and failure of the technique. Sclerosing-encapsulating peritonitis can also occur (➔ see 'Sclerosing peritonitis').
* Glucose exposure depends on the total dialysate volume and the glucose concentration in the dialysate. The lowest possible glucose concentration should always be used.
* Peritoneal membrane toxicity also results from glucose degradation products (GDPs), which develop during sterilization of dialysate if the pH is >3.5, and attach to the proteins of the mesothelial cells of the peritoneal membrane. GDPs may also contribute systemically to the pro-oxidative state of CKD stage 5.
* High-glucose solutions contribute to obesity, hyperinsulinism, and dyslipidaemia.

The buffer and pH

Lactate-based solutions

* The conventional buffer is lactate in supraphysiological concentrations.
* This is because bicarbonate in peritoneal dialysate will cause precipitation of magnesium and calcium carbonate.
* Lactate is metabolized to bicarbonate in the liver. Bicarbonate then diffuses into the dialysate.
* Lactate has similar toxic properties to the peritoneal membrane as glucose.
* The pH of lactate-based solutions is low (5.5–6.5) and this causes pain on filling. Pain usually settles as equilibrium occurs.

Bicarbonate-based solutions

These solutions have less toxicity but principally due to cost are not used worldwide.

* Separate bags mean that the bicarbonate can be mixed at inflow so that lactate is not necessary and therefore the toxicity associated with lactate is reduced.

- Separate bags also enable the glucose to be sterilized at low pH and therefore GDPs do not form.
- The pH of the mixed solution is physiological.
- This results in less abdominal pain and less injury to the peritoneum.

Icodextrin

- Icodextrin can be used for sustained high osmotic pressure (via the small pores) during a long dwell, either the daytime dwell or as one CAPD exchange.
- It consists of glucose polymers that are too large to diffuse across the peritoneal membrane but are absorbed into the lymphatics. In the blood it is hydrolysed to maltose. Therefore, its use is limited to a once-daily prescription.
- GDPs and osmolality are low but lactate is high and the pH is 5.5.
- Sodium removal is relatively greater, so care must be taken to not induce hypovolaemia.
- Glucose-specific assays are needed to measure serum glucose to not measure maltose as well.
- Measurement of serum amylase is affected, giving falsely low results. Lipase should be used to determine pancreatitis.

Amino acid solutions

- Amino acids can also be used as osmotic agents; the osmolality is equivalent to 1.36% glucose dialysate.
- GDPs are low, lactate is high, pH is 6.7, and there is toxicity to the peritoneal membrane.
- They provide a source of nutrition but may increase plasma urea and acidosis. Optimum oral nutrition is preferable.

Electrolytes

- Sodium in dialysate is usually 132–134 mmol/L.
- Most sodium is lost by convection (solvent drag), unless short exchanges are used, when free water removal increases relative to sodium.
- The shorter dwells and higher UF rates in infants may result in sodium depletion and the need for sodium supplementation, particularly if there are ongoing renal tubular sodium losses or diarrhoea. Fluid overload predominates in older children.
- Dialysate may contain calcium of 1.75 mmol/L or 1.25 mmol/L (equivalent of ionized calcium levels). Diffusion of calcium into and out of the blood will depend on the plasma calcium level and can be prescribed according to the need to remove calcium or promote its absorption from dialysate.
- Dialysate magnesium levels are 0.25–0.5 mmol/L.

Reference

Schmitt CP, Bakkaloglu SA, Schröder C, et al. Solutions for peritoneal dialysis in children: recommendations by the European Pediatric Dialysis Working Group. *Pediatr Nephrol* 2011;26:1137–1147.

Monitoring of the effects of the peritoneal dialysis prescription

The following need to be monitored each day:
- Weight, BP, and temperature pre and post dialysis.
- Initial drain (from the daytime dwell).
- UF overnight.
- Alarms and lost dwell time.
- Dialysate glucose concentration used.
- Appearance of PD drain effluent—is it cloudy? Any fibrin present?

Parents need to be given instructions as to when to contact their managing centre:
- Some families may need frequent (even daily) contact initiated by their centre, others can be given the following criteria to call in:
  - Fever ± cloudy dialysate ± abdominal pain.
  - Deviation from parameters set for the upper and lower limit for BP and weight.
  - If there is negative UF overnight, i.e. retention of dialysate.
  - If PD drain effluent is not transparent, i.e. if fibrin is seen, or effluent is cloudy or blood stained.
  - Drain problems overnight, often seen with frequent alarms or large lost dwell times (if using smart dwell setting).
  - If the child has not opened their bowels for 2 days.

An example of a monitoring form for a week is shown in Fig. 19.1. With new cyclers, this information can be retrieved and transmitted through the Internet from home to the managing centre.

Peritoneal equilibrium test

The PET gives two measures of membrane function during a 4 h dwell:
Small solute transport:
- How easily does creatinine cross from the plasma to the peritoneal cavity? This is measured by the ratio of dialysate creatinine (D) to plasma creatinine (P) (ratio D/P creatinine).

Ultrafiltration:
- How easily does glucose cross from the peritoneal cavity to the blood? This is measured by the ratio of dialysate glucose at 4 h to dialysate glucose at time 0 (D4/D0 glucose).

The 'leakier' the peritoneal membrane:
- the higher D/P creatinine.
- the lower D4/D0 glucose.

Solute transport varies between individuals and affects the dialysis prescription. It can change with time and is the commonest cause of failure of UF and the peritoneal dialysis technique.

The procedure
- Measures the rate at which creatinine and glucose reach equilibrium between the blood and dialysate. Patients are divided into high (rapid movement of creatinine into the peritoneum and elimination of glucose), high average, low average, and low transporters.

	Weight before	Weight after	BP before	BP after	Temp before	Temp after	initial drain	Average dwell	UF	Lost Dwell	Number of 2.27%	Number of 1.38%	Bowels open?	Fluids drank?
Monday														
Tuesday														
Wednesday														
Thursday														
Friday														
Saturday														
Sunday														

Dialysis Programme

Total therapy volume		time		fill volume		last bag fill		cycles		dwell	

Observation ranges: Outside of these ranges call the hospital on the numbers you have

	Weight before	Weight after	Blood pressure before	Blood pressure after	Temperature	UF	Lost Dwell
					36.0 – 37.5		Below 1 hr

Fig. 19.1 Monitoring form for a week.

- The patient must empty the peritoneal cavity as completely as possible before the test dwell.
- The peritoneum is filled with 1100 mL/m^2 of 2.5% dextrose dialysate. Dialysate and plasma samples are obtained at 0, 2, and 4 h into the exchange.
- There are standard curves available (see Fig. 19.2) for the ratio of dialysate to plasma for creatinine and glucose against time. These can be used for comparison to determine if a child is a high, high average, low average, or low transporter for creatinine and glucose.
- Roughly, the dialysate/plasma creatinine ratio at the end of 4 h dwell (D/Pcr) grades the patient's transport status as high if >0.77, high average if >0.64, low average if >0.51, and low if <0.5.
- Those with a very high or high average transport (high D/Pcr) have a rapid decline in dialysate glucose concentration and less UF, whereas those with average low and low transport (low D/Pcr) have a high 4 h dialysate glucose level and normal to high UF.
- UF failure may be due to excessive salt and water ingestion, excessive fluid absorption during the long dwell exchange, non-compliance with dialysis prescription, after recurrent peritonitis, and peritoneal sclerosis and/or adhesions.

Although ideally a PET will guide the prescription, in most cases PD will start without this information.

High transporters
- Reach small solute equilibration more quickly.
- Solutes and UF are reabsorbed.

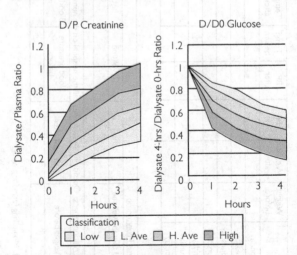

Fig. 19.2 (Left) Dialysate creatinine versus plasma creatinine at 4 h (D/P creatinine). (Right) Ratio of dialysate glucose at 4 h versus dialysate glucose at time zero (D/D0); H. Ave = high average, L. Ave = low average.

- Treat with:
  - short dwell times: APD.
  - icodextrin in day.
- Short cycles must be balanced against a relative reduction in dwell time as a greater proportion of the cycle will be spent filling and draining, and dialysis time will be lost.

Low transporters

- Solute D/P ratio increases linearly.
- UF continues during the dwell.
- Treat with long dwell times: CAPD or APD, so the glucose osmotic force remains present for longer and UF is maintained.

In general

- Infants and young children are high transporters.
- Older children and young adults are low transporters.

Peritoneal membrane changes over time

Anatomical changes:

- Increased thickness of the mesothelial layer.
- Local vasculopathy with neoangiogenesis (increased VEGF).
- Impaired host defences (decreased phagocytosis and bactericidal activity).

These changes result in fibrosis, progressing to sclerosis and calcification. ~50% of children have peritoneal sclerosis after 5 years on PD.

Functional changes:

- Increased glucose absorption.
- Decreased net UF.
- Increased small solute clearance.

= change to high transporter status.

High transporter status is associated with:

- increased dialysate protein losses.
- rapid progression to peritoneal membrane failure.
- greater risk of sclerosing peritonitis.
- increased mortality:
  - low albumin.
  - increased prevalence of vascular disease.

Transporter status may increase after peritonitis and with time on PD.

Delivered dialysis dose (creatinine clearance and Kt/Vurea) and dialysis adequacy

Classical measures of dialysis adequacy are based on small solute clearance using urea and creatinine and are defined as the minimum urea clearance and nutritional intake that prevent adverse outcomes. Measures used in PD are creatinine clearance and Kt/Vurea. One of the most important factors influencing adequacy is residual renal function, which can decrease with time (➔ see 'Haemodialysis: adequacy').

Creatinine clearance

Creatinine clearance is obtained from 24 h collections of dialysate and urine normalized to 1.73 m^2 BSA. Ideally the average of renal creatinine and urea nitrogen clearance (since at lower GFR creatinine clearance over estimates GFR because it is secreted by the tubules) is added to the peritoneal clearance. Creatinine clearance can be calculated by measuring the plasma creatinine at the midpoint of a timed dialysate collection by:

$$\text{Clearance of creatinine (Cr)} = \frac{\text{Cr in dialysate} \times \text{drained dialysis flow rate}}{\text{plasma Cr}}$$

$$\text{Weekly creatinine} = \text{total drain volume} \times \frac{\text{dialysate Cr}}{\text{plasma Cr}} \times 7$$

The result is normalized to body BSA and the total creatinine clearance = peritoneal + renal clearance

Weekly creatinine clearance =

$$\frac{Cr\ in\ dialysate \times dialysate\ volume \times 1.73 \times 7}{plasma\ Cr \times BSA}$$

It has been suggested that values should be >40 L/week/1.73 m^2 in infants, >50 L/week/1.73 m^2 in 12–24-month-olds, and >60 L/week/1.73 m^2 in those >2 years of age. It is easier to achieve creatinine clearance targets in high transporters, although these patients may have unsatisfactory UF.

Kt/V urea

Kt/V is the clearance of urea divided by the urea distribution volume (V, total body water).

K = based on standard clearance formula UV/P.

V = volume of distribution of urea = 0.6 × weight.

t = the number of dialysis days per week.

$$Weekly\ urea\ Kt/V = \frac{drain\ volume}{0.6 \times weight} \times \frac{dialysate\ urea \times 7}{plasma\ urea}$$

Total Kt/V = peritoneal + renal Kt/V

The minimum weekly goal for adult patients is a Kt/V urea of 2.1 (including contributions by residual renal function) and it is likely that the dose for children should at least equal this.

Kt/V and Ccr may not correlate. This is because urea is cleared better in low transporters so that Kt/V may be higher than in high transporters, whereas high transporters with high convective clearance and high UF have better Ccr.

Measures of dialysis adequacy other than small solute clearance

As well as small solute clearance, additional ways to assess the success of dialysis include:

- dialysis access complications and longevity.
- preservation of residual kidney function.
- fluid balance, BP, left ventricular function.
- biochemical and haematological control.
- nutrition and growth.
- discomfort, BP changes, and UF rates during the dialysis process.
- psychosocial adjustment, hospitalization, and school attendance.

These criteria need to be balanced against a dialysis programme that has the least possible adverse effects on quality of life (Table 19.2).

Complications

- Abdominal pain, particularly on filling and draining.
- Abdominal distension due to the presence of dialysate may cause vomiting, constipation and decreased appetite; and have an adverse effect on self-perception of body image.
- Exit site infections (➜ see 'Care of the exit site and exit site infection').
- Peritonitis (➜ see 'Peritonitis in patients on chronic peritoneal dialysis').

Table 19.2 What ways do we have to improve the dialysis process and how can we assess whether optimum dialysis has been achieved?

Optimum dialysis	How can this be assessed?
Well-functioning, long-lasting access with no complications	Compliance with 'fistula first' policy Access infection; access failure
Maintaining residual kidney function	Urine output; use of diuretics
Target weight maintained, with normal BP without antihypertensives and no left ventricular hypertrophy	BP SDS, echocardiogram, number of antihypertensive medications
No discomfort during dialysis or intradialytic hypotension	Percentage with pain interfering with PD. Intradialytic weight gains, UF rates <13 mL/kg/h for HD
No anaemia, acidosis, or potassium, calcium, phosphate, or PTH disturbance	Audit of haematological and biochemical control
Good nutrition and growth	Urea, albumin, Ht SDS, weight SDS, head circumference SDS, pubertal development
No hospitalizations for complications	Hospitalization rates
Psychosocial care provided. Educational input	Access to social workers, psychologists, and play therapists. Assessment of health-related quality of life Targeted educational needs and good school attendance

- Sclerosing peritonitis (➔ see 'Sclerosing peritonitis').
- Hydrocoeles, with scrotal fluid accumulation due to a patent processus vaginalis.
- Hernias are common. As well as the uncovering of congenital hernias there may be new hernias in the abdominal wall due to the raised abdominal pressure when dialysis fluid is in the abdominal cavity.
- Pleuro-peritoneal fistula may allow the passage of dialysate into the pleural cavity. Diagnosis can be made by US or the instillation of radioisotope into the peritoneal cavity. A significant leak will need a change to HD. Repair may be difficult as the defect can be small. Pleurodesis may be an alternative approach.
- Intra-abdominal adhesions.
- High intake of glucose may lead to insulin resistance and hyperlipidaemia.
- Parental/carer stress and burn out.

Peritonitis in patients on chronic peritoneal dialysis

The peritoneum can be infected by skin organisms at the time of connection/disconnection to the dialysis bag or cycler, by damage to the line, or via the Tenckhoff tunnel if the exit site is infected. *Staphylococcus aureus* and *S. epidermidis* and *Pseudomonas aeruginosa* are the most common causative bacteria. They may adhere to the catheter (biofilm) making eradication difficult, predisposing to recurrent infection. More rarely, organisms from the bowel may cause peritonitis.

Important general points
- Symptoms and outcome are usually worse with *Staphylococcus aureus* and Gram-negative infections, particularly *Pseudomonas*, and fungi.
- Prolonged use of broad-spectrum antibiotics may result in fungal peritonitis.
- Treatment should be aimed at preservation of the peritoneal membrane rather than the catheter.
- UK Renal Association standards state that units should not have more than one episode of peritonitis per 14 patient months averaged over 3 years.

Clinical presentation
- Cloudy dialysate fluid—needs urgent dialysate microscopy (menstruating girls may develop cloudy or blood-stained PD fluid).
- Abdominal pain.
- Fever.
- History of line break/contamination.
- Septic shock.
- The exit site and tunnel should be evaluated and any exudate swabbed and cultured.

Assessment
May present either as a local infection with minor systemic signs or associated severe systemic illness.
- Obtain a PD sample as soon as possible. The optimum dwell time is 2 h, minimum 1 h. If the abdomen is dry (e.g. patient on NIPD) manually fill with the normal PD fill volume and dwell for 1 h before draining.
- Send 50–100 mL of PD fluid effluent (to increase the chances of detecting the organisms) for cell count and differential, Gram stain, and culture (MC&S).
- WBC and differential, CRP.
- Blood cultures.

Diagnosis
- Treatment should be initiated if there are >100 WBC × 10^6/L PD effluent, or if there are 50–100 WBC × 10^6/L and symptoms/signs are suggestive of peritonitis.
- If between 50 and 100 WBC × 10^6/L and the patient is asymptomatic, hold dialysis and repeat a specimen after a repeat 2 h dwell.
- The WBCs are usually >50% neutrophils. If the cell count is persistently high, but the differential is predominantly lymphocytes or mononuclear cells, fungal peritonitis should be considered.
- Polymorphonuclear leucocytes may also be associated with visceral inflammation, such as appendicitis; monocytes are associated with gastroenteritis and icodextrin use; and eosinophils may be associated with allergy.
- Most laboratories report the total polymorphonuclear leucocyte count, without distinguishing between neutrophils and eosinophils in response to a request for routine microscopy of peritoneal dialysate effluent. If there is a possibility of eosinophilic peritonitis, an eosinophil count must be specifically requested.
- Organisms may be seen on Gram stain, although this may only be positive in ~30% of cases.
- A positive PD fluid culture usually develops within 24 h, and in the majority (75%) the diagnosis can be established within 72 h.
- No growth from PD fluid in the presence of other evidence of peritonitis (culture-negative peritonitis) should only occur in <15% of cases (UK Renal Association standards). It may be due to culture methods of low sensitivity, small culture volume, causative microorganisms that need special culture methods, in patients already on antibiotics, and non-infectious peritonitis. Culturing a large volume of dialysate improves the accuracy of diagnosis. Most methods presently use concentration methods, filtration, or centrifugation.

Eosinophilic peritonitis
Eosinophilic peritonitis is a response of the peritoneum to foreign substances (e.g. a component of the dialysis system, air, the dialysate (particularly icodextrin), and intraperitoneal medications). The child is usually asymptomatic, although the dialysate effluent is cloudy, sometimes with visible fibrin strands. It may be misdiagnosed as infection because not all laboratories report the eosinophil count, giving only the total polymorphonuclear cells.
- It should be considered if there is culture-negative peritonitis.
- It is defined as >100 white cells/mL of PD effluent, of which eosinophils constitute >10% of the total white cell count.
- There may also be a peripheral blood eosinophilia.
- It occurs most often after catheter insertion or during the treatment phase of peritonitis.
- It is more common in the very young.
- Rarely it may occur in association with fungal and parasitic infections.
- It may be persistent and may mask genuine infection.
- It is benign and usually resolves spontaneously over 2 to 6 weeks, although occasionally it may be so severe that catheter obstruction occurs due to fibrin, particularly in infants. Intraperitoneal heparin may be necessary.

Table 19.3 Dose of oral sodium cromoglicate for eosinophilic peritonitis

Age (years)	Weight (kg)	Dose
< 2	<5	50 mg three times daily
	>5 to <10	50 mg four times daily
2–14		100 mg four times daily
14–18		200 mg four times daily

- It may occur post surgery.
- Usually no treatment is necessary but oral antihistamines or sodium cromoglicate or intraperitoneal hydrocortisone may be helpful.

Dose of oral sodium cromoglicate for eosinophilic peritonitis (maximum dose 40 mg/kg/day), see Table 19.3.

Post-surgical peritonitis (within 2 weeks of procedure)

- A raised PD fluid white cell count is often found following placement of a PD catheter or other intraperitoneal procedures, or even post nephrectomy, but symptomatic peritonitis is uncommon.
- The white cells may be eosinophils.
- The operative procedure should be covered with IV antibiotics (e.g. amikacin 10 mg/kg and teicoplanin 10 mg/kg stat). The catheter is flushed frequently (10 mL/kg) until the dialysate is clear and then capped off.
- The catheter is flushed weekly (10 mL/kg) before use but a PD fluid sample should only be sent for microscopy and culture if the child is symptomatic. Treatment will be indicated in a symptomatic child with a rising WBC on serial PD fluid samples.

Line break/contamination of catheter

- Obtain 50–100 mL of PD fluid; if <100 WBC × 10⁶/L present add vancomycin and ciprofloxacin (➔ see 'Treatment of peritonitis') to dialysis bags for 48 h but continue usual dialysis regimen. If >100 WBC × 10⁶/L noted then treat as peritonitis.

If line break/contamination occurs before PD has commenced:
- Perform a line change.
- Give IV antibiotics (➔ see 'Treatment of peritonitis') for 48 h and continue as clinically indicated.

Treatment of peritonitis

General management

- IV antibiotics may be necessary if there is severe systemic involvement or if the child is immunosuppressed.
- Intraperitoneal antibiotics with broad-spectrum Gram-positive and Gram-negative cover should be given until cultures are available. An example of an antibiotic regimen is shown in the following section.
- Continuous cycling (CCPD) should be started for 48 h and continued until the dialysate WBC count, which should be checked daily, is <100 × 10⁶/L, then the usual regimen can be reinstated, with antibiotics into the dialysis bags.

- The usual total therapy volume but with a total therapy time of 24 h can be used for CCPD. This will give the same number of cycles per day but with increased dwell times and should be continued for 2 days. Intraperitoneal antibiotics and heparin should be added to all of the dialysis fluid bags.
- Close observations of fluid balance and plasma potassium levels are necessary.
- Oral antifungal therapy such as nystatin 100,000 U four times a day should be given while on antibiotics.
- Samples of PD fluid effluent should be sent daily for microscopy and culture to monitor treatment response. Allow at least 2 h between the last exchange and sampling.
- If the WBC count is <100 × 10⁶/L after 48 h continue on usual dialysis regimen adding antibiotics to PD fluid as previously described (including last bag fill if on CCPD).
- If the WBC count is >100 × 10⁶/L after 48 h, continue cycling regimen.
- In most cases the child can go home after 48 h to continue treatment.
- Continue for a minimum of 2 weeks, depending on the organism. 4 weeks of treatment may be necessary for *S. aureus*.

Antibiotics
(➔ See Chapter 22.)

- If there is only minor systemic illness, treatment can be intraperitoneal without IV antibiotics. Some centres use an intraperitoneal loading dose.
- Intraperitoneal antibiotics giving broad-spectrum Gram-positive and Gram-negative cover should be given until cultures are available. A common regimen would be to start with both intraperitoneal vancomycin and ciprofloxacin until Gram stain/culture of PD fluid is available. Then modify treatment accordingly:
  - Gram +ve organisms: vancomycin (25 mg/L) intraperitoneally.
  - Gram −ve organisms: ciprofloxacin (20 mg/L) intraperitoneally.
  - No organisms seen but >100 WBC × 10⁶/L: vancomycin (25 mg/L) plus ciprofloxacin (20 mg/L) intraperitoneally.
  - Plus heparin 400 U/L intraperitoneally (for 48 h cycling and continue as clinically indicated).
  - Plus nystatin oral suspension 100,000 U four times day while on antibiotics.
- If there is severe systemic illness or the child is immunocompromised, IV and intraperitoneal therapy is recommended. Initially use both IV vancomycin and ciprofloxacin until Gram stain/culture of PDF available. Then modify treatment accordingly:
  - Gram + ve organisms: vancomycin 10 mg/kg stat IV. If the 24 h level is <10 mg/L give further dose.
  - Gram −ve organisms: ciprofloxacin 5 mg/kg dose 12-hourly IV (maximum dose 400 mg 12-hourly).
  - No organisms seen but >100 WBC × 10⁶/L: vancomycin 10 mg/kg stat IV (if 24 h level <10 mg/L give further dose) plus ciprofloxacin 5 mg/kg dose 12-hourly IV (maximum dose 400 mg 12-hourly).
  - Plus heparin 200 U/L intraperitoneally (for 48 h cycling and continue as clinically indicated).
  - Plus nystatin oral suspension 100,000 U four times a day while on antibiotics

- Continuing antibiotic therapy can be modified according to the identity and sensitivity of the organisms cultured. Flucloxacillin 50 mg/L can be substituted for sensitive Gram-positive organisms if there is concern about the development of resistance to vancomycin; and gentamicin 5 mg/L or amikacin 25 mg/L can be substituted for possible ciprofloxacin resistance. When no bacteria are isolated, both antibiotics are continued.

Indications for removal of the catheter

- Fungal peritonitis.
- Severe intra-abdominal sepsis and septicaemic shock.
- Exit site or tunnel infection due to the same organism as that causing the peritonitis.
- This is a recurrence with the same organism within 4 weeks of stopping therapy (i.e. relapsing peritonitis). *Pseudomonas* is particularly difficult to eradicate and is the commonest cause of catheter removal.
- Persistently raised WBC count after 3–4 days if infection severe, or 7 days if infection mild.
- Child remains symptomatic after 3–4 days.

After the catheter has been removed:
- Antibiotics should be continued for another 5–7 days.
- A new catheter can be inserted at a minimum of 1 week after all clinical evidence of peritonitis has subsided, providing *S. aureus* carriage has been eliminated and any infection in the Tenckhoff tunnel has resolved.

Fungal peritonitis

Children at risk:
- Frequent broad-spectrum antibiotic usage.
- Immunosuppressed post transplant with PD catheter *in situ*.

Treatment:
- Start treatment with liposomal amphotericin—1 mg/kg as a daily dose IV changing if possible after 48 h (following fluconazole sensitivity testing and identification) to fluconazole 12 mg/kg IV as a daily dose for 48 h decreasing to 6 mg/kg/day (maximum dose 200 mg daily) for a total of at least 2 weeks.
- If the child still has a PD catheter *in situ* following a renal transplant, the dose must be adjusted based on renal function (remember that fluconazole increases calcineurin inhibitor levels).
- Continue with oral fluconazole for further 4 weeks. Most *Candida albicans* are sensitive to fluconazole.
- Catheter removal as soon as possible (particularly if not being used, e.g. if not removed at the time of transplant) as adhesions precluding future PD develop rapidly.
- Re-initiation of PD is usually possible following successful early treatment of fungal peritonitis as long as it was treated promptly. However, it is wise to rest the peritoneum for 3 months if possible.

Complications of peritonitis

- Catheter removal and need for HD.
- Loss of UF.
- Malnourishment due to catabolism, poor nutritional intake, and high dialysate protein losses.
- Fungal peritonitis.
- Persistent intra-abdominal sepsis requiring laparotomy and peritoneal washouts.
- Adhesions and failure of future peritoneal dialysis.
- Ileus and pancreatitis.
- Death.

Reference

Warady BA, Bakkaloglu S, Newland J, et al. Consensus guidelines for the prevention and treatment of catheter-related infections and peritonitis in pediatric patients receiving peritoneal dialysis: 2012 update. *Perit Dial Int* 2012;32(Suppl 2):S32–86.

Sclerosing peritonitis

The peritoneum becomes thickened and fibrosed, affecting gut peristalsis and leading to gut obstruction and malnutrition.

Causes

- Prolonged period on PD. Although time on PD is important, not all children will inevitably develop sclerosing peritonitis.
- Recurrent peritonitis.
- Prolonged use of peritoneal dialysate fluid with high glucose concentrations.

Presentation

- Episodes of sterile peritonitis, fever, abdominal pain, high CRP, and/or ascites (which can be haemorrhagic).
- Poor UF and decreasing small solute clearance.
- Adhesions may cause gut obstruction.
- Adhesions may cause the dialysis catheter to move out of the pelvis, resulting in poor drainage.

Diagnosis

- No easy screening test (other than biopsy) so a high index of suspicion is necessary.
- Thickened bowel loops may be seen on US.
- Peritoneal calcification may be present.
- Diagnosis is ultimately dependent on biopsy of the peritoneum.

Treatment

- Transfer to HD (although the process may continue).
- Immunosuppression has been used but there is limited evidence of efficacy.
- Surgery to remove the thickened membrane if gut obstruction occurs. This should only be undertaken by specialized teams.
- Total parenteral nutrition may be necessary.
- Tamoxifen has been used in adults; the concomitant administration of corticosteroids in many trials makes the specific effect of tamoxifen difficult to ascertain.

Outcome

- Mortality is high due to the complications of surgery and malnutrition.
- Subsequent intraperitoneal transplantation, if necessary, is technically difficult.

Reference

Shroff R, Stefanidis CJ, Askiti V, et al. Encapsulating peritoneal sclerosis in children on chronic PD: a survey from the European Paediatric Dialysis Working Group. *Nephrol Dial Transplant* 2013;28:1908–1914.

Sclerosing peritonitis

The peritoneum becomes thickened and fibrosed, affecting gut transit and leading to gut obstruction and malnutrition.

Extracorporeal treatment

Haemodialysis: principles

* A semipermeable membrane allows the passage of water and small-molecular-weight molecules, and inhibits the movement of larger molecules.
* Solute transfer occurs by diffusion and convection.
* Water is removed by ultrafiltration (UF).

Diffusion is movement down a concentration gradient and is affected by:
* membrane permeability.
* membrane surface area.
* solute molecular weight.
* solute charge.
* transmembrane concentration gradient is therefore maximized by high flow rates of blood and dialysate in opposite directions (countercurrent).
* temperature of the dialysate.

Convection (solute drag)
* Passive movement of solute 'dragged' by water moving down an osmotic or pressure gradient.
* It is independent of the concentration gradient but dependent on the UF rate and the dialyser.

Ultrafiltration
* The process whereby water is moved across the membrane by convective flow down a pressure gradient, which is created by generating a transmembrane pressure within the dialysate compartment by the dialysis effluent pump. Large-molecular-weight molecules are removed better by convection than diffusion.
* The net rate of UF is affected by the surface area, structure, and thickness of the dialyser, and the transmembrane hydrostatic pressure and osmotic pressure.

Haemodiafiltration (HDF)
The combination of dialysis and UF. This may be needed when large volumes of fluid need removal.

Mass transfer
* Toxins in the intravascular space will be rapidly removed.
* Intracellular toxins need time to move into the intravascular space as concentration gradients change, so are removed more slowly.
* Molecular size will also affect removal (see Table 20.1).
* Large numbers of biochemically active, potentially toxic 'middle molecules' have been identified: e.g. peptides that may contribute to poor appetite, anaemia, inflammation, and CVD.
* The best known is beta-2-microglobulin, which can cause dialysis-related amyloid.
* Some protein-bound middle molecules may also be toxic, e.g. leptin, and are particularly difficult to remove by any dialysis technique.

Table 20.1 Uraemic retention solutes by molecular weight, and their method of removal during haemodialysis

Solute	MW	Example (MW)	Method of removal
Small solutes	<500	Urea (60), creatinine (113)	Diffusion
Middle molecules	300–5000	Vitamin B12 (1355)	Diffusion/convection
Low-MW proteins	5000–50,000	Beta-2-microglobulin (11,800)	Diffusion/convection
Large proteins	>50,000	Albumin (60,000)	Convection

MW, molecular weight, in Da.

Haemodialysis: the machine, dialysate, and water

There are two circuits—for blood and dialysate, which run in opposite directions, separated by the semipermeable membrane of the dialyser. Fig. 20.1 illustrates the important elements of a HD circuit.

A paediatric HD machine needs:
* a volumetric fluid removal system, i.e. one where the in- and outflow volumes from the dialyser are measured so that UF volume is measured directly.
* the ability to measure and remove very small amounts of fluid.
* to be capable of low blood flow speeds.
* to be able to use lines of varying blood volumes.
* to have a bicarbonate dialysate delivery system.

HD machines can have systems for continuous online monitoring of the haematocrit, converting this to blood volume. They also measure oxygen saturation, BP, pulse, and Kt/V urea.

New machines are able to combine diffusive and convective solute transport (HDF) and are able to generate ultrapure dialysate and infusion fluids 'online'.

The Cardio-Renal Pediatric Dialysis Emergency Machine (CARPEDIEM®) and Newcastle Infant Dialysis Ultrafiltration System (NIDUS®) HD machines are designed for acute HD and can be a bridge for chronic HD in very small infants (down to 800 g) until conventional machines can be used.
* CARPEDIEM® machine: dual-lumen catheters as small as 4–4.5 Fr can be used with a minimal line volume of 27 mL. Dialyser surface areas range from 0.075 to 0.25 m^2 and miniature roller pumps deliver flow rates of 5–50 mL/min.
* NIDUS® machine: a single-lumen catheter allows for better flows with an extracorporeal circuit volume of <10 mL. Blood is aspirated and is then passed repeatedly through a high-flux polysulphone 0.045 m^2 hollow-fibre haemofilter before being returned to the patient.

Portable home HD machines use dialysate that can be pre-prepared as 5 L bags or prepared by the system from tap water. This offers families the freedom of a portable machine that does not rely on plumbing of the home water supply for children >10 kg.

Dialysate

* Is a solution of purified water, Na, K, Mg, Ca, Cl, dextrose, and bicarbonate.
* Electrolytes are mixed and proportionated by the dialysis machine.
* Bicarbonate is the dialysate buffer: the dialysis solution contains acetic or citric acid, which lower the pH of the final mixture and prevents precipitation of Ca and Mg carbonate. Bicarbonate is added by a second proportionating pump.
* The dialysis machine monitors the electrical conductivity of the dialysis solution to ensure the correct proportion of water to concentrate is being used.
* Standard dialysate flow is 500 mL/min (range 300–800 mL/min).
* Dialysate is warmed to 35–37.5°C.

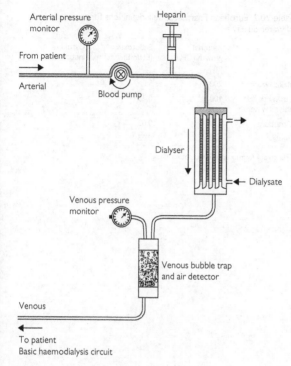

Fig. 20.1 The important elements of a haemodialysis circuit.

Water

- A system of progressively smaller filters, activated carbon and water softeners, culminating in a reverse osmosis unit in the machine, purify water so it is of a quality suitable for dialysate production by removing particulates, dissolved inorganic and organic substances, microorganisms, and toxins.
- Water quality standards (bacterial, endotoxin, and chemical content) should be checked monthly (ℜ see https://www.ncbi.nlm.nih.gov/pmc/articles/PMC4596525/ and ℜ http://www.renal.org/docs/default-source/guidelines-resources/RA_and_ART_Guideline_on_Water_Treatment_Facilities_and_Water_Quality_for_Haemodialysis_26_06_11.pdf?sfvrsn=0).
- Ultra-pure water is ideal, but is essential for HDF.
- Even very low levels of endotoxin in the water can cause cytokine-mediated inflammation that, in turn, may contribute to the increased risk for CVD seen in patients on dialysis (Table 20.2).

Table 20.2 European Pharmacopoeia definitions for the upper limit of water quality

	Bacterial growth (CFU/mL)	Endotoxin (EU/mL)	Cytokine induction
Mains water	200	5	+
Conventional dialysis water	100	0.25	+
Ultra-pure	0.01	0.03	–
Sterile	10^{-6}	0.03	–

CFU, colony-forming units; EU, endotoxin units.

Haemodialysis: factors affecting the prescription

The extracorporeal circuit

- The extracorporeal circuit is composed of an arterial ('A', red) line and a venous ('V', blue) line. The 'A' line carries blood out of the child to the haemodialyser, while the 'V' line takes dialysed blood back to the child.
- Pressures are monitored in the arterial and venous segments. Low-pressure alarms indicate insufficient blood flow ('sucking'). High venous pressure alarms indicate reduced return of blood to the patient. If an alarm activates, the blood pump is stopped and the lines are clamped.
- Sample ports in either side of the circuit allow blood samples to be obtained while the child is on the machine.
- The lines and the haemodialyser are selected on the basis that a child can usually tolerate 8% (up to a maximum of 10%) of their total blood volume (80 mL/kg estimated dry weight) in the extracorporeal circuit.
  - *Example*: a child weighing 10 kg has a total blood volume of 800 mL (10 × 80 mL); therefore, the extracorporeal circuit is 64–80 mL, so the total volume of the lines and haemodialyser must not exceed 64–80 mL. There are lines that are made in a variety of sizes (Gambro®; Kimal® for neonatal) by different companies. Some examples are shown in Table 20.3.
- Lines are primed with saline.
- If it is necessary to exceed the safe extracorporeal volume because the smallest available circuit volume is still >10% of the child's circulating volume, then the circuit must be primed with blood. The blood is not washed back into the child at the completion of dialysis to prevent haemoconcentration.

The haemodialyser

- The haemodialyser is composed of two compartments, one for blood and one for dialysate, which are separated by the semipermeable membrane. A hollow fibre configuration achieves the maximal membrane surface area over which blood and dialysate make contact.
- The membrane can be modified cellulose or a synthetic material. Unmodified cellulose membranes are the least biocompatible, and may cause activation of complement and leucocytes, or a severe allergic reaction within minutes of starting dialysis. Sterilizing solutions (e.g. ethylene oxide) may also cause allergic reactions.
- The dialyser size is selected on the basis of its surface area and the priming volume. Roughly, the surface area should be equal to, but not exceed that of the child. At present, haemodialyser surface areas range from 0.25 m^2 up to 1.7 m^2 and above. The greater the surface area, the greater the clearance of water and solutes.
- The ultrafiltration coefficient, KUf, describes the dialyser's ability to remove water. For example, a KUf of 2.0 means that 2 mL/h of UF will occur for each 1 mmHg of transmembrane pressure (TMP).
- Dialysers with KUfs of <10 mL/h/mmHg are referred to as low flux and those with a rate of 15–60 mL/h/mmHg are called high flux. Synthetic membranes tend to be high flux.

Table 20.3 Volumes of haemodialysis lines

	Venous (mL)	Arterial (mL)	Total (mL)
Mini-neonatal (<6 kg)	21	8	29
Neonatal (6–12 kg)	22	18	40
Paediatric	42	30	72
Adult	70	62	132

- Solute transport properties of dialysate membranes are expressed as the mass transfer-area coefficient (KoA) for urea (mL/min).
- Dialysers of usual efficiency (for removal of small solutes) have a KoA of 300–500 mL/min; high-efficiency dialysers may have a KoA of >700 mL/min.
- Clearance of creatinine, urea, vitamin B12, and phosphate are given for all dialysers. Refer to the specific manufacturer specification sheet for precise clearance values.
- Some molecular weights (Da): urea, 60; creatinine, 113; vitamin B12, 1355; and albumin, 60,000.
- Dialysers may be sterilized with irradiation, steam, or ethylene oxide. Priming the circuit with 1–2 L of saline to expel air and prepare the capillaries for use will also help flush out remaining ethylene oxide and other soluble compounds in the circuit, which may be toxic or cause allergic reactions at the commencement of dialysis.

Types of haemodialysis

- Conventional HD uses a low-flux (small pore size) membrane and solute removal is primarily by diffusion.
- High-efficiency HD uses a low-flux membrane with a high efficiency (KoA) for removal of small solutes. It is also achieved by using a larger surface area membrane and a high blood flow.
- High flux HD utilizes high-flux membranes. It is more efficient in removing solutes that are substantially larger than urea (middle-sized and large molecules such as vitamin B12 and beta-2 microglobulin respectively), but may not be more efficient than conventional HD in removing small solutes.
- Because conventional HD is principally diffusive based, even when using high-flux dialysers it is limited in clearing middle-sized molecules (molecular weight 200–20,000 Da), which are better removed by convection.
- HDF superimposes convection upon standard diffusive blood purification. It is possible to use a high-flux haemofilter to ultrafilter up to 30% of the blood volume passing through it. The desired volume of replacement fluid is then infused into the blood circuit. Better clearance of beta-2-microglobulin may reduce the risk of amyloidosis. Ultrapure dialysate is necessary. Care must be taken that excess fluid removal does not occur.
- High-flux dialysers or HDF are becoming the norm even in small children particularly if they are likely to be on HD for an unpredictable time, and those showing evidence of amyloidosis.

Length of session

- 4 h is standard for chronic HD.
- Shorter sessions will adversely affect clearance of large molecules.
- Long (or frequent short) sessions (e.g. overnight) improve fluid balance and phosphate clearance, both of which have a positive effect on mortality.
- Increasing the number of hours per week on dialysis is the most important factor that can improve outcome.
- For acute dialysis:
  - If the plasma urea is >30 mmol/L then the session should last no more than 1–2 h.
  - Patients with tumour lysis syndrome may need a very long session.
  - For acute correction of hyperkalaemia, 1–1.5 h may be sufficient.

Frequency of sessions

- Chronic HD is conventionally performed three times a week.
- More intensified regimens are beneficial to BP, growth, bone health, quality of life, and life expectancy. Such regimens may be daily for 3 h or slow overnight.
- Intensified regimens may be performed in HD centres—some centres offer short daily, nocturnal intermittent, or daily nocturnal HD or HDF. Medication requirements are reduced, including phosphate binders, erythropoietin, and antihypertensive agents. Fluid limitations and dietary restrictions can also be lifted.
- Acute HD is performed as often as necessary (usually daily), but with an aim to achieve a target of three times a week.

Blood pump speeds

The speed at which the blood is pumped out of the child and around the circuit is equivalent to their extracorporeal volume total, i.e. up to body weight (kg) × 8 mL/min. Thus, the 10 kg child, with an extracorporeal circuit of 64–80 mL can have blood speeds of up to 80 mL/min.

Estimation of target weight

- In chronic HD, the aim is to end the session with the child at their target/desired weight, i.e. the weight below which the child will become symptomatically hypotensive.
- Target weight can only be determined by careful, persistent fluid removal to achieve normal BP after dialysis.
- Target weight needs to be reassessed at least monthly, and more often in very small children.
- The child who is always hypertensive is likely to be above their target weight; antihypertensives can usually be discarded when this is achieved.
- However, attainment of target weight with conventional three-times-a-week dialysis can be difficult in the child who has high interdialytic weight gains requiring large UF volumes. Much better results have been obtained with daily dialysis, with most children no longer needing antihypertensives at all.

Fluid removal

- The fluid loss required is calculated by the interdialytic weight gain, the volume of saline required for the 'wash back', and any drinks consumed

during the session. The HD machine will adjust the TMP accordingly, depending on the time (in hours), and the venous pressure (affected by the blood speed and peripheral resistance), to give an hourly UF rate.
- The greater the TMP that is set, the greater the amount of fluid that will be removed from the child, and the more likely that the child will feel unwell.
- High UF rates while diffusion is occurring are not well tolerated. To counteract this, isolated UF can be performed, in which the flow of dialysate is halted, therefore diffusion and hence dialysis ceases. This allows more fluid to be removed more quickly from the child, and is useful when there are large volumes for UF.
- The amount each child will tolerate losing per hour varies, but 10 mL/kg/h is a safe starting point. Up to 600 mL/hour can be removed in children ≥40 kg, who are consistently volume overloaded.
- No more than 5% of body weight should be removed in one session, or 0.2 mL/kg/min.
- Fluid loss (UF) can only be achieved if the fluid is in the vascular space. As the vascular space empties, refilling must occur from the other compartments, to allow UF to continue. The child will show signs of hypovolaemia if UF (from HD or isolated UF) continues unchecked.
- If hypovolaemia occurs, the UF rate should be decreased and the child given a drink or bolus of saline to correct hypotension, if necessary:
  - Many patients collapse having had no prior warning of feeling unwell, therefore close monitoring of BP and other observations (including peripheral temperatures) is important during isolated UF.
  - Chronic HD children are often able to recognize the early warning signs and can prevent such episodes.
- A child undergoing acute HD should be treated with caution, as their target weight will not have been established and their response to extracorporeal treatments is unknown.
- As dialysis does not occur during isolated UF, the length of time on the dialysis machine will increase.

Anticoagulation
- Heparin is given at a rate of 5–50 U/kg/h through the arterial side of the circuit to prevent the blood clotting. For the child with AKI with no bleeding disorders, a rate of 10 U/kg/h can be given.
- LMWH is an alternative, given as a bolus of 1 mg/kg at the beginning of the session.
- The heparin infusion should stop 30 min prior to the end of dialysis if a fistula is being used, to prevent bleeding after the needles have been removed.
- The formation of clots, particularly in the bubble trap, should be monitored. A bolus of 50–100 mL of saline flushed through the circuit with the arterial lines clamped may reveal clot formation. UF will need to be increased to remove the extra saline. The heparin dose may be increased and/or a bolus of heparin given. The venous side of the blood circuit can be changed during the session to prevent total clotting.
- The heparin dose will need to be adjusted in the patient with abnormal clotting or low platelets. Heparin-free dialysis can be used; the circuit can be primed with heparinized saline (3000–5000 U/L) (and then

flushed) as this will bind to the dialyser. The dialyser must be checked regularly for signs of clotting. High blood flow will help prevent clotting.
• Heparin may induce thrombocytopenia in some patients, which resolves on stopping treatment.

Clots will form when there is:
• slow blood flow because of access flow problems.
• inadequate heparinization.
• a raised haematocrit.
• a long period of UF, as the warmed dialysate flow is lost, and the haematocrit is raised as fluid is removed.
• if a circuit clots off completely, the blood in the lines is lost. This will not have an immediate detrimental effect on the child, providing the rules on extracorporeal volume have been observed.
• if clotting problems persist, aspirin and/or dipyridamole or warfarin or treatment may be considered.

Biochemistry

• *Na*: the dialysate Na must be within 10 mmol of the child's plasma Na to avoid disequilibrium. The Na dialysate concentrate level can be altered on the machine within preset parameters (➔ see discussion of Na ramping in 'Haemodialysis: complications').
• *K*: as the usual concentration of K in dialysate is 1–2 mmol/L, adjustment may be needed for children with low plasma K levels or in those requiring a long dialysis session, when a dialysate K of 3–3.5 mmol/L can be used; if the child has a very high K level, a zero-K dialysate can be used for a short period of time, before reverting to the normal K dialysate. There is a danger of severe hypokalaemia if a zero-K is used for too long. The use of plasma K monitoring equipment (ionometer) is recommended to facilitate management of hyperkalaemia. Although immediately after HD K levels are very low, they rebound rapidly.
• *Bicarbonate*: the dialysate level can be adjusted on the machine, within preset limits. The level is usually ~35 mmol/L.
• *Urea*: a rapid reduction in serum urea, usually if >40 mmol/L for chronic patients and 30 mmol/L for acute patients, can result in disequilibrium syndrome (➔ see 'Haemodialysis: complications', p. 561). Mannitol can be infused (1 g/kg), during HD, through the bubble trap to counteract this. The best way to avoid disequilibrium is to keep the dialysis session short, <2 h.
• *Creatinine*: will fall rapidly during the session as there is none in the dialysate, but it will rebound and rise rapidly following the end of dialysis.
• *Ca*: the standard dialysate level is 1.75 mmol/L. This is equivalent to the blood-ionized Ca, so results in an influx of Ca into the patient and a rise in serum Ca post dialysis. Dialysates containing Ca concentrations from 1.25 mmol/L (which is equivalent to the blood in the normal child) are available, and can be used in hypercalcaemia, in order to remove Ca from the patient.
• PO_4: after an initial fall in the first 1–2 h, movement from the intracellular compartment is slow; therefore, long dialysis sessions (e.g. overnight) result in the best phosphate clearance.

Administration of blood products

- *Albumin*—low serum albumin will result in oedema and difficulty in removing excess fluid:
  - If the child is oligoanuric, 20% albumin should only be given when on dialysis, as the resultant fluid shifts can cause pulmonary oedema.
  - It must be given in small boluses through the arterial infusion port at the beginning of the session, to allow time for movement of fluid into the intravascular compartment.
- *Blood*: should only be required to prime the lines if the dialyser and lines volume exceeds the safe extracorporeal circuit volume, i.e. in infants. This blood prime is not washed back into the child at the end of the session.
- If blood is required for the treatment of anaemia, the calculation for number of millilitres of blood required = weight (kg) × 3 × number of g/dL that the Hb is to be raised.
- The blood is infused in small boluses at the beginning of dialysis, through the arterial infusion port, so that K will be dialysed out. Resulting fluid shifts may lead to the need for UF towards the end of the session.

Haemodialysis: complications

Common complications

- Nausea, vomiting, itching, pains, and cramps.
- Intradialytic hypotension due to:
  - intravascular volume depletion due to slow refilling from the extravascular space.
  - shifting of fluid from the extracellular to intracellular space due to a decrease in serum osmolality due to urea removal and use of a dialysate Na lower then plasma, as this leads to hyponatraemia in blood returning to the patient.
  - excessive UF requirements because of a high interdialytic salt and water intake.
  - impaired sympathetic activity.
  - vasodilation in response to warm dialysate.
  - splanchnic pooling of blood while eating during dialysis.
  - use of antihypertensive agents.

Treatment of intradialytic hypotension

- Acutely, normal saline 5 mL/kg and cessation of UF.
- The daily fluid allowance and target weight must be reassessed.
- UF separate from dialysis.
- *Na ramping*: the machine can be programmed to deliver a Na concentration higher than that of the plasma at the beginning of the session so that Na diffuses into the plasma and balances the change in osmolality caused by diffusive urea removal. The Na concentration in the dialysate is then progressively reduced. Although this technique helps intradialytic hypotension, the danger is that there is inadequate Na removal, hence contributing to chronic fluid overload and hypertension.
- Newer machines are able to monitor circulating blood volume by determining changes in haematocrit. A decrease in blood volume of >8% in the first 90 min or >4% thereafter is likely to lead to hypovolaemia.

Less common complications

- *Disequilibrium*—due to the plasma urea concentration falling more rapidly than brain cell urea concentration, with the resultant movement of water into brain cells by osmosis:
  - It can present with headache, nausea, and dizziness, and progress to disorientation, seizures, and coma.
  - Symptoms resolve spontaneously, but if severe can be treated with IV mannitol using 1 g/10% of body weight.
  - Mannitol can also be used prophylactically when initiating HD in someone with a high urea.
- *Haemolysis*: may present with pains and nausea, and a dark appearance to venous blood. It may be due to overheating, contamination or hypotonicity of dialysate, kinking of the lines, or a malfunctioning pump. Dialysis should be stopped and the K must be checked immediately. Haemolysis may continue for some hours.
- *Urticaria*: can be treated with an antihistamine or hydrocortisone if severe.

- *Air embolism*: rare as air detectors will clamp the return lines. 1 mL/kg may be fatal:
  - Presents with fitting or coma in the upright patient, and chest symptoms if recumbent.
  - Treatment is to clamp the lines, stop the pump, place the patient head down in the left lateral position, give 100% oxygen (to enhance nitrogen diffusion out of air bubbles), and resuscitation as necessary.
  - Air may need to be aspirated from the ventricle.
- *Anaphylactic reaction to the dialyser*—can occur at any time and necessitates a change of dialyser:
  - 'First-use syndrome' occurs soon after the start of dialysis and disappears with dialyser reuse and predialysis rinsing or can occur at any time. Both cause hypotension (sometimes hypertension), angio-oedema, pulmonary symptoms, chest and abdominal pain, vomiting, fever, urticaria, and pruritus.
  - Reactions can result from activation of plasma complement or kinin systems by the dialysis membrane; or the release of noxious materials as contamination of the dialyser may have occurred during manufacture or the sterilization process (e.g. with ethylene oxide).
  - Dialysis must be stopped and blood should not be returned to the patient.
  - Normal saline for hypotension, adrenaline SC or IM (1:1000 concentration), and/or hydrocortisone may be necessary.
- *Dialysis-related amyloidosis*—symptoms are typically first reported after 7–10 years of dialysis:
  - A disabling, progressive condition caused by the polymerization within tendons, synovium, and other tissues of beta-2-microglobulin, a large (molecular weight 11,600 Da) molecule, released into the circulation as a result of normal cell turnover.
  - Clearance is improved by longer dialysis sessions and HDF.

Haemodialysis: adequacy

The clearance of urea is used as the basis for all calculations of dialysis adequacy, and is the minimum urea clearance and nutritional intake that prevents adverse outcomes. However, it has to be remembered that:
- urea clearance represents small molecule clearance.
- it does not measure clearance of larger and more important molecules that move more slowly.
- clearance figures for optimal dialysis have not been established.
- studies in adults suggest that residual renal function is more important for survival than measured 'adequacy'.

Small solute clearance (urea kinetic modelling (UKM), Kt/V, urea reduction ratio (URR)):
- UKM uses pre- and post-dialysis samples over two sessions to measure urea clearance and generation rates. It takes into account residual renal function, predicted dialyser clearance, blood and dialysate flow, time on dialysis, and fluid removal. It can be used to assess protein intake as well, but is not commonly used because of its complexity.
- Kt/V (K = urea clearance of dialyser, t = treatment time, V = volume of distribution = $0.6 \times$ body weight) can be predicted from the pre- and post-dialysis urea, weight loss, and duration of dialysis. There are several different formulae available for the calculation. Most would use the Daugirdas II formula (also discussed in this section).
- URR underestimates the dose of dialysis as it does not take into account convective losses or residual renal function. It is calculated as follows:

$$\left[(\text{Pre} - \text{dialysis urea} - \text{post} - \text{dialysis urea}) / \text{Pre} - \text{dialysis urea}\right] \times 100$$

- Errors can occur by incorrect blood sampling:
  - If the sample is contaminated by blood from the dialyser, or heparin, or if there is recirculation, the urea result will be underestimated, giving a falsely high Kt/V.
  - The earlier the blood is drawn after the completion of dialysis, the higher the apparent delivered dose, as urea rises rapidly post dialysis.
  - Methods of standardization of post-dialysis sampling are the slow-flow and stop-flow methods.
  - Stop dialysate flow is the most commonly used, but gives higher results.
  - *Stop-dialysate-flow method*—stop dialysate flow, but keep blood pump running for 5 min; take sample from anywhere in circuit.
- Kt/V (Daugirdas II) can be calculated as follows:

$$Kt/V = -\ln(C_1/C_0 - 0.008 \times t) = (4 - 3.5 \times C_1/C_0) \times UF/W$$

where C_0 and C_1 = pre- and post-dialysis blood urea (mg/dL), respectively; t = time (h); UF = ultrafiltration volume (kg); W = post-dialysis weight (→ see 'Appendix', p. 681 for urea conversion figures).
- Urinary creatinine clearance can be calculated using the standard formula:

$$(\text{Urine creatinine} \times 24\,\text{h urine volume}) / \text{serum creatinine}$$

- Problems include collecting a timed urine collection and that the true GFR is overestimated (due to increased tubular secretion of creatinine at low GFRs, resulting in a 25% day-to-day variation in the same patient.
- Measures of adequacy in children have not been defined, but consensus standards propose that they should be equal to or better than adult recommendations of >1.2 for Kt/V and >65% for URR.

For measures of dialysis adequacy other than small solute clearance, ➔ see Chapter 19.

Haemodialysis: vascular access

Acute HD will require either a temporary percutaneous dual-lumen catheter (e.g. vascath or GamCath®) or a tunnelled cuffed catheter (e.g. Permcath®). Access for chronic HD is by tunnelled line, arteriovenous (AV) fistula, or rarely shunts or grafts.

Tunnelled lines

Used in children who are too young for an AV fistula or who are not expected to be on dialysis long; e.g. awaiting a living-related transplant. Such lines have a greater risk of poor function, infection, and hospitalization, and are associated with increased mortality in adults.

- Superior to non-tunnelled lines, but inferior to an AV fistula.
- The internal jugular vein is the preferred site. Lines should preferably not be sited in the subclavian veins as this may lead to vascular stenosis and, therefore, the inability to create a fistula in the future.
- Stenoses typically occur at the catheter entry site into the vein and at the catheter tip site.
- Vascular access problems are indicated by arterial or venous pressure alarms:
  - Low arterial pressure alarms indicate there is an insufficient blood flow reaching the blood pump.
  - Commonly referred to as 'sucking' and is usually a result of poor access position in the vessel.
  - Low venous pressure alarm also indicates poor blood flow.
  - High venous pressure alarm indicates that there is an occlusion to the flow of returning blood.
  - Due either to poor access position, fistula stenosis, or the presence of clot formation. Alteplase (tPA) can be used to dissolve suspected clots in the central line. A solution of 1 mg/mL is instilled in the dead space of the catheter and left for at least 1 h, preferably overnight or between dialysis sessions, after which it is aspirated. It can also be used as a line lock post dialysis as prophylaxis against line clotting and infection.
- In order to achieve satisfactory blood flow rates, the larger the gauge of the access the better. Catheter sizes range from 6.5 to 14 Fr in differing lengths (12 or 18 cm or 12–40 cm for smaller or larger gauges, respectively) and are chosen according to the size of the child and their vessels (see Table 20.4).
- Most lines are dual lumen, but HD can also be achieved using single-lumen access:
  - In infants, single-lumen access may be more appropriate, as a catheter with a larger lumen can be inserted, remembering that flow is proportional to the fourth power of the radius.
  - In order to obtain two-directional blood flows with a single lumen line, the dialysis circuit has to be modified.
  - This can be achieved by the double-pump method, using two blood pumps which pump alternately, or by using a single pump that pumps intermittently, using gravity to let blood flow back in to the child.
  - Both methods require an expansion chamber in the circuit to allow for the pressure changes.

Table 20.4 Catheter size and positioning according to the weight of the child

Size of child	Catheter size (Fr)	Siting
Neonate	5 (single lumen)	Femoral vein
3–6 kg	7	Internal or external jugular or femoral vein (preferably not subclavian)
6–15 kg	8	
>15 kg	9	
>30 kg	≥10	

- This results in an increased volume of blood in the circuit and a larger degree of recirculation.
- Recirculation occurs when blood that has been dialysed returns to the dialyser inlet, i.e. the access flow rate is less than the blood pump. It can be a marker of venous stenosis.
- Recirculation >10% requires further access investigation.
- *Measurement of recirculation*:
  - Take arterial and venous samples from the access lines 30 min after the start of dialysis (without UF).
  - Halve the pump speed then switch it off.
  - Clamp arterial line above the port and take a sample from it (this is the sample representing systemic circulation).
  - Restart dialysis.
  - Measure urea in arterial (A), venous (V) and systemic (S) circulations:

$$\text{Recirculation}(\%) = \left[(S-A)/(S-V) \right] \times 100$$

Vascular access infection

Catheter-related infections

Infections may be at the exit site, the SC tunnel, or in the catheter, with development of biofilm and difficulty eradicating the bacteria. Line sepsis may present as a rigor soon after starting dialysis, fever with raised CRP or septicaemic collapse.

Definitions

- *Exit site infection*: erythema, tenderness, and discharge within 2 cm of the exit site.
- *Tunnel infection*: tenderness, erythema, and induration along the SC tract >2 cm from the exit site.
- *Catheter colonization*: repeated growth of the same organism without signs of sepsis.
- *Catheter infection*: septicaemia, bacteraemia, or fungaemia with:
  - at least one positive culture of the same organism from the catheter and a peripheral vein.
  - clinical signs of infection (fever, hypotension).
  - no other cause of infection.
  - a raised CRP.

Prevention
- Strict attention to aseptic technique.
- Monthly culture of the exit site, and nose of child and carers, and treatment for 5 days every month with nasal or exit site mupirocin if *Staphylococcus aureus* grows.
- There is no evidence that the type of dressing or the use of lines impregnated with antimicrobials is superior in children.
- Post-dialysis heparin into the line decreases clot formation, which may lead to infection. Alteplase may be more effective, but is more expensive, although a recent study suggests that once-a-week administration may be enough to reduce line blockage and sepsis.

Factors increasing the risk of catheter infection
- Exit site and/or tunnel infection or contamination of the hub.
- Failure of aseptic technique, frequent catheter access, and long duration of use.
- Use of non-tunnelled, rather than tunnelled lines.
- Immunosuppression, hypoalbuminaemia, and diabetes.
- Nasal and cutaneous colonization with *Staphylococcus aureus*.

Treatment of exit site, tunnel, and catheter infections
- Fig. 20.2 demonstrates the steps in the management of exit site, tunnel, and catheter infections.
- Antibiotic locks, using an antibiotic to which the organism is sensitive and instilled into the line after dialysis, may be effective at treating line colonization. The antibiotic is then removed at the start of the next dialysis session.
- Antibiotic locks must be instilled into each lumen. Usual instilled volume would be 1.2 mL. If the lumen is smaller, the calculated amount of antibiotic would be less, as the amount of heparin cannot be reduced. One schedule would be to start empirically with:
  - amikacin 55 mg (i.e. 1.1 mL amikacin) + 0.1 mL preservative-free heparin 1000 U/mL 12-hourly. If initial cultures grow Gram-positive cocci at 24–48 h, change to:
  - teicoplanin 146 mg (i.e. dilute 200 mg teicoplanin with 1.5 mL water and take 1.1 mL) + 0.1 mL preservative free heparin 1000 U/mL once daily.
  - the catheter can be recultured by omitting an antibiotic dose, and instilling heparinized saline (10 U/mL) into the line instead, leave for 8 h and then send the fluid for culture.
  - locks can be continued until a 48 h culture is clear.
- Empiric treatment of septicaemia is usually with vancomycin in units with a significant incidence of MRSA. If there is severe systemic illness, two antibiotics are used. For example, initially use both IV vancomycin and ciprofloxacin until Gram stain/culture available. Then modify treatment accordingly:
  - Gram-positive organisms = vancomycin 10 mg/kg stat IV.
  - Repeat dose daily if 24 h post-dose level <10 mg/L.
  - Gram-negative organisms = ciprofloxacin 5 mg/kg dose 12-hourly IV (maximum dose 400 mg 12-hourly).
- Antibiotics can be more specific when culture results are available.

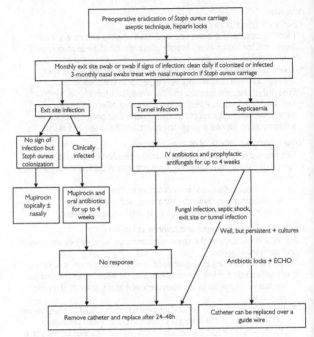

Fig. 20.2 Prevention and treatment of haemodialysis catheter-related infection.

- Prophylactic antifungal agents are recommended, e.g. oral nystatin, when on antibiotics.
- Antibiotic therapy (IV) would usually be continued for 2 weeks, but may need to be longer if there is endocarditis (all patients with proven line infection need an echocardiogram). Fungal infection also requires a prolonged treatment course.

Removal of the catheter associated with septicaemia

Necessary if:
- it is not needed.
- it is not tunnelled.
- there is septic shock.
- it is associated with an exit site or tunnel infection.
- there is fungal infection.
- there is persistence of fever after 48 h of therapy.

Replacement of the line
- With ongoing positive growths from the line, but none of the conditions associated with septicaemia (➔ see 'Removal of the catheter associated with septicaemia', p. 568), it has been shown to be safe and effective (in adults) to replace the line over a guide wire, as long as antibiotics have been started.
- With ongoing positive blood cultures and any of the conditions associated with septicaemia (➔ see 'Removal of the catheter associated with septicaemia', p. 568), the line should be removed and replaced, preferably after a minimum time of 48 h.

Fistulae

An AV fistula is the preferred method of vascular access in children on chronic HD because of the decreased infection risk (in comparison to a line) and preservation of vessels for future use. It can be used in children who are able to cooperate with needling; education and play therapy may enable this even in children with a needle phobia. Children on short-term dialysis (e.g. awaiting a date for a living-related transplant) may elect to be dialysed via a tunnelled line.

Preoperative assessment
- A fistula should be created at least 6 weeks before it is needed as it takes some time to mature.
- The child who has had previous lines will need upper limb venography to establish patency of the vessels. A thrombosed subclavian vein will preclude a fistula being created in that arm as venous return may be obstructed. US is unreliable as collaterals may be mistaken for patent upper limb vessels and the veins cannot be seen under the clavicle.
- Children must be prepared for the use of the fistula using appropriate educational tools (play therapy, etc.).
- May be created at the wrist (radiocephalic or radiobasilic), the elbow (brachiocephalic), or by basilic vein transposition (brachiobasilic). It is preferable to start distally to preserve more proximal vessels for future use.
- *Allen test*: occlude the radial artery by pressure to ensure that the ulnar artery supply to the hand is adequate.

The surgery
- The child must be well hydrated or left at slightly above usual target weight if already on dialysis.
- Antihypertensives should be stopped if possible.
- Ensure IV fluids started when fasting begins preoperatively.
- Studies in children show a primary failure rate varying from 0% to 30% (highest risk in small vessels, particularly radiocephalic), patency 61% at 1 year and 34% at 2 years.

Postoperative care of the fistula
- Elevate the arm to reduce swelling and keep it warm with a padded dressing.
- Assess the fistula thrill using finger tips or stethoscope; check for bleeding and the circulation of the hand every 30 min for the first 24 h.

- Loss of thrill requires an emergency Doppler US and urgent intervention if the fistula has clotted.
- Clots can be removed by catheter, surgery, or locally instilled tPA.
- Clot removal after 48 h is rarely successful in restoring flow.
- Dialysis should be delayed by at least 24 h if possible, and usual target weight increased for the next week.
- The arm should not be used for BP measurement or venepuncture thereafter.
- Dehydration should be avoided.
- Tight clothing and watches on the fistula arm should be avoided.
- After discharge, the fistula should be checked for a thrill every day; if the thrill is lost, this is an emergency that should be managed as perioperatively.
- Prophylactic antiplatelet doses of aspirin (1–5 mg/kg/day) may reduce the risk of clotting.

Cannulation of the arterialized veins when the fistula is mature

- Veins are rarely adequately arterialized ('mature') before 4 weeks.
- The skin should be cleaned before use and sterile topical analgesic creams can be applied.
- Single needling may be used at first.
- Needles should be placed proximal to the fistula, with the arterial needle distal to the venous one, which should be as far away as possible. The arterial needle can point in either direction, but the venous needle should be towards the heart.
- Fistula needle sizes range from 15 to 17 G.
- The needle sites should be changed as repeated needling in the same place will cause weakness of the vessel wall and aneurysm formation.
- It is also possible to use the 'buttonhole technique'. Two sites (one for each needle) are selected and needles are inserted in exactly the same spots at exactly the same angle. Over 8–10 cannulations, scar tissue will form creating a tunnel at each site. The scab is then removed prior to inserting special blunt needles. This is less painful and aneurysms are less likely to form. Cleaning of the area before needling must be scrupulous.

Fistula stenoses

- Stenoses can occur proximal to, distal to, or within the fistula, due to turbulent blood flow and intimal damage. The commonest site is a few centimetres distal to the anastomosis. They can also occur where the vein passes through the cribriform fascia.
- Venous stenosis will result in slow blood flow through the fistula and, therefore, a predisposition to thrombosis.
- The fistula should have an easily compressible pulse and a continuous thrill, which is palpable with blood flows >450 mL/min.
- If there is a stenosis, the thrill is distal to the pressure drop. The risk of the fistula clotting increases when the flow is <650 mL/min.
- *Elevation test evaluates outflow*: the fistula should collapse on elevation of the arm if there is no downstream stenosis.

- *Augmentation test evaluates inflow*: a finger is used to cause complete occlusion of the access several centimetres beyond the arterial anastomosis. If the fistula flow is normal, the portion of fistula upstream from the occluding finger demonstrates augmentation of the strength of the pulse.
- Fistulae should be screened 3–6-monthly using Doppler US to look for blood flow rates and the presence of stenoses. Blood flow is reduced if <200–300 mL/min (400 mL/min for adults).
- Failed augmentation test, low blood flow, or low arterial pressure suggests stenosis at the inflow to the fistula. Arteriography is necessary to examine the arterial flow into the fistula.
- Failed elevation test, increased venous pressure, or thrombosis needs a fistulogram, when X-ray contrast is used to demonstrate the blood flow into and out of the fistula.
- In the presence of low flow or increased venous pressure, recirculation should be checked.
- Recirculation occurs when dialysed blood returning from the venous line to the circulation is taken back into the arterial line for redialysis. If >10–15%, this suggests venous stenosis.
- Stenosis >50% of vessel diameter needs angioplasty, stenting, or surgical repair.
- Central vein obstruction with swelling of the arm and neck will occur if there are stenosed central veins (particularly subclavian).

Other complications
- Thrombosis.
- Infection.
- Ischaemia of the hand or 'steal syndrome'.
- Aneurysm.
- Pseudoaneurysm, due to communication of the fistula with an enclosed area of surrounding tissue. It may lead to prolonged bleeding and needs to be repaired.
- Extravasation injury.
- High cardiac output.
- Cosmetic.

Grafts and shunts
- An artificial conduit can be inserted between an artery and vein SC (graft), where it can be needled, or may be brought out externally (shunt) where the loop can be disconnected to attach to dialysis lines.
- They should only be used if AV fistulae or tunnelled lines are not possible.
- Pre- and postoperative care is as for AV fistulae. Risks are:
  - infection that can be difficult to eradicate.
  - stenosis at the anastomosis site.
  - thrombosis.
  - disconnection and blood loss (with shunts).
- US screening should be more frequent than for AV fistulae. Blood flows <600 mL/min are considered significant, or a 20% reduction in flow in <3 months.

Haemodialysis: blood-borne viruses

* HD unit patients and staff are at risk from blood-borne viruses, particularly hepatitis B, hepatitis C, and HIV.
* A number of outbreaks of hepatitis B were reported in HD units during the 1960s in the UK and elsewhere.
* Transmission may result from percutaneous exposure to blood or other fluids, via droplets or through contaminated equipment.
* Universal precautions should be followed as for all patients, and the entire dialysis circuit should be decontaminated after each use by heat or chemical disinfection. External surfaces should be wiped over between patients using a Cl-based disinfectant.
* All staff and patients should be immunized and/or show immunity to hepatitis B (➲ see 'Management: immunization schedule for infants and children').
* If a patient is exposed to hepatitis B or has been to an endemic area, such as the Middle East and Far East, and has antibody titres <100 IU/ L in the last year, then hepatitis B immunoglobulin and vaccine should be given by IM injection, and the patient should be screened weekly for HBsAg for 3 months. Patients who are or who might become HBsAg positive should be dialysed in a separate room with their own machine.
* Although screening for hepatitis C or HIV is not universally recommended at present, many units do so. Hepatitis C can be spread nosocomially, so a separate room is recommended for the patient who is hepatitis C positive, but a dedicated machine is not necessary. HIV is less infectious, but the same criteria apply. Testing for hepatitis C antibody 3-monthly and for HIV annually is a reasonable compromise.

Reference

Rees L. Haemodialysis. In: Avner ED, Harmon WE, Niaudet P, et al., Eds. *Pediatric Nephrology*, 7th edn. Berlin: Springer-Verlag, 2014:2433–2454.

Continuous renal replacement therapy

Background

Continuous renal replacement therapy (CRRT) is a technique used in the intensive care unit for the management of AKI. In the commonest type, blood is pumped from a vein, through the filter and back to a vein (continuous veno-venous haemofiltration (CVVH)), but an artery to a vein can also be used (CAVH). Solute movement is principally by convective flow so high UF rates are needed (➔ see 'Haemodialysis: principles'). A countercurrent circuit can be used to haemodialyse too, thereby adding in diffusive solute clearance (CVVHD, CAVHD). CVVHDF employs both dialysis and UF. The UF contains electrolytes in a concentration similar to that of the plasma, so the larger the UF volume, the greater the clearance. The UF is returned as 'replacement fluid', which is designed to correct abnormal biochemistry. The proportion of the UF that is replaced is adjusted in order to achieve or maintain euvolaemia. Slow, continuous UF (SCUF) can be used to remove fluid (UF) in smaller quantities, such that replacement is not required.

Advantages

- It is best for patients with cardiovascular instability as it allows slow fluid removal so that major fluid shifts do not occur.
- Episodes of hypotension are less likely to occur than with HD, decreasing the risk of further ischaemic insult if the kidneys are recovering.
- Therapeutic drug levels are more easily maintained than with HD.

Disadvantages

- Clearance is less than for HD, but can be increased by maximizing blood flow, UF, and/or dialysate flow rate, depending on the type of CRRT.
- Rough comparative urea clearance ratio for daily treatment is:

  $$HD = CVVHD = 3 \times CVVH = 4 \times PD$$

- In patients with inborn errors of metabolism with very high ammonia levels (>400 µmol/L), CRRT may not provide adequate clearance, and HD is preferable until the ammonia levels are <200 µmol/L (➔ see 'Emergency renal management of inborn errors of metabolism', p. 299).
- K and PO_4 losses may be excessive, but can be replaced in the replacement fluid or IV.

The prescription

- Standard blood flow is 3–5 mL/kg/min, but can increase to 8–10 mL/kg/min when high clearances are required.
- The extracorporeal circuit volume should not be >10% of the child's blood volume (as for HD).
- If the circuit is >10% of blood volume, the lines must be blood primed. If the haematocrit of the packed cells to be given is high, they must be reconstituted with saline to a haematocrit ~30% to prevent blood clotting in the filter.
- Filtrate is replaced with commercially available solutions containing Na, K, Ca, Mg, Cl, and lactate (see Table 20.5), or bicarbonate via a separate infusion.

Table 20.5 Ranges of electrolyte concentrations in replacement fluid

Electrolyte	Concentration (mmol/L)
Na	132–140
K	0–2
Ca	1.6–1.8
Mg	0.5–1.5
Cl	100–115
Lactate	30–45

- Lactate is a better buffer than bicarbonate when the solution is stored in plastic bags, as plastic is soluble to CO_2. Lactate is stable, whereas bicarbonate will break down over time to H_2O and CO_2, and lose its buffering capacity. However, lactate will be delivered to the patient, making patient levels difficult to interpret. Bicarbonate is, therefore, preferable in children.
- Standard dialysate flow is 1–2 L/h.
- UF rates of 35 mL/kg/h may be used.
- Patient water loss = [UF + urine output + insensible losses + other losses (e.g. gut, drains)] – fluid replacement.
- Fluid removal of 0.5–2 mL/kg/h can be tolerated, depending on need.
- The fluid is replaced before entry into the filter as it decreases blood viscosity and decreases the chance of clotting in the filter.

Anticoagulation

- Clotting of the filter is a common problem, often caused by mechanical problems and added to by slow blood flows and high UF rates.
- The use of anticoagulation must be carefully considered in the child with abnormal clotting, such as disseminated intravascular coagulation, as the potential for bleeding has to be balanced against clotting of the filter, which will be a particular risk in the child who is receiving fresh frozen plasma (FFP) and platelets.
- Heparin is given as a loading dose of 20 U/kg and a prefilter infusion of 10–30 U/kg/h to keep the partial thromboplastin time (PPT) at 60–90 s or the activated coagulation time (ACT) at 130–170 s.
- Epoprostenol may also be infused through the filter to prolong its life.
- Some centres prefer to use Na citrate pre filter, which binds Ca thereby stopping the coagulation cascade. Ca then must be infused post filter to prevent hypocalcaemia.

Reference

Sutherland SM, Alexander SR. Continuous renal replacement therapy in children. *Pediatr Nephrol* 2012;27:2007–2016.

Plasmapheresis and immunoadsorption

Plasma exchange

During plasma exchange, the patient's plasma is exchanged for albumin or FFP. It may be undertaken by a centrifugal cell separator (when there is no limit to the molecular weight of the proteins that can be removed) or a membrane plasma filter (which may not remove large immune complexes).

The process

* Machines have large extracorporeal volumes (>200 mL), so the lines need to be primed with blood in children <20 kg in weight.
* The amount of plasma exchanged is related to the circulating plasma volume, such that 'one volume' is approximately two-thirds of the total blood volume, i.e. ~50 mL/kg.
* A one-volume exchange (50 mL/kg) will remove 60% of plasma macromolecules, and five one-volume exchanges will remove 90% of the total immunoglobulin.
* Usually the amount of plasma exchanged is two volumes, i.e. 100 mL/kg daily for 5 days, and may be followed by five further daily sessions.
* Fluid replacement is with warmed 4.5% albumin or FFP or Octaplas®, which contain potentially missing complement and clotting factors. Dilution of albumin may be needed to prevent fluid shifts.
* Clotting must be checked before and after each session as clotting factors are depleted. Commonly by the third day fibrinogen levels have fallen to <2 g/dL, so FFP can be added at the end of the exchange at a dose of 150–300 mL, depending on the weight of the child.
* If the Ca is <2.0 mmol/L, 1 g of Ca can be added per litre of albumin.
* Anti-coagulation is usually with heparin, but citrate can be used.
* Chlorphenamine can be given if allergic reactions are seen. Reactions are often related to the speed at which the FFP is delivered.
* Immunosuppression is used after the course to prevent the return of the immunological abnormalities if the exchange has been performed for immunological reasons.

Complications

* Coagulation disturbances.
* Infection.
* Allergic reactions to plasma, particularly FFP.
* Fluid imbalance.

Renal diseases for which it has been used

* Anti-GBM disease.
* ANCA-associated vasculitis with crescentic nephritis and/or pulmonary haemorrhage or other life-threatening complications.
* Crescentic nephritis due to other causes.
* HUS/thrombotic thrombocytopenic purpura with cerebral involvement.
* Recurrent FSGS post transplantation.
* Acute antibody-mediated transplant rejection.
* *SLE*: severe lupus nephritis resistant to conventional therapy, cerebral lupus, or other fulminant multisystemic manifestation.

Immunoadsorption

Protein A columns selectively remove immunoglobulin (principally IgG) from plasma. They have been used to remove human immunoglobulins in diseases associated with pathogenic antibodies. Currently, they are being tried in membranous nephropathy; the removal of human leucocyte antigen antibodies in highly sensitized transplant recipients; and for removal of ABO antibodies to allow blood group incompatible transplantation. Results so far are encouraging.

Transplantation

Renal transplantation immunology

Background

The immune response in the context of transplantation consists of the following:

* Recognition of foreign antigens.
* Activation of antigen-specific lymphocytes.
* The effector response.
* The major histocompatibility complex (MHC) located on chromosome 6 consists of a linked set of genetic loci containing many genes involved in the immune response.
* The human MHC includes the human leucocyte antigen (HLA) genes—the products of these genes are expressed on the cell surface as glycoproteins.
* There are three classes within the MHC region:
  * Class I region—includes the HLA genes *HLA-A*, *HLA-B*, and *HLA-C*.
  * Class II region—includes HLA genes *HLA-DR*, *HLA-DQ*, and *HLA-DP*.
  * Class III region—includes the genes for components of the complement cascade and cytokines, e.g. tumour necrosis factor, lymphotoxin alpha.
* Class I molecules are expressed on nearly all nucleated cells.
* Class II molecules are only expressed on B cells, antigen-presenting cells (APCs), and on activated endothelial cells (that can act as APCs).
* APCs are a group of cells (such as dendritic cells) that process antigens and present them, in association with HLA molecules, to T cells.
* Donor APCs may migrate out of the graft to a secondary organ and stimulate T cells directly (direct recognition) or host APCs may pick up donor antigens that have been shed from the graft and stimulate host T cells indirectly (indirect recognition).
* T-cell receptors recognize peptides bound to HLA molecules.
* CD4 T cells (T helper cells) interact with class II molecules, resulting in the production of cytokines which leads to a cascade of cellular and humoral reactions that are responsible for the effector responses important in transplant rejection.
* CD8 T cells (T killer cells) are cytolytic, directly interacting with cells expressing class I and may be toxic to the cell to which they bind.

Blood group

* Although blood group O is the universal donor and AB the universal recipient, for reasons of equity, in the UK, and in most organ allocation systems, donor kidneys are first allocated on the basis of blood group identity, i.e. patients are only offered kidneys from donors of the same blood group as themselves.
* Transplantation can take place across the blood group barrier if the recipient titres of anti-A or -B are low. The levels of titres vary from undetectable to high and this influences the ability to go ahead and the treatment used to prevent a reaction. Such treatments include rituximab, plasma exchange, and/or immunoadsorption. Overall it is

preferable to choose a donor who is blood group compatible, crossing the blood group barrier only if there is no alternative.
- The rhesus antigen is not expressed on kidney cells and plays no role in organ matching.

Histocompatibility and immunogenetics laboratories

These laboratories support renal transplant programmes by providing three main services:
- HLA (tissue) typing.
- Detection and definition of HLA-specific antibodies.
- Pre-transplant cross-matching.

HLA typing

HLA (tissue) typing refers to the series of DNA-based laboratory tests whereby an individual's HLA genes are characterized and hence the HLA molecules expressed on the surface of their cells identified. HLA molecules are on the surface of all the nucleated cells (i.e. in humans, all cells apart from RBCs) but for ease of sampling, DNA from peripheral blood lymphocytes is routinely used.
- The DNA-based tests used for HLA typing are referred to as PCR-SSP (sequence-specific primer) and LABType® SSO (sequence-specific oligonucleotide).
- Historically, HLA typing used a microcytotoxicity test whereby HLA antigens were identified using known HLA antibodies. The HLA antigens have been allocated numbers as they have been recognized. Subsequently, new antisera have demonstrated narrower specificities, which are conventionally shown in brackets, e.g. HLA-A9 has been split into HLA-A23 and HLA-A24 so is written as HLA-A23(9) and HLA-A24(9). These are called split antigens, and can usually be treated similarly in the matching process. This form of nomenclature is referred to as the serological HLA type.
- DNA technology has led to the identification of many more alleles so that at least two fields separated by a colon and a minimum of four digits are now used. The first field denotes the antigen family or allele group, e.g. HLA-A*01 where the * denotes that DNA technology has been used and the second field denotes the allele, e.g. HLA-A*01:01.
- The most common HLA antigen is HLA-A2, which is found in almost 50% of Caucasian people. 90% of Caucasians with HLA-A2 have HLA-A*02:01, although other ethnic groups may have different alleles. Frequencies of other HLA antigens vary with ethnicity, e.g. HLA-B8 is present in 30% of Irish people; HLA-B54 is unique to Far Eastern populations, such as Japan; and HLA-A36 is found in the Black (Afro-Caribbean) population.
- Some antigens are inherited together more often than would be expected by chance, e.g. HLA-A1, HLA-B8 HLA-DR17 and HLA-A2, HLA-B44, HLA-DR7. This is known as linkage disequilibrium.
- Individuals may be homozygous for a HLA antigen, i.e. they will appear to only have one HLA antigen at any locus, rather than two as they have inherited the same antigen from each parent. For example, if they had only one HLA-A antigen, which was HLA-A2, and only one HLA-B, which was B44, together with DR1 and DR2 their HLA type would be recorded as follows: HLA-A2,-;B44,-;DR1,DR2.

Detection and definition of human leucocyte antigen-specific antibodies

* Sensitization is the development of antibodies to HLA antigens, which can result as a consequence of exposure to non-self HLA. This can occur three ways:
  * Previous transplantation.
  * Blood or platelet transfusion or FFP.
  * Pregnancy, when the mother is exposed to paternal HLA antigens.
* HLA antibodies may be unique to a specific allele or limited group (private) or recognize an epitope that is shared by more than one HLA molecule (public) resulting in cross-reactivity. HLA antibodies do not develop to one's own HLA antigens, except in rare cases where a HLA allele is not expressed on the cell surface.
* The term calculated reaction frequency (cRF) is an indicator of the level of sensitization for a patient. The result given for a particular patient is the percentage of blood group identical, HLA-incompatible donors in the pool of 10,000 UK donors, i.e. if the cRF is 50%, then half of donors would be expected to give a positive cross-match and be unacceptable.
* Antibodies specific for HLA are now usually defined using microbead array or ELISA techniques that have proved more sensitive than cytotoxicity.
* IgM antibodies are usually autoantibodies, of little relevance to tissue reactivity (in the context of transplantation biology), and can be ignored, unless directed at HLA.
* If a patient does not develop an antibody to a mismatched antigen on regular post-transplant checks, it is likely that they have not responded to that antigen and may be given it again in a subsequent graft.
* If a patient has HLA specific antibodies to a potential living donor, antibody removal may be considered. This can be attempted in many ways, although none are guaranteed effective, and the procedure must be considered as of increased immunological risk (ⓘ http://www.bts.org.uk).
* The production of *de novo* donor HLA-directed antibodies (donor-specific antibodies (DSAs)) post transplant has been shown to be associated with both acute and chronic graft rejection.
* The presence of concurrent DSA forms part of the Banff criteria for diagnosis of antibody-mediated rejection.
* Indicators for DSA testing include evidence of graft dysfunction, suspected/confirmed non-compliance, and at the time of transfer to another unit.
* There is currently uncertainty regarding the management of the entirely asymptomatic patient with stable graft function who develops DSA. For this reason, routine measurement of DSA is not recommended outside of research settings.

Pre-transplant cross-matching

* The donor/recipient cross-match is an essential pre-transplant test performed to confirm the absence of donor-directed HLA antibodies, which could initiate severe rejection in the recipient.

- HLA-specific antibodies should have been defined prior to transplant, decreasing the chances of a positive cross-match.
- The complement-dependent cytotoxic cross-match is the most common test, where donor lymphocytes are incubated with recipient serum in the presence of complement. A positive cross-match is a contraindication for transplantation.
- Flow cytometry cross-match is a more sensitive cross-match test. It is particularly useful in patients who are sensitized or where the cell source for cross-matching is peripheral blood.
- Serum tested must have been collected within the previous 6 weeks and preferably one taken on the day of transplant. If the child has been transfused since the most recent sample, a fresh serum sample must be provided.
- The T-cell cross-match identifies antibodies to HLA class I, whereas the B-cell cross-match identifies antibodies to both HLA class I and class II.
- Historic positive, current negative cross-matches may be acceptable for transplantation if the sensitization event is blood transfusion, the antibody was transient or extra immunosuppression can be tolerated.
- A virtual cross-match (VXm) can be performed pre transplant for selected patients who meet strict criteria, whereby the donor HLA type is reviewed against the patient's HLA antibody profile to determine whether the patient has donor-directed antibodies that would cause a positive cross-match test result. A VXm can be performed before cross-match material is available and allows the transplant team to proceed to theatre before the cross-match test. The purpose of this approach is to reduce the cold ischaemia time (CIT) without compromising the safety of transplantation. For these patients, a cross-match test must be carried out retrospectively to confirm the negative VXm

Human leucocyte antigen matching and organ allocation

- After blood group, kidneys are allocated according to the degree of HLA mismatching, those recipients with the lowest degree of mismatching to the donor being given priority. This is because:
  - HLA (particularly class II) mismatching is associated with worse graft outcome
  - the development of antibodies to mismatched antigens will prejudice the chances of finding subsequent grafts.
- It is convention to count the number of donor HLA antigen mismatches, as this is a reflection of antigen dose. Three loci are considered—HLA-A, HLA-B, and HLA-DR. Each individual has two antigens at each locus, and there can be 0, 1, or 2 mismatches at each locus. This mismatching is abbreviated to a three-number code, whereby 000 is no mismatch at any locus, i.e. a perfect match and 222 is two mismatches at each locus, i.e. a complete mismatch.
- Deceased donor organs are allocated in the UK by NHS Blood and Transplant (NHSBT) using an evidence-based computer algorithm based on five ranked tiers of recipients. Paediatric patients are prioritized throughout. Tiers A and B both refer to 000 mismatched paediatric patients where Tier A is the highly sensitized patients and Tier B is all other 000 paediatric patients. Patients are prioritized within Tiers A and B according to their accrued waiting time.

- In the event of a tie in waiting time, the recipient at the closest unit to the offering/retrieval centre, based on transport time, will receive the offer. Tier D refers to 'favourably matched' paediatric recipients (i.e. 100, 010, or 110 mismatched) and Tier E is all other eligible patients. Tier C refers to adult patients only. Within Tiers D and E, patients are prioritized according to a points-based system of seven elements, the most influential being waiting time (ℜ www.odt.nhs.uk).
- The chance of a patient receiving a graft that is well matched for their HLA antigens will depend on the frequency of their antigens in the deceased donor population, which also reflects their ethnic background in comparison with the donor population, as well as the presence of any anti-HLA antibodies. A 'matchability' score for a patient's antigens can be calculated from the deceased donor population and used to generate a score of 1–10, so that 1 is easiest to match and 10 is hardest to match.
- It may be considered unwise to mismatch at a common antigen, e.g. HLA-A2, particularly in children, to avoid sensitization to half the potential donors which would compromise retransplantation.
- As well as HLA, the major histocompatibility barrier, there are many minor histocompatibility loci. This means that only identical twins can be transplanted without immunosuppression, even if all HLA antigens are matched.

Parental donation

- Most children will share three antigens with each parent as they have inherited the genes found on one chromosome (e.g. 1A, 1B, 1DR antigen, often referred to as a haplotype). Even so, graft survival has been found to be very good and equivalent to a 0 mismatched deceased donor graft. If parents have HLA antigens in common they could be better than 1 haplotype match.
- Parents must be made aware that tissue typing may identify potential non-paternity, but this is not a paternity test.
- All living donor transplants require approval from a representative of the Human Tissue Authority.
- If a relative is considering donation to a patient that is active on the waiting list for a deceased donor kidney, it is a useful strategy to ensure the potential living donor's antigens that are mismatched with the recipient are registered as unacceptable for any deceased donor kidney. If the deceased donor transplant then fails, this approach limits the chance of antibodies developing which would prevent future living donation.

Further reading

Dyer P, Little A-M, Turner D. Testing for histocompatibility. In: Forsythe JLRF, Ed., *Transplantation: A Companion To Specialist Surgical Practice*, 5th edn. St Louis, MO: Elsevier Saunders, 2013:57–69.

Vaccination in transplant patients

Background

- Prior to transplantation, children should be fully up to date with all routine childhood vaccines and additionally receive varicella zoster, pneumococcal (if transplanted before this vaccine was routine), Bacille Calmette–Guérin (BCG; where and when available), and hepatitis B vaccines (➔ see 'Immunization schedule for children with chronic kidney disease').
- After transplantation, children should be given non-live vaccines normally according to the routine childhood immunization schedule, but should *not* receive live vaccines.

Vaccines that are not recommended post transplant

- Oral polio vaccine (OPV/Sabin), including the vaccination of household contacts (this is now only rarely offered as the inactivated vaccine is given in a combined diphtheria, tetanus, pertussis, polio, and *Haemophilus* type b conjugate vaccine as part of the routine immunization schedule).
- MMR or rubella vaccine.
- BCG, BCG SSI vaccine.
- Yellow fever vaccine (Arilvax®, Stamaril®).
- Oral typhoid vaccine (Vivotif®).
- Varicella vaccine (Varivax®, Varilrix®).
- All other live vaccines.

Vaccines that can be administered post transplant

- Diphtheria, tetanus, pertussis (acellular, component), poliomyelitis (inactivated), and *Haemophilus* type b conjugate vaccine (adsorbed).
- *Haemophilus influenza* type B (Hiberix®) vaccine.
- Hepatitis A vaccine (Avaxim®, Havrix Monodose®).
- Hepatitis B vaccine (Engerix B®, HB-Vax Pro®).
- Inactivated polio vaccine (IPV/Salk).
- Meningococcal group C conjugate vaccine (Meningitec®, Menjugate®).
- Meningococcal polysaccharide A, C, W135, and Y vaccine (ACWY Vax®).
- Meningococcal group B vaccine (Bexsero®)
- Pneumococcal polysaccharide unconjugated vaccine (Pneumovax® II).
- Pneumococcal polysaccharide conjugated vaccine (Prevenar® 13).
- Rabies vaccine.
- Vi capsular polysaccharide typhoid vaccine (Typherix®, Typhim Vi®).
- Influenza vaccine is recommended annually.
- Bivalent, quadrivalent, or nine-valent HPV vaccine. In most countries, routine vaccination is only recommended in girls. There is a strong argument to support the vaccination of boys undergoing transplantation in view of their significantly increased risk of HPV-driven malignancies.

Further reading

Danzinger-Isakov L, Kumar D, AST Infectious Diseases Community of Practice. Guidelines for vaccination of solid organ transplant candidates and recipients. *Am J Transplant* 2009;Suppl 4:1600–6143.
Joint Formulary Committee. *British National Formulary 2016–2017*. London: BMJ Group and Pharmaceutical Press, 2016.

Kidney transplantation: the surgery

Living donation

Although many adults wish to donate a kidney to a child, many find they are unable because of one or more of the following:

* Antibody incompatibility (either incompatible blood group with significant titres of anti-A or anti-B antibodies, or the presence of anti-HLA antibodies in the child). Kidney sharing schemes and antibody-incompatible transplants are likely to make these issues less problematic.
* Diagnosis of renal disease or other morbidity of which they were previously unaware.
* Obesity (a donor body mass index of <30 kg/m^2 is usually required).
* Anatomical variants or abnormalities (e.g. multiple renal arteries to both kidneys, bilateral kidney stones, and the detection of a single kidney).
* Social or financial reasons.

Most children are able to undergo successful transplantation using an adult live donor kidney once they have reached 8–10 kg in weight.

Advantages for the recipient
* The ability to plan the timing of transplantation, which can be before dialysis becomes necessary (pre-emptive transplantation).
* Graft survivals after live donor kidney transplantation is better than after deceased donor kidney transplantation even if the degree of HLA matching match is inferior.

Disadvantages
* Mortality risk for the donor of 0.03%, requirement for donor blood transfusion 1%, risk of conversion to open surgery from the laparoscopic approach 1%, and risk of venous thromboembolism 1%.
* Postoperative pain, which may be minimized by laparoscopic donor nephrectomy. May need up to 3 months to return to normal activity.
* Two studies report a higher risk of CKD stage 5 among donors than among a healthy age-matched control population; however, the absolute 15-year incidence of CKD stage 5 is <1%.
* All-cause mortality and the risk of cardiovascular events are similar among donors and a healthy age-matched control population, although one study provides evidence for a 5% increase in all-cause mortality after 25 years that is attributable to donation.
* The risks of gestational hypertension or pre-eclampsia seem to be 6% higher in pregnancies among donors than in pregnancies in a healthy, age-matched control population.

Deceased donors

* In general, children receive the highest quality kidneys from deceased donors in order to optimize the chances of prolonged graft survival. Kidneys with several adverse factors are called 'marginal' kidneys and are not often used in children. Careful discussion of the risks and benefits of using 'marginal' kidneys should be had with relevant clinical colleagues, and the patient and their family.
* Kidneys from deceased donors <5 years of age are generally not used for paediatric recipients as they are associated with an increased risk of technical problems and graft thrombosis.

- Kidneys from deceased donors aged >55 years are generally not used in children (although a living donor over this age may be acceptable).
- Prolonged hypertension or hypotension may damage the donor kidney.
- Disseminated malignancy is a contraindication to transplantation. Deceased donors with selected primary CNS tumours, non-melanoma skin cancers, carcinomas *in situ*, or malignancies treated >5–10 years ago may be able to donate kidneys to children. Careful discussion is needed with oncology colleagues on a case-by-case basis to determine risks of tumour transmission.
- Kidneys from patients with CKD or cortical necrosis on biopsy should not be used.
- Kidneys from deceased donors who are hepatitis B core antibody-positive and hepatitis B surface antigen-negative can be used in paediatric recipients, but discussions should be had with virology colleagues, and consideration given to the use of antiviral medications in the recipient (e.g. lamivudine). Recipients should be immunized against hepatitis B pre transplant.
- Hepatitis C (HCV)- and HIV-positive donors can be considered for use in HCV- and HIV-positive recipients but experience in paediatric recipients is limited and careful discussion with virology colleagues is essential.
- Diabetes mellitus for >5 years or other donor diseases that might affect the kidney are relative contraindications to donation.
- Donors who have died from sepsis can be accepted if the infection has been satisfactorily treated and the causative organism has been identified: some centres will not accept organs from donors with meningococcaemia who have had <48 h of antibiotics. Potential donors are likely to be rejected if there is concern about undiagnosed infections.
- Kidneys can be used from donation after circulatory death (DCD) donors. A rapidly increasing body of data suggest that short- to medium-term graft survival is no different from donation after brain death (DBD) donors, however it is recognized that donation after circulatory death is associated with an increased risk of delayed graft function (DGF) in the recipient.
- Trauma may occur to the kidney or its vessels during its removal. This is usually repairable, but sometimes may lead to organ discard.
- Kidneys are removed with a 'patch' of donor aorta attached to the renal artery or arteries. Those with multiple renal arteries may need 'bench' surgery to anastomose a small artery to a larger one if the patch is unsatisfactory.

Warm and cold ischaemia times, and anastomosis time

- Warm ischaemia time (WIT) can be defined as the time between circulatory arrest in the donor and the start of perfusion with cold preservation solution. In DBD donors, the warm ischaemia time is effectively zero, as the surgeon at organ retrieval controls the time of circulatory arrest. With kidneys from DCD donors, a period of warm ischaemia is inevitable and is likely to contribute to higher rates of DGF post transplant. It is likely that warm ischaemic periods of >20–30 min increase the risk of non-function of the transplanted kidney.

- Organ preservation fluids are used to minimize cellular injury associated with ischaemia. There is considerable variation nationally in the preservation fluid used; these include Marshall's (hyperosmolar citrate), and University of Wisconsin solutions. In deceased donor transplantation the donor kidneys are perfused *in situ* prior to removal and then packed in preservation solution at 4°C for transportation. In living donation, the kidney is perfused on the bench following removal.
- Cold ischaemia time (CIT) is usually defined as the time from start of cold perfusion to the restoration of blood flow in the recipient. Prolonged CIT results in endothelial activation and graft outcome worsens with longer CITs. For a kidney from a DBD donor, graft survival deteriorates with a CIT of >20–24 h; kidneys from DCD donors seem to have a CIT threshold of 12–16 h.
- Anastomosis time is the time between removal from cold storage and restoration of warmed blood flow within the kidney. This usually takes 25–35 min. Prolonged anastomosis times are associated with reduced graft survival and increased rates of DGF.

Ischaemic injury and acute tubular necrosis

Donor factors, WIT, CIT, anastomosis times, and reperfusion injury contribute to ischaemic injury and DGF (acute tubular necrosis):

- DGF can only be definitively diagnosed after exclusion of technical causes of non-function and acute rejection. DGF is diagnosed in retrospect, i.e. after the kidney functions. If 'DGF' continues for >3–4 months, it is considered to be permanent, e.g. primary non-function. There are many definitions of DGF; the most widely used is 'the need for dialysis (for any reason) within the first week post transplantation'.
- There may be no urine output or relative oliguria with a slowly falling plasma creatinine. Alternatively, there may be significant urine output, often from the native kidneys.
- Cytokine release in the kidney during acute tubular necrosis may make rejection more likely.

DGF masks diagnosis of other complications including acute rejection (which occurs with a higher incidence in the setting of DGF) and recurrent disease, making weekly US, DTPA, or MAG3 and biopsy necessary.

The operation

- The external iliac artery and vein are used in older children, and the common iliac vessels or aorta and IVC in smaller ones. An arbitrary cut-off weight for the use of the aorta and IVC would be <20 kg. The right side is preferable as it is easier to expose the common iliac vein.
- If the aorta is used, the incision is midline or paraumbilical, and oblique if the iliac vessels are used.
- The transplant may be intraperitoneal in small children, although there is an increasing tendency to perform extraperitoneal surgery, even in the smallest recipients.
- If the kidney is large in comparison with the child, a right nephrectomy may be necessary.
- The ureter is usually anastomosed to the bladder. A stent is usually left through the new vesicoureteric junction (VUJ) to reduce the risk of transplant ureteric stenosis, or urine leak.

- Some children with abnormal bladders may require a transplant ureterostomy or ureteric implantation into an augmented bladder or ileal conduit.

Surgical complications

- Wound infection (5%), usually treated with antibiotics alone although wound drainage may be needed.
- Lymphocoele (5–10%), due to leakage from lymphatics that are cut during dissection around the blood vessels:
  - Appears to be more common with the use of sirolimus and everolimus.
  - Presentation may depend on size—may present with obstruction to transplant drainage, swollen leg due to obstruction of venous return, or alternatively be an incidental US finding.
  - Diagnosis by US and aspiration, when the biochemistry of the fluid is found to be similar to plasma, although the protein content may be higher.
  - Treatment may be non-operative (e.g. small collections without graft or venous obstruction), or by external percutaneous drainage, or by 'marsupialisation', where the lymphocoele cavity is opened into the peritoneal cavity.
- Bleeding (5–10%), particularly as most centres would use heparin or aspirin as prophylaxis against graft thrombosis.
- Urinary leaks (1–2%) can be at the VUJ, from the ureter due to compromised ureteric blood flow, or occasionally from a ruptured calyx. This may present with:
  - abdominal pain
  - an abdominal collection on US
  - a rising plasma creatinine due to reabsorption
  - a falling plasma creatinine with relative oliguria (urine leakage within abdominal cavity):
    - diagnosis is by aspiration and biochemical analysis, when the creatinine concentration in the aspirated fluid is similar to urine; or by imaging by cystogram (for a bladder leak), DTPA scan, or IV pyelogram
  - treatment is often by bladder catheterization to allow the leak to heal, although surgery may be necessary if there is a large volume leak, or if bladder catheterization fails to heal the leak.
- Ureteric obstruction (2–4%):
  - Early may be acute post surgery due to clots.
  - Later may be due to VUJ obstruction or to ureteric stenosis, which is predisposed to by the tenuous blood supply to the ureter.
- A lymphocoele may compress the ureter:
  - Ureteric stenosis may also be due to BK virus infection.
  - Rarely due to calculi or tumour.
  - Diagnosis is by US (hydronephrosis), DTPA/MAG3 with furosemide. Definitive diagnosis is often with antegrade contrast studies down a nephrostomy tube.
  - It may be possible to dilate a short (<2 cm), narrowed segment endoscopically; surgical repair is usually favoured as endoscopically

dilated stenoses often recur. Treatment for other causes vary by underlying cause (e.g. calculi, tumours, etc.).

* Renal artery stenosis (2–5%) generally presents after the third month post transplantation. It may result from:
  * technical issues at the time of transplantation (unrecognized damage to the renal artery or recipient vessels, poor anastomosis technique)
  * some studies suggest that donor age and other co-morbidities (e.g. hypertension), and the presence of anti-HLA antibodies in the recipient, are associated with renal artery stenoses
  * diagnosis is suggested by Doppler US findings. Definitive diagnosis requires formal arteriography, though CT and/or MR angiography is increasingly useful
  * treatment is by balloon dilatation if feasible or surgery.

Graft thrombosis (2–3%)

This may originate in the arterial or more commonly the venous system, and usually occurs within the first 5 days post transplant. Most centres use perioperative prophylaxis with either LMWH (particularly if there is a positive procoagulant screen (➔ see 'Preparation for renal replacement therapy', p. 497) or aspirin. This is started at surgery; thereafter protocols vary, but LMWH is usually continued until the child mobilizes. Aspirin 1 mg/kg body weight/24 h as a single daily dose (maximum 75 mg) is more commonly used in the child with a normal procoagulant screen and is continued for 4–12 weeks post transplant.

* Causes of graft thrombosis may be:
  * slow blood flow due to surgical technique or decreased circulating blood volume
  * procoagulant state (which should be excluded pre transplant)
  * severe rejection
  * external compression of vessels, e.g. by haematoma or limited space within the abdomen or pelvis.
* Presentation is with:
  * sudden reduction of urine output and rising creatinine
  * macroscopic haematuria if venous
  * graft swelling and pain or tenderness.
* *Investigations:* no flow will be seen through the transplant on imaging by urgent Doppler US.
* There should be a low threshold for a return to theatre to explore the graft. Rarely, early graft thrombosis can be successfully treated with graft removal, flushing, and re-implantation. More commonly, the graft is not salvageable.

The failing graft

Most kidney transplants fail many years post transplantation, and deterioration happens slowly. British Transplant Society guidelines on the management of slowly failing grafts are as follows:

- Patients with a failing graft need routine CKD care (anaemia, metabolic disturbances, hypertension), including early consideration of retransplantation.
- Immunosuppression can be reduced in the late stages of graft dysfunction. Complete withdrawal of immunosuppression has the benefits of removal of its side effects but this must be balanced against the risk of *de novo* allosensitization:
  - Immunosuppressive therapy can be continued to avoid immunological sensitization if a living kidney donor is available and there is the prospect of retransplantation pre-emptively or within 1 year of starting dialysis.
  - Immunosuppressive treatment should be withdrawn after graft failure when there are immunosuppression-related complications and an anticipated delay in retransplantation.
- All immunosuppression apart from steroids should be stopped immediately after transplant nephrectomy, with subsequent gradual withdrawal of steroids.
- If withdrawal of immunosuppression is followed by acute rejection, steroid therapy should be restarted, followed by transplant nephrectomy when acute inflammation has settled.
- If the graft is left *in situ,* azathioprine/mycophenolate can be stopped immediately, followed by gradual taper of the calcineurin inhibitor (CNI) or mammalian target of rapamycin (mTOR) inhibitor, e.g. dose reduction of 25% per week. Steroids should be withdrawn last.
- Serum samples should be obtained for HLA-specific antibody screening 4 weeks after any changes in immunosuppression, or surgery.

Indications for graft nephrectomy in a failed graft

- Localizing symptoms (pain, infection, bleeding) resistant to medical therapy.
- To create space for retransplantation.
- To enable complete withdrawal of immunosuppression.
- Risk of graft rupture.
- Graft malignancy.
- Refractory anaemia with raised CRP

The role of graft percutaneous embolization pre surgery has been suggested as a way to reduce the need to support blood transfusion (and subsequent HLA sensitization) during the surgery itself, but there is no clear evidence for its use at present.

References
℧ https://bts.org.uk/guidelines-standards/
℧ https://www.odt.nhs.uk/transplantation/tools-policies-and-guidance/sabto/

Immunosuppressive therapy in renal transplant patients

Immunosuppressive therapy is given following renal transplantation to prevent rejection of the graft and to treat episodes of acute rejection. The exception to this is where the donor is an identical twin of the recipient.

General principles

* Most paediatric kidney transplant recipients in Europe and North America are commenced on a CNI (most commonly tacrolimus) in conjunction with a corticosteroid and an antiproliferative immunosuppressant drug (MMF or less frequently azathioprine).
* Following the results of large multicentre studies in the USA and Europe, an increasing number of centres now either avoid corticosteroids or withdraw these after 5 days.
* An induction antibody may be added in a number of different circumstances, including where corticosteroid withdrawal is planned, where ciclosporin is used as the CNI, and where the risk of rejection is thought to be greater (e.g. second or subsequent transplants or the less well-matched kidney). In Europe, this is most frequently the anti-CD25 monoclonal antibody basiliximab. In the USA, where the use of induction antibodies is generally greater, the polyclonal anti-T-cell antibody antithymocyte globulin (ATG) was used in around 18% of patients, with a further 40% receiving an anti-CD25 monoclonal antibody or the monoclonal anti-T-cell antibody OKT3 (North American Pediatric Renal Trials and Collaborative Studies (NAPRTCS) 2014 report). OKT3 is no longer manufactured.
* 2017 NICE guidelines have recommended the use of tacrolimus, MMF, and basiliximab as initial immunosuppressive therapy.
* Relatively intense immunosuppressive therapy is given in the early post-transplant period when the risk of acute rejection is greatest, with a subsequent tapering (reduction in corticosteroid dose and target CNI level) to reduce the risk of adverse effects in the long term.
* Because of concerns about the long-term nephrotoxicity of the CNIs, a number of regimens aim to reduce the dose of or remove these agents at various time intervals post transplantation. These regimens have generally incorporated the use of the mTOR inhibitors.
* Very few prospective RCTs have been performed in the field of paediatric renal transplantation and there is no good evidence to support the use of any particular regimen.
* While all of the agents discussed in this chapter have specific individual adverse effects, immunosuppressive drugs are, in general, associated with an increased risk of infection (bacterial, viral, and fungal) and malignancy. The more potent immunosuppressive agents will reduce the risk of acute rejection at the price of an increased risk of adverse effects. The goal of optimal immunosuppressive therapy is to balance these risks and benefits.

- Non-adherence with therapy is a major cause of morbidity and graft loss, particularly in the adolescent population. Therapeutic regimens should be kept as simple as possible, with the use of once-daily medication where feasible. The importance of cosmetic side effects of therapy should not be underestimated.

Calcineurin inhibitors: tacrolimus and ciclosporin

- These agents modify T-cell function, inhibiting IL-2 production by activated T cells.
- Both drugs are licensed for use in children in Europe and North America.

Tacrolimus

- Available as a twice-daily immediate release preparation (Prograf® capsules or Modigraf® granules). Generic versions are also available.
- A granular soluble twice-daily preparation is available for administration to smaller children and those who cannot swallow capsules. This allows predictable dosing and should be used in preference to extemporaneous liquid preparations.
- A newer prolonged-release preparation of tacrolimus (Advagraf®) allows once-daily administration.
- Paediatric studies are currently ongoing to determine whether Prograf® and Advagraf® can be used interchangeably.
- There have been a number of instances where Prograf® and Advagraf® have been dispensed interchangeably with adverse patient outcomes. It is therefore recommended that the drug is prescribed using the appropriate brand name.
- Prograf® is started at 0.15 mg/kg/dose 12-hourly (oral). Subsequent dosing is altered in response to trough tacrolimus levels, the dose being adjusted upwards or downwards to achieve desired target trough levels. Many centres will reduce the starting dose to 0.1 mg/kg/dose (adult starting dose) in young adults.
- Advagraf® is given at same total daily dose, i.e. 0.3 mg/kg daily or 0.2 mg/kg daily. Advagraf® capsules are large and must be taken whole—as such, they are generally only suitable for children of around 8 years and above.
- Monitoring of trough (concentration at 12 h, C_{12} for Prograf and Modigraf and at 24h, C_{24} for Advagraf) levels is mandatory:
  - Typical target ranges are 10–12 micrograms/L for first 1–2 months and 5–10 micrograms/L thereafter.
  - Many centres will progressively reduce target tacrolimus levels with increasing time post transplantation, particularly in stable patients.
  - The Symphony study showed excellent outcomes in adults using a combination of low-dose tacrolimus (target levels 3–7 micrograms/L), MMF, and corticosteroids. Many paediatric centres are following this regimen.
  - Levels <2 microgram/L cannot be reliably measured using conventional assays.
- Diarrhoeal illness may result in increased tacrolimus levels due to enhanced enterohepatic circulation and careful monitoring should take place when this develops.

* Food decreases the rate and extent of absorption of the drug with high-fat meals producing the most pronounced effect—around a 35% reduction in area under the curve.
* Where IV tacrolimus needs to be given, one-fifth of the oral dose should be administered over a 2 h period:
  * The drug interacts with polyvinyl chloride (PVC) and needs to be infused via non-PVC tubing.
  * Experience with IV tacrolimus is limited and there is anecdotal evidence of the drug causing severe hypertension; oral tacrolimus is very well absorbed and there are very few instances in which IV therapy should prove necessary.

Ciclosporin

* Dose 3–5 mg/kg/dose given 12-hourly (oral) with subsequent dose adjustment to achieve target levels.
* Monitoring of drug levels is mandatory. Typical target ranges at 12 h after dose (C12) are 150–250 micrograms/L for the first 3–6 months and 75–150 micrograms/L thereafter.
* There has previously been some interest in monitoring drug levels at 2 h post dose (C2 levels), as this has been shown to be a better estimate of exposure to the drug in the first 4 h following oral administration. No paediatric data has shown improved graft outcome using such an approach.
* Where IV ciclosporin needs to be given, one-third of the oral dose should be administered over a 2 h period.

Adverse effects of calcineurin inhibitors

* Many adverse effects are common to both agents including:
  * nephrotoxicity (reversible vasoconstriction in the short term, but also irreversible interstitial fibrosis in the long term)
  * hypertension
  * headache
  * tremor
  * hepatic dysfunction
  * diabetes mellitus (more common with tacrolimus)
  * hypomagnesaemia
  * hyperkalaemia.
* Ciclosporin-specific cosmetic side effects include:
  * hypertrichosis (worse in dark-skinned, dark-haired individuals)
  * gingival overgrowth (worse where dental hygiene is poor and improves with careful tooth brushing. May respond to azithromycin, occasionally requires gingivectomy).

Important drug interactions with calcineurin inhibitors

* Tacrolimus or ciclosporin levels should be very carefully monitored when a number of drugs are used in conjunction with them (see Box 21.1). Interactions may result in either high levels risking drug toxicity or low levels risking under-immunosuppression that increases the risk of the development of rejection.
* Dose adjustments should be made in response to high or low levels.

Box 21.1 Drugs affecting calcineurin inhibitor levels and increasing risk of nephrotoxicity

The following increase CNI levels:
- Grapefruit juice [T+ C].
- Allopurinol [C].
- Erythromycin [T + C].
- Chloramphenicol [T + C].
- Doxycycline [C].
- Clotrimazole [T].
- Fluconazole [T + C].
- Ketoconazole [T + C].
- Ritonavir [T + C].
- Nelfinavir [T + C].
- Nifedipine [T].
- Verapamil [C].
- Diltiazem [T + C].
- Omeprazole [T].
- Chloroquine [C].
- Methylprednisolone [C].
- Metoclopramide [C].
- Progestogens [C].
- Cimetidine [C].
- Tacrolimus [C].
- Clarithromycin [T + C].

The following reduce CNI levels:
- Rifampicin [T + C].
- Griseofulvin [C].
- Carbamazepine [C].
- Phenobarbital [C].
- Phenytoin [C].
- St John's wort [C].

The following increase the risk of nephrotoxicity:
- Ibuprofen and other NSAIDs [T + C].
- Amphotericin [T + C].
- Aminoglycosides [C].
- Co-trimoxazole and trimethoprim [C].
- Vancomycin [C].

The following increase the risk of hyperkalaemia:
- ACE inhibitors and ACE II antagonists [C].
- K sparing diuretics [T + C].

C = ciclosporin; T = tacrolimus.

- Oestrogens and progestogens: efficacy of oral contraception possibly decreased with tacrolimus.
- Increased risk of myopathy with statins and ciclosporin: avoid rosuvastatin.

Antiproliferative agents: azathioprine, mycophenolate mofetil, and mycophenolic acid

- These agents inhibit purine synthesis.
- Azathioprine has been used since the earliest days of solid organ transplantation and remains in routine use as initial immunosuppressive therapy in ~20% of centres in the USA (NAPRTCS 2014 report) and a number of UK centres.
- Its use has been superseded by MMF in the USA and many European countries, particularly when used in combination with ciclosporin.
  - A 2015 Cochrane meta-analysis of 23 adult studies showed that compared with azathioprine, MMF results in a 30% reduced risk of acute rejection and 20% reduction in graft loss; however, there was no improvement in patient survival or graft function.
- No prospective paediatric RCTs have directly compared the two agents.
- Both drugs are licensed for use in childhood following renal transplantation in Europe and the USA.

Azathioprine
- Dose 1–3 mg/kg daily.
- Principal adverse effect is myelosuppression:
  - Most pronounced in those with genetically determined low levels of thiopurine methyltransferase (TPMT), an enzyme with a major role in azathioprine catabolism.
  - TPMT activity is controlled by a common genetic polymorphism and 1:300 patients have very low enzyme activity.
  - Patients can be screened for TPMT levels or for the presence of genetic polymorphisms.
  - Regular monitoring of FBC is mandatory.
  - Where neutropenia occurs, the dose should be halved (absolute neutrophil count $0.5–1.5 \times 10^9/L$) or stopped ($<0.5 \times 10^9/L$). Isolated lymphopenia is not an indication for dose reduction.

MMF
- Dose 600 mg/m^2 per dose given twice daily with ciclosporin. Maximum dose 2 g daily.
- Dose reduced to 300 mg/m^2 per dose when used in conjunction with tacrolimus.
- Metabolized to mycophenolic acid (MPA), which is the active drug.
- There is a tenfold interindividual variability in plasma MPA levels following a standard dose of MMF.
- There is uncertainty as to whether MPA levels should be measured to guide dosing. This is not, at present, standard practice in most UK centres. Studies in adult patients investigating whether monitoring MPA levels improves outcomes have produced conflicting results.
- Risk of leucopenia and invasive viral infection is greater than with azathioprine.
- Monitoring of FBC is mandatory at every clinic visit.

- Principal adverse effects are upper and lower GI symptoms: diarrhoea, vomiting, constipation, nausea, and dyspepsia, often necessitating a dose reduction to 50–75% of the previous dose, or the administration of the same daily dose given as four divided doses (beware adherence issues).
- There is increasing evidence that adverse effects may be linked to high MPA levels.

Mycophenolate sodium
- Metabolized to the active compound MPA.
- Not licensed for use in children; there is little paediatric experience with this agent.

Corticosteroids
- The corticosteroids are potent immunosuppressants.
- Prednisolone is the most widely used agent in the UK, but its precursor Prednisone is used in the USA and much of Europe.
- Prednisolone dosing schedules vary greatly, although most units will use relatively high doses in the early post-transplant period with a rapid taper. An example is as follows:
  - Intraoperative: 600 mg/m^2.
  - Day 1: 60 mg/m^2 daily.
  - Days 2–7: 40 mg/m^2 daily.
  - Days 8–14: 30 mg/m^2 daily.
  - Days 15–21: 20 mg/m^2 daily.
  - Days 22–28: 15 mg/m^2 daily.
  - Days 29–42: 10 mg/m^2 daily.
  - >Day 42: <10 mg/m^2 daily.
- In the TWIST study, only five doses of corticosteroid were administered (300–600 mg/m^2 day 0, 60 mg/m^2 day 1, 40 mg/m^2 day 2, 30 mg/m^2 day 3, 20 mg/m^2 day 4, then discontinued); this resulted in improved growth and metabolic profile with no increase in the rate of acute rejection. The Stanford protocol avoids all use of corticosteroids with similar good outcomes.
- Methylprednisolone IV is often used in place of prednisolone in the first few postoperative days (1 mg methylprednisolone = 1.25 mg prednisolone).
- Where an early corticosteroid withdrawal regimen is not used, daily therapy can be converted to alternate-day therapy at around 2–3 months post transplant if rejection has not been a problem to improve growth velocity and reduce other adverse effects. German studies have shown the safety and efficacy of corticosteroid withdrawal as late as 1–2 years post transplantation.
- The adverse effects of corticosteroids include obesity, growth disturbance, Cushingoid features, acne, reduced bone mineral density, striae, cataracts, diabetes, adrenal suppression, hypertension, gastrointestinal upset, myopathy, and hirsutism.

Antibody therapies

Anti-CD25 monoclonal antibodies: basiliximab and daclizumab

* These agents bind to the IL-2 receptor (CD25) on T cells and prevent the IL-2-mediated proliferation of activated T cells. They may also be cytotoxic to regulatory T cells, which also express CD25—the significance of this is not yet known.
* Their use reduces the incidence of acute rejection, this effect being more pronounced with ciclosporin-based regimens.
* There are very few adverse effects, although acute anaphylaxis has been reported to occur, albeit rarely.
* Daclizumab is no longer produced, though was used in a number of RCTs, including the TWIST study. While there is no good evidence to show that basiliximab and daclizumab can be used interchangeably, for pragmatic reasons this has occurred.

Basiliximab

* Dose 10 mg if patient <40 kg and 20 mg if patient ≥40 kg.
* Can be given via a central or peripheral vein.
* A total of two doses are given: one immediately prior to transplant surgery and the second on postoperative day 4.

Antithymocyte globulin

* Antithymocyte polyclonal antibody produced in rabbits.
* Dose 1.0–1.5 mg/kg/day given daily for 3–9 days, starting on day of transplantation. Should be administered over 6 h.
* May produce a cytokine release syndrome, and premedication with paracetamol, steroids, and an antihistamine is recommended.
* Other reported side effects include diarrhoea, 'flu-like' symptoms, hypotension, nausea, dysuria, dyspnoea.

Mammalian target of rapamycin inhibitors: sirolimus (rapamycin) and everolimus

* These agents inhibit T-cell proliferation through binding to mTOR (the mammalian target of rapamycin (sirolimus), the prototypic drug in this group).
* They are not currently licensed for use in paediatric transplantation in the UK and global experience in paediatric transplantation is limited, though growing. In the UK, NICE did not approve their use as initial immunosuppressive therapy.
* Studies in adult patients show promising results and these agents are theoretically attractive as they are non-nephrotoxic and appear to have a beneficial effect on atherosclerosis
* A recent paediatric study reported similar short-term results with the use of basiliximab, ciclosporin, and prednisolone with the introduction of everolimus and reduction of ciclosporin dose at 2 weeks followed by the withdrawal of prednisolone when compared with ongoing ciclosporin, MMF, and prednisolone therapy.

- Adverse effects include poor wound healing and lymphocoele, blood dyscrasias (anaemia, thrombocytopenia, and leucopenia), mouth ulcers, elevation of transaminases, proteinuria, and dyslipidaemia (hypercholesterolaemia and hyperlipidaemia).
- mTOR inhibitors should be temporarily discontinued around the time of elective surgery to avoid wound complications
- Sirolimus and everolimus have been used both as primary immunosuppressants in cases of CNI toxicity and also as rescue therapy in cases of acute rejection.

Sirolimus

- The drug half-life appears to be shorter in children than in adults and many have recommended a twice-daily dosing regimen, particularly in children <5 years of age.
- Increased clearance of sirolimus occurs in the presence of ciclosporin.
- Black patients may require higher doses; whether this also applies to children is not known.
- At present, there are insufficient data to make clear dosing recommendations, though published regimens have used doses of 1–3 mg/m^2 once daily to achieve levels of 5–15 micrograms/L when used in conjunction with CNIs and 15–25 micrograms/L in CNI-free regimens.

Everolimus

- A dose of 0.8 mg/m^2 twice daily has been recommended with target trough levels of 3–6 ng/mL.

Newer agents

Belatacept

- Biological agent which binds to C5 and blocks the terminal complement pathway. Also indirectly inhibits antigen-specific antibody production by B lymphocytes.
- Given by IV infusion; following initial induction therapy, maintenance dose is given every 4 weeks. Therefore of great potential benefit in the non-adherent patient.
- No significant experience of the use of this agent in children and its use should be confined to properly conducted clinical trials.

Eculizumab

- Biological agent which blocks the alternative complement pathway. Well-established therapy for aHUS.
- Growing interest in using eculizumab to prevent complement-mediated injury in kidney transplantation.
- No significant experience of the use of this agent in children and its use should be confined to properly conducted clinical trials.

Further reading

Ganschow R, Pape L, Sturm E, et al. Growing experience with mTOR inhibitors in pediatric solid organ transplantation. *Pediatr Transplant* 2013;17:694–706.

Acute T-cell-mediated and antibody-medicated rejection and chronic allograft nephropathy: diagnosis and management

Acute rejection: introduction

- Acute reduction in renal function secondary to specific pathological changes in the transplanted kidney.
- Important cause of early graft dysfunction.
- Occurs most frequently between 1 week and 3 months post transplantation, though may occur at any time, particularly with immunosuppression failure (e.g. non-adherent patients), or iatrogenically, through the weaning of immunosuppression regimens. The importance of non-adherence cannot be overestimated, particularly in the teenage years; where acute rejection occurs beyond the first year post transplantation, non-adherence should be considered to be the cause unless proved otherwise.
- Most commonly asymptomatic and detected through a rise in plasma creatinine following routine measurement. In severe cases, symptoms may include mild fever, oliguria, and malaise. Hypertension and graft tenderness may be detected. Urine inspection may detect macro- or microscopic haematuria, proteinuria, and pyuria.
- Should be suspected where plasma creatinine rises ≥25% from previous baseline or where the rate of fall in creatinine is less than anticipated. This is however only a rough guideline, and there should always be an awareness of the possibility of rejection with any rise in creatinine.
- Diagnosis is made by renal biopsy after structural causes for acute graft dysfunction have been excluded by US.
- In the modern immunosuppression era, incidence has fallen to <10% in the first year post transplant.
- Risk factors include the sensitized patient with DSAs, high number of HLA mismatches, prolonged CIT, DGF, treatment non-adherence, African American ethnicity, and second or subsequent transplants.
- Acute rejection occurs at a lower frequency following living donation compared with deceased donation.
- There has been much debate regarding the long-term impact of episodes of acute rejection. The current consensus is that overall, acute rejection negatively impacts on graft survival and is a predictor for chronic allograft nephropathy, otherwise known as interstitial fibrosis/tubular atrophy (➔ see 'Chronic allograft nephropathy (interstitial fibrosis and tubular atrophy)'). However, in cases where acute rejection is mild and there is a full response to treatment, long-term graft survival may be unaffected.

Histological forms of acute rejections

- Acute T-cell-mediated rejection (TCMR), previously known as cellular rejection:
  - Infiltration of the tubules and interstitium by lymphocytes.
- Acute antibody-mediated rejection (ABMR):

- Evidence of acute tissue injury, the presence of circulating DSAs, and histological evidence of an antibody-mediated process (e.g. C4d deposition).
- TCMR and ABMR may coexist. This may occasionally lead to undertreatment or incorrect treatment.
- Subclinical rejection is defined as the presence of either TCMR or much more rarely ABMR where there has not been evidence of deterioration in graft function. Diagnosed following routine protocol biopsy; this practice is less prevalent in paediatric recipients than in adults. As such, there are no good data on the prevalence of subclinical rejection in paediatric recipients.
- Borderline rejection is diagnosed when changes including tubulitis and mononuclear cell interstitial infiltration are present, but the Banff criteria (➔ see 'Banff classification for T-cell-mediated rejection') for TCMR are not met. The significance of this category is unknown with no good evidence on which to base treatment decisions. Empiric treatment before the biopsy may convert true TCMR into this category.

Differential diagnosis of allograft dysfunction

First 7 days after transplantation

- Acute tubular necrosis/reperfusion injury—linked to prolonged (>24 h) CIT or anastomosis time, or donor morbidities (AKI, vascular disease).
- Hyperacute antibody-mediated rejection (➔ see 'Acute antibody-mediated rejection').
- Hypovolaemia.
- Acute obstruction of the transplant ureter (e.g. by clot).
- Renal vascular thrombosis (➔ see 'Kidney transplantation: the surgery').
- Surgical complications e.g. lymphocoele, urinary leak (➔ see 'Kidney transplantation: the surgery').

7 days to 3 months plus after transplantation

- Acute rejection—both T-cell-mediated and antibody-mediated (➔ see 'Acute T-cell-mediated rejection' and ➔ 'Acute antibody-mediated rejection').
- Infection—commonly urine infection (➔ see 'Infection post-transplantation').
- CNI toxicity
- Thrombotic microangiopathy (TMA)—as a result of recurrence of aHUS (➔ see 'Recurrence and de novo disease post-transplantation') or secondary to CNI exposure or phospholipid syndrome. Acute ABMR will also show features of TMA
- Viral infection—including CMV and BK virus (BKV) (➔ see 'Infection post-transplantation').
- Recurrent or de novo glomerular disease (➔ see 'Recurrent and de novo disease post-transplantation').
- Renal artery stenosis (➔ see 'Kidney transplantation: the surgery').
- Ureteric obstruction (➔ see 'Kidney transplantation: the surgery').
- Bladder dysfunction.
- Chronic allograft nephropathy (➔ see 'Chronic allograft nephropathy (interstitial fibrosis and tubular atrophy)').

Acute T-cell-mediated rejection

(See Fig. 21.1.)
* T-cell infiltration of graft reacting to non-self HLA antigens present within tubules, interstitium, vessels, and glomeruli.
* Defined histologically by the presence of interstitial inflammation comprising >25% of the unscarred compartment (classified as an i-score ≥2—➔ see 'Quantitative criteria for tubulitis ('t') score') and tubulitis with more than four mononuclear cells per tubular cross-section or group of ten tubular cells (classified as a t-score ≥2). Alternatively, a diagnosis of TCMR can be rendered in the presence of any degree of arteritis (so-called v-lesion).

Banff classification for T-cell-mediated rejection

* Borderline—mild interstitial inflammation (<25% of non-sclerotic cortical parenchyma; i0 or i1) plus any tubulitis (t1, t2, or t3) or significant interstitial inflammation (>25% of non-sclerotic cortical parenchyma; i2 or i3), plus foci of mild tubulitis (t1).
* Type 1A—significant interstitial infiltration (>25% of non-sclerotic parenchyma; i2 or i3) and foci of moderate tubulitis (t2).
* Type IB—significant interstitial infiltration (>25% of non-sclerotic parenchyma affected; i2 or i3) and foci of severe tubulitis (t3).
* Type IIA—mild-to-moderate intimal arteritis (v1) with or without interstitial inflammation and tubulitis.
* Type IIB—severe intimal arteritis comprising >25% of the luminal area (v2) with or without interstitial inflammation and tubulitis.
* Type III—transmural arteritis and/or arterial fibrinoid change and necrosis of medial smooth muscle cells with accompanying lymphocytic inflammation (v3).

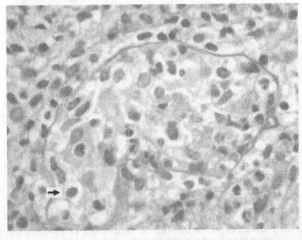

Fig. 21.1 Tubulitis. Lymphocyte nuclei seen within tubular epithelium inside tubular basement membrane. See also Plate 14.

Acute antibody-mediated rejection

(See Fig. 21.2.)

- Binding of circulating antibodies to donor antigens (predominantly HLA class I and/or II) on endothelial cells, resulting in inflammation and cellular damage.
- Very rarely may present in the immediate postoperative period due to the presence of pre-existing donor specific HLA antibodies. Modern antibody screening and cross-matching techniques have virtually eliminated this form of rejection, although it remains high on the differential diagnosis list in patients undergoing desensitization protocols, those presenting with vascular thromboses, and those with C4d-positive staining with acute tubular necrosis on biopsy or deteriorating graft function.
- Diagnostic criteria recently revised (2016). For the diagnosis of acute/active ABMR, the following three features must be present;

1. Histologic evidence of acute tissue injury, including one or more of the following; microvascular inflammation (glomerulitis (g) >0 and/or peritubular capillaritis score (ptc) >0), intimal or transmural arteritis (v >0), acute thrombotic microangiopathy without other cause, acute tubular injury without other cause.

2. Evidence of current or recent antibody interaction with vascular endothelium, including at least one of the following; linear C4d staining in peritubular capillaries (C4d2 or C4d3 by IF on frozen sections, or C4d >0 by immunohistochemistry on paraffin sections), at least moderate microvascular inflammation ([g + ptc] ≥2); molecular markers, if properly validated.

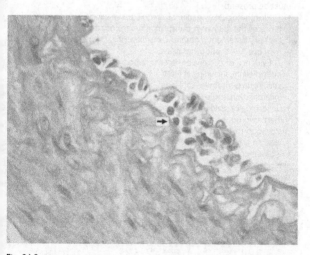

Fig. 21.2 Endothelialitis. Lymphocytes seen within intima of artery—a histological change suggestive of acute ABMR. See also Plate 15.

3. Serological evidence of donor specific antibodies.
- Where two out of three criteria are present, this is considered 'suspicious' for ABMR and depending on clinical circumstances treatment may be instituted (see below)
- C4d is a degradation product of the classical complement pathway. Deposition of C4d in the peritubular capillaries is indicative of anti-donor complement activity.
- Donor specific antibodies should be measured whenever acute rejection is suspected or diagnosed. Children with pre-existing DSA at the time of transplantation (from previous transplantation, blood transfusion etc.) have an increased risk of ABMR and graft loss. Where de novo DSA develop after transplantation this places the patient at increased risk of late-onset ABMR. The presence of de novo donor-directed HLA specific antibodies is recognized to be strongly predictive of graft failure in adult studies. Reduction in DSA titres by desensitization techniques has been shown to stabilize or improve graft function; however, serial monitoring of DSAs is not yet routine practice.

Chronic antibody-mediated rejection

- Defined in 2001 and now a formal category within the Banff classification system.
- Distinct process resulting from repetitive thrombotic events and inflammatory changes leading to endothelial cell injury and allograft matrix remodelling. Manifests as transplant glomerulopathy.
- Results in a slow and progressive decline in graft function
- For the diagnosis of chronic active ABMR, all three of the following must be present;
  - 1. Morphological evidence of chronic tissue injury, including one of more of the following; transplant glomerulopathy, severe peritubular capillary basement membrane multilayering, arterial intimal fibrosis of new onset without other cause.
  - 2. Evidence of current or recent antibody interaction with vascular endothelium, including at least one of the following; linear C4d staining in peritubular capillaries, at least moderate microvascular inflammation, molecular markers, if properly validated
  - 3. Serological evidence of donor specific antibodies
- Where two out of three criteria are present, this is said to be 'suspicious' for chronic ABMR
- The term transplant glomerulopathy describes thickening/duplication of the basement membrane with occasional double contour appearance similar to that seen in membranoproliferative disease but without the dense deposits.

Treatment of transplant rejection

No randomized controlled trial of treatment for acute transplant rejection has ever been performed. Management strategies are based entirely upon practice in adult kidney recipients.

Treatment of acute T-cell-mediated rejection

- First-line treatment is generally with IV methylprednisolone:
  - The dose given in most centres is 600 mg/m^2 up to a maximum of 1 g daily for 3–5 days, although there is no evidence for any particular regimen with some units giving the drug in lower doses or on alternate days.
  - The dose should be administered in 50 mL 0.9% saline over 2–4 h with ECG and BP monitoring.
- There may be an initial further rise in plasma creatinine though a response to treatment typically occurs within 5 days or so, with a fall in the plasma creatinine back to or close to baseline values in the majority.
- In ~40%, the plasma creatinine remains elevated above baseline, indicating either chronic damage or ongoing rejection.
- Following successful IV treatment, some centres return patients to their original steroid dose (including no steroid therapy in those on steroid-free protocols), while other centres increase maintenance steroid therapy for a period of time before tapering the dose back to pre-rejection levels. The intensity of other non-steroid immunosuppression may be increased, e.g. by running higher CNI trough levels or switching from ciclosporin to tacrolimus or azathioprine to MMF.
  - These strategies depend upon the severity of the rejection, the completeness of the response to steroids, and local practice.
  - It is also important to ascertain whether there have been any issues with non-adherence. In such cases, escalation of maintenance immunosuppressive therapy is probably not warranted; the focus should be on ensuring adherence.
- Where there is no response to IV steroids by day 7–10, a diagnosis of steroid-resistant rejection is made. This is generally an indication for the commencement of a lymphocyte-depleting antibody, though some may try a further course of IV methylprednisolone, e.g. where there appears to have been a partial response.
  - ATG, derived from rabbit (thymoglobulin), or equine (ATGAM®) serum are the commonest lymphocyte-depleting agents in routine use.
- Indications for use of an antilymphocyte preparation include:
  - induction therapy
  - TCMR refractory to steroid treatment
  - recurrent TCMR
  - type IIa, IIb, or III rejection (in some units).
- ATG 2 mg/kg is given daily for a total of 7–10 days. Patients should be administered IV hydrocortisone and antihistamine 30 min prior to dose:
  - Must be diluted in a large volume (500 mL in adults and older children) of either 0.9% saline or 5% glucose and given through a central venous catheter.
  - If leucopenia (<2.5 × 10^9/L) or thrombocytopenia (<80 × 10^9/L) occur, the dose should be halved.
  - If severe leucopenia (<1.5 × 10^9/L) or thrombocytopenia (<50 × 10^9/L) occur, treatment should be discontinued and recommenced at half the dose when the count has improved up to day 10, when treatment should be discontinued.
  - Maintenance immunosuppression is usually discontinued for the duration of treatment.

* All patients should receive co-trimoxazole prophylaxis against *Pneumocystis jirovecii* for 3 months.
* Valganciclovir prophylaxis against CMV should be given for 3 months to all patients (American Society of Transplantation (AST) 2013 and Renal Association 2015 guidelines).
* *Complications*:
  * Massive T-cell depletion lasting months to years.
  * Minor allergic reactions are very common.
  * Minor and major infections during therapy or after.
  * PTLD and other malignancies, particularly viral related.
* Following successful treatment, most centres return patients to their original maintenance immunosuppression or augment it.

Treatment of antibody-mediated rejection
The general principles behind the treatment of all forms of ABMR are the elimination of circulating anti-allograft antibodies, immunomodulation, and the inhibition of the complement system. No adequately powered prospective RCTs have ever been conducted in children with ABMR and all management is based upon that in adult transplant recipients.

Acute antibody-mediated rejection
* Conventional first-line treatment is with plasma exchange in conjunction with low-dose intravenous immunoglobulin (IVIG) ± rituximab.
* Removal of circulating anti-allograft antibodies using plasma exchange/ plasmapheresis:
  * Most frequently utilized initial therapy.
  * 1.5–2 volume exchange performed daily for 3–5 days in first instance followed by thrice-weekly therapy.
  * Patient plasma replaced with 5% albumin ± FFP.
  * Success rate as monotherapy is ~50%, increasing to 80–90% when used in combination with IVIG and rituximab.
* IVIG.
  * Fixes HLA antibodies at low dose (0.5–1 g/kg), preventing complement activation.
  * At higher doses (2 g/kg) has been shown to also decrease DSA levels.
* Rituximab:
  * B-cell depleting anti-CD20 monoclonal antibody.
  * Most frequently used dose in acute ABMR is 375 mg/m^2 (➔ see p. 640).
* Other concomitant therapeutic strategies:
  * In addition to the above-mentioned strategies, baseline immunosuppression should be optimized, including increasing the tacrolimus or MMF dose or the addition of steroids.
  * Where TCMR exists alongside acute ABMR, the former should be treated as described above.
  * BP and proteinuria should be controlled with the use of RAS blockade.

Second-line strategies for acute antibody-mediated rejection
* Where the above is unsuccessful or suboptimal, a number of more experimental therapies have been used in children, though experience is limited.

- Bortezomib:
  - Protease inhibitor which induces apoptosis in mature plasma cells, thus reducing DSA production. Designed and licensed for the treatment of lymphoma and multiple myeloma.
  - Promising results in studies in adult transplant recipients with acute ABMR.
  - However, serious haematological, GI, and neurological adverse effects have been reported.
- Belatacept:
  - Inhibits co-stimulatory blockade by binding to CD86/CD80 complex.
  - Developed as a non-nephrotoxic alternative to CNIs.
  - Growing successful use in adult transplant recipients with acute ABMR.
  - Concerns about high risk of PTLD have limited its use in children with ABMR.
- Eculizumab:
  - Monoclonal antibody which binds to C5. Inhibits membrane attack complex deposition and tissue destruction.
  - Reports of its successful use in treating children with refractory acute ABMR.
  - Increased risk of infection with encapsulated organisms (➔ see 'Atypical haemolytic uraemic syndrome').
- Alemtuzumab:
  - Anti-CD52 monoclonal antibody which depletes T and B lymphocytes, monocytes, macrophages, and other leucocyte populations.
  - Most commonly used as an induction agent, however there are reports of successful treatment of adults with acute ABMR.
- Splenectomy:
  - Reserved for severe resistant cases.
  - Removes peripheral reactive B cells.
  - Places recipient at significantly increased lifetime risk of infections from encapsulated bacteria.

Treatment of chronic antibody-mediated rejection
- Extremely challenging disorder with no proven effective therapy.
- General approach to treatment is as for acute ABMR, though success rate much lower.
- Bortezomib and splenectomy have both been shown to be effective in difficult adult cases.

Chronic allograft nephropathy (interstitial fibrosis and tubular atrophy)
- Poorly understood condition, previously known as chronic rejection.
- No universally accepted diagnostic criteria; however, it is generally accepted to mean graft dysfunction at >3 months following transplantation without evidence of acute rejection, CNI toxicity, or recurrent or de novo glomerular disease.

- The Banff 2005 system introduced the term interstitial fibrosis and tubular atrophy (IF/TA) without any specific aetiology. This distinguished the disorder from, e.g. chronic antibody-mediated rejection, where evidence of ongoing rejection was present.
- Banff classification:
  - Grade I—mild fibrosis of the interstitium (i.e. affecting 6–25% of the cortical area) and mild atrophy of the tubules (i.e. up to 25% of the area of the cortical tubules), either with or without specific glomerular or vascular findings suggestive of chronic allograft nephropathy.
  - Grade II—moderate interstitial fibrosis (i.e. affecting 25–50% of the cortical area) and moderate tubular atrophy (i.e. involving 26–50% of the area of the cortical tubules), with or without specific changes as in grade I.
  - Grade III—severe interstitial fibrosis (i.e. affecting >50% of the cortical area) and tubular atrophy (i.e. involving >50% of the area of the cortical tubules), with or without specific changes as in grade I.
- Common cause of graft failure after first year of transplantation (in adult patients the commonest cause is death with a functioning graft).
- Progressive deterioration in graft function associated with proteinuria and hypertension.
- Diagnosis is made by graft biopsy; this excludes other disorders such as recurrent disease, rejection, etc.
- No proven therapy to delay the inevitable decline in renal function necessitating dialysis and/or re-transplantation. Most would continue immunosuppressive therapy with a CNI and MMF/azathioprine ± prednisolone. BP should be well controlled; an ACE inhibitor or ARB will additionally reduce proteinuria. Other CKD-specific treatment should be commenced (➔ see 'Chapter 18').
- Chronic allograft nephropathy or 'creeping creatinines' were previously treated with reduction or elimination of CNIs with a view to reducing long-term CNI toxicity:
  - Evidence for this approach is seriously flawed in the modern era of good antibody detection techniques.
  - ~90% of graft failures can now be attributed to either glomerulonephritis or ABMR, with the ABMR accounting for almost two-thirds of cases.
  - Reducing immunosuppression in the face of an undetected ABMR is likely to speed disease progression.

Quantitative criteria for tubulitis ('t') score

- t0: no mononuclear cells in tubules.
- t1: foci with 1–4 cells/tubular cross-section (or 10 tubular cells).
- t2: foci with 5–10 cells/tubular cross-section.
- t3: foci with >10 cells/tubular cross-section, or the presence of at least two areas of tubular basement membrane destruction accompanied by i2/i3 inflammation and t2 tubulitis elsewhere in the biopsy.

Quantitative criteria for intimal arteritis ('v') score

- *v0:* no arteritis.
- *v1:* mild to moderate intimal arteritis in at least one arterial cross-section.
- *v2:* severe intimal arteritis with at least 25% luminal area lost in at least one arterial cross-section.
- *v3:* transmural arteritis and/or arterial fibrinoid change and medial smooth muscle necrosis with lymphocytic infiltrate in vessel.

Quantitative criteria for mononuclear cell interstitial inflammation ('i') score

- *i0:* no or trivial interstitial inflammation (<10% of unscarred parenchyma).
- *i1:* 10–25% of parenchyma inflamed.
- *i2:* 26–50% of parenchyma inflamed.
- *i3:* >50% of parenchyma inflamed.

Quantitative criteria for early allograft glomerulonephritis ('g') score

- *g0:* no glomerulonephritis.
- *g1:* glomerulonephritis in <25% of glomeruli.
- *g2:* segmental or global glomerulonephritis in 25–75% of glomeruli.
- *g3:* glomerulonephritis (mostly global) in >75% of glomeruli.

Quantitative criteria for interstitial fibrosis ('ci')

- *ci0:* interstitial fibrosis in up to 5% of cortical area.
- *ci1:* mild—interstitial fibrosis in 6–25% of cortical area.
- *ci2:* moderate—interstitial fibrosis in 26–50% of cortical area.
- *ci3:* severe—interstitial fibrosis in >50% of cortical area.

Quantitative criteria for tubular atrophy ('ct')

- *ct0:* no tubular atrophy.
- *ct1:* tubular atrophy in up to 25% of cortical tubules.
- *ct2:* tubular atrophy in 26–50% of the area of cortical tubules.
- *ct3:* tubular atrophy in >50% of the area of cortical tubules.

Quantitative criteria for allograft nephropathy ('cg')

- *cg0:* no glomerulopathy—double contours in <10% of peripheral capillary loops in most severely affected glomerulus.
- *cg1:* double contours affecting up to 25% of peripheral capillary loops in the most affected of non-sclerotic glomeruli.
- *cg2:* double contours affecting up to 26–50% of peripheral capillary loops in the most affected of non-sclerotic glomeruli.
- *cg3:* double contours affecting up >50% of peripheral capillary loops in the most affected of non-sclerotic glomeruli.

Quantitative criteria for mesangial matrix increase ('mm')

- *mm0:* no mesangial matrix increase.
- *mm1:* up to 25% of non-sclerotic glomeruli affected (at least moderate matrix increase).
- *mm2:* up to 26–50% of non-sclerotic glomeruli affected (at least moderate matrix increase).
- *mm3:* >50% of non-sclerotic glomeruli affected (at least moderate matrix increase).

Quantitative criteria for vascular fibrous intimal thickening ('cv')

- *cv0*: no chronic vascular changes.
- *cv1*: vascular narrowing of up to 25% of luminal area by fibrointimal thickening of arteries ± breach of internal elastic lamina or presence of foam cells or occasional mononuclear cells.
- *cv2*: increased severity of changes described for cv1 with 26–50% narrowing of vascular luminal area.
- *cv3*: severe vascular changes with >50% narrowing of vascular luminal area.

Quantitative criteria for arteriolar hyaline thickening ('ah')

- *ah0*: no PAS-positive hyaline thickening.
- *ah1*: mild to moderate PAS-positive hyaline thickening in at least one arteriole.
- *ah2*: moderate to severe PAS-positive hyaline thickening in more than one arteriole.
- *ah3*: severe PAS positive hyaline thickening in many arterioles.

Quantitative criteria for peritubular capillaritis (ptc)

- *ptc0*: no significant cortical ptc or <10% of PTCs with inflammation.
- *ptc1*: ≥10% of cortical peritubular capillaries with capillaritis, with max 3–4 luminal inflammatory cells.
- *ptc2*: ≥10% of cortical peritubular capillaries with capillaritis, with max 5–10 luminal inflammatory cells.
- *ptc3*: ≥10% of cortical peritubular capillaries with capillaritis, with max >10 luminal inflammatory cells.

Further reading

Ng YW, Peräsaari J, Lauronen J, et al. Antibody-mediated rejection in paediatric kidney transplantation; pathophysiology, diagnosis and management. *Drugs* 2015;75:455–472.

Recurrent and *de novo* renal disease following renal transplantation

Introduction

- Primary disease recurrence accounts for 7–8% of graft losses in children.
- More common in children than in adults undergoing transplantation.
- This may be an underestimate as there may be further additional undiagnosed cases.
- Rates of graft loss associated with recurrent disease are high with FSGS, MPGN/C3 glomerulopathy, primary hyperoxaluria, and aHUS, and lower with IgA nephropathy, HSP, ANCA vasculitis, and SLE.
- A primary diagnosis of a disease with a high risk of recurrence may influence whether a living donor transplant is performed.
- Careful post-transplant monitoring is required to diagnose recurrent disease early. Targeted treatment strategies are available for certain diseases.
- Table 21.1 summarizes the recurrence risk and incidence of graft loss according to primary renal disease.

Focal segmental glomerulosclerosis

- Variable incidence according to population studied, but most studies quote a recurrence rate of 20–40%.
- There is a 50% rate of graft loss associated with recurrent FSGS.

Table 21.1 Recurrent disease post transplant

	Recurrence risk (%)	Graft loss where recurrent disease develops (%)
FSGS	20–40[a, b]	40–60
C3GN (formerly MCGN type 1)	20–30	33
Dense deposit disease (formerly MCGN type 2)	70–100	25
aHUS	50	80
Membranous nephropathy	30	8–15
Alport syndrome (anti-GBM)	10	>50
IgA/HSP	60	5
SLE	30	Rare
ANCA + vasculitis	17	?
CNS	25	50

[a] Risk of recurrence 4% for genetic causes of FSGS (*NPHS2* mutations etc.).

[b] 60–100% where previous kidney is lost through recurrent disease.

- Where the first graft is lost to recurrent disease, the risk of recurrence in the next graft rises to 60–100%.
- There may be a link with the presence of an unidentified circulating factor which increases capillary permeability.
- Typically occurs early in the post-transplant period with heavy proteinuria, and progressive renal insufficiency and graft failure. Most graft losses occur in the first year after transplantation.
- Risk factors for recurrence:
  - Short time from initial disease presentation to development of CKD stage 5 (consistent finding across most studies).
  - Previous history of steroid-sensitive nephrotic syndrome, which subsequently became steroid resistant.
  - Recurrent FSGS in a previous transplant (subsequent risk 60–100%).
  - Presence of mesangial proliferation on initial native biopsy.
  - Children experience recurrent disease more frequently than adults.
  - Risk appears to be greater in older children.
  - Risk lower in US African Americans (who have a higher incidence of primary disease). Higher risk in white and Asian children.
  - Multiple other risk factors have been inconsistently reported, including pre-transplant nephrectomy, dialysis duration, however these remain controversial.
- Children with FSGS secondary to genetic mutations (both non-syndromal and syndromal) appear to be at very low risk (~4%) of developing recurrent disease. This observation is consistent with the theory that the defect is intrinsic and specific to the kidney.
- Some patients with genetic disease (typically with null mutations, i.e. no expression of protein) may experience disease recurrence due to an immune response against the protein in the transplant kidney that the patient was deficient of (e.g. Nephrin, or type 4 collagen). Because of the absence of the protein in the native tissue, the patient's immune system did not develop tolerance to it during development.
- Risk is not increased with the use of living donors. However, data from the USA report that the graft survival benefit of living donor transplantation is lost in the adolescent population, living donor transplant survival in FSGS patients equating to deceased donor graft survival in non-FSGS patients.
- Some would recommend not using a living donor for transplantation into a patient with FSGS except for those cases where a genetic mutation has been detected.
- Recurrent FSGS is associated with an increased risk of acute tubular necrosis and acute rejection.
- While there is conflicting evidence to support the theory that pre-transplant nephrectomy reduces the risk of disease recurrence, this is frequently performed because where heavy proteinuria persists this increases the risk of renal venous thrombosis. Where nephrectomy has been performed, if post-transplant proteinuria is detected one can be certain that this originates from the transplanted rather than the native kidneys.
- Diagnosis of recurrent FSGS is clinical:
  - Recurrent disease will be indicated by the development of heavy (nephrotic range) proteinuria within days to weeks following

engraftment, which may be associated with a progressive fall in plasma albumin. This may be accompanied by hypertension and deterioration of kidney function.
- The urine should therefore be tested daily for proteinuria, commencing on the day of transplantation. KDIGO 2009 guidelines recommend testing the urine daily for 1 week, weekly for 4 weeks, 3-monthly for the first year, and then annually. In practice, most will monitor for proteinuria more regularly than this.
- occasionally, immediate recurrence can manifest as primary non-function.
- early renal biopsy will not show any significant change on light microscopy, but podocyte foot process fusion may be seen on electron microscopy; it may take weeks to months for the characteristic FSGS lesions to develop.

Pre-emptive strategies and treatment of established recurrent FSGS

No single therapy or regimen has been shown to be superior and a variety of different regimens have been reported. None have been subjected to RCTs.
- Some have advocated the commencement of immunosuppression 5–7 days prior to transplantation, using combinations of high-dose ciclosporin (levels 250–350 micrograms/L) and prednisolone and prednisolone or tacrolimus, rituximab, and pre-transplant plasma exchange. There has never been a prospective randomized trial of any of these therapies; given the rarity of the clinical problem, it would be difficult to conduct an adequately powered trial without major international collaboration.
- Proposed strategies for the treatment of established disease include:
  - plasma exchange—this should be started as soon as the diagnosis is established
  - two-volume plasma exchange for 10 days (2-day break after fifth exchange), then once weekly for 8 weeks, with individualization of regimen according to response and the presence of breakthrough proteinuria upon weaning
  - IV methylprednisolone 250 mg/m^2 for 3 days then return to existing post-transplant steroids
  - oral cyclophosphamide 2 mg/kg daily in place of azathioprine/MMF for 8 weeks
  - high-dose IV ciclosporin (levels 250–350 micrograms/L). This may be due to direct action on the podocyte
  - rituximab and immunoadsorption using protein-A columns (which remove antibodies) have also both also been used, with encouraging results
  - these are reports of the use of abatacept, ofatumumab, and galactose and lipid apheresis.

C3 glomerulopathy (C3GN) and dense deposit disease (membranoproliferative glomerulonephritis (MPGN))

- This disease has now been reclassified as C3GN; however, all of the existing literature describes outcomes following patients diagnosed with MPGN.

- Recurrence occurs later than with FSGS, typically later in the first year or in the second year after transplantation. Proteinuria, which may reach nephrotic range, is the commonest manifestation.
- MPGN type I recurs in 20–30% of adults and children. Recurrence is manifested by proteinuria, which may initially be low level. Progressive deterioration of renal function leading to graft loss is common, occurring in around one-third.
- MPGN type II recurs in 70–100% of patients, though only 12–25% will develop heavy proteinuria and renal impairment and ultimately lose their grafts to recurrent disease.
- KDIGO 2009 recommendations propose testing for proteinuria at least monthly initially then every 3 months for the first year and annually thereafter. Most children will have their proteinuria quantified more frequently than this.
- There is no good evidence for any effective treatment of recurrent type I or II MPGN. There are reports of encouraging outcomes in type 1 MPGN with eculizumab, rituximab, plasmapheresis, and cyclophosphamide. No successful treatment exists for recurrent type II MPGN.

IgA nephropathy/Henoch–Schönlein purpura

- Recurrence at a histopathological level (mesangial IgA deposition) occurs in up to 60% of adult patients. Such recurrence was initially thought to be benign, although more recent studies have shown that ~13% will lose some function and ~5% lose their grafts secondary to this. Good paediatric data are not available.
- Significant recurrence (proteinuria, haematuria, and deterioration of renal function) generally has a late onset, often several years after transplantation
- Risk of graft loss is increased where a previous graft has been lost to recurrent disease.
- Recurrence is thought to be less common where MMF is used for immunosuppression as opposed to azathioprine.
- HSP nephritis recurrence rate is ~20%.
- There is no good evidence for any form of therapy for the prevention or treatment of recurrent IgAN or HSP nephritis. ACE inhibitors should be used to reduce proteinuria.
- KDIGO guidelines (2009) recommend screening IgAN transplant recipients for microscopic haematuria during the first month after transplantation, 3-monthly for the first year, and annually thereafter.

Membranous nephropathy

- ~30% recurrence rate in adults at 3 years with graft loss of 8%.
- Presents with proteinuria of varying degrees.
- Renal function is generally preserved in the early stages, although patients with heavy proteinuria and early recurrence progress rapidly towards graft failure.
- In contrast to idiopathic membranous nephropathy in the native kidney, the rate of spontaneous remission is very low.
- The use of IV methylprednisolone has been shown to be effective in one series of adult transplant recipients.

- Where recurrence is associated with the identification of anti-PLA2R antibodies, treatment with rituximab may be effective.
- General measures should be instituted, similar to those for any patient with proteinuria, including the use of ACE inhibitors and ARB, control of BP, and use of lipid-lowering therapy where indicated.
- It is important to distinguish recurrent membranous nephropathy from de novo membranous nephropathy, which can develop in association with late allograft dysfunction.

Crescentic glomerulonephritis of multiple aetiologies
- Risk is 3–10%.
- Treatment should comprise plasma exchange in combination with cyclophosphamide.

Primary hyperoxaluria
- Where isolated kidney transplantation is performed for infantile primary hyperoxaluria, the risk of graft loss is generally very high because of rapid deposition of oxalate in the transplanted kidney (strictly this is due to persistence of primary disease rather recurrent disease). This results in graft loss in ~90% of cases and there is no effective therapy.
- However, a small number of patients with pyridoxine responsive disease may benefit from isolated renal transplantation with ongoing pyridoxine therapy.
- Liver transplant followed by kidney transplant or combined kidney–liver transplantation will restore both renal function and the missing enzyme, allowing normal oxalate production and clearance (see 'Transplantation in special circumstances').
- Urinary oxalate levels may remain high for some time after combined liver–kidney transplantation (CLKT) despite normalization of plasma oxalate levels, placing the transplanted kidney at risk of recurrent nephrocalcinosis. This can be ameliorated by a high fluid intake and the use of potassium citrate or other crystallization inhibitors. The use of haemodialysis in this situation remains controversial (see 'Primary hyperoxaluria').

Haemolytic uraemic syndrome
- The cause of CKD stage 5 in 2–5% of children.
- In contrast to diarrhoea and pneumococcal-associated HUS, where the risk of recurrence is very low (probably <1%) unless there is a coexisting genetic mutation, children with aHUS have a high rate of recurrence post transplantation and this is frequently associated with graft loss. Overall the risk is ~50%
- Most recurrences occur early, usually within a month of transplantation.
- Presentation of recurrence is with thrombocytopenia, microangiopathic haemolytic anaemia, and graft dysfunction.
- Renal biopsy demonstrates typical HUS glomerular changes including endothelial cell swelling, widened subendothelial spaces, and glomerular capillary fibrin deposits.

- Mutations in genes encoding complement regulatory proteins and secondary disorders of complement regulation play a central role in many cases of aHUS. Endothelial damage occurs through an unregulated complement cascade. Increased understanding of the disease process has transformed therapy and outcomes.
- Gene mutations are identified in at least 50% of cases:
  - complement factor H (CFH, 20–30% of mutations), membrane co-factor protein (MCP, 10–15%), complement factor I (CFI, 10–15%);
  - mutations in genes encoding complement factor B (CFB), C3, and thrombomodulin have also been reported (see 'Atypical haemolytic uraemic syndrome').
- The risk of disease recurrence varies significantly according to the genetic abnormality:
  - MCP mutations: transplantation restores normal MCP levels and the risk of recurrence is very low. Living donation can therefore be considered.
  - CFH, CFI, and CFB mutations: high rates of recurrence (66–80%). Graft loss rates following disease recurrence are particularly high (60–80%). There appears to be a lower risk for recurrence where mutations occur in the first 15 short consensus repeats of CFH. If living donation is contemplated, the donor must be screened to ensure they do not carry the mutation themselves as asymptomatic carriers are described.
  - Disease recurrence with DGKE mutations is extremely rare.
  - A number of cases with combined mutations have been reported with variable outcomes.
  - Other causes include anti-factor H antibodies (5–10% of cases) and methylmalonic aciduria.
- The development of eculizumab has transformed outcomes in this disease group, both with regard to the management of the initial episode and also the prevention and management of recurrent disease.
- KDIGO guidelines (2009) recommend that screening for microangiopathy takes place post transplantation by measuring LDH, haptoglobins, platelet count, and blood films.
- Recurrence generally occurs early, within the first month or two after transplantation, though later recurrences have been reported. The risk seems to be increased where there is DGF, acute rejection, or infection.
- Previously the very high-risk patients (those with CFH, CFI, and CFB mutations) would be managed with intensive plasma exchange and/ or CLKT, the donor liver serving as the source of these previously missing proteins. Isolated kidney transplantation was recommended where there was no evidence of CFH, CFI, CFB, or C3 mutations and could be safely performed with MCP mutations, or where any mutation was present and another family member had previously successfully undergone isolated renal transplantation. Plasma exchange was recommended pre- and postoperatively.
- The efficacy of eculizumab means that these aggressive, high-risk strategies can generally be avoided.

- It has been suggested that eculizumab should be used prophylactically at the time of transplant in those at high risk of relapse, i.e. mutations in CFH, CFI, C3, or CFB, combined mutations, no indented mutations but CFH polymorphisms, or autoantibodies against CFH; although not routinely in those at low risk of relapse, i.e. mutations in *MCP*, *DGKE*, or no polymorphisms found and no antibodies against CFH.
- However, more information is required about dosing and duration of therapy.
- Plasma exchange may be of benefit when there are antibodies against CFH.

Treatment of established recurrent HUS

- Biological agents blocking complement activity, e.g. eculizumab.
- Plasma exchange therapy, if no response to eculizumab.
- Purified factor H may prove to be effective in the future.

Systemic lupus erythematosus

- Series of adult patients report histological recurrence rates of 2–30%, though graft loss secondary to recurrent disease appears to be relatively rare.
- A NAPRTCS series reported one case of disease recurrence resulting in graft loss in 94 children with SLE undergoing 100 transplants.
- The common misconception that 'SLE burns itself out' after the kidneys fail should be dispelled.
- The use of IV methylprednisolone and increased doses of MMF has been reported as a successful treatment for recurrent SLE nephritis

ANCA-associated vasculitis

- The number of transplanted patients is small, although recurrences of the large majority of the vasculitides are reported, and has been reported as high as 17% for ANCA-associated vasculitides in adults. There are no good paediatric data.
- ANCA positivity at the time of transplantation is thought to be associated with the development of vascular lesions in the graft, but is not a risk factor for graft loss.
- It is generally agreed that the systemic disease should be in stable remission at the time of transplantation.
- KDIGO guidelines (2009) recommend screening for proteinuria and haematuria during the first month post transplantation, 3-monthly during the first year, and annually thereafter.
- Treatment is with corticosteroids and cyclophosphamide or MMF with or without additional plasma exchange as in *de novo* disease. Rituximab is being used with increasing frequency.

Cystinosis

- Cystinosis does not recur in the transplanted kidney. Occasionally, cystine crystals can be seen on a transplant biopsy, reflecting recipient lymphocytes in the graft. These crystals do not affect graft survival or function. In fact, many series show superior graft survival in cystinosis patients compared with those with other causes of CKD stage 5.
- Treatment with cysteamine must be continued to prevent deposition of cystine in other organs (➔ see 'Cystinosis').

Diabetes mellitus

- The histological changes of diabetic nephropathy may recur in the transplanted kidney, though graft loss as a result of this is most unusual.

Alport syndrome

- The number of children undergoing renal transplantation with a diagnosis of Alport syndrome is relatively small.
- An anti-GBM nephritis may develop following de novo exposure to normal type IV collagen, resulting in RPGN.
- Risk is 3–10%.
- Risk is increased with large truncating mutations in the COL4A5 gene.
- Treatment is as for RPGN, with cyclophosphamide ± plasma exchange.
- Graft prognosis is poor with graft loss over weeks to months in at least 50% of cases.

Finnish-type congenital nephrotic syndrome

Nephrotic syndrome may recur in up to 25% of children with Finnish type CNS following transplantation:

- Related to the production of anti-nephrin antibodies due to an immune response against the nephrin protein that the patient was deficient of in the transplant kidney, rather than recurrent disease per se. Because of the absence of the protein in the native tissue, the patient's immune system did not develop tolerance to it during development.
- Most common in those with null mutations.
- May respond to treatment with cyclophosphamide ± plasma exchange and rituximab has also been used in this clinical situation.
- Up to 50% graft loss may occur due to recurrence.

De novo disease

De novo membranous nephropathy

- More common than recurrent membranous nephropathy.
- Probably due to antibodies directed against glomerular antigens in the graft.
- Occurs late post transplant with worsening of renal function and heavy proteinuria.
- Treatment with diuretics will improve oedema. There are reports of disease remission being induced with the use of corticosteroids.

Further reading

Bacchetta J, Cochat P. Primary disease recurrence – effects on paediatric renal transplantation outcomes. Nat Rev Nephrol 2015;11:371–384.

Van Stralen K, Verrina E, Belingheri M, et al. Impact of graft loss among kidney diseases with a high risk of post-transplant recurrence in the paediatric population. Nephrol Dial Transplant 2013;28:1031–1038.

Urinary tract infection post transplantation

Introduction

- Bacteriuria is a common complication of renal transplantation, occurring in 20–88% of childhood transplant recipients.
- The wide-ranging reported incidence may reflect differences in the rate of reporting of both symptomatic infections and apparently asymptomatic bacteriuria.
- Febrile UTI may cause significant morbidity and is usually associated with acute graft dysfunction.
- A number of episodes of seemingly asymptomatic bacteriuria are associated with a transient deterioration of graft function, implying the presence of asymptomatic parenchymal involvement warranting antibiotic therapy:
  - In such cases it must be assumed that any symptoms have been masked by the immunosuppressive therapy.
  - For this reason, many centres recommend that all transplant recipients should undergo regular routine urine microscopy and culture as part of their follow-up. Treatment should only be given for a positive culture if the child is symptomatic or where there is an otherwise unexplained rise in the plasma creatinine (see later in this topic).
- UTI within the first 6 months post transplantation, particularly when febrile, negatively affects long-term graft survival through both renal scarring and interstitial injury.
- UTI may precipitate an episode of acute rejection.

Specifics

- UTI is most common in the first month after transplantation when immunosuppression is heaviest and ureteric stents and urethral catheters may be *in situ*.
- The most common infecting organisms are:
  - *Escherichia coli*
  - *Pseudomonas aeruginosa*
  - enterococci (*Enterobacter cloacae*, *Streptococcus faecalis*, and *Proteus* spp.).
- Risk factors for post-transplant UTI include:
  - abnormal bladders (posterior urethral valve bladders with and without augmentation, neuropathic bladders)
  - vesicoureteric reflux (VUR) into the native kidneys, dilated native urinary tracts (the native urinary tract may be an important source of infection)
  - VUR into the graft (see later in this topic)
  - pre-transplant history of UTI
  - the presence of a ureteric or other stent
  - diabetes mellitus
  - sex—twice as common in boys.

Investigations

- Urine microscopy and culture.
- CRP.
- Blood culture.
- Plasma creatinine.

Treatment

- While there is no good evidence to support this strategy, the authors recommend that antibiotics should be given IV in the early period post transplantation where immunosuppression is heaviest or where there is significant fever or systemic upset. Choice of antibiotic should be determined by local guidelines based upon patterns of sensitivities.
- There may be an additional case for the administration of IV therapy where there is a significant rise in the plasma creatinine, even if the infection is seemingly asymptomatic.
- Symptomatic afebrile UTI may be treated with oral antibiotics unless specific risk factors (renal dysfunction etc.) are present.
- If there are no symptoms and the plasma creatinine is entirely stable (asymptomatic bacteriuria), then conservative management is recommended. The repeated treatment of asymptomatic bacteriuria encourages the growth of resistant organisms.
- If there is a transplant ureteric stent *in situ*, early removal must be considered.
- *Candida* UTIs should be treated with oral fluconazole in the first instance, although IV therapy (fluconazole, amphotericin, or flucytosine) may be required if this is not effective or if the child is significantly unwell (⟳ see 'Infection post-transplantation'). *Caution*: fluconazole will increase the levels of CNIs.
- There is no broad agreement about the use of prophylactic antibiotics in at-risk patients and no RCTs have been conducted. Most units will use co-trimoxazole for the first 6 months post transplantation, principally as prophylaxis against *Pneumocystis* infection: this will additionally provide some prophylaxis against UTI. Where this is not used, most would use a prophylactic antibiotic such as trimethoprim for 3–6 months, particularly where there is underlying urological abnormality as the cause of CKD stage 5 or where there is known to be VUR into the graft.

Subsequent investigation and management

Children should undergo imaging of their graft following a UTI:
- Many centres perform a DMSA scan to determine whether renal parenchymal scarring has developed. Long-term data suggest that febrile UTI may lead to focal defects on DMSA scanning, however identical changes may also result from renal biopsy and vascular complications, making interpretation difficult.
- Where parenchymal scarring is detected, controversy exists as to whether a micturating cystourethrogram should be performed. This is an invasive unpleasant procedure with a significant radiation burden. The majority of centres have abandoned this practice.
- VUR occurs in >50% of transplanted kidneys: most transplant surgeons perform an antireflux procedure when anastomosing the allograft ureter to the native bladder though it is unknown if this procedure is beneficial.

- The importance of VUR is controversial. There is some evidence that it increases the risk of acute pyelonephritis and subsequent scarring of the graft and it has been suggested that children with progressive scarring should receive antibiotic prophylaxis.
- Some have advocated the use of antireflux procedures (e.g. STING when VUR is clinically significant), although this has never been formally studied and is not without risk as the distal ureteric blood supply is precarious.

Further reading

John U, Kemper MJ. Urinary tract infections in children after renal transplantation. *Pediatr Nephrol* 2009;24:1129–1136.

New-onset diabetes after transplantation

Introduction

* New-onset diabetes after transplantation (NODAT) has been reported as a complication in 4–25% of adults and 3–20% of children and adolescents.
* There is much variation in the definition of NODAT (ranging from transient hyperglycaemia to long-term requirement for insulin or oral hypoglycaemic agents), variability in duration of follow-up, etc., hence the wide variation in reported incidence.
* In many instances there is unidentified abnormal glucose tolerance prior to transplant, which worsens following transplantation.
* Around 2–7% of children develop significant NODAT requiring insulin or oral hypoglycaemic therapy. The incidence appears to be increasing.
* The significance of NODAT has previously been underestimated.

Aetiology

The aetiology of NODAT is multifactorial:
* Corticosteroids are known to increase peripheral insulin receptor resistance and may inhibit beta-cell insulin secretion.
* The CNIs are known to be toxic to beta cells; the risk appears to be somewhat greater with tacrolimus than ciclosporin.

Risk factors

Reported risk factors:
* Ethnicity (African Americans and Hispanics).
* Family history of diabetes mellitus.
* Abnormal glucose metabolism pre transplant or other components of the metabolic syndrome (e.g. dyslipidaemia, hypertension, and hyperuricaemia).
* Use of corticosteroids.
* Use of CNIs, particularly tacrolimus.
* Use of sirolimus
* Higher degree of HLA mismatch (related to a need for more intensive immunosuppression).
* High body mass index.
* Treatment for acute rejection.
* Cystinosis, ADPKD, Bardet–Biedl syndrome, Alstrom syndrome, HUS, or the *HNF1B* mutation as a cause of CKD stage 5.
* Hepatitis C positivity.

NODAT is associated with a significantly poorer long-term outcome for both the patient and the graft:
* NODAT is a major determinant of the increased cardiovascular morbidity and mortality seen in transplant recipients.
* Associated with reduced patient survival, increased risk of graft loss, and increased risk of infection.
* Adult series have shown survival with NODAT to be comparable with that observed in patients with pre-transplant diabetes mellitus, emphasizing the importance of strategies to avoid the development of NODAT where possible.

Investigation

Avoidance

- Centres that have used steroid-free immunosuppressive regimens have reported very low rates of NODAT (see Stanford data and TWIST study).
- There may be a case for avoiding the use of tacrolimus in those patients with a strong family history of diabetes mellitus and other significant risk factors.
- A number of fasting blood glucose (FBG) measurements should be made as part of the transplant work-up.
- Screening for known risk factors for NODAT.
- Some have proposed performing formal glucose tolerance tests on all children awaiting renal transplantation to identify those at risk of NODAT and to alter the immunosuppressive regimen accordingly. This has been shown to increase the diagnosis rate compared with the use of FBG levels only.

Identification and investigation of NODAT

- Early detection and appropriate treatment of transplant recipients who have developed NODAT can ameliorate the long-term consequences of the condition.
- However, it is important to be aware that transient hyperglycaemia relating to stress, corticosteroids, and other factors is very common in the first few days post transplant and often settles spontaneously.
- KDIGO guidelines for adult patients recommend monitoring of FBG levels, oral glucose tolerance test, and/or HbA1c in patients post transplant at least weekly in the first 4 weeks, then at 3, 6, and 12 months, then annually.
- This may be difficult to achieve in smaller children, in whom random blood sugars should be measured. Furthermore data are not available to determine whether these recommendations are appropriate for children.
- Random blood sugar levels of >11 mmol/L, the presence of glycosuria, or other symptoms should prompt measurement of a fasting blood sugar:
  - FBG <6.1 mmol/L is normal.
  - FBG 6.1–6.9 mmol/L represents prediabetes (glucose intolerance): an oral glucose tolerance test should be performed; fasting insulin, anti-glutamic acid decarboxylase (GAD) antibodies and anti-islet cell antibodies should be measured.
  - FBG >7 mmol/L is diagnostic of NODAT: fasting insulin, anti-GAD antibodies, and anti-islet cell antibodies should be measured.
- An oral glucose tolerance test is performed by measuring blood glucose levels 2 h after administration of 75 g of glucose—NODAT is known to be underdiagnosed if only the FBG is used:
  - 2 h blood glucose <7.8 mmol/L is normal.
  - 2 h blood glucose 7.9–11.0 mmol/L represents pre-diabetes (glucose intolerance).
  - 2 h blood glucose >11 mmol/L is diagnostic of NODAT.

Treatment

- Expert endocrinological advice should be sought.
- Every attempt should be made to reduce immunosuppressive therapy in an attempt to reverse the NODAT. This should be achievable in the long-term in 50–75% of patients:
  - Steroid dose should be lowered to the minimum acceptable and discontinuation of steroid therapy considered.
  - Where tacrolimus is used, the target trough level should be reduced to around 3–5 micrograms/L.
  - A switch from tacrolimus to ciclosporin might be considered.
  - There is a clear risk of inducing an episode of rejection with these strategies and there is a strong case for increasing other immunosuppressive therapy to try and prevent this, e.g. replacing azathioprine with MMF.
- Adult guidelines recommend a stepwise approach to treatment, beginning with non-pharmacological therapy (weight loss, exercise, stopping smoking), progressing to oral agent monotherapy, oral combination therapy, then insulin therapy, with or without oral agents. These may be appropriate in the young adult population.
- Some children (particularly those with low serum insulin levels) will require insulin therapy, although many (particularly those with significant obesity, evidence of peripheral insulin resistance, and negative antibody status) resemble patients with type 2 diabetes and should be treated with oral hypoglycaemic agents. Metformin is the only agent licensed in children. This reduces hepatic glucose production and increases insulin-mediated glucose uptake in peripheral tissues. Its use is associated with the development of lactic acidosis and contraindicated in CKD.
- Careful attention should be paid to weight loss, exercise, and smoking avoidance.
- Patients should be carefully monitored:
  - Lipid levels measured regularly.
  - Annual screening for retinopathy.
  - Aggressive treatment of hypertension.

Further reading

Garro R, Warshaw B, Felner E. New onset diabetes after kidney transplant in children. *Pediatr Nephrol* 2015;30:405–416.

Infection post transplantation

General points

- Infections are an important cause of morbidity and mortality following kidney transplantation. The 2014 NAPRTCS report indicates that infection was responsible for 28.5% of post-transplant deaths (12.7% bacterial, 8% viral, and 7.8% non-specific).
- The type of infection can be predicted by its timing post transplantation:
  - In the first 4 weeks, infections are most likely to be bacterial and related to the transplant surgery.
  - Between 1 and 6 months, opportunistic infections predominate as well as reactivation of latent viral infections previously present in the recipient.
  - After 6 months, infection is most commonly with community-acquired viruses as well as infections associated with chronic graft dysfunction.
- Risk factors for post-transplant infection:
  - Young age at transplantation.
    - Less likely to have been exposed to viruses that may reactivate following intense immunosuppression.
    - However lack of prior exposure increases disease severity following infection with CMV, respiratory syncytial virus, influenza, and other viruses.
    - Reduced likelihood of exposure to EBV pre transplant significantly increases risk of post-transplant EBV and PTLD.
    - Reduced likelihood of having received full course of routine childhood immunizations—risk of vaccine-preventable infections. It is, however, essential that immunization status is assessed as part of the pre-transplant evaluation and immunizations should be updated using expedited regimens where necessary.
  - Intraoperative factors:
    - More potent immunosuppression increases the risk of all infections, particularly the transplant-associated viruses CMV, EBV, and BKV but also community-acquired pathogens, e.g. respiratory syncytial virus and influenza.
    - Reduces efficacy of all vaccines administered post-transplantation.
  - Use of organs from adult donors increases the likelihood of mismatching for CMV and EBV, thereby increasing potential disease severity.
  - The multiple intravascular lines and catheters that are used to monitor the transplant recipient increase the bacterial and fungal infection risk.
  - Immunosuppression post transplant:
  - Malnutrition.

Bacterial infections

- The use of a broad-spectrum antibiotic for 1–3 days as perioperative prophylaxis against common bacterial postoperative infections is relatively common practice.
- UTI is the most common bacterial infection (➔ see 'Urinary tract infection post-transplantation').
- Other common infections include surgical wound infections.

- Catheters and intravascular lines increase risk of infection and should be routinely removed as early as possible postoperatively. Infection related to catheters and lines should almost invariably result in their immediate/early removal.
- Consideration should be given to removal of the Tenckhoff catheter at the time of transplant, particularly if there is infection of the exit site or if there has been recent peritonitis. Infection of a peritoneal catheter is difficult to diagnose as flushing it may introduce infection so it should be removed if infection is suspected.
- It is standard practice to culture a sample of the preservation fluid used for the transport of deceased donor kidneys. Where this is positive, antibiotic cover should be given.
- Multidrug bacterial resistance is commonly observed.

Diarrhoea

- May be infectious or related to medications, particularly MMF.
- Infectious causes include bacterial (*Campylobacter jejuni*, *Salmonella* spp., and *Clostridium difficile*) viral (CMV—see **➔** 'Viral infections', rotavirus, norovirus) or parasitic (*Cryptosporidium*, *Giardia*, amoebiasis).
- Infection with C. difficile may lead to pseudomembranous colitis. Treatment is initially with metronidazole.

Fungal infections

Colonization of the skin and gut with fungi can occur post transplantation. Growth from urine, particularly if recurrent, or blood may signify invasive disease, and will be unlikely to clear if associated with an in-dwelling catheter, which should be removed if clinically possible.

- Patients being treated with broad-spectrum antibiotics or high doses of immunosuppressants (particularly corticosteroids) are at greatest risk, so some centres use antifungal prophylaxis, such as oral nystatin 100,000 units four times daily (to prevent fungal infection in the gut and shedding in stool) or fluconazole (see Table 21.2) in these situations.
- Commonest are *Candida* species. Infection can be anywhere, but oesophagitis and cystitis are the commonest sites. *Candida* in the urine should be treated to prevent ascending infection, which can result in fungal balls and obstruction to urinary drainage.

Table 21.2 Dose of fluconazole according to age and infection type

	<2 weeks	2–4 weeks	4 weeks to 11 years	12–18 years
Mucosal *Candida* and for prophylaxis in the immunocompromised patient	3–6 mg/kg on day 1 then 3 mg/kg every 72 h	3–6 mg/kg on day 1 then 3 mg/kg every 48 h	3–6 mg/kg on day 1 then 3 mg/kg daily. Maximum 100 mg daily	50 mg daily (up to 100 mg daily with difficult infections)
Invasive disease	6–12 mg/kg every 72 h	6–12 mg/kg every 48 h	6–12 mg/kg daily. Maximum 800 mg daily	

- *Aspergillus* is the second commonest fungal infection. It may be isolated from sputum, and on chest X-ray appears as opacities or empyema.
- Fluconazole should generally be given as first-line therapy for invasive candidiasis. This can be given orally (the drug is well absorbed) or by IV infusion over 10–30 min. The dose is the same orally and IV.
- Fluconazole increases CNI levels, so if their levels are already high, it is advisable to make a small (e.g. 10%) reduction in the dose of tacrolimus or ciclosporin and check drug levels within 48–72 h.
- Fluconazole dose should be halved if the GFR is <50 mL/min/1.73 m^2.
- Duration of treatment will vary with severity of infection, varying between 7 days and 8 weeks.
- Liposomal amphotericin (a potentially less nephrotoxic preparation of amphotericin) is indicated in severe candidal infection. This is also first-line treatment for *Aspergillus* infection.
- Other agents, including flucytosine, itraconazole, and voriconazole, can be used in refractory cases or for resistant organisms.

Pneumocystis jirovecii pneumonia

- Usually presents during the first 6 months of intensive post-transplant immunosuppression with fever, cough, oxygen desaturation with exercise, and a diffuse interstitial infiltrate on chest X-ray. Diagnosis is by bronchoalveolar lavage.
- *Pneumocystis* may coexist with CMV.
- Co-trimoxazole should be used as prophylaxis and is particularly useful in the first 6 months post transplant (see Table 21.3). It is usually given at night. Some centres administer treatment daily, though others follow oncology practice and give the drug three times weekly, e.g. Monday, Wednesday, and Friday.
- Patients with glucose-6-phosphate dehydrogenase deficiency (or other situations where co-trimoxazole is contraindicated) can receive nebulized pentamidine as prophylaxis, although this drug requires specialized facilities for administration because it is teratogenic and potentially toxic to those administering it.
- 480 mg of co-trimoxazole contains sulfamethoxazole 400 mg and trimethoprim 80 mg.

Table 21.3 Dosage for co-trimoxazole for the first 6 months post transplant

Weight	Dose of co-trimoxazole, mg, once daily
10–15 kg	240 mg (1/2 tablet or 5 mL of paediatric suspension
15–30 kg	360 mg (3/4 tablet or 7.5 mL of paediatric suspension
30–60 kg	480 mg (1 tablet or 10 mL of paediatric suspension)
>60 kg	960 mg (2 tablets)

Co-trimoxazole will additionally provide prophylaxis against post-transplantation UTI. Patients requiring long-term UTI prophylaxis should be restarted on their routine antibiotic prophylaxis, e.g. trimethoprim when the co-trimoxazole is stopped.

UK practice is to discontinue co-trimoxazole after 6 months; however, others recommend indefinite use given the ongoing increased risk of *Pneumocystis* infection.

Viral infections

Viral infection can be a particular problem in children post-transplant because:

* vaccines are not currently available for all viruses
* natural immunity is ordinarily acquired with increasing age
* children are more likely to be immunologically naïve to viruses transmitted in the donor kidney.

Once infected, certain viruses may lie dormant (latent) and can be reactivated.

Immunosuppressive medications profoundly affect cell-mediated immunity, increasing the risk of severe viral infection (primary or reactivation).

Antiviral therapy is effective for CMV and BKV, but not EBV.

Cytomegalovirus

* Major cause of morbidity in children undergoing renal transplantation.
* Infection may be primary (typically acquired from an infected donor organ) or secondary (due to reactivation of latent infection or superinfection with a new strain in a seropositive individual), asymptomatic (asymptomatic CMV infection), or symptomatic (CMV disease). Primary infection is associated with the highest morbidity and mortality rates. Secondary infection tends to result in milder illness.
* Symptomatic CMV disease typically occurs in the early period following transplantation; however, time to onset can be significantly later if chemoprophylaxis is used.
* Prior to the availability of ganciclovir, CMV disease was commonly fatal.

Risk factors

* Those most at risk are the antibody negative recipient (R−) of a positive donor (D+), although disease can also occur with R+ D− and R+ D+ combinations, but not with R− D− unless infection is acquired from a source other than the transplant. CMV may also be transmitted by blood products containing leucocytes.
* Intensive immunosuppressive protocols, especially the use of antilymphocyte products for induction or treatment of rejection.
* Co-infection with related viruses (human herpesvirus (HHV)-6 and -7).

Classification (American Society of Transplantation 2013)

CMV infection

* Presence of CMV replication regardless of symptoms.
* CMV infection without any symptoms should be labelled asymptomatic CMV infection.

CMV disease (CMV infection accompanied by clinical signs and symptoms) is divided into CMV viral syndrome and tissue invasive disease.

CMV viral syndrome

Evidence of CMV infection plus one or more of the following:
- Fever >38°C for at least 2 days.
- New or increased malaise.
- Leucopenia.
- >5% atypical lymphocytes.
- Thrombocytopenia.
- Transaminases >2× ULN.

CMV tissue invasive disease
- Pneumonia.
- GI disease.
- Hepatitis.
- CNS disease.
- Retinitis.
- Others (nephritis, cystitis, myocarditis, pancreatitis).

Indirect effects of CMV infection
- Acute and chronic allograft injury (with increased risk of rejection). Important role in chronic graft vasculopathy.
- Depressed immune response (with increased risk of opportunistic infection).
- Increased risk of EBV-related PTLD.

Diagnosis
- CMV DNA viral load assay by quantitative PCR.
- The pp65 antigenaemia assay is an alternative, although less frequently used.
- Histological examination of involved organs remains the gold standard for diagnosis of invasive disease.

Management

Substantial efforts should be made to prevent infection occurring and to treat early where invasive disease occurs:
- Pre-transplant antibody status of donor and recipient must be established.
- All seronegative recipients should receive CMV negative or leucodepleted blood products.
- Management options include:
  - the use of anti-CMV prophylaxis in all at-risk individuals, *or*
  - regular surveillance post transplantation with prompt pre-emptive treatment where evidence of infection develops.
- Both strategies have advantages and disadvantages, which need to be considered in the context of the patient and the allograft.
- Many US authorities prefer prophylaxis for the higher risk D+ R− group, while recognizing the utility of pre-emptive therapy in the R+ group.
- There is a real lack of large, multicentre RCTs comparing the two strategies in children. The small number of adult RCTs which have been performed have shown that both strategies are equally effective at preventing CMV, but long term graft survival rates were better with prophylaxis.

Prophylaxis
* Proven efficacy in a large number of clinical trials.
* Easy to coordinate.
* Higher drug costs.
* Potential for greater drug toxicity, e.g. neutropenia in early stages post transplantation when immunosuppressed and receiving other drugs associated with neutropenia, e.g. co-trimoxazole.
* Theoretical advantage of preventing replication of other viruses, including HHV-6.
* Theoretically more likely to prevent indirect effects of CMV.
* Late-onset CMV (disease occurring after discontinuation of prophylaxis) may be a significant problem.
* Potential for emerging drug resistance.

Surveillance and pre-emptive treatment
* Fewer trials, particularly in children.
* May reduce drug costs and toxicity.
* Higher laboratory costs.
* Requires excellent logistic coordination.
* Can be difficult if families live a distance from the transplant centre.

Antiviral prophylaxis against CMV
* British Transplantation Society (BTS) guidelines (2015) recommend that prophylaxis should be given to CMV-negative patients (R–) receiving CMV-positive organs (D+) and also where donor and recipient are CMV positive and treatment with ATG/ALG/OKT3 is being given.
* AST guidelines (2013) recommend prophylaxis for D+/R– and also all R+ kidney transplants and also in all patients receiving anti-lymphocyte therapies as prophylaxis or for treatment of rejection.
* Valganciclovir, the valine ester prodrug of ganciclovir, has improved bioavailability (ten times that of oral ganciclovir), allowing once-daily dosing. It has proven efficacy in preventing CMV disease in adults and is most units' agent of first choice for chemoprophylaxis against CMV, recommended in both AST and BTS guidelines:
  * Available as 450 mg tablets and 50 mg/mL oral solution.
  * Not licensed in the UK, but approved in the USA by the Food and Drug Administration from 4 months to 16 years for prophylaxis against CMV in solid organ recipients.
  * Dose (mg) = 900 × BSA (m²)/1.73 × eGFR (mL/min/1.73 m²)/125 once daily for 3 months (Royal Manchester Children's Hospital protocol).
  * An alternative dosing schedule has been recommended by Vaudry et al. (2009). Dose (mg) = 7 x BSA × eGFR (pharmacokinetics (PK) studies performed using this dose showed very similar exposure to that reported in adult patients receiving 900 mg daily).

Treatment is generally administered for the first 3 months post transplantation.

A number of adult studies have shown a benefit in increasing duration of valganciclovir prophylaxis to 6 months. AST guidelines (2013) recommend 6 months of prophylaxis in D+/R– transplants but 3 months of prophylaxis in other situations. Most UK centres continue to administer 3 months of prophylaxis.

No high-quality paediatric RCTs have compared 3- and 6-month prophylaxis:

- CMV Ig has been investigated in a small number of trials with contradictory findings. It has a potential role as additive therapy, though further studies are required.
- Aciclovir has poor *in vitro* activity.
- Ganciclovir has been investigated and shown to be effective in many clinical trials and a Cochrane meta-analysis found it to be superior to aciclovir in preventing CMV disease. It is generally administered IV because oral administration results in lower serum levels (low bioavailability and increased weight-adjusted clearance). This requires continuous IV access and is expensive.
- Valaciclovir, the valyl ester of aciclovir, has improved bioavailability, and has been shown to be effective against CMV disease and to reduce the incidence of acute rejection.

Surveillance for CMV

- On day 1 post-transplant and weekly thereafter for 12 weeks screen for CMV DNA by PCR.
- If CMV DNA is detected in the blood by PCR, treatment (pre-emptive therapy) should be commenced as 60% will go on to develop disease within 10 days.
- There has been international standardization of the measurement of viral load; however, the viral load threshold level for initiation of treatment varies between centres. At Great Ormond Street Hospital, London, UK, when a CMV viral load of >3000 IU/mL is detected on two occasions, valganciclovir is commenced and the dose of MMF or azathioprine is reduced. Where the viral load continues to rise despite this therapy, then IV ganciclovir is commenced.
- AST guidelines recommend treatment with either IV ganciclovir (adult dose 5 mg/kg twice daily) or valganciclovir (adult dose 900 mg twice daily). This should continue until the PCR is negative. Most authorities recommend that two negative results be obtained prior to treatment discontinuation.

Treatment of CMV disease

CMV viral syndrome and invasive disease

IV ganciclovir is the mainstay of treatment in children.

- Has been shown to be efficacious in many uncontrolled studies in adult patients.
- Dose is 5 mg/kg twice daily, though dose needs reducing if GFR reduced (see Table 21.4). Ganciclovir is removed by HD, therefore doses must be given post dialysis.
- Initial clinical response is usually observed in 5–7 days.
- Duration of therapy is 2–4 weeks, although uncertainly exists regarding optimum duration:
  - BTS guidelines recommend at least 2 weeks of therapy and complete resolution of clinical symptoms.
  - PCR results can tailor duration of therapy.

Table 21.4 Intravenous ganciclovir dosing

Creatinine clearance (mL/min/1.73 m²)	Dose of IV ganciclovir (mg/kg)	Dosing interval
>80	5	Twice daily
50–80	2.5	Twice daily
10–50	1.25–2.5	Once daily
<10 and haemodialysis	1.25	Once daily post dialysis

- Risk of relapse is lower in those where PCR is negative at the end of therapy.
- Treatment should continue until there is clinical resolution of symptoms, negative PCR, and at least 2 weeks of therapy have been administered (AST guidelines).
- The child treated for rejection is more likely to remain PCR positive and may need a longer course of IV ganciclovir.
- Where the child improves clinically, it is possible to change to oral valganciclovir (see later in this topic).
- May be associated with leucopenia and thrombocytopenia, although it must be remembered that this may be a manifestation of the CMV disease.
- The blood count should be regularly monitored and consideration given to dose reduction if cause of leucopenia and/or thrombocytopenia felt to be ganciclovir.

Studies in adult patients with mild to moderate CMV disease have shown oral valganciclovir to be comparable in efficacy to IV ganciclovir, and AST guidelines endorse the use of this agent in mild to moderate CMV disease. A number of paediatric centres use oral valganciclovir in this situation; however, there are very limited data on this strategy in children.

Immunosuppression should be reduced in the presence of CMV disease unless there is evidence of concurrent acute rejection.

- The removal of MMF/azathioprine alone may be sufficient where there is only minor organ, e.g. marrow involvement:
  - If more major organ involvement, halving of CNI dose is conventional.
- CMV Ig may be used in serious infection in conjunction with IV ganciclovir. While there is no good evidence to support its use, many would consider in life-threatening disease and pneumonitis.
- Care should be taken to exclude other opportunistic infections.
- Ganciclovir resistance may develop after the first course of treatment, so persistence of a positive PCR needs to be investigated for drug resistance.
- If there is resistance to ganciclovir, cidofovir or foscarnet can be used:
  - Cidofovir is nephrotoxic—this is heightened in the presence of CNIs.
  - Foscarnet is also nephrotoxic, neurotoxic (seizures), and may cause electrolyte disturbance, including hypocalcaemia.
- A number of new therapies are under investigation, including letermovir and cyclopropavir.

Varicella zoster virus

VZV infection is associated with a high morbidity and mortality in immuno-suppressed children.

- All children should have anti-varicella IgG antibody titres measured on entry to a CKD stage 5 programme.
- If blood products have been given in the preceding 3 months, antibody titres may be falsely positive so need to be rechecked.
- Children without antibodies are assumed to be at risk from chickenpox, even when there is a history of the disease.
- Varicella vaccine is now available and should be given to all varicella naïve children prior to transplant (➔ see 'Immunosuppressive therapy in renal transplant patients').
- If the child has been documented as being antibody positive, there is no need to re-check antibodies if the child is in contact with chickenpox post transplantation.
- Those receiving valganciclovir prophylaxis against CMV infection will be protected against VZV while this is ongoing.
- If the child who is varicella naïve (antibody negative) post transplantation (e.g. where transplantation has taken place before chickenpox exposure or vaccination) is exposed to varicella infection:
  - check anti-varicella IgG antibody status
  - human varicella zoster immunoglobulin (VZIG) should be given if antibody negative
  - VZIG should be given as soon as possible after exposure; it must be given within 10 days of contact. Protection from VZIG may only last for 3 weeks and, therefore, if a second exposure occurs a further dose is required.
- VZIG dosage:
  - <5 years: 250 mg IM.
  - 5–10 years: 500 mg IM.
  - >10 years: 750 mg IM.
- The incubation period is 8–21 days after contact, but add 7 days to incubation period if VZIG is given = 8–28 days after contact. Patients are contagious for 1–2 days prior to the rash appearing and until the spots have scabbed over. Varicella spots can crop several times, so careful examination is necessary.
- If chickenpox or shingles develops, treatment is with high-dose oral aciclovir for 7 days with dosage adjustment where the GFR is reduced.
- Children who develop severe chickenpox should be given IV aciclovir for 7 days.
- The course of IV aciclovir can be reduced or changed to oral treatment dependent on the severity of the illness.
- Dosing information is in Tables 21.5 and 21.6.
- It is not usually necessary to stop or reduce immunosuppression, but this can be done (e.g. reduction of the MMF or azathioprine dose) if presentation is severe.
- Once the course of aciclovir has finished, return to normal maintenance immunosuppression if the azathioprine/MMF has been changed.
- Serum antibody titres should be checked after 3 months to confirm future immunity.

Table 21.5 Oral aciclovir

Age	Dose	Dose interval
<2 years	200 mg	× 4 daily for 5 days
2–6 years	400 mg	× 4 daily for 5 days
6–12 years	800 mg	× 4 daily for 5 days
>12 years	800 mg	× 5 daily for 7 days
If the eGFR is <10 mL/min/1.73 m²		
<2 years	100 mg	Twice daily for 5 days
>2 years	200 mg	Twice daily for 5 days

Table 21.6 Intravenous aciclovir

Age	Dose	Dose interval
<3 months	10–20 mg/kg	× 3 daily for 7 days
3 months–12 years	500 mg/m²	× 3 daily for 5 days
>12 years	10 mg/kg	× 3 daily for 5 days
Reduced creatinine clearance, mL/min/1.73 m²		
25–50	As above	Twice daily
10–25	As above	Once daily
<10	125 mg/m²	Once daily or after dialysis

BK virus

BK is a polyoma virus. It is so called because BK were the initials of the first patient it was described in. BKV infection, as with CMV, may be primary or secondary (due to reactivation or infection with a new strain) and asymptomatic or symptomatic. Primary infection may be asymptomatic or present with mild pyrexia, malaise, vomiting, respiratory illness, pericarditis, and transient hepatic dysfunction. BKV is important in immunosuppressed patients because after primary infection BKV remains latent in the kidney and urinary tract where it may be reactivated. BKV infection in transplant recipients is associated with:
* polyomavirus-associated nephropathy (incidence 1–10% of kidney recipients)
* polyomavirus-associated haemorrhagic cystitis (though this is mainly a problem in bone marrow transplantation)
* rarer manifestations include ureteric stenosis, pneumonitis, encephalitis, retinitis, multiorgan failure, and leucoencephalopathy.

Diagnosis
* Presentation may be inconspicuous, with no clinical or laboratory signs other than high-level viruria as defined by decoy cell (urinary epithelial cells infected with BKV) shedding, and the detection of BKV by PCR in the urine and blood.

- Diagnosis of BKV nephropathy is by transplant biopsy. Non-specific cytopathic changes are seen—these may mimic rejection or drug toxicity, and should be confirmed by an ancillary technique such as immunohistochemistry for BKV protein or by *in situ* hybridization for BKV nucleic acids.
- All children with acute rejection refractory to conventional treatment should have their biopsies re-evaluated to ensure that evidence of BKV-associated nephropathy has not been overlooked.
- Acute rejection and BKV-associated nephropathy may occur concurrently. This requires expert diagnosis.
- Diagnosis of BKV-induced ureteric stenosis and cystitis is by tissue biopsy.
- Risk factors for BKV infection include use of ureteric stents, acute rejection and antirejection treatment, steroid exposure, lymphocytedepleting antibodies, higher immunosuppressive drug levels, tacrolimus-MPA compared to ciclosporin-MPA or to mTOR inhibitor-combinations, and low or absent BKV-specific T-cell responses as well as retransplantation after graft loss due to BKV-associated nephropathy.

Screening
- AST guidelines (2013) recommend that screening for BKV should occur to identify patients at increased risk of BKV-associated nephropathy:
  - 3-monthly for the first 2 years post transplantation and then annually to 5 years.
  - Urine should be screened by PCR or cytology for decoy cells—those with evidence of high-level urinary replication should undergo blood BKV PCR assessment.
  - Blood PCR studies should also be performed in all patients undergoing a renal biopsy for allograft dysfunction or surveillance.
  - Where viral loads are consistently high, consideration should be given to renal biopsy to diagnose or exclude BKV-associated nephropathy.

Management
Where blood BKV PCR studies are persistently positive, immunosuppressive therapy should be reduced. AST 2013 guidelines recommend the following:
- Reduce dose CNI by 25–50% in one or two steps, then reduce antiproliferative agent (MMF or azathioprine) by 50% then discontinue the latter if necessary.
Or
- Reduce antiproliferative drug by 50% then reduce CNI by 25–50% followed by discontinuation of the antiproliferative drug if necessary.

These strategies have been shown to be safe and effective in children, but are associated with an 8–12% risk of acute rejection. This is generally corticosteroid sensitive.

Nephropathy

- A definitive diagnosis of BKV-associated nephropathy can only be made by renal biopsy. A minimum of two cores should be taken. Diagnosis should be sought by demonstrating BKV cytopathic changes in allograft tissue, and confirmed by immunohistochemistry or *in situ* hybridization.
- Concurrent acute rejection may be present. This is indicated by the presence of endarteritis, fibrinoid vascular necrosis, glomerulonephritis, or C4d deposits along peritubular capillaries.

Management

- Treatment of nephropathy is with reduction of immunosuppression as outlined previously in management of persistently elevated PCR studies. In the longer term, it is recommended (AST guidelines) that baseline immunosuppression is maintained at lower exposure levels (tacrolimus <6 micrograms/L, ciclosporin <150 micrograms/L, sirolimus <6 micrograms/L, and MMF dose <1000 mg in adults).
- In those with sustained high-level BKV PCR values despite these measures, antiviral agents should be considered. However, no studies have shown these agents to be superior to immunosuppression reduction alone.
- Cidofovir has been shown to be effective in a number of adult series: adverse effects include nephrotoxicity and anterior uveitis (12–35%).
- Leflunomide has immunosuppressive as well as antiviral properties and this therefore a potentially attractive option:
  - Significant toxic effects have been described including hepatitis, haemolysis, thrombotic microangiopathy, bone marrow suppression, and fungal pneumonia.
  - Data regarding use in children are very sparse.
- Where acute rejection occurs following reduction of immunosuppression, this should be treated according to standard protocols.

Epstein–Barr virus and post-transplant lymphoproliferative disease

Key points

- EBV is an important cause of morbidity and mortality in paediatric kidney recipients.
- EBV disease ranges from a non-specific viral illness to PTLD including lymphoma (incidence 1–2% in children).
- Over-immunosuppression leading to breakdown of cytotoxic T-cell (CD8+) surveillance for EBV allows latently infected cells to undergo lytic replication and ultimately B-cell transformation.
- Variation in severity of disease is related to the degree of immunosuppression and the adequacy of the host immune response.
- Symptomatic EBV infection and PTLD are more common after primary EBV infection.
- Onset of EBV infection/PTLD most frequently occurs in the first year post transplantation.

- EBV infection/PTLD should be suspected in the child with protracted fever, diarrhoea, exudative tonsillitis, lymphadenopathy, organomegaly, leucopenia and atypical lymphocytosis.
- Up to one-third of late cases of PTLD are not related to EBV.

Risk factors for the development of PTLD
- Primary EBV infection.
- Seronegative recipient status.
- The use of potent immunosuppressive agents (particularly antilymphocyte globulin).
- Coexistent CMV disease.
- Young recipient age.

PTLD should be considered with the following symptoms and signs:
- Sore throat and tonsillar enlargement, particularly if associated with a tonsillar membrane.
- Lymphadenopathy, hepatosplenomegaly.
- Fever, weight loss, and night sweats.
- Malaise and lethargy.
- Chronic sinus congestion.
- Abdominal symptoms, e.g. pain, change in bowel habit, bowel obstruction.
- GI bleeding.
- Respiratory symptoms, dyspnoea, or stridor.
- Headache.
- Focal neurological symptoms.
- A fulminant illness, often accompanied by high LDH and uric acid blood levels, which may lead to urate nephropathy.
- Headache.

Although the most concerning EBV-related disease after transplantation is PTLD, children may experience non-PTLD-related EBV disease. Features include infectious mononucleosis manifestations (fever, malaise, pharyngitis, lymphadenopathy, etc.). Many of these features are similar to those seen in PTLD.

Histology
- EBV positive neoplastic PTLD is a B-cell lymphoproliferative process. Mono- or oligoclonal cell populations replace the underlying tissue structure. With benign hyperplasia (infectious mononucleosis) nodular architecture is preserved; with polymorphic PTLD there is polyclonal proliferation and local invasion with destruction of the nodal architecture; with monomorphic PTLD, neoplastic transformation of the tissue occurs. Although the first two are more likely to respond to reduction of immunosuppression, monomorphic PTLD may also, so treatment must be guided by specific histopathology (see Box 21.2 below).
- The presence of EBV in the cells can be demonstrated by *in-situ* hybridization for Epstein–Barr Early RNA (EBER) on fixed tissues and EBNA-CFT on fresh tissue. EBV latent membrane proteins (LMPs) may be found on immunostaining (but not always) and may be useful in diagnosing Hodgkin's type PTLD.

Box 21.2 Categories of PTLD

* Early lesion:
  * Plasmacytic hyperplasia.
  * Infectious mononucleosis-like lesion.
* Polymorphic PTLD.
* Monomorphic PTLD (classified according to lymphoma they resemble).
* B-cell neoplasms:
  * Diffuse large B-cell lymphoma.
  * Burkitt lymphoma.
  * Plasma cell myeloma.
  * Plasmacytoma-like lesion.
  * Other.
* T-cell neoplasms:
  * Peripheral T-cell lymphoma
  * Hepatosplenic T-cell lymphoma
  * Other.
* Classical Hodgkin lymphoma-type PTLD.

* PTLD can be confused with transplant rejection unless the cells are identified by B-cell markers such as CD19, CD20, CD21 or CD22 (although B cells can be present with rejection in the absence of PTLD).

Prevention of PTLD

* Recipient EBV antibody status must be established pre-transplant. Donor status must be obtained with living donors and can be requested for deceased donor kidneys. EBV seropositive children under 18 months of age should be considered as seronegative for purposes of risk stratification.
* Patients at risk of primary CMV infection should also be recognized as being at significantly increased risk of PTLD.
* There have been trials of a vaccine, but no licenced product is available.
* At risk patients should be monitored carefully for symptoms/signs suggestive of PTLD and where these are detected, appropriate investigations should be urgently pursued. Where biopsies are performed because of dysfunction, PTLD should always be considered in the differential diagnosis.
* Anti-viral therapy (aciclovir and ganciclovir) inhibits the lytic-replicative cycle of EBV, but has no effect on the latent or oncogenic virus. There is no good evidence to support or refute the use of these agents as a preventative strategy.

EBV surveillance: the use of viral load

Regular surveillance post-transplant for the development of EBV viraemia and an immune response to it can be useful in the prevention of PTLD. This is best restricted to high-risk seronegative recipients; monitoring of low risk seropositive children is not routinely recommended. Reduction of immuno-suppression should be considered in those without pre-existing immunity, rising EBV loads and symptoms.

Viral load (EBV DNA by PCR)

- Viral load should be measured every 1–2 weeks in the first 6 months and monthly thereafter to one year. However, in the post-transplant immunosuppressed state intermittent low grade viraemia with circulating EBV-DNA may be detected in whole blood at all times. The presence of EBV-DNA in plasma implies a higher viral load and is more suggestive of ongoing viral replication.
- There is considerable variation between laboratories in EBV viral load testing.
- The viral load that represents potential progression to PTLD is not known, but a rising titre at any level is likely to represent over immunosuppression, particularly if accompanied by CMV and/or BKV. Even viral loads as low as 200 copies/mL whole blood may be significant. In the normal individual with mononucleosis the EBV viral load is around 2,000 copies/mL. Current views are that an EBV load >20,000 copies/mL whole blood by real-time PCR on 2 occasions, even if stable, is cause for concern, and that if >100,000 reduction of immunosuppression is indicated. These figures must be viewed in the context of pre-transplant immune status, the clinical presentation and the level of immunosuppression.

Reduction of immunosuppression

- This is the best documented strategy to prevent PTLD development. There are insufficient data to determine the efficacy of anti-viral agents, rituximab or adoptive immunotherapy in this situation

Investigation of suspected PTLD

If symptoms persist or develop, full investigation is necessary and a histological diagnosis is essential in order to guide future management. Histopathology remains the gold standard for the diagnosis of PTLD:

- EBV DNA quantitative assay and EBV serology (VCA IgM, EBNA IgG).
- Immunoglobulins and T and B cell subsets.
- US looking for lymphadenopathy and US of the renal transplant as the transplanted organ is commonly involved in PTLD.
- Biopsy of the most accessible site likely to yield a diagnosis.

Investigations at diagnosis of PTLD

- Uric acid, LDH.
- Chest X-ray.
- Whole-body CT with contrast.
- MRI of the head if there are any neurological signs and symptoms.
- Bone marrow aspirate and trephine for morphology, immunophenotyping, and cytogenetics.
- Lumbar puncture if Burkitt lymphoma or T-cell lymphoma.

Treatment of established PTLD

Progressive reduction of immunosuppression is continued until there is

- an effective antiviral cytotoxic T-cell response
- marked reduction of the EBV genome copy number
- resolution of any masses
- acute rejection, in which case, if there are still significant masses, cytotoxic therapy is necessary
- EBV load should not be ignored because the child is otherwise well.

Slow and gradual reduction of immunosuppression is effective (~two-thirds will respond to this strategy) and safe if

* the patient is not acutely sick. Life-threatening illness (often accompanied by elevated LDH, increased age, fever, night sweats, and weight loss), organ dysfunction, extra-lymphoid and multiorgan involvement by PTLD are independent prognostic factors for lack of response to reduction in immunosuppression and poor survival. Faster reduction of immunosuppression, rituximab, cytotoxic T cells, and/or early chemotherapy are usually necessary
* the patient does not deteriorate clinically
* the tumour bulk does not increase during the process
* the histology is not Hodgkin or Burkitt lymphoma, when specific chemotherapy is necessary.

A suggested schema for reduction of immunosuppression for established PTLD

* Stop azathioprine, MMF, and sirolimus
* Leave steroids unchanged.
* Reduce the CNI depending on clinical symptoms as per Table 21.7.
* If the patient is not deteriorating clinically and the disease bulk is not increasing, slow reduction of immunosuppression can continue.
* Complete response is likely by 6 months, but may take longer.
* Immunosuppression should be restarted if rejection occurs, unless PTLD becomes life-threatening.
* If the PTLD is within the first 2 years, immunosuppression will need to be restarted after remission, but at a lower dose. If after 2 years, the patient may not need reintroduction of immunosuppression.
* If the patient has progression of disease, the immunosuppression can be withdrawn faster. If this is not effective, rituximab (anti-CD20 antibody) may be necessary, followed by cytotoxic T cells and/or chemotherapy if this fails.
* Complete or partial surgical resection as well as radiotherapy have been used as adjunctive therapy along with reduced immunosuppression.

Table 21.7 Reducing the calcineurin inhibitor

Weeks post-diagnosis	0	1	2	3	4	5	6	7	8	9	10	11	12
% Dose remaining													
Clinically stable	90		75		60		45		30		15		0
Progressive rise in tumour size	90	75	60	45	30	15	0						
Life-threatening disease	40	30	20	15	0								

A suggested schema for the response to persistence of EBV positivity or the development of symptoms in Fig. 21.3.

Clinical assessment of remission
The aim is complete remission:
- The clinical response must be assessed every week by checking for fever, lymphadenopathy, tonsillar enlargement, respiratory symptoms, organomegaly, and size of any masses, which can often be measured by US or chest X-ray.
- A follow-up CT with contrast should be done 4 weeks after the initial assessment.
- If clinical and radiological response occurs, continue monitoring fortnightly until complete remission is achieved. After this patients should be evaluated monthly for 1 year and 2-monthly for a further year.

Rituximab
The anti-CD20 monoclonal antibody, rituximab, is safe and relatively effective in studies so far, but there are no controlled trials. It is therefore currently the best second-line therapy (unless there is fulminant disease). Approximately two-thirds of those who fail to respond to reduction in immunosuppression will respond to this agent.
- The CD20 antigen is expressed on >90% of PTLD cells, but also on B lymphocytes. Rituximab will not work if CD20 is not present on the PTLD cells.

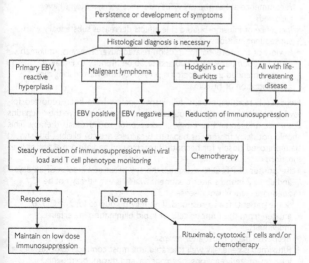

Fig. 21.3 Response to persistence of EBV positivity or development of symptoms.

- Rituximab causes lysis of the B cells expressing CD20 and thus aborts the lytic-replicative phase of EBV-driven lymphoproliferation. As serum immunoglobulin levels are maintained by persisting plasma cells, infection risk is low, although a cytokine release syndrome and/or tumour lysis syndrome can occur for bulky PTLD.
- Rituximab is given in a dose of 375 mg/m^2/dose/week IV × 4.

Guidelines for the administration of rituximab in PTLD

Note: differs from its use in SLE.

- Dosage: 375 mg/m^2 as an IV infusion, weekly for 4 weeks.
- For patients <10 kg a dose of 12.5 mg/kg is recommended.
- Premedicate with chlorphenamine and paracetamol 1 h prior to the infusion.

Comments

- Vials are available as 500 mg and 100 mg units.
- Dilute the required dose with NaCl 0.9% or glucose 5% to a final concentration of 1–4 mg/mL.
- Initial infusion rate is 25 mg/h then increase rate by increments of 25 mg/h every 30 min up to a maximum of 200 mg/h, according to tolerance. Consider halving the rate for patients <10 kg.
- Infusions have been associated with a cytokine release syndrome of fever and rigors which usually present within the first 2 h. Other reported symptoms include pruritus and rashes, dyspnoea, bronchospasm, angio-oedema, and transient hypotension.
- Consider stopping antihypertensives 12 h prior to administration due to risk of hypotension.
- In the event of an infusion-related adverse event, stop infusion and recommence at half the previous rate once the symptoms have resolved.
- Incidence of infusion-related side effects decreases substantially with subsequent infusions.
- In view of the potential for infusion-related adverse events, rituximab must be given between 09.00 and 17.00 on Monday to Friday. It is recommended that a doctor is present on the ward during the administration of rituximab.

Hepatitis B reactivation and fulminant hepatitis have been reported following rituximab therapy. All patients should therefore have their hepatitis B surface antigen and serology checked prior to rituximab therapy. This should not delay therapy as hepatitis B carriers are still eligible, but should be monitored closely for hepatitis B reactivation and abnormalities of liver function.

- Responses of PTLD to rituximab therapy occur at a median of 25 days and up to 2 months after treatment, which is why it may not be adequate in fulminant disease.
- Some patients fail to respond. This may be due to loss of CD20 antigen from the tumour cells or rapid elimination in certain individuals.
- Response may be lost after relapse.
- Rituximab is generally well tolerated, the most common toxicities being infusion-related reactions, neutropenia, and thrombocytopenia.

- Check clinical response, viral DNA load, and graft function weekly.
- IVIG replacement is not routinely recommended in patients who receive rituximab after solid organ transplant. However, immunoglobulin levels should be checked after completion of therapy. Consider immunoglobulin replacement in patients with a history of recurrent chest infections or significant hypogammaglobulinaemia.

Follow-up

- Restaging with clinical examination, EBV viral load, LDH, and repeat CT scans with contrast should be performed 2–3 weeks after the last dose of rituximab.
- If the patient goes into complete remission after rituximab then no further treatment need be given.
- The child should be followed up monthly for the first year after diagnosis and 2-monthly for a further year with radiological imaging as appropriate. EBV DNA viral loads should be performed monthly for the first year.
- Immunosuppression should be kept at the minimum that maintains satisfactory graft function.

Cytotoxic T cells

Passive immunization using *in vitro* expanded EBV-specific cytotoxic T lymphocytes has been used to successfully treat EBV-driven lymphoproliferation. However, this approach currently remains experimental, and takes some time to be prepared, which affects its usefulness.

Chemotherapy

The following patient groups need treatment with chemotherapy. The type of chemotherapy should be that which is appropriate for the underlying histology.

- Patients with aggressive disease or worsening despite reduction of immunosuppression may need chemotherapy together with the first two doses of rituximab, to gain more rapid disease control.
- Patients with bone marrow involvement and cytogenetic rearrangements.
- Patients who relapse after or fail to respond to rituximab.
- Patients with Hodgkin lymphoma or Burkitt lymphoma.
- Monomorphic PTLD occurring late after transplantation and patients with T-cell or CNS PTLD.

Prognostic indicators

The following have been shown to be associated with poorer outcomes in PTLD:

- Severe clinical symptoms.
- Multisite disease.
- CNS disease.
- T- or NK-cell PTLD.
- Spindle cell PTLD
- EBV-negative PTLD.
- Co-infection with hepatitis B or C.
- Monoclonal disease.
- Presence of mutation of proto-oncogenes or tumour suppressor genes.

Further reading

Green M, Michaels M. Infections in pediatric solid organ transplant recipients. *J Ped Infect Dis Soc* 2012;1:144–151.

The American Society of Transplantation Infectious Diseases Guidelines 3rd Edition. *Am J Transplant* 2013;13:1–371.

Vaudry W, Ettenger R, Jara P, et al. Valganciclovir dosing according to body surface area and renal function in pediatric solid organ transplant recipients. *Am J Transpl* 2009;9:636–643.

Malignancy in dialysis patients and following renal transplantation

- There is evidence that dialysis patients who have yet to undergo transplantation are at increased risk of malignancy:
  - Up to four times that of expected rates in general population for some malignancies.
  - Risk appears highest for renal cell carcinoma (four times that of the general population), bladder cancer (1.5 times that of the general population), and thyroid and other endocrine cancers.
  - Explanation for this is unclear, though postulated factors include CKD stage 5-associated immunodeficiency, suboptimal nutrition, and interaction between uraemia and dialysis-associated immune dysfunction and cancer risk factors including smoking;
  - Malignancies may not manifest until post-transplant period.
  - Patients with genetic mutations increasing the risk of renal and gonadal malignancies, e.g. those with *WT1* mutations should undergo bilateral nephrectomy or gonadectomy prior to transplantation.
- The long-term use of immunosuppressive therapy to prevent graft rejection increases the risk of malignancy in the transplanted patient. In general, more potent immunosuppressive therapy further increases risk.
- Overall, the increased risk of malignancy in adults is 2.1 times that in the general population. A number of malignancies, many of which are linked to viral infection, occur with a >fivefold increased risk. These included Kaposi sarcoma, skin cancer, non-Hodgkin lymphoma, liver, anal, vulval, cervical, and lip cancers.
- Other malignancies with an increased incidence include lung, kidney, colorectal, pancreatic cancers and Hodgkin lymphoma.
- There exist a number of guidelines (e.g. AST guidelines), which recommend enhanced screening/surveillance for malignancy in the transplant recipient, e.g. more frequent cervical cytology, skin surveillance, etc.
- While data on PTLD are well reported in children (see 'Infection post transplantation'), there are fewer data available regarding non-PTLD malignancies in children. However, these consistently show that paediatric kidney recipients are also at increased risk.
- A large NAPRTCS registry study observed a non-PTLD malignancy incidence rate of 72 per 100,000 patient years; a 6.7-fold risk compared with the general paediatric population:
  - The most commonly detected malignancies were renal cell carcinoma, thyroid carcinoma, melanoma, Wilms tumour, and hepatocellular carcinoma.
  - Median time to diagnosis was 23.9 months post transplantation.
  - On long-term follow-up, of the 35 children who developed malignancies, 40% were alive with a functioning graft. Nine died with a functioning graft.
  - Increased risk was seen regardless of age, sex, race, primary renal disease, and transplant era. The specific induction or maintenance immunosuppression type was not identified as a risk factor.

- A Swedish study of 536 paediatric solid organ transplant recipients reported a 12.5-fold increased risk of any malignancy, including PTLD compared with the general population:
  - Non-Hodgkin lymphoma was the commonest malignancy followed by renal cell carcinoma.
- A series of 884 paediatric kidney recipients from Minnesota with follow-up into adult life reported 235 malignancies in 136 (15.4%) recipients at a median age of 29 years.
- Despite the increased risk of renal malignancy, there are currently no recommendations for screening paediatric kidney recipients.

Reference

Smith JM, Martz K, McDonald RA, et al. Solid tumors following kidney transplantation in children. *Pediatr Transplant* 2013:17:726–730.

Graft survival in transplant recipients

Graft survival

- The outcomes of kidney transplantation continue to improve.
- Results for living donor recipients are superior to those receiving deceased donor grafts (see Tables 21.8–21.10).
- Longer-term follow-up data report graft survival of 23–95% at 10 years, 35% at 15 years, and 21–36% at 20 years.

Prognostic variables affecting graft survival

- NAPRTCS 2014 registry data report the following as being the most influential adverse prognostic variables of graft survival for recipients of living donor grafts (see Box 21.3):
  - Black race.
  - Previous transplantation.
  - No induction antibody therapy.
- Among recipients of deceased donor organs, factors associated with adverse graft survival include:
  - recipient age >24 months (compared with <24 months)
  - prior transplantation
  - more than five blood transfusions
  - black race
  - prior dialysis
  - cold storage time >24 h.

These 2014 data show a graft survival advantage in living and deceased donor recipients with no HLA-B mismatches and living donor recipients with no HLA-DR mismatches. The large majority of global registry data shows that the degree of HLA mismatching is associated with long-term graft survival, but not acute rejection. The best results are generally seen in HLA-identical living donor transplants and the worst in poorly matched kidneys from deceased donors.

- Adolescence is associated with an increase in graft loss secondary to non-adherence.
- Results are superior with pre-emptive transplantation, although any analysis is complicated because many such transplants will be from living related donors.
- Graft survival and CIT have a reciprocal relationship.

Further reading

NHS Blood and Transplant (NHSBT). Annual Report 2015. ⅍ https://www.gov.uk/government/publications/nhs-blood-and-transplant-annual-report-and-accounts-2015-to-2016

North American Pediatric Renal Trials and Collaborative Studies. NAPRTCS 2014 Annual Transplant Report. 2014. ⅍ https://web.emmes.com/study/ped/annlrept/annualrept2014.pdf

Rees L. Long-term outcome after renal transplantation in childhood. Pediatr Nephrol 2009;24:475–484.

Table 21.8 USA graft survival data by year of transplant (NAPRTCS report 2014)

	1 year (%)	3 year (%)	5 year (%)	7 year (%)
Living donor 1987–1995	91.2	84.6	78.9	72.4
Living donor 1996–2004	95.2	90.9	85.6	80.2
Living donor 2005–2013	96.9	93.4	83.8	82.4
Deceased donor 1987–1995	80.7	70.5	62.4	56.3
Deceased donor 1996–2004	93.5	84.1	78.1	67.3
Deceased donor 2005–2013	95.0	87.3	83.0	76.6

Box 21.3 Causes of graft failure (3045 graft losses following 12189 transplants, NAPRTCS 2014 report)

Chronic rejection: 35.6%
Other/unknown: 13.8%
Acute rejection: 13.0%
Vascular thrombosis: 9.6%
Death with functioning graft: 9.1%
Recurrent disease: 7.0%
Patient discontinued medication: 4.4%
Primary non-function: 2.1%
Bacterial/viral infection: 1.7%
Accelerated acute rejection: 1.4%
Malignancy: 1.2%
Other technical: 1.1%
Hyperacute rejection: 0.7%
Renal artery stenosis: 0.5%
Ciclosporin toxicity: 0.5%
De novo kidney disease: 0.3%

Table 21.9 UK graft survival data by year of transplant (NHSBT annual report 2015)

Year of transplant	No. at risk on day 0	% Graft survival (95% confidence interval)							
		1 year		2 year		5 year		10 year	
2002–2004	200	93	(88–95)	91	(86–94)	80	(74–85)	69	(62–75)
2005–2007	187	92	(88–95)	90	(85–94)	85	(79–90)		
2008–2010	184	97	(93–99)	92	(87–95)	82	(76–87)		
2011–2014	200	97	(93–99)						

Table 21.10 Graft survival after first paediatric living donor kidney transplant

Year of transplant	No. at risk on day 0	% Graft survival (95% confidence interval)			
		1 year	2 year	5 year	10 year
2002–2004	119	97 (92–99)	96 (91–99)	92 (84–96)	80 (70–86)
2005–2007	139	98 (93–99)	98 (93–99)	95 (89–98)	
2008–2010	182	96 (91–98)	94 (90–97)	87 (81–91)	
2011–2014	251	97 (94–98)			

Suggested renal transplant recipient discharge follow-up

See Table 21.11.

Table 21.11 Suggested renal transplant recipient discharge follow-up

Time	Until 2 weeks	2–4 weeks	4–8 weeks	8–12 weeks	3–5 months	5–12 months	Annual review
Visit[a]	Daily	×3/week	×2/week	Weekly	Fortnightly	Monthly	Yes
FBC	×3/week	×3/week	×2/week	Weekly	Fortnightly	Monthly	Yes
Biochemistry	Daily	×3/week	×2/week	Weekly	Fortnightly	Monthly	Yes
Tac/Ciclo levels	×3/week	×3/week	×2/week	Weekly	Fortnightly	Monthly	Yes
Additional tests[b]	Once	Once	Once	Once	Once	6, 9, 12 months	Yes
Urine ACR or PCR	A (below)	A (below)	A (below)	Once	Once	6, 9, 12 months	Yes
EBV/CMV PCR DNA	Twice	Twice	Twice	Twice			
HLA antibodies[c]	Once	Once	Once				Yes
Transplant renal US	Week 1					6 + 12 months	Yes
DTPA/MAG3	B	B	B	B	B	B	B
DMSA		3 weeks				C	C
GFR						6 + 12 months	Yes
24 h ABPM	D	D	D	D	D	D	Yes

(Continued)

Table 21.11 (Contd.)

a Minimum visits or more frequently if any clinical concerns.

b Additional tests = ferritin, iCa, PTH, urate, fasting glucose, and lipids:

A = once or if proteinuria on dipstick or daily if primary disease is FSGS or CNS.

B = perform DTPA/MAG3 to exclude obstruction (e.g. primary non-function/renal allograft dysfunction if increased creatinine ± transplant hydronephrosis).

C = at 3 weeks post transplantation if abnormal bladder, recurrent UTIs, blood vessel sacrificed at transplantation plus 3 months after transplant pyelonephritis/UTI.

D = when severe hypertension to improve BP control and help in investigation.

NB: there are some centres which will perform protocol biopsies, e.g. at 3 months and 12 months, though there is no good evidence that this practice improves clinical outcomes in children and further research is required.

c HLA antibodies also measured if develop acute rejection or renal biopsy performed for graft dysfunction.

Transplantation in special circumstances

Combined liver–kidney transplantation

There are a small number of situations where CLKT is performed in preference to kidney transplantation alone. This accounts for ~2% of all liver transplants in children. The commonest indications for CKLT in adults are polycystic kidney and liver disease, primary hyperoxaluria, and advanced liver failure with concomitant significant renal disease. In children however, the commonest indications are ESKD due to inherited metabolic diseases where the transplanted liver serves as the major source of the missing enzyme which has caused the renal failure

- Primary hyperoxaluria type 1. Here the transplanted liver becomes the source of the missing enzyme glyoxylate reductase/hydroxypyruvate reductase and the transplanted kidney restores normal renal function. CLKT is currently the generally accepted treatment of first choice in this disease (➔ see 'Primary hyperoxaluria' and ➔ 'Recurrent and *de novo* disease following renal transplantation').
- Methylmalonic acidaemia. Caused by the complete or partial deficiency of the mitochondrial enzyme methylmalonyl-CoA mutase or by defects in the synthesis of adenosylcobalamin. CKD is an early complication. There is significant controversy over the management of these patients, though many would now recommend CLKT; the amount of replacement enzyme produced by a transplanted liver and kidney is significantly greater than that produced by a kidney alone. Despite this, there is considerable experience with isolated kidney transplantation in some centres.
- Atypical haemolytic uraemic syndrome (aHUS). CLKT in conjunction with intensive plasma exchange was previously the treatment of first choice of those with CFH, CFI and CFB mutations. With the development of and growth in experience with the use of eculizumab, isolated kidney transplantation can now be performed (➔ see 'Atypical haemolytic uraemic syndrome' and 'Recurrent and *de novo* disease following renal transplantation').
- Autosomal recessive polycystic kidney disease. Associated with hepatic ductal plate malformation which can result in congenital hepatic fibrosis and Caroli disease. Liver function is generally well preserved in younger children, though where advanced liver disease is present in the setting of CKD stage 5 a number of successful CLKTs have been performed (➔ see 'Polycystic kidney disease').
- Alpha-1 antitrypsin deficiency. The commonest genetic cause of chronic liver disease in children. A membranoproliferative glomerulonephritis is well described in this population with a small number progressing to CKD stage 5. Timely liver transplantation may prevent progression of CKD, however where CKD stage 5 and chronic liver disease coexist, CLKT has been successfully performed.
- Other indications for CLKT include glycogen storage disease 1a and tyrosinaemia.

The results of CLKT are very dependent upon the precise indication; however, in general, they are comparable with those obtained from isolated liver transplantation. The amount of immunosuppression required is often less than with isolated kidney transplantation.

ABO-incompatible transplantation

* Kidney transplantation has traditionally been performed using basic principles of blood transfusion, with O being the universal donor and AB the universal recipient. ABO antigens are expressed on most epithelial and endothelial cells.
* However, the growing discrepancy between the number of organs available and the number of patients requiring transplantation has resulted in ABO-incompatible transplantation becoming increasingly prevalent in adults over the past decade.
* There is also a small but growing experience of ABO-incompatible transplantation in children.
* Pre-transplant conditioning in children remains challenging and should be restricted to centres with a large volume of patients and significant experience of the technique in adult patients.
* One protocol utilized in London, UK, recommends the pre-transplant treatment of all children with an antibody (anti-A or anti-B) titre of >1 in 8 using a range of desensitization strategies. Those with antibody titres of 1 in 8 to 1 in 16 receive rituximab, those with titre of 1 in 16 to 1 in 64 receive rituximab and double filtration plasmapheresis and those with titres >1 in 64 receive rituximab and immunoadsorption. Maintenance immunosuppression is with tacrolimus and MMF, which is commenced 1 week preoperatively.
* Short- and medium-term results appear to be good with rates of rejection and graft survival comparable to ABO-compatible patients. There is, however, a real paucity of long-term outcome data.

Transplantation of highly sensitized patients

* Children awaiting kidney transplantation may be sensitized (the presence of anti-HLA antibodies) because of previous transplants or blood and platelet transfusions. The presence of these antibodies and memory B and T cells create an immunological barrier, linked to an increased risk of antibody-mediated rejection and poorer graft survival.
* Where there are anti-HLA antibodies against a broad array of HLA antigens, this significantly reduces the likelihood of obtaining a deceased donor kidney, as the potential donor pool becomes smaller.
* There may be living donors available and willing to donate, though prevented from doing so using conventional immunosuppressive strategies because of the presence of anti-HLA antibodies directed against antigens present in the donor resulting in a positive cross-match.
* UNOS (United Network for Organ Sharing) data suggest that while the number of highly sensitized adult patients is significantly increasing, the number of highly sensitized children remains quite stable. In the UK, children with a calculated reaction frequency of >85% (meaning antibodies are present against 85% of the last 10,000 UK deceased donors) account for 8% of the waiting list and wait on average 3.5 years for a deceased donor organ.

- In this situation, desensitization is one possible approach to allow successful living donor transplantation to take place, however alternative strategies, including paired donor matching schemes should be considered. In the UK, the National Living Donor Kidney Sharing Scheme, organized by NHSBT matches donors and recipients from different families so that the donor from a family where transplantation is not possible because of a positive cross-match can donate to a recipient from a similarly affected family, with the other donor and recipient being paired in the same manner.
- Desensitization should only take place in high-volume centres donors with considerable experience in the technique.
- There is some experience in adult transplantation of desensitizing patients to increase the likelihood of donors organ becoming available and to increase the potential pool of donor available through a paired donor matching scheme.
- The general principle is to reduce the antibody titre to achieve an acceptable cross-match to avoid early antibody-mediated rejection.
- Recognized strategies to remove anti-HLA antibodies include the use of lymphocyte-depleting agents (e.g. ATG or alemtuzumab), IVIG, plasmapheresis, bortezomib as well as a number of newer more experimental agents including tocilizumab, belimumab, and eculizumab.
- There is little published data on desensitization strategies and outcomes in children.

Transplantation in the presence of proteinuria

- The risk of renal venous thrombosis is significantly increased by the presence of significant proteinuria around the time of transplantation.
- In patients with congenital nephrotic syndromes, nephrectomy and early dialysis is frequently performed prior to transplantation, though in some a conservative course is adopted with the expectation that proteinuria will fall as CKD progresses. This latter approach is also adopted in those patients with steroid-resistant nephrotic syndrome who have developed CKD stage 5.
- Where significant proteinuria (Upr:Ucr >100 mg/mmol is still present at the point at which transplantation is being planned, most would recommend nephrectomy being performed.
- As well as reducing the risk of venous thrombosis, elimination of native urine output allows the early definitive diagnosis of recurrent disease in patient with FSGS (➔ see 'Steroid-resistant nephrotic syndrome' and ➔ 'Recurrent and de novo disease following renal transplantation').

Drug prescribing

Basic principles

Varying degrees of AKI and CKD will result in reduced clearance of drugs and their metabolites which are excreted primarily by the kidney:

* Great care needs to be taken when prescribing in AKI and CKD.
* Details of necessary dose adjustments are available in the *British National Formulary for Children* and other texts.
* Where uncertainty exists, consultation with an expert paediatric renal pharmacist should take place.
* Dose modification is generally only necessary where drugs or their metabolites are >90% renally excreted.
* Drugs that are nephrotoxic and renally excreted, e.g. the aminoglycosides, are most likely to cause problems.
* Wherever possible, drug levels should be measured in AKI and CKD.
* The GFR may alter in both AKI and CKD. It is therefore important that drug doses are regularly reviewed.

Drug handling is altered in AKI and CKD

* Bioavailability may be altered by reduced GI motility, nausea, vomiting, and anorexia. Phosphate binders may form insoluble products with some drugs, e.g. sodium bicarbonate.
* Volume of distribution may be altered by the presence of volume overload (oedema and ascites), and reduced in volume depletion or muscle wasting.
* Protein binding is altered by acidosis, malnutrition, and inflammation. This can result in high levels of the free drug despite normal blood levels (e.g. phenytoin).
* Renal clearance of drugs and metabolites is reduced in the presence of AKI and GFR, the reduction in clearance being linked to the reduction in GFR. It may be the metabolites that produce the adverse reaction because of their accumulation, e.g. morphine glucuronides, which accumulate to prolong analgesia and respiratory depression.
* Patients with AKI and CKD are often taking multiple medications, thus increasing the risk of drug interactions.
* Many drugs will be cleared by haemodialysis. This depends on the molecular weight and the degree of protein binding of the drug:
  * Drugs with a large volume of distribution are generally lipid soluble and not confined to the circulation; they are not well cleared by haemodialysis.
* Peritoneal dialysis is less efficient at clearing drugs unless they have a low volume of distribution and low protein binding.

Important calculations

* Body surface area (m^2) = $\sqrt{}$(height in cm × weight in kg/3600).
* Estimated GFR (mL/min/1.73m^2) = height in cm × 36.5/plasma creatinine in μmoL/L.
* Normal GFR values are low in infancy and increase to adult values by 1–2 years of age.

Drug dosing in patients on haemodialysis

- Compared with adult patients, there is little published information on drug dosing in children on haemodialysis.
- Much of the existing adult data on drug clearance on haemodialysis is based on older dialysis technologies and clearance by modern filters will be significantly greater.
- It is logical to administer drugs known to be cleared by haemodialysis immediately at the end of the dialysis sessions.

Drug dose adjustment

- Where AKI or CKD necessitates a reduction in drug dosage, this can be achieved by either reducing the dose and keeping the dosing interval the same, or maintaining the same dose and increasing the dosing interval.
- Increasing the dosing interval is advantageous with drugs with long plasma half-lives and may help with compliance.
- However, increasing the dosing interval may result in wide variation in the plasma concentration and for drugs with a narrow therapeutic window, dose reduction may be a preferable strategy.
- Where dose reduction is performed, there is a smaller difference between Cmax (peak) and Cmin (trough) levels.
- Where there is an increase in the half-life of a drug because of reduced renal clearance, this results in an increased time until steady-state blood levels are reached

Further reading

Aronoff GR, Bennett WM, Berns JS. *Drug Prescribing in Renal Failure: Dosing Guidelines for Adults and Children*, 5th edn. Philadelphia, PA: American College of Physicians, 2007.
Daschner M. Drug dosage in children with reduced renal function. *Pediatr Nephrol* 2005;20:1675–1686.
Paediatric Formulary Committee. *British National Formulary for Children*. London: Pharmaceutical Press, 2017.

Intraperitoneal drug doses

A number of antibiotics can be administered intraperitoneally for the treatment of peritonitis. Here, drugs are dosed per litre of dialysis fluid, and will reach equilibrium with the blood so that the level in the dialysate will be the same as the blood. Some centres use an intraperitoneal loading dose. Where there is severe systemic illness or the child is immunocompromised, an IV loading dose is recommended.

Further reading

Aronoff GR, Bennett WM, Berns JS. *Drug Prescribing in Renal Failure: Dosing Guidelines for Adults and Children*, 5th edn. Philadelphia, PA: American College of Physicians, 2007.
Daschner M. Drug dosage in children with reduced renal function. *Pediatr Nephrol* 2005;20:1675–1686.
Paediatric Formulary Committee. *British National Formulary for Children*. London: Pharmaceutical Press, 2017.

Specific drug issues of importance

Opiate analgesics

- Certain active opiate metabolites (e.g. morphine-3-glucoronide and morphine-6-glucoronide) are renally excreted and can therefore accumulate in AKI and CKD, resulting in depressed conscious level and respiratory depression.
- IV infusions of morphine should be run at up to a maximum of 50% of the standard dose where the GFR is <10 mL/min/1.73 m^2 and at 75% of the standard dose when 10–50 mL/min/1.73 m^2. Great care needs to be taken with long-term oral dosing, where the dose should be similarly reduced.
- Pethidine has a potent active metabolite (norpethidine), which accumulates where the GFR is moderately to severely reduced, and may cause seizures.

Antibiotics and other anti-infective agents

- Gentamicin and other aminoglycosides (e.g. tobramycin and amikacin) need to be used with great care in AKI and CKD as they are significantly nephro- and ototoxic. The risk of nephrotoxicity is increased by the presence of volume depletion, pre-existing renal impairment, hypokalaemia, hypomagnesaemia, and the concomitant administration of other nephrotoxic drugs (e.g. calcineurin inhibitors, diuretics, etc.).
  - Gentamicin should be dosed at 60% of the daily dose divided into two doses where the GFR is <40 mL/min/1.73 m^2 and at 10% of the total daily dose given once daily where the GFR is <10 mL/min/1.73 m^2.
  - Levels should be accurately measured—target trough levels should be <2 mg/L (<1 mg/L for endocarditis) and peak levels 5–10 mg/L (3–5 mg/L in endocarditis, and 8–12 mg/L in cystic fibrosis).
  - Aminoglycosides are extensively cleared by haemodialysis and dosing should take place post dialysis.
- Vancomycin is used quite frequently in haemodialysis patients for the treatment of dialysis catheter infections. The drug is not extensively cleared by haemodialysis and dosing may only be required once every 5–7 days. Random levels should be checked and a repeat dose administered once the trough falls below 10 mg/L.
- The third-generation cephalosporins require dose reduction in severe AKI and CKD (50% dose reduction when GFR <10 mL/min/1.73 m^2).

Table 22.1 Drugs that do not require dose alteration at all levels of renal failure including patients receiving renal replacement therapy

Alfacalcidol	Levothyroxine
Amiodarone	Mesna
Amitriptyline	Metolazone
Amlodipine	Micafungin
Atorvastatin	Minocycline
Azithromycin	Mycophenolate mofetil (accumulation of metabolites possible)
Calcium channel blockers	
Caspofungin	Omeprazole
Chloramphenicol	Ondansetron
Clindamycin	Pantoprazole
Clonidine	Paracetamol
Clonazepam	Phenoxymethylpenicillin
Diltiazem (may exacerbate hypokalaemia)	Phenytoin
Dipyridamole	Pravastatin
Disodium pamidronate (though rate of infusion should be reduced)	Rifampicin
	Simvastatin
Domperidone	Sirolimus
Doxazosin	Sodium valproate
Furosemide (not haemodialysis)	Steroids
Fusidic acid	Tacrolimus
Imipramine	Terfenadine
Itraconazole	Verapamil
Labetalol	Voriconazole
Lansoprazole	Warfarin

Table 22.2 Drugs to be avoided in severe renal failure including patients receiving renal replacement therapy

Amphotericin (excluding liposomal preparation)
Cidofovir
Chlorothiazide/hydrochlorothiazide (not effective)
Disodium etidronate
Foscarnet
Gaviscon® and similar alginate preparations (high Na content)
Glibenclamide
Lithium
Nitrofurantoin
NSAIDs (see also Table 22.3)
Pethidine
Spironolactone
Sucralfate
Tenofovir
Tetracycline

Table 22.3 Drugs that if necessary should be started at lower doses, with monitoring of response and/or levels

ACE inhibitors	Ibuprofen
Beta blockers	Indometacin
Chlorphenamine	Mesalazine and sulfasalazine
Diazepam	Nitrazepam
Enoxaparin/dalteparin	Temazepam

- Amphotericin is significantly nephrotoxic. The liposomal preparation does not need dose adjustment and is associated with a lower risk of nephrotoxicity; this should be used in the presence of AKI or CKD if no alternative agent is suitable.
- Aciclovir, valaciclovir, valganciclovir, and ganciclovir: ➲ see 'Infection post transplantation' for information about dose reduction.

Information on drugs that do or do not require dose alteration, or need to be commenced at lower starting doses, at all levels of reduced GFR, including patients receiving renal replacement therapy, as well as those to be avoided are listed in Tables 22.1–22.5.

Table 22.4 Drugs where dose alteration is necessary

Anti-infective agents	Other drugs
Aciclovir	*Anticonvulsants (monitor levels):*
Amikacin	Carbamazepine
Amoxicillin	Clonazepam
Amoxicillin/clavulanic acid	Ethosuximide
Ampicillin	Gabapentin
Benzylpenicillin	Lamotrigine
Carbamazepine	Levetiracetam
Cefalexin	Midazolam
Cefotaxime	Phenobarbital
Cefradine	Topiramate
Ceftazidime	*Antihistamines:*
Ceftriaxone	Cetirizine
Cefuroxime	*Gout therapies:*
Chlorambucil	Allopurinol
Chloroquine	Colchicine
Ciprofloxacin	*Antineoplastic agents:*
Clarithromycin	Cisplatin
Co-trimoxazole	Cyclophosphamide
Doxycycline	Ifosfamide
Erythromycin	Methotrexate
Ethambutol	*Antiviral agents:*
Flucloxacillin	Didanosine
Fluconazole	Lamivudine
Flucytosine	Stavudine
Ganciclovir	Zidovudine
Gentamicin	*GI drugs:*
Imipenem/cilastatin	Cimetidine
Isoniazid	Metoclopramide
Mefloquine (use with caution)	Ranitidine
Meropenem	*Opiates:*
Metronidazole	Codeine phosphate
Pentamidine	Diamorphine
Piperacillin/tazobactam	Digoxin
Pyrazinamide	*Bisphosphonates:*
Rifampicin	Disodium pamidronate
Teicoplanin	Sodium clodronate
Tobramycin	
Valaciclovir	
Valganciclovir	
Vancomycin	

Table 22.5 Drug loading doses

Drug	Intraperitoneal loading dose (mg/L)	Intraperitoneal maintenance dose (mg/L)
Amikacin	25	12
Cefotaxime	500	250
Ceftazidime	250	125
Cefuroxime	500	15
Ciprofloxacin	50	25
Clindamycin	300	150
Gentamicin	8	4
Teicoplanin	400	125
Tobramycin	8	4
Vancomycin		12.5–25

Further reading

Aronoff GR, Bennett WM, Berns JS. *Drug Prescribing in Renal Failure: Dosing Guidelines for Adults and Children*, 5th edn. Philadelphia, PA: American College of Physicians, 2007.

Daschner M. Drug dosage in children with reduced renal function. *Pediatr Nephrol* 2005;20:1675–1686.

Paediatric Formulary Committee. *British National Formulary for Children*. London: Pharmaceutical Press, 2017.

Psychosocial issues

Ethical issues

Ethics provides a means of evaluating and choosing between different, often competing options and is about analysing values, rather than facts. Contemporary bioethics utilizes four principal axioms upon which arguments may be developed:

- Respect for autonomy.
- Beneficence.
- Non-maleficence.
- Justice.

The aim is to determine whether, for any particular decision, harm is outweighed by benefit and that any decision is made in the best interests of the child. Advances in the field of RRT allow the provision of life-sustaining therapy for virtually any child, including the newborn and children with other severe co-morbidities, who previously would have succumbed to their renal disease. This raises a number of key ethical issues, the following of which are frequently recurring themes in all paediatric nephrology units:

- The commencement of RRT in infants, children, and adolescents with significant co-morbidities.
- The commencement of RRT in the newborn.
- The withdrawal of RRT in infants, children, and adolescents.
- The management of non-adherence with prescribed therapy and the impact of non-adherence on subsequent decisions regarding listing for renal transplantation.
- Identification of non-paternity following tissue typing.
- Families who wish to travel abroad to purchase a kidney.
- Live related transplantation when there is a significant risk of disease recurrence in the graft.
- The use of siblings who offer themselves as donors, but may be considered too young.
- Parental discord over management, e.g. live donor transplant from a 'separated' partner.

These scenarios all create ethical dilemmas because:

- clinical facts alone do not determine what course of action should follow
- there may be disagreements between parties (team members, parents, parents and children, parents and professionals) as to what is the right course of action
- applying ethical principles may produce conflicting outcomes
- the law is ambiguous or silent in directing what must be done.

In trying to resolve dilemmas, it is important to analyse the moral basis of the dispute and determine how the application of ethical theories (e.g. utility, duty) or principles (e.g. beneficence, non-maleficence, respect for autonomy, justice) may help.

The moral basis of medicine requires that professionals offer treatments that are in the best interests of their patients. In practice, this means that professionals should offer treatment that is intended to produce more benefit than harm, and respect as much capacity for self-determined choice (autonomy) as their patients are capable of. The latter is more problematic in children because they may lack the capacity to make an informed choice about their treatment. Their parents have the ethical and legal right to make such choices on their behalf provided they act in their child's best interests. Disputes about best interests and who should decide them are at the heart of many of the themes identified in the provision of RRT. What follows is a practical approach to decision-making in RRT cases. It is important to recognize and separate facts from values:

- Establish and agree which consultant is leading the care for the family.
- Check that the family have read and understood available information about their child's disease and the treatment and complications, or had access to explanations (on more than one occasion) including long-term outcome data.
- The lead consultant should discuss the child with other members of the nephrology subspecialty team, including clinical nurse specialists, dieticians, play therapists, psychologists, teachers, and social workers to obtain relevant information, and ascertain their views.
- Other consultants managing co-morbidities need to be part of discussions.
- If discussions involve transplantation, discuss with the transplant surgeon and anaesthetist.
- The lead consultant or appropriate member of the renal team should inform and discuss with the local team (paediatrician) and GP; this will provide more information about family background, co-morbidities, etc.
- It may be necessary to convene a multidisciplinary team meeting, to be chaired by the lead consultant to share information and to clarify issues.
- It is important to ensure good note-keeping.
- Consideration should be given as to whether a second independent opinion would be useful:
  - Offer to facilitate, but allow the family to also select independently should they wish.
  - It is important to be clear as to the purpose of the second opinion, i.e. whether to clarify clinical facts or to provide an opinion of what should be done (the latter involves value judgements, rather than pure clinical facts).
- Once appropriate background clinical, psychological, and social facts have been obtained and controversy about further proceedings remain, either within the team or between the team and the family, a formal, full clinical ethical committee review should be considered to facilitate the decision-making process.
- The time frame over which the decision needs to be made (and by whom) should be defined. Where possible, take time to come to a decision. In an emergency and in the presence of a critical ethical problem, consider a second opinion from a consultant.
- Consider whether legal services should be involved.
- The family should be provided with advance notice of important meetings. There should be due consideration of timing and place (e.g. out of clinic/ward, 'neutral' area), so as to maximize freely informed decision-making. Attendance is best limited to preserve the privacy/intimacy of the occasion.

- Consideration should be given as to how the views of the child (in accordance with their age, experience, and capacity) are obtained and what weight is placed upon those views.
- Ensure all relevant professionals (inside and outside the hospital) are aware of decisions, and that the latter are recorded properly:
  - Staff may need support (often led by the psychosocial team).
  - Consider meeting to reflect or debrief (usually after an appropriate interval).
  - The decision-making process should be transparent inclusive, accountable, responsive, and reasonable.

Further reading

Dionne JM, d'Agincourt-Canning L. Sustaining life or prolonging dying? Appropriate choice of conservative care for children in end-stage renal disease: an ethical framework. *Pediatr Nephrol* 2015;30:1761–1769.

Non-adherence in paediatric renal disease

Non-adherence

- Defined by the WHO as 'the degree to which the person's behaviour corresponds with the agreed recommendations from a health care provider'.
- Is a common problem with particularly severe consequences after renal transplantation:
  - Systematic review in adult subjects has shown that 22% of organ recipients are non-adherent with treatment and that a median of 36% of graft losses are associated with prior non-adherence.
  - The odds of graft failure increase sevenfold where non-adherence occurs.
  - A review of paediatric studies investigating non-adherence following solid organ transplantation revealed a prevalence of medication non-adherence of 32% for kidney recipients (31% for liver recipients and 16% for heart recipients).

Consequences of non-adherence

Post transplant

- Aetiological factor in graft loss in 14% of paediatric kidney recipients.
- Increased risk of late acute rejection resulting in additional hospital admissions, clinic visits, time absent from school/parental employment, and a significant risk of loss of renal function.

In chronic kidney disease

- Phosphate binders are commonly omitted, resulting in an increased risk of hyperphosphataemia and therefore chronic kidney disease–mineral bone disorder (CKD-MBD).

Risk factors for non-adherence

- Adolescence is a major risk factor for non-adherence and rates are much higher in this population than in adults. This is reflected in:
  - the poorest long-term graft survival compared with all other age groups.
  - higher rates of late acute rejection in this age group.
- Demographic and socioeconomic factors:
  - Low socioeconomic status.
  - Ethnicity (increased non-adherence reported in African Americans).
  - Single-parent families.
  - Family instability.
  - Poor communication within family.
  - Insufficient family social or emotional support.
- Patient-related factors:
  - Poor knowledge of medications/disease.
  - Low self-esteem.
  - Forgetfulness.
  - Learning difficulties.
  - History of non-adherence.
  - Prior history of child abuse.

- Condition-related factors:
  - Longer time post transplantation.
  - Longer on dialysis.
- Treatment-related factors:
  - Cosmetic adverse effects of drugs.
  - Number of drugs and number of doses per day.
  - Taste/palatability.
  - Cost of drugs.
- Healthcare setting and healthcare provider-related factors:
  - Poor communication between multiprofessional team and patient.
  - Authoritarian consultation style.
  - Lack of understanding of non-adherence.
  - Family lack of trust in healthcare providers.

Methods of documenting non-adherence

- Self-reporting.
- Observation by parents or other family members.
- Physical or biochemical markers:
  - Absence of adverse cosmetic or other effects (e.g. non-Cushingoid when on high doses of corticosteroids).
  - Unrecordable or low blood drug levels.
  - Persistent biochemical abnormalities, particularly phosphate.
- Adverse events related to non-adherence, e.g. acute rejection, graft loss.
- Electronic monitoring: microchip inserted into medicine container/ bottle top records each time the container/bottle is opened. This can be downloaded onto a PC by the doctor or the patient.
- Monitoring of pill usage or dispensing records.

Strategies to improve adherence

- *Simplification/modification of drug regimen*:
  - Reducing number of drugs and doses.
  - Use of once-daily medications.
  - Use of drugs with longer half-lives requiring less strict adherence with timing.
  - More palatable drugs.
  - Drugs with fewer cosmetic adverse effects.
- *Patient education*:
  - Understanding of medication purpose.
  - Understanding of medication dose.
  - Understanding of importance of adherence, medication adverse effects, etc.
- *Behavioural strategies*:
  - Use of medication intake records with reward system.
  - Use of cues (meals, teeth cleaning, etc.).
  - Monitored dosage boxes into which all drugs are inserted for the coming week.
  - Alarms (watch, mobile phone prompts, etc.).
- *Strategies to improve social support*:
  - Involvement of family.
  - Peer support groups.

- *Other:*
  - Practical help with cosmetic issues (make-up and hair removal strategies).
  - Regular discussion about/monitoring of non-adherence.
  - Early intervention by psychologist/psychiatrist where problems detected with patient and/or family.

Further reading

Steinberg EA, Moss M, Buchanan CL, et al. Adherence in pediatric kidney transplant recipients: solutions for the system. *Pediatr Nephrol* 2018;33:361–372.

Long-term growth

- ~50% of children requiring RRT before their 13th birthday have a final height below the normal range.
- Height is below the normal range in some children with CKD too: growth rate and GFR decline in parallel.
- The Ht SDS declines in parallel with age at the start of RRT: those born with CKD have the worst height prognosis.
- Growth in children on dialysis is particularly difficult to maintain. In the North American Pediatric Renal Trials and Collaborative Studies (NAPRTCS) registry, Ht SDS on dialysis decreased from −1.64 to −1.71 after 1 year and −1.84 after 2 years.
- The mean Ht SDS on commencing PD is −2.35 SD, and is below normal worldwide, but there is a large variation, ranging in 21 countries from −1.3 to −3.5. Regional variations in resources are likely to contribute to these differences.
- Height prognosis has improved during the last decades due to better management of the complications of CKD, better dialysis machines and programmes, reduction of steroid use post transplant, and the use of rhGH. In the NAPRTCS registry, Ht SDS at the time of transplant has improved from −2.4 in 1987 to −1.4 in 2007.
- The improvement in growth seems to be the greatest during the peripubertal years.
- Factors associated with a better height prognosis are older age at start of RRT, a more recent era for the start of RRT, cumulative percentage time with a transplant (particularly if immunosuppression is steroid free), use of rhGH, and greater Ht SDS at initiation of RRT. Post transplant, the youngest children and those with the greatest pre-transplant height deficit show the best growth.
- Factors associated with a worse height prognosis are young age and earlier start of RRT, metabolic disorders (e.g. hyperoxaluria), cystinosis, co-morbidities, and longer duration of dialysis.
- Improved growth parallels an improvement in patient survival.

Reference

Rees L. Growth hormone therapy in children with CKD after more than two decades of practice. *Pediatr Nephrol* 2016;31:1421–1435.

Long-term survival of children on renal replacement therapy

Survival on dialysis

- After 5 years is:
  - ~60% for 0–1 year of age.
  - ~80% for 2–5 years of age.
  - ~85% for >6 years of age.
- Co-morbidity increases the mortality risk sevenfold, and is commonest in the youngest children.
- There is no difference in outcome in infants who do not have other co-morbidities in comparison to older children.
- Mortality increases with increasing duration of dialysis.
- The presence of residual renal function improves outcome.
- There is no difference between PD and HD with respect to survival.
- There has been no significant improvement since the 1990s.
- Causes of death on dialysis:
  - Co-morbidity.
  - Treatment withdrawal (± co-morbidity).
  - Failure to obtain or maintain dialysis access.
  - Infection, cardiopulmonary or cerebrovascular events.
  - CVD in up to 38%—arrhythmias, valve disease, cardiomyopathy, and arteriosclerosis.
  - CVD is more common after 10 years of RRT, with a risk for a young adult in their 20s 800-fold greater than for the normal population.

Survival post transplant

- 1-year patient survival is 96–100% and 5-year survival is 90–99%.
- Longer-term follow-up data report patient survival of 75–95% at 10 years, 83–94% at 15 years, 54–86% at 20 years, and there is one report of 81% 25-year patient survival.
- Survival is improving, particularly in the very young.
- Age does not affect mortality in most recent studies.
- There is a small benefit from pre-emptive transplantation.
- There is a small benefit from living donation, particularly in the very young.
- The risk of death from CVD is increased by 1.6 in African Americans.
- Principal causes of death following transplant are:
  - infection.
  - malignancy.
  - CVD.

The average additional years of life expectancy at age 20–25 years are:
- 55–60 years in the normal population.
- 35–40 years with a renal transplant.
- 10–15 years on dialysis.

Compared with normal children, the lifespan of a child on dialysis is reduced by 40–60 years and a child with a transplant reduced by 20–25 years.

Reference

The North American Pediatric Renal Trials and Collaborative Studies (NAPRTCS). NAPRTCS 2014 Annual Report. ♪ https://web.emmes.com/study/ped/annlrept/annlrept.html

Palliative care

Background

The decision to focus on palliative care and not treatment aimed to cure or prolong life often evolves gradually. Different members of staff and members of the family may be working towards the decision at different rates and time, and discussion is essential for the transition. This time can also be helpful in providing an opportunity for planning.

Palliative care for the sick child and their family needs to be comprehensive and consider medical and nursing needs, psychosocial and spiritual care, and the practical needs of the family wherever care will be taking place. If available, the local palliative care team should be consulted early on and, if the family agrees, involved in discussions with the family. As they have experience with symptom care, staff to follow the patient outside the hospital, and a network of contacts in the local community (hospices, community nurses, etc.), their help is invaluable.

Symptom management

The following points are important:
- Assessment of the child's symptoms and their likely cause.
- Development of a management plan for each symptom, including both pharmacological and non-pharmacological approaches.
- How these symptoms are likely to progress and what the plans are for management when this occurs.
- What new symptoms may arise—consider probable ones, possible ones, and even those which are unlikely.
- Develop a clear management plan for each of these.
- Consider prescription and availability of drugs, and appropriate routes of administration now, and later in the illness.
- Consider any equipment that will be needed such as syringe pumps, catheters, special mattresses, oxygen, etc.

Liaison and planning care

- If the family is keen to care for their child at home, the earlier links can be developed with the community and the closer these are, the easier the discharge will be.
- Since community services vary, arrangements need to be made individually for each family, according to their circumstances.
- Family doctors, community nursing teams, local shared-care hospitals, and hospices are likely to be involved.
- The role of each care group needs to be decided before the child's discharge. In particular, who will be available at nights and over weekends, and how the family has access to them needs to be planned. A key worker, usually one of the nursing staff either from the hospital or community, should take on the role of coordination of care.
- Often a system develops whereby local carers, such as the GP and community nurses, take on routine 24 h care, but they need back-up and access to experience and advice in paediatrics and paediatric palliative care, also on a 24 h basis.

- Information about symptom management and the network of carers should be clearly communicated both to the family and all those involved in their management.

Support for the child and family

- This needs to be ongoing as the illness progresses.
- If the family are taking on the responsibility of care in the home setting, they need as much information and confidence as possible in managing the child's symptoms and the likely progress of the disease. As the illness progresses, they will also need information about how the child may die and what to do after the child has died in relation to a death certificate, registration, funeral, etc.
- They may need information and support in talking about illness and the child's death with siblings, grandparents, and with the sick child themselves.
- Families need the opportunity to talk about their own feelings and the wide range of emotions they are likely to be experiencing at this time.
- The sick child needs the opportunity to talk about their understanding of what is happening to them, their fears, and their feelings.
- All the family may need to think about their immediate aims and also plan short-term goals both in relation to care and also socially.

Palliative care checklist

The following should be involved in discussions regarding discharge and subsequent care:

Within the hospital

- Consultant in charge.
- Counsellor.
- Ward sister.
- Ward registrar.
- Consultant in palliative care.
- Psychologist.
- Social worker.
- Religious representative.
- Pharmacist.
- Dietician.

Outside the hospital

- Paediatric community nurse.
- Local paediatrician.
- GP.
- Health visitor.

Discharge plans

These must begin as soon as possible, preferably before the final decision to discharge has been made. The child may be discharged either to his/her home, to the local hospital, or to a children's hospice.

Potential problems

Checklist to be reviewed at least weekly:
- Mobility.

- Weakness.
- Anorexia, nausea and vomiting, and weight loss.
- Sore mouth.
- Diarrhoea or constipation.
- Cough or dyspnoea.
- Headache.
- Fits.
- Abnormalities of micturition.
- Bone pain.
- Abdominal pain.
- Skin (itching, sweating).
- Oedema.
- Anaemia.
- Bleeding.
- Infection, fever.
- Behaviour/sleep disturbance/anxiety/depression.

Symptom management

- A number of drugs used in symptomatic care are excreted renally and therefore the drug levels may be affected. As the illness progresses, the use of individual drugs needs to be considered in relation to the goals of the treatment and the priority of the child's comfort and dignity.
- It is essential to aim for high-quality symptom management throughout the child's illness. The suffering they experience from treatment and its side effects will be what the child remembers.
- For those children who unfortunately cannot be cured, palliative care, including rigorous attention to symptom management, will help to provide as good a quality of life as possible for the time that remains.
- Although pain may not be a prominent problem for children dying from renal disease, it will be a fear for parents and its management should be anticipated and planned for. Pain is a complex sensation related not only to physiological insult to the tissues, but also influenced by psychological, social, and cultural factors.
- Pain assessment tools, according to the child's age and ability, are available. Body charts are helpful for all ages to locate and identify sites of pain, while colour, faces, numeric, and visual analogue scales can be used to measure severity. Parents usually interpret their child's feelings reliably, but may sometimes under- or overestimate the pain because of their own attitudes.
- Physical and psychological management includes education, explanation, distraction, relaxation and hypnosis, physical care (including attention to warmth and cold), massage, and physiotherapy.

Drug management

- Pharmacological management of pain includes non-opioids, mild opioids, strong opioids, NSAIDs, amitriptyline, and anticonvulsants.
- In most situations, analgesics of gradually increasing strength can be used, according to the WHO's concept of an analgesic ladder (Fig. 23.1).

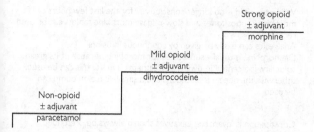

Fig. 23.1 The WHO analgesic ladder.

- Paracetamol is helpful in mild to moderate pain and has few side effects. When pain is no longer relieved by regular paracetamol, a mild opioid can be introduced. Side effects are similar to the strong opioids (➔ see 'Opioid side effects', p. 678). The analgesic effect of codeine has a ceiling and when pain is no longer relieved, a strong opioid is needed.
- Morphine sulfate is the strong opioid of choice and 4-hourly or 12-hourly (slow-release) preparations are available. When using slow-release preparations, always also provide a short-acting preparation, to use for breakthrough pain.

Doses and frequency

- The initial dose should be calculated according to the child's weight and then increased, in increments, to provide adequate analgesia. In most situations pain is constant and analgesics should be given regularly, not as required.
- Strong opioids are metabolized in the liver and eliminated via the kidneys:
  - Accumulation may occur with renal disease, and lower doses given less frequently may be appropriate; this must be determined for each patient individually depending on their need for pain relief, the progress of the disease, and where palliative care is occurring (i.e. home, hospital).
  - Good analgesia should remain the primary aim, but may be achieved more gradually by starting with half the recommended dose/kg and giving subsequent doses only when pain recurs, observing carefully, and working out a personal dose and dosing schedule for each individual.

Routes of administration

- The route of choice is oral, with increasing doses as necessary.
- If the oral route is not possible, e.g. because of nausea and vomiting, difficulty swallowing, or gradual loss of consciousness, another route is needed.
- During palliative care, some children tolerate rectal medication well, and prefer it to the thought of any needles.

- When the child is no longer conscious or for the last few hours of life, morphine suppositories and slow-release morphine tablets can be used rectally.
- Analgesics can easily be given by continuous infusion.
- Diamorphine is usually substituted for morphine because of its greater solubility. If a central in-dwelling IV catheter is *in situ* this can be used, otherwise the needle is placed SC and a simple infusion pump can be used.

Opioid side effects

- Constipation is invariable. Laxatives should always be prescribed prophylactically.
- Drowsiness is also common at first, but this almost always wears off within 2–3 days. It is useful to warn parents about this or they may worry that the disease has suddenly progressed.
- Nausea and vomiting may be managed with intermittent or prophylactic antiemetics.
- Some children experience itching; this usually also wears off, but if not, antihistamines are helpful.
- Respiratory depression does not appear to cause problems in children being treated with opioid drugs for pain, as there is a wide margin between the dose causing respiratory failure and that required for analgesia.
- Sometimes parents are reluctant to consider the use of morphine for their child's pain. In order to overcome this, reasons for their concern need to be explored:
  - Often it is not the use of morphine itself, but that it represents an acknowledgement that the child is actually dying.
  - Parents may also be confused about addiction and need reassurance that psychological addiction does not seem to occur in children requiring opioids for severe pain.
  - Although tolerance will develop, should the pain be relieved then the morphine dose can easily be tapered and then stopped.

Bone pain

- Bone pain may be related to renal osteodystrophy. Adjustment of phosphate binders and activated vitamin D may help. These drugs may also be important in the prevention of hypocalcaemia and its symptoms.
- Although NSAIDs can be helpful for bone pain, careful consideration is necessary in children with renal failure because of potential problems from GI bleeding and further renal impairment.

Nausea and vomiting

- There are many causes of nausea and vomiting. Identifying the cause can help in making a logical choice of antiemetics. If initial choices are unsuccessful then combining a number of drugs, which work through different mechanisms, may improve the situation.

Constipation

Constipation may be due to inactivity, poor nutrition, poor fluid intake, hypercalcaemia, and hypokalaemia, as well as a side effect of opioid therapy. A suggested treatment schedule is shown in Fig. 23.2.

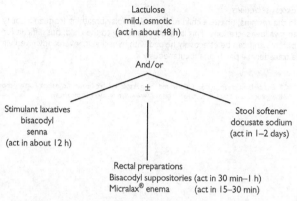

Fig. 23.2 Treatment of constipation.

Convulsions

Convulsions are a risk for a child dying from renal disease, and parents should be warned and prepared. Occasional, short fits may not require medication, although rectal or buccal diazepam should be available, either in hospital or at home, in case they are more prolonged. Regular oral anticonvulsants may be appropriate for some children having frequent convulsions over a prolonged period. SC midazolam (which is compatible with diamorphine and can be mixed in the same syringe) is helpful for children being cared for at home and requiring regular parenteral medication for convulsions.

Anxiety and agitation

Anxiety as the disease progresses may reflect a patient's need to talk about their fears and can be helped by discussion and reassurance. Low-dose oral diazepam may also be helpful. Restlessness and agitation are common in the final stages of life and can be treated with haloperidol, levomepromazine, or midazolam, all of which are compatible with diamorphine in SC infusions.

Itching

Itching may be a problem from increasing uraemia and as a side effect of opioids. Oral antihistamines may help relieve opioid-related itching. Topical preparations, such as calamine, can also be used. In some uraemic patients, itching is the major problem and the following practical advice can be useful in this specific context:
- Avoid excessively warm baths.
- When drying the skin, dab with a towel, rather than rub.
- Dietary measures that help to control uraemia may help with itching.

Hiccups

These may be helped by chlorpromazine.

Excess secretions

In the terminal phase, a child may develop noisy breathing from an inability to swallow secretions. This is rarely distressing to the child, but difficult for parents and can be effectively helped with hyoscine, conveniently given via a transdermal patch or subcutaneously.

Further reading

NICE. *End of Life Care for Infants, Children and Young People with Life-Limiting Conditions: Planning and Management.* London: NICE, 2016. ℘ https://www.nice.org.uk/guidance/ng61

Supplementary information

Furosemide test of urinary acidification

Indication

Assessment of urinary acidification (e.g. in a child with suspected RTA). The furosemide test can be used as an alternative to ammonia loading, which is often poorly tolerated in children as it is highly emetic. Usually, a child with RTA will present with metabolic acidosis and the urine can be analysed directly. In that case, there is no need for a further test of urinary acidification. The test can be considered if a 'subclinical RTA' is suspected, i.e. a mild RTA that is apparent only when the system is stressed.

A major problem in assessing urinary acidification in children is the method of obtaining the sample: if exposed to air, CO_2 will diffuse out of the sample, resulting in an artificial increase in pH (➡ see 'Disorders of acid–base balance: acidosis', p. 155). Thus, urine obtained by bag or from cotton balls in the nappy is useless for acid–base assessment. Ideally, the urine is collected under oil to avoid any diffusion of CO_2 and assessed immediately (i.e. not sent in an air-filled container to the laboratory).

Contraindications

If the child has marked electrolyte imbalance, in particular, hypokalaemia (K <3.5 mmol/L), furosemide may potentiate the abnormality. Obstruction of the urinary tract may be accentuated by furosemide.

Basis

Furosemide causes volume depletion, which in turn up-regulates distal Na reabsorption, which is in exchange for K and H ions, thus increasing urinary H concentration and lowering urinary pH (➡ see 'Disorders presenting with hypokalaemic alkalosis', p. 173). Furosemide inhibits the Na/K/Cl pump in the thick ascending limb of the loop of Henle, thereby increasing Na delivery to the distal tubule.

Protocol

- Ensure the child is not on bicarbonate (or citrate) supplements.
- Fast from midnight (not essential, e.g. in infants).
- *Baseline biochemistry*: urine Na, K, pH (by glass electrode), creatinine, plasma Na, K, TCO_2, urea, and creatinine.
- Give an oral (or IV) dose of furosemide, 1 mg/kg.
- Collect urine every 30 min for 3 h (or each specimen) and measure the urine pH straight away.
- After 3 h, recheck plasma Na, K, TCO_2, urea, and creatinine.
- Prior to discharge, ensure the child is not clinically dehydrated.

Results

Normal children and adults will lower urine pH to <5.5, usually by 2 h, always by 3 h. Any urine pH <5.5 indicates normal urine acidification and the test can be stopped. Failure to achieve a urine pH <5.5 suggests a distal tubular acidification defect.

Further reading

Rodriguez Soriano J, Vallo A. Renal tubular hyperkalaemia in childhood. *Pediatr Nephrol* 1988;2:498–509.

DDAVP® test

Aim

To assess the capacity of the kidneys to maximally concentrate urine.

Background

Final concentration of urine is achieved by the action of ADH (also known as vasopressin) acting on the collecting duct cells within the kidney tubule. Vasopressin, secreted by the posterior pituitary gland, binds to a receptor (V2R) and through a number of steps causes aquaporin 2 (AQ2) water channels to be localized on the luminal surface of the tubular cells. This allows water to pass from the urinary lumen into the cells, thereby concentrating urine.

Inability to concentrate urine may be congenital (usually due to mutations in the genes encoding V2R or AQ2). In these situations, babies have adequate vasopressin, but no renal response (congenital nephrogenic diabetes insipidus, usually X-linked).

Acquired defects may affect the secretion of vasopressin, in which case there is insufficient hormone to act on the kidney (central diabetes insipidus), or be due to a variety of kidney diseases or drugs damaging or affecting the V2R pathway (secondary nephrogenic diabetes insipidus).

Assessment of urinary concentration includes:

* history.
* examination.
* routine investigations (include early morning urine osmolality).
* *water deprivation test:* ➔ see 'Water deprivation test and DDAVP® test', p. 182, not safe in babies in whom congenital nephrogenic diabetes insipidus considered.
* 1-desamino-8-D-arginine vasopressin (DDAVP®) test.

Basis of DDAVP® test

A pharmacological dose of synthetic vasopressin (desmopressin) will maximally stimulate the V2R, thereby driving the kidney to maximally reabsorb water.

Potential hazards

The major risk of this test is water overload, which can occur if a child is given fluid in excess of the volume of fluid passed in urine. This occurs when desmopressin 'works', i.e. a positive test (➔ see 'Interpretation of test', p. 684). The risk can be avoided, by strict control of fluid input by carers and health professionals.

Procedure

* Ensure child has been assessed (as described, and check this test is appropriate).
* Inform biochemistry laboratory of the test.
* Take baseline plasma biochemistry (Na, K, TCO$_2$, urea, creatinine, osmolality) and collect baseline urine (this can be done up to 4 h before test).
* Withhold feeds and other fluids for 2 h before test commences.

- Thereafter, the child should only receive a fluid input (milk/juice/water) equivalent to the volume of urine passed for the next 4 h (if test negative, i.e. no significant urinary concentration) or 6 h (if test positive, i.e. significant urinary concentration).
- A notice stating 'Do not feed this child water/feed/juice without nurse approval' should be placed over the cot and explained to carers.
- At start of test, give an intramuscular injection of desmopressin. The dose is 0.4 micrograms (400 ng) in infants and children <2 years of age and 2 micrograms in children >2 years of age.
- Collect and send every urine sample to laboratory for urgent urine osmolality. Note times urine was collected carefully (see Table 24.1 for sample information sheet).
- After 4–6 h repeat the plasma biochemistry and osmolality. Urine collection can stop at 6 h.
- Return to normal feeds by 6 h unless plasma biochemistry is abnormal.

Interpretation of test

Babies with a genetic defect in urinary concentration typically have a urine osmolality between 30 and 100 mOsm/kg. Most will show no significant increase after the desmopressin, but a few (with milder mutations) may increase the urine osmolality to perhaps 200 mOsm/kg.

A normal response would be a value >1000 mOsm/kg (older children/adults) or >600 mOsm/kg (infants, <1 year). Typically, a normal individual will stop passing urine after the injection for a few hours, but the effect should wear off after 4–6 h.

The 'Bichet' protocol

Background

In selected children, IV application of desmopressin at a higher dose will need to be considered. Typically, this will be in children who had an intermediate response to the standard DDAVP® test. Reasons for an intermediate response include incomplete absorption or so-called partial nephrogenic diabetes insipidus (NDI). In partial NDI, patients have mutations in the gene encoding the vasopressin receptor (V2R) that lower its sensitivity, thus requiring higher doses to initiate urinary concentration ('shift in the dose–response curve'). To assess these patients, IV desmopressin is

Table 24.1 Information required for sampling

Sample	Time	Urine osmolality	Plasma osmolality	Plasma sodium
Baseline				
Last sample				

Table 24.2 Observation flow sheet

Time (mins)	-30	-15	0	10	15	20	30	40	50	60	80	90	100	120	140
Actual time (eg: 09:00)	|..|	|..|	|..|	|..|	|..|	|..|	|..|	|..|	|..|	|..|	|..|	|..|	|..|	|..|	|..|
DDAVP® infusion			|...|												
Blood pressure (mmHg)															
Pulse (beats/min)															
Fluid intake (mL)															
Urine: volume (mL)															
Urine: osmolality															
Na															
Plasma: U&E															
Plasma: osmolality															

The open cells indicate times of observations. The suggested times for urine measurements are for patients with a urinary catheter only. In patients without a catheter, a urine sample should be obtained before the desmopressin infusion and then every void during the observation period. If no urine is produced during this time, the first void after the test should be used. It is important to measure the volume of urine as accurately as possible and to limit fluid intake of the proband during the observation period to the volume of urine produced during that time.

administered at a dose of 0.3 micrograms/kg (the same dose used in von Willebrandt disease), according to a protocol developed by D. Bichet. This protocol has been used for >20 years in several hundred children without serious complications. However, as with the standard protocol, patients are at risk of hyponatraemia if they respond to the desmopressin and they keep on drinking fluids.

Patients with a normal thirst mechanism will stop drinking, when their kidney conserves water, but patients with psychogenic polydipsia are at risk as are infants who keep on being fed by their carers. It is therefore of paramount importance to closely monitor the fluid intake of the patient during the observation period, so that it not exceed the amount excreted during this time. Desmopressin at this dose will also lead to a slight drop in BP (~10 mmHg) 30–60 min after the infusion with a concomitant increase in heart rate (~25 bpm).

The effect of desmopressin wears off after ~60–90 min. Thus, the observation period needs to be only 2 h after finishing the infusion.

Preparation and procedure

- Continue hydrochlorothiazide or amiloride, but discontinue indometacin at least 3 days in advance (if the patient receives any of these medications).
- Admit the patient to the ward.
- Do not dehydrate, but stop fluids 2 h prior to infusion to avoid absorption of fluid from the gut during the test. Start IV (with a large-bore catheter) with a three-way stopcock to be able to repeat blood samples.
- Note all observations (BP, pulse, urine volume, fluid given) on the flow sheet (see Table 24.2 for a sample).
- *Before the infusion*: three periods of observation of 15 min each (–30, –15, and 0 min) for BP, pulse, and urine volume. On each urine sample, obtain volume and osmolality.
- It is important that the child voids before desmopressin is given. This will prevent the mixing of urine produced after desmopressin with that already present in the bladder. It will also provide a baseline urine osmolality.
- Infuse desmopressin 0.3 micrograms/kg of body weight in 1 mL/kg of saline over 20 min.
- Observe for 2 h after finishing the infusion (Table 24.2).

Reference

Bichet D, Razi M, Lonergan M, et al. Hemodynamic and coagulation responses to 1-desamino[8-D-arginine] vasopressin in patients with congenital nephrogenic diabetes insipidus. *N Engl J Med* 1988;318:881–887.

Disodium pamidronate infusion

May be used for the treatment of hypercalcaemia (when the PTH is normal) resistant to conventional therapy (➔ see 'Disorders of calcium: hypercalcaemia', p. 138). Other indications include osteoporosis and for the calcinosis of juvenile dermatomyositis (anecdotal).

During the infusion

- Check temperature, pulse, and respiratory rate prior to, and at end of, infusion.

The infusion
- The dose is 1 mg/kg/day to a maximum of 60 mg on three successive days.
- Dilute pamidronate initially in water, but infuse in saline or 5% dextrose.
- Final concentration should not exceed 12 mg/100 mL of diluent.
- Give infusion over 4 h on first occasion. Thereafter, pamidronate can be given over 2–4 h.
- Give a 30 mL flush over 20 min.
- Time interval between doses is 12–36 h.

Expected side effects

Side effects are more prominent during the first infusion. Approximately half of the children undergoing their first infusion may experience temporary flu-like 'symptoms' including fever, musculoskeletal aches, and pains and vomiting, but side effects become less marked over time. Treat with paracetamol.

Pamidronate is reported to cause asymptomatic hypocalcaemia, hence, its use for hypercalcaemia. Although calcium supplementation is recommended for those receiving pamidronate for osteoporosis, this is not recommended when it is being used to treat hypercalcaemia. The manufacturer advises avoiding use if GFR <30 mL/min/1.73 m².

Intravenous cyclophosphamide

Cytotoxic drugs such as cyclophosphamide act predominantly on rapidly dividing cells, such as T lymphocytes, and are therefore immunosuppressive and anti-inflammatory, as well as having anticancer properties. Pulse IV cyclophosphamide may be used for the treatment of some vasculitic disorders: polyarteritis, SLE, and dermatomyositis.

Potential adverse effects

* Includes bone marrow suppression, GI symptoms, haemorrhagic cystitis, and hair loss. Males may be rendered azoospermic. Amenorrhoea and female infertility can occur with an increase in risk with increasing age over 25 years.
* Cyclophosphamide is contraindicated in pregnancy.
* Contact with infectious diseases should be avoided as far as possible during the period of cyclophosphamide therapy and infections should be treated vigorously.

Dose

Cyclophosphamide IV 500–1000 mg/m^2 per dose (based on National Institutes of Health (NIH) protocol, usual starting dose 500 mg/m^2; maximum dose 1.2 g).

Investigations

Each dose is preceded by a FBC, U&Es, LFTs, and creatinine. Dosage should be reduced or delayed if there is evidence of bone marrow suppression, particularly if neutrophils are <1.5 × 10^9/L. Bone marrow suppression is most likely to occur 7–10 days following administration of the dose so the FBC should be checked at this time. Urine should be monitored for haematuria and proteinuria throughout the treatment period.

INTRAVENOUS PRESCRIPTION CHART								WARD
CHEMOTHERAPY								

SURNAME	FIRST NAME	HOSP NUMBER	D.O.B.	WEIGHT:	DATE:	HEIGHT	SURF AREA	ALLERGIES?
			AGE	WEIGHT:	DATE:			

DATE	IV FLUID	VOLUME	ADDITIVES	RATE	DURA-TION	DRS SIG	DATE & TIME	NURSE UNIT	NOTES
–0:15	CYCLOPHOSPHAMIDE		Ondansetron_____mg	Slow IV bolus					5 mg/m^2 (max 8 mg)
–0:15			Mesna_____mg	Slow IV bolus	Over 15 min				20% Cyclo-phosphamide dose
0:00			Cyclophosphamide___mg	Slow IV bolus	Over at least 10 min				Give via 3-way tap into hydration fluids
0:00	Glucose 2.5%/ Sodium Chloride 0.45%	mL	Mesna_____ (_____mg per 500 mL bag or_____mg per 1000 mL bag)	mL/h	12 h				Hydration rate = 85 mL/m^2/h Mesna dose =100% Cyclophosphamide dose

Fig. 24.1 Cyclophosphamide infusion chart.

Administration

- The dose is given with sodium 2-mercapto-ethanesulphonate (mesna) cover (120% of cyclophosphamide dose) with IV hydration, to reduce the incidence of haemorrhagic cystitis, and with ondansetron to reduce nausea.
- Mesna is a sulphydryl-containing compound that is excreted in the urine. Co-administration with alkylating agents, such as cyclophosphamide significantly reduces their urotoxic effects by reacting with the metabolites in the urinary system.
- For patients with a history of haemorrhagic cystitis, the total mesna dose may be increased in 20% increments up to 180%. Administration time for the cyclophosphamide is increased, and the hydration time may also be increased to 16–20 h.
- For those patients who have an allergic reaction to mesna, a revised protocol is used: give IV cyclophosphamide over 1 h. Omit mesna, but ensure patient is adequately hydrated and increase hydration fluids to 125 mL/m^2/h for 12 h.

Sequence of administration

See cyclophosphamide infusion chart, Fig. 24.1.

- 15 min before cyclophosphamide, a slow IV bolus of ondansetron 5 mg/m^2 (maximum 8 mg), *and*
- Mesna (20% cyclophosphamide dose) IV bolus over 15 min.
- Cyclophosphamide (20 mg/mL concentration) given over at least 10 min via three-way tap into hydration fluids, with the patient supine.
- *Hydration with*: mesna (100% cyclophosphamide dose) in 2.5% glucose/ 0.45% NaCl run over 12 h at 85 mL/m^2/h.
- Ondansetron 4 mg (4–12 years) or 8 mg (>12 years) orally twice a day for 2 days if required.
- If emesis is a problem, an IV dose of dexamethasone 100 micrograms/ kg (maximum 4 mg) may also be given.

Take care to ensure that the IV cannula is correctly sited and that saline flushes in easily before administering cyclophosphamide. If extravasation occurs, the duty plastic surgery team is contacted (Fig. 24.1).

Personal protective equipment

Personal protective equipment is necessary when preparing, handling, and administering cytotoxic drugs, to minimize the risk of accidental contamination.

Further reading

Boumpas I, Austin HA 3rd, Vaughan EM, et al. Risk for sustained amenorrhea in patients with systemic lupus erythematosus receiving intermittent pulse cyclophosphamide therapy. *Ann Intern Med* 1993;119:366–369.

Brogan PA, Dillon MJ. The use of immunosuppressive and cytotoxic drugs in non-malignant disease. *Arch Dis Child* 2000;83:259–264.

Guidelines for the use of basiliximab

Background

Basiliximab is indicated for the prophylaxis of acute organ rejection in *de novo* allogeneic renal transplantation. It is a murine/human chimeric monoclonal antibody that is directed against the interleukin-2 receptor alpha chain (CD25 antigen), which is expressed on the surface of T lymphocytes in response to antigenic challenge. Basiliximab specifically binds to the CD25 antigen on activated T lymphocytes expressing the high-affinity interleukin-2 receptor and thereby prevents binding of interleukin-2, the signal for T-cell proliferation. Complete and consistent blocking of the interleukin-2 receptor is maintained as long as serum basiliximab levels exceed 0.2 micrograms/mL (4–6 weeks). As concentrations fall below this level, expression of the CD25 antigen returns to pretherapy values within 1–2 weeks. Basiliximab does not cause cytokine release or myelosuppression.

The current marketing authorization for basiliximab is for use in adults and for concomitant use with ciclosporin and corticosteroids only, although there is data to support its use in children over the age of 2 years and with other immunosuppressive agents.

Patient selection

Patients receiving a second or third transplant

* Patients who may have developed antibodies precluding further administration of a monoclonal antibody.
* Patients who are deemed unable to tolerate standard triple therapy.
* Patients receiving steroid-free immunosuppressive protocols.
* Patients will be given two infusions of basiliximab.

Dose

* <40 kg: 10 mg infused on day 0 within 2 h prior to surgery and on day 4 after transplantation.
* >40 kg: 20 mg infused on day 0 within 2 h prior to surgery and on day 4 after transplantation.

Reconstitution and administration

* Basiliximab is provided as:
  * a vial containing 20 mg basiliximab powder.
  * plus an ampoule of water for injections.
* Add 5 mL water for injection to the vial containing 20 mg basiliximab powder.
* Shake the vial gently to dissolve the powder. After reconstitution the solution should be used immediately (at least within 24 h if stored in a refrigerator).

The reconstituted solution is isotonic and must be further diluted:
* 10 mg dose must be diluted to at least 25 mL (20 mg to at least 50 mL) with NaCl 0.9% or glucose 5% for infusion.
* Infuse over 20–30 min.
* Do not mix with any other preparation.

Contraindications

Known hypersensitivity to basiliximab or any other component of the formulation.

Undesirable effects

- Basiliximab did not increase the incidence of serious adverse events observed in organ transplantation when compared with placebo.
- Acute adverse events suggestive of hypersensitivity were not reported in 363 patients who received basiliximab in two randomized trials:
  - Infections occurred at similar rates in patients who received basiliximab or placebo and so did CMV infections.
  - Post-transplant lymphoproliferative disorders occurred in 0.3% and 0.6%, respectively, of basiliximab and placebo patients.
  - In these trials, a total of 13 patients (5 basiliximab and 8 placebo recipients) developed various malignancies in the first 12 months after transplant.
- One study of paediatric renal transplant patients showed a marked decrease in ciclosporin levels within the first 6 weeks when combined with basiliximab, possibly due to interaction at the cytochrome P450 metabolism level. This indicates that children receiving basiliximab need to be closely monitored for decreasing ciclosporin levels.

Further reading

Kahan BD, Rajagopalan PR, Hall M. Reduction of the occurrence of acute cellular rejection among renal allograft recipients treated with basiliximab, a chimeric anti-interleukin-2-receptor monoclonal antibody. United States Simulect Renal Study Group. *Transplantation* 1999;67:276–284.

Administration of blood to patients with or approaching chronic kidney disease stage 5

The administration of blood products to patients who will need RRT should be avoided as far as possible because HLA sensitization can occur following transfusion of blood and platelets. Possible options to reduce this risk are as follows:

- Children awaiting planned surgery should have their haemoglobin boosted with erythropoietin, raising it to the upper limit of the normal range, to reduce the risk of the need for blood transfusion.
- Ensure that the iron stores are replete.
- Post-transplant CMV-negative blood should be prescribed for patients who are CMV negative.
- Anti-HLA antibodies should be measured 10 days after blood products have been given.

Protocol for percutaneous transluminal angioplasty

Introduction

Balloon dilation of stenosed renal arteries is a form of treatment utilized in childhood renovascular hypertension. Most patients who undergo an angioplasty procedure have been fully investigated previously in terms of renal function, differential kidney function by isotope scanning, delineation of significant vascular pathology affecting a kidney or the kidneys via Doppler US, renal arteriography, and renal vein renin studies. In addition, the patients will be receiving antihypertensive therapy, usually with several agents involved.

Pre-angioplasty checklist

- Detailed history of condition, anatomical sites of pathology, differential renal function, renal vein renin data, site to be dilated, presence or absence of cerebrovascular or other non-renal vascular disease, and cardiac status.
- Details of all drugs being administered, especially antihypertensives, their dosages, and schedules of delivery. It is particularly important to identify drugs that might modify cardiovascular responsiveness, such as beta blockers.
- Details of BP control, i.e. levels of BP usually maintained and requirements concerning range of BP to be aimed at—especially relevant if cerebrovascular disease is also present.
- All previous isotope, ultrasonographic, and angiographic imaging must be reviewed.
- If no renal isotope study (DMSA or MAG3) has been undertaken within 3 months of the procedure, a repeat must be undertaken prior to the proposed angioplasty.
- Consent must be obtained and risks of the procedure explained in detail to parents.

Bloods

- Haemoglobin, white blood count, and platelet count.
- Clotting screen.
- U&Es and plasma creatinine.
- Group and cross-match 1 unit of blood.

Drugs

- Establish the protocol for each individual child concerning drug administration preoperatively with the anaesthetist and the nephrologist involved with the case. Usually, antihypertensives are given at approximately the usual time prior to the procedure, but this may need individual modification.
- Make sure the anaesthetist is aware of each agent, especially those that interfere with cardiovascular responsiveness and if the child has cerebrovascular disease, and agree BP levels to be maintained during the procedure and in the recovery area.
- *NB*: beta blockers may mask the signs of blood loss, i.e. inappropriate bradycardia and other drugs might be associated with tachycardia when volume replete.

Post procedure

- Postoperative BP and pulse rate agreed limits will have been determined for the individual child prior to the procedure being undertaken. Hypotension with or without tachycardia, pallor, or abdominal pain may indicate haemorrhage, and would necessitate urgent evaluation and action. Adequate vascular access must be available for IV fluid administration and/or blood if necessary, as well as for the administration of parenteral antihypertensive therapy.
- A follow-up renal isotope scan (DMSA or MAG3 should be undertaken 24–48 h following the procedure.
- Further management (e.g. prescription of aspirin) should be decided on an individual basis.

Travel information: guidance for renal patients

It is most important that renal patients are advised to contact their doctor, nurse, or pharmacist before they consider travelling to a country that requires specific vaccinations and/or malaria prophylaxis. For patients on ciclosporin or tacrolimus, it is wise to start antimalarials at least 2 weeks before travelling so that levels can be checked and any dosage adjustments made.

For the most up-to-date information on vaccines and antimalarials, refer to the *British National Formulary* for telephone numbers and websites.

Vaccines

A list of vaccines that may or may not be recommended for immunosuppressed patients may be found in the chapter on renal transplantation (⊃ see 'Vaccination in transplant patients', p. 583).

Antimalarials for prophylaxis

The correct antimalarial for the part of the world visited must be prescribed. In addition, patients must be told to avoid mosquito bites, take their prophylaxis medicines regularly, and must visit their doctor immediately if they fall ill within 1 year and especially within 3 months of return from holiday.

If mefloquine recommended

The dose is adjusted for age, but no dose changes are required for renal patients.

Tablets 250 mg

Started 2–3 weeks before entering endemic area and continued for 4 weeks after leaving:
- 5–19 kg: 62.5 mg once a week.
- 20–30 kg: 125 mg once a week.
- 31–45 kg: 187.5 mg once a week.
- >45 kg and adults: 250 mg once a week.

If doxycycline recommended

The dose is adjusted for age, but no dose changes are required for patients on PD or HD. For transplant patients, doxycycline can alter ciclosporin or tacrolimus levels.

Capsules 50 mg, 100 mg, dispersible tablets 100 mg

Started 1 week before entering endemic area and continued for 4 weeks after leaving. (If on ciclosporin or tacrolimus, start 2 weeks before so that levels can be checked and any dose adjustments made.)
- >12 years, 25–45 kg: 75 mg once a day.
- Adult: 100 mg once a day.

If chloroquine and proguanil recommended

Chloroquine

The dose is adjusted for age, but no dose changes are required for renal patients unless they are in CKD stage 5.

* *Tablets (chloroquine base) 150 mg*: started 1 week before entering endemic area and continued for 4 weeks after leaving.
* Dose 5 mg chloroquine base/kg once a week. Equivalent to:
  * 1–4 years: half a tablet once a week.
  * 5–8 years: one tablet once a week.
  * 9–15 years: one-and-a-half tablets once a week.
  * adults: two tablets once a week.
* *Renal impairment*: no dose reduction until GFR <10 mL/min/1.73 m²— give 50% dose.

Proguanil

The dose is adjusted for age and for renal function.

Tablets 100 mg

Started 1 week before entering endemic area and continued for 4 weeks after leaving.

* Infants up to 12 weeks, bodyweight <6 kg: 25 mg once daily.
* 12 weeks to 11 months, 6–10 kg: 50 mg once daily.
* 1–3 years, 10–16 kg: 75 mg once daily.
* 4–7 years, 16–25 kg: 100 mg once daily.
* 8–12 years, 26–45 kg: 150 mg once daily.
* >13 years, >45 kg, adult dose: 200 mg once daily.

In renal impairment

* GFR >60 mL/min/1.73 m²: standard dose.
* GFR 20–59 mL/min/1.73 m²: 50% dose.
* GFR 10–19 mL/min/1.73 m²: 25% dose every second day.
* GFR <10 mL/min/1.73 m²: 25% dose once a week.

If proguanil with atovaquone (Malarone®) recommended

The dose is adjusted for age and renal function. Started 1–2 days before entering endemic area and continued for 1 week after leaving.

Tablets proguanil 100 mg, atovaquone 250 mg
* Adult and child >40 kg: one tablet once daily.

Paediatric tablets proguanil 25 mg, atovaquone 62.5 mg
* Child 11–20 kg: one tablet once daily.
* 21–30 kg: two tablets once daily.
* 31–40 kg: three tablets once daily.

In renal impairment
* Malarone® should not be given if GFR <30 mL/min/1.73 m².
* For GFR 30–60 mL/min/1.73 m² suggest 50% dose, although there is no data for this.

Miscellaneous

Calculation of body surface area

$$BSA\,(m^2) = \sqrt{[height\,(cm) \times weight\,(kg)\,/\,3600]}$$

Fractional excretion

(→ See also 'Management: fluid and electrolytes', p. 463.)

This is most commonly used in calculation of the fractional excretion of sodium (FENa), which may be useful in the assessment of volume status (→ see Chapter 17).

$$FEx = [(Ux\,/\,Px) \times (Pcr\,/\,Ucr)] \times 100$$

where FEx = fractional excretion of solute x (expressed as %); Ux = urine concentration of solute x; Px = plasma concentration of solute x; PCr = plasma concentration of creatinine; and UCr = urine concentration of creatinine.

Ux, Px, PCr, and UCr should be in the same units.

Clinical relevance: FENa

In a well child, FENa simply reflects Na intake. It is also important to note that FENa increases as GFR decreases: if GFR is halved, the exact same amount of sodium in the urine will represent a doubled percentage of the filtered load. Thus, numbers below assume a previously normal GFR. In the setting of acute oliguria, FENa can be used to define the aetiology: FENa >2.5% suggests established acute tubular necrosis, whereas FENa <1% suggests renal hypoperfusion (pre-renal AKI) and the patient would probably benefit from volume expansion. It is important to obtain the urine sample before diuretics are used to increase urine output. While a low FENa after a furosemide challenge would still be consistent with pre-renal AKI, an elevated FENa could be due to the drug or acute tubular necrosis.

Conversion to SI units

Table 24.3 gives the conversion factor required to change from mg/dL (used in North America) to SI units.

Table 24.3 Conversion factor to change from mg/dL to SI units

	Conversion factor
Creatinine	88.4
Urea	0.357
Calcium	0.2495
Phosphate	0.3229
Glucose	0.05551
PTH (pg/mL)	0.106 (pmol/L)

Recipe for 0.45% saline/5% glucose

To a 500 mL bag of 5% glucose add 7.5 mL of 30% NaCl. NB: in some instances, e.g. the neonate, this recipe can be used to make 0.45% saline/10% glucose by adding the same NaCl to a similar volume of 10% glucose.

Blood pressure (BP) by age and height

Data provided are from National High Blood Pressure Education Program Working Group on High Blood Pressure in Children and Adolescents. (2007) A pocket guide to blood pressure measurements in children. Copyright © 2007 US Department of Health and Human Services. Available at: ℘ https://www.nhlbi.nih.gov/files/docs/bp_child_pocket.pdf

There are also revised BP categories and stages available from the American Academy of Pediatrics Clinical Practice Guidelines from 2017 (Pediatrics. 2017;140(3):e20171904 or ℘ http://pediatrics.aappublications.org/content/140/3/e20171904..info).

See Tables 24.4 and 25.5.

Table 24.4 Girls' SBP by age and height (heights given for age at mid year)

Age	BP Classification	Systolic BP (mmHg)						
3	Height (cm)	91	92	95	98	100	103	105
	Prehypertension	100	100	102	103	104	106	106
	Stage 1 HTN	104	104	105	107	108	109	110
	Stage 2 HTN	116	116	118	119	120	121	122
4	Height (cm)	97	99	101	104	108	110	112
	Prehypertension	101	102	103	104	106	107	108
	Stage 1 HTN	105	106	107	108	110	111	112
	Stage 2 HTN	117	118	119	120	122	123	124
5	Height (cm)	104	105	108	111	115	118	120
	Prehypertension	103	103	105	106	107	109	109
	Stage 1 HTN	107	107	108	110	111	112	113
	Stage 2 HTN	119	119	121	122	123	125	125
6	Height (cm)	110	112	115	118	122	126	128
	Prehypertension	104	105	106	108	109	110	111
	Stage 1 HTN	108	109	110	111	113	114	115
	Stage 2 HTN	120	121	122	124	125	126	127
7	Height (cm)	116	118	121	125	129	132	135
	Prehypertension	106	107	108	109	111	112	113
	Stage 1 HTN	110	111	112	113	115	116	116
	Stage 2 HTN	122	123	124	125	127	128	129
8	Height (cm)	121	123	127	131	135	139	141
	Prehypertension	108	109	110	111	113	114	114
	Stage 1 HTN	112	112	114	115	116	118	118
	Stage 2 HTN	124	125	126	127	128	130	130

Table 24.4 *(Contd.)*

Age	BP Classification	Systolic BP (mmHg)						
9	Height (cm)	125	128	131	136	140	144	147
	Prehypertension	110	110	112	113	114	116	116
	Stage 1 HTN	114	114	115	117	118	119	120
	Stage 2 HTN	126	126	128	129	130	132	132
10	Height (cm)	130	132	136	141	146	150	153
	Prehypertension	112	112	114	115	116	118	118
	Stage 1 HTN	116	116	117	119	120	121	122
	Stage 2 HTN	128	128	130	131	132	134	134
11	Height (cm)	136	138	143	148	153	157	160
	Prehypertension	114	114	116	117	118	119	120
	Stage 1 HTN	118	118	119	121	122	123	124
	Stage 2 HTN	130	130	131	133	134	135	136
12	Height (cm)	143	146	150	155	160	164	166
	Prehypertension	116	116	117	119	120	120	120
	Stage 1 HTN	119	120	121	123	124	125	126
	Stage 2 HTN	132	132	133	135	136	137	138
13	Height (cm)	148	151	155	159	164	168	170
	Prehypertension	117	118	119	120	120	120	120
	Stage 1 HTN	121	122	123	124	126	127	128
	Stage 2 HTN	133	134	135	137	138	139	140
14	Height (cm)	151	153	157	161	166	170	172
	Prehypertension	119	120	120	120	120	120	120
	Stage 1 HTN	123	123	125	126	127	129	129
	Stage 2 HTN	135	136	137	138	140	141	141
15	Height (cm)	152	154	158	162	167	171	173
	Prehypertension	120	120	120	120	120	120	120
	Stage 1 HTN	124	125	126	127	129	130	131
	Stage 2 HTN	136	137	138	139	141	142	143
16	Height (cm)	152	154	158	163	167	171	173
	Prehypertension	120	120	120	120	120	120	120
	Stage 1 HTN	125	126	127	128	130	131	132
	Stage 2 HTN	137	138	139	140	142	143	144
17	Height (cm)	152	155	159	163	167	171	174
	Prehypertension	120	120	120	120	120	120	120
	Stage 1 HTN	125	126	127	129	130	131	132
	Stage 2 HTN	138	138	139	141	142	143	144

Source: data from National High Blood Pressure Education Program Working Group on High Blood Pressure in Children and Adolescents. (2007) *A pocket guide to blood pressure measurements in children.* Copyright © 2007 US Department of Health and Human Services. Available at: https://www.nhlbi.nih.gov/files/docs/bp_child_pocket.pdf

Table 24.5 Boys' SBP by age and height (heights given for age at midyear)

Age	BP Classification	Systolic BP (mmHg)						
3	Height (cm)	92	94	96	99	102	104	106
	Prehypertension	100	101	103	105	107	108	109
	Stage 1 HTN	104	105	107	109	110	112	113
	Stage 2 HTN	116	117	119	121	123	124	125
4	Height (cm)	99	100	103	106	109	112	113
	Prehypertension	102	103	105	107	109	110	111
	Stage 1 HTN	106	107	109	111	112	114	115
	Stage 2 HTN	118	119	121	123	125	126	127
5	Height (cm)	104	106	109	112	116	119	120
	Prehypertension	104	105	106	108	110	111	112
	Stage 1 HTN	108	109	110	112	114	115	116
	Stage 2 HTN	120	121	123	125	126	128	128
6	Height (cm)	110	112	115	119	122	126	127
	Prehypertension	105	106	108	110	111	113	113
	Stage 1 HTN	109	110	112	114	115	117	117
	Stage 2 HTN	121	122	124	126	128	129	130
7	Height (cm)	116	118	121	125	129	132	134
	Prehypertension	106	107	109	111	113	114	115
	Stage 1 HTN	110	111	113	115	117	118	119
	Stage 2 HTN	122	123	125	127	129	130	131
8	Height (cm)	121	123	127	131	135	139	141
	Prehypertension	107	109	110	112	114	115	116
	Stage 1 HTN	111	112	114	116	118	119	120
	Stage 2 HTN	124	125	127	128	130	132	132
9	Height (cm)	126	128	132	136	141	145	147
	Prehypertension	109	110	112	114	115	117	118
	Stage 1 HTN	113	114	116	118	119	121	121
	Stage 2 HTN	125	126	128	130	132	133	134
10	Height (cm)	130	133	137	141	146	150	153
	Prehypertension	111	112	114	115	117	119	119
	Stage 1 HTN	115	116	117	119	121	122	123
	Stage 2 HTN	127	128	130	132	133	135	135
11	Height (cm)	135	137	142	146	151	156	159
	Prehypertension	113	114	115	117	119	120	120
	Stage 1 HTN	117	118	119	121	123	124	125
	Stage 2 HTN	129	130	132	134	135	137	137
12	Height (cm)	140	143	148	153	158	163	166
	Prehypertension	115	116	118	120	120	120	120
	Stage 1 HTN	119	120	122	123	125	127	127
	Stage 2 HTN	131	132	134	136	138	139	140

Table 24.5 *(Contd.)*

Age	BP Classification	Systolic BP (mmHg)						
13	Height (cm)	147	150	155	160	166	171	173
	Prehypertension	117	118	120	120	120	120	120
	Stage 1 HTN	121	122	124	126	128	129	130
	Stage 2 HTN	133	135	136	138	140	141	142
14	Height (cm)	154	157	162	167	173	177	180
	Prehypertension	120	120	120	120	120	120	120
	Stage 1 HTN	124	125	127	128	130	132	132
	Stage 2 HTN	136	137	139	141	143	144	145
15	Height (cm)	159	162	167	172	177	182	184
	Prehypertension	120	120	120	120	120	120	120
	Stage 1 HTN	126	127	129	131	133	134	135
	Stage 2 HTN	139	140	141	143	145	147	147
16	Height (cm)	162	165	170	175	180	184	186
	Prehypertension	120	120	120	120	120	120	120
	Stage 1 HTN	129	130	132	134	135	137	137
	Stage 2 HTN	141	142	144	146	148	149	150
17	Height (cm)	164	166	171	176	181	185	187
	Prehypertension	120	120	120	120	120	120	120
	Stage 1 HTN	131	132	134	136	138	139	140
	Stage 2 HTN	144	145	146	148	150	151	152

Source: data from National High Blood Pressure Education Program Working Group on High Blood Pressure in Children and Adolescents. (2007) *A pocket guide to blood pressure measurements in children.* Copyright © 2007 US Department of Health and Human Services. Available at: https://www.nhlbi.nih.gov/files/docs/bp_child_pocket.pdf

Index

Figures, tables and boxes are indicated by an italic *f*, *t* or *b* following the page number.

W

X

Z